AF738826

SYSTEMIC LUPUS ERYTHEMATOSUS

Edited by **Hani Almoallim**

Systemic Lupus Erythematosus
Edited by Hani Almoallim

Published by InTech
Janeza Trdine 9, 51000 Rijeka, Croatia

Copyright © 2012 InTech
All chapters are distributed under the Creative Commons Attribution 3.0 license, which allows users to download, copy and build upon published articles even for commercial purposes, as long as the author and publisher are properly credited, which ensures maximum dissemination and a wider impact of our publications. After this work has been published by InTech, authors have the right to republish it, in whole or part, in any publication of which they are the author, and to make other personal use of the work. Any republication, referencing or personal use of the work must explicitly identify the original source.

As for readers, this license allows users to download, copy and build upon published chapters even for commercial purposes, as long as the author and publisher are properly credited, which ensures maximum dissemination and a wider impact of our publications.

Notice
Statements and opinions expressed in the chapters are these of the individual contributors and not necessarily those of the editors or publisher. No responsibility is accepted for the accuracy of information contained in the published chapters. The publisher assumes no responsibility for any damage or injury to persons or property arising out of the use of any materials, instructions, methods or ideas contained in the book.

Publishing Process Manager Bojan Rafaj

Technical Editor Teodora Smiljanic

Cover Designer InTech Design Team

Additional hard copies can be obtained from orders@intechopen.com

Systemic Lupus Erythematosus, Edited by Hani Almoallim
p. cm.
ISBN 978-953-51-0266-3

We are IntechOpen, the world's leading publisher of Open Access books

Built by scientists, for scientists

4,000+
Open access books available

116,000+
International authors and editors

120M+
Downloads

151
Countries delivered to

Our authors are among the
Top 1%
most cited scientists

12.2%
Contributors from top 500 universities

CLARIVATE ANALYTICS BOOK CITATION INDEX INDEXED

WEB OF SCIENCE™

Selection of our books indexed in the Book Citation Index in Web of Science™ Core Collection (BKCI)

Interested in publishing with us?
Contact book.department@intechopen.com

Numbers displayed above are based on latest data collected.
For more information visit www.intechopen.com

For EU product safety concerns:
IN TECH d.o.o., Prolaz Marije Krucifikse Kozulić 3, 51000 Rijeka, Croatia,
info@intechopen.com or visit our website at intechopen.com.

Meet the editor

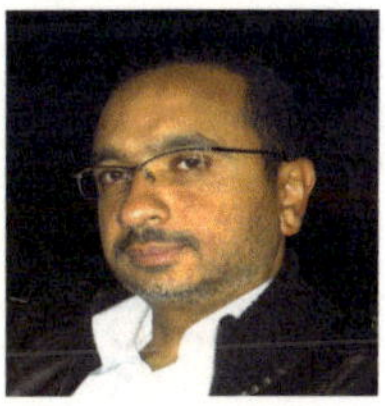

Hani Almoallim, an Associate Professor of Medicine, Umm Alqura University (UQU), Makkah, Saudi Arabia, has completed his training in Internal Medicine and Rheumatology at University of British Columbia, Vancouver, Canada. He is currently the head of Department of Medicine at UQU. He is also consultant rheumatologist at King Faisal Specialist Hospital, Jeddah, Saudi Arabia. He has made major changes in the filed of medical education in his department particularly curriculum design and assessment methods. He published most of his work through the American Association of Medical Colleges – MedEdPORTAL. He was appointed recently as the Supervisor of Alzaidi's Chair of Research in Rheumatic Diseases at UQU. He is supervising several educational and research work on the national level. He has multiple publications in rheumatology. Research interests: SLE, muscuoloskeletal examination, use of ultrasound in rheumatology and rheumatoid arthritis.

Contents

Preface

Systemic lupus erythematosus (SLE) is a multi-systemic disease characterized by a wide variety of autoantibodies leading to highly heterogeneous clinical manifestations. SLE, or lupus, the Latin name for wolf is a unique, complex disease that comes with its own challenges; a challenge in diagnosis as lupus has a broad scope of symptoms, various clinical presentations & often does not follow a predictable course.

Another challenge is the management of Lupus; a healthcare professional maybe able to control the symptoms and disease activity with treatment, but it is not uncommon for health care professionals to encounter a lupus patient with numerous severe symptoms that are difficult to control. These challenges drove our efforts to write this book.

SLE book provides an overview of lupus and the elements involved in caring for patients with this disease. It addresses primarily healthcare professionals who deal with lupus patients. Each chapter of this book deals with a specific aspect of the disease. We addressed new advances in the pathogenesis of SLE. At the same time, we provided a comprehensive clinical guide for dealing with this disease.

Today, the prognosis for people with lupus is better than it was two decades ago; advances in research, improved treatments and the evolution in information resources helped many lupus patients to remain active and involved with life, family, and work. We hope that this book can provide healthcare professionals with a solid grounding in this important disease so that they can provide the care to make an active and involved life a reality for women and men with lupus.

At the end, we would like to express our gratitude by thanking the team of internationally recognized authors who participated with us in the process of writing this book.

Dr. Hani Almoallim
MBBS, ABIM, FRCPC, DipMedEd
Head Department of Medicine, Medical College, Umm Alqura University(UQU)
Associate Professor, Medical College, UQU
Consultant Rheumatologist, King Faisal Specialist Hospital and Research Center
Saudi Arabia

Part 1

The Scientific Basis of SLE

1

Genetics and Epigenetic in Systemic Lupus Erythematosus

Suad M. AlFadhli
Kuwait University
Kuwait

1. Introduction

Systemic lupus erythematosus (SLE) (OMIM #152700) is the prototype of a multiorgan autoimmune disease and still considered as a disease with an ambiguous etiology. The disease predominantly affects women during the reproductive years at a ratio of eight women per one man (Lopez, 2003). Its pathogenesis is multifactorial lying on genetic and environmental factors in which it occurs in genetically-predisposed individuals who have experienced certain environmental triggers resulting in an irreversible loss of immunologic self-tolerance. The nature of these environmental triggers is largely unknown. It is most likely that it requires a number of environmental triggers occurring together or sequentially over a limited period of time. The concept has therefore emerged of 'threshold liability' in which disease develops when a threshold of genetic and environmental susceptibility effects is reached (Jönsen,2007). Epigenetics, the control of gene packaging and expression independent of alterations in the DNA sequence, is providing new directions linking genetics and environmental factors. It has become clear that besides genetics, epigenetics plays a major role in complex diseases with complex immunological pathogenesis like lupus. Convincing evidence indicates that epigenetic mechanisms, and in particular impaired T cell DNA methylation, provide an additional factor. Interpreting the precise contribution of epigenetic factors to autoimmunity, and in particular to SLE, has become an active research area.

Herein, we will discuss our current understanding of SLE as an autoimmune disease and as a complex genetic disorder. Through the review of the current list of best validated SLE disease susceptibility candidate genes, in particular considering how the known and potential function of these genes may allow us to articulate the genetic of SLE pathogenesis. In addition we will review the effect of epigenetics on SLE pathology.

1.1 SLE, the disease

This complex autoimmune disease results on defects of multiple immunologic components of both the innate immune system and the adaptive immune system including altered immune tolerance mechanism, hyperactivation of T and B cells, decreased ability to clear immune complexes and apoptotic cells, and failure of multiple regulatory networks (Firestein, 2008). Moreover it is likely that immunological dysfunction precedes the onset of clinical disease by many years, making it a particularly challenging disease to study (Arbuckle, 2003).

SLE is a heterogeneous disease that has a diverse range of clinical symptoms, resulting from a widespread immune-mediated damage and it is presented differently from patient to patient (Arnett, 1988). The most common clinical manifestations of this disease include an are erythematous rash, oral ulcers, polyarthralgia, polyserositis, nonerosive arthritis, renal, hematologic, neurologic, pulmonary and cardiac abnormalities. Eleven criteria were identified for SLE clinical presentation, at least four of the 11 coded criteria need to be present for a clinical diagnosis of SLE (Arnett, 1988; Hochberg, 1997; Tan, 1982). Ethnic and genetic heterogeneity contributes to the complexity in SLE clinical presentation. Differently from Multiple sclerosis and although the disease is progressive in nature, no severity criteria have been developed to subgroup SLE patients (with the exception of kidney disease) (Tsao, 1998). A more detailed classification of SLE this heterogeneous disease would significantly help in its genetic analysis. Analyses conditioned on specific disease traits suggest that genetic effects arising from particular linkage regions may contribute to specific clinical or immunological features of SLE (i.e. the presence of haemolytic anaemia or the production of dsDNA antibodies) (Ramos, 2006; Hunnangkul, 2008). A similar picture has arisen from the study of mouse models. However, now it is widely accepted that SLE occurs in phases during a period of time that can be also of years. Therefore, the following steps in the development process of SLE have been suggested: i) genetic predisposition, ii) gender as an additional predisposing factor, iii) environmental stimuli which start immune responses, iv) appearance of autoantibodies, v) regulation of the autoantibodies, T and B cell fails with the development of the clinical disease, vi) chronic inflammation and oxidative damage as causes of tissue damage influencing morbidity (Gualtierotti, 2010).

1.2 Genetic contribution in the pathology of lupus

A genetic contribution to human lupus is well established. The strong genetic contribution to the development of SLE is supported by the high heritability of the disease (>66%), a higher concordance rate for SLE in monozygotic twins than in dizygotic twins or siblings (24–56% versus 2-5%, respectively) which was observed over 30 years ago, and the high sibling recurrence risk ratio of patients with SLE (between eightfold and 29-fold higher than in the general population) and up to 10% of SLE patients have a relative with lupus (Deapen, 1992). Clustering of SLE is fairly rare occurring only in 1/1000-2000 cases. Except in the rare cases of complement deficiency, the inheritance pattern of SLE does not follow simple Mendelian rules as we would expect for a single major gene effect, instead a polygenic model of susceptibility provides the best explanation for the familial clustering. Suggesting that genetic risk in most lupus patients arises from the combination of a number of relatively common variations in several different genes, each of these variations have a modest effect size, contribute to disease genesis. Despite this knowledge, however, it is a challenge to fully understand the genetic pathogenesis of the disease. This is essentially because SLE features a polygenic genetic model, which according to today's evidence may involve as many as 100 genes, and every gene only has a moderate effect size. Genetic studies can enhance our understanding of disease pathogenesis better. During the past few years, progress in biomedical science, bioinformatics, and experimental technology has given us new tools rapidly advanced our understanding of the genetic basis of systemic lupus erythematosus (SLE) and allowed a deeper investigation of SLE genetics and genomics. High throughput genotyping/sequencing platforms, high-throughput expression-level study technologies, etc., have brought forth many new insights. In particular, the genome-wide association study (GWAS) approach, with its ability to screen hundreds of thousands of SNPs across the genome without previous knowledge of candidate regions or genes, has not only supported some findings from previous candidate gene studies, but also discovered convincing evidence for novel genetic loci that may be implicated in SLE (Hardy, 2009; Hirschhorn, 2009). Although the number of genes involved in susceptibility to SLE is increasing in number with the advances in research and technology, however, the complete list of genes that fully account for disease susceptibility is not completed yet. Table1 represents the top SLE candidate genes categorized by chromosomal location.

Most of the genes proven to be associated with susceptibility to SLE are involved in three types of biological process: 1) immune complex processing, 2) toll-like receptor function and type I interferon production, and 3) immune signal transduction in lymphocytes. Several genes without an obvious immunologic function in SLE have been discovered from recent GWA studies such as: KIAA1542, PXK, XKR6, ATG5, etc. (Harley, 2008). These novel gene (loci) discoveries, which are assumed the most powerful and interesting results from GWA studies, can lead us to new pathways or mechanisms that we previously didn't know. The genetic heterogeneity between ethnic populations has been suggested to be important in SLE risk (Yang, 2009), showing the need for further GWAS in the various populations. Genetic loci for SLE in an ethnic group are not always replicated in the other ethnic groups, especially between Whites and Asians (Kim, 2009). However, some loci have been shown consistent associations across ethnicities such as; HLA-DRB1, FCGRs (FCGR2A and FCGR3A), STAT4, and IRF5, BLK, TNFAIP3, BANK1, and MECP2, providing common mechanisms in the development of SLE across ethnic groups. For example: In a large collection of different ethnic groups including European American, Korean, African American, and Hispanic American, relatively high-density genotyping across STAT1 and STAT4 genes has confirmed the association of multiple STAT4 SNPs and common risk haplotypes with SLE in multiple racial groups (Namjou, 2009).

The ethnical diversity in gene association with SLE can be explained due to various reasons: *First*, different genetic backgrounds in the various populations from different ancestries result in the different genetic risk factors for the same disease (Namjou, 2009; Kochi 2009; Tian , 2008). *Second*, SLE as most of the complex traits in human are developed by combined genetic factors and environmental factors for a long period of time. *Third*, the other explanation of inconsistency in genetic association among populations is that disease-associated SNP is unlikely to be the causal variant and rather is more likely to be in strong LD with the biologically relevant variant (Hardy, 2009; Graham, 2009). To date, since it is not feasible to test all variants of human genome even in a GWA study, the aforementioned reasons as reasonable explanation of non-reproducible genetic studies between populations.

1.3 SLE and Copy Number Variation (CNV) and Mendelian forms of SLE

1.3.1 Copy Number Variation (CNV)

CNV is exhibited in up to 12% of the human genome (Ku, 2010). Therefore, it is increasingly believed that large-scale deletion or duplication of DNA segments is a major source of human genetic variation (Ku, 2010). CNVs appear to play an important role in several common diseases (International Schizophrenia Consortium, 2008; Sebat, 2007). The relative contribution of CNVs, to the genetic component of SLE is unclear. Comprehensive studies of CNVs in SLE are expected in the coming years. Although evidences of the involvement of CNVs in SLE susceptibility are accumulating, for example; CNV was found in various genes involved in the pathology of SLE such as: the Fc receptor region (Fanciulli, 2007), Complement Factor 4 in the HLA class III region (Yang,2007), the histamine H4 receptor (HRH4) (Yu, 2010), however, a definitive role for the CNV has not been convincingly disentangled from nearby, linked risk variants (Fanciulli, 2007; Yang,2007).

1.3.2 Mendelian manner of SLE

A number of rare variants that cause SLE in a Mendelian manner have been identified throughout the years, including disruption of several complement pathway components (Harley, 1998). The Mendelian forms of SLE shed light onto pathways critical in pathogenesis, but account for only a small portion of the overall disease incidence (Harley, 1998).

2. Genes involved in the susceptibility to SLE

Herein we will describe the involvement of the key genes involved in the susceptibility to SLE. The genes will be introduced according to their location on the chromosomes.

2.1 Chromosome 1

There is considerable evidence supporting that multiple genes on this chromosome contribute to the development and expression of SLE (Tsao, 2000).

2.1.1 Fcγ receptors: FCGR2A, FCGR3A, FCGR2B and FCGR3B, (1q23-24)

The Fragment crystallizable receptors (FcRs) Fcγ receptor family (FCGRs: FCGR2A (CD32a); FCGR2B (CD32b); FCGR3A (CD16a) and FCGR3B (CD16b)) are a heterogeneous group of hematopoeitic cell surface glycoproteins that bind to the Fc region of immunoglobulins and facilitate the efficiency of antibody-antigen interactions with effector cells of the immune system. These receptors regulate a variety of cellular and humoral immune responses including phagocytosis, immune complex clearance, degranulation, antibody-dependent cellular cytotoxicity, transcriptional regulation of cytokine and chemokine expression, and B cell activation. The cellular distribution and Ig isotype (IgA, IgD, IgE, IgG and IgM) specificity influence the regulatory roles of Fc receptors. In broad terms, FcγRs can be classified into high or low affinity receptors based on their affinity for IgG or into activating (FcγRI, FcγRIIA/C, FcγRIII) or inhibitory (FcγRIIB) receptors based on their signaling activity and associated functions as they stimulate or inhibit immune functions such as phagocytosis, cytotoxicity, degranulation, antigen presentation and cytokine production via immune tyrosine activating or inhibitory motifs (ITAM or ITIM). In humans, three major classes of IgG-receptor have been described; FcγRI (CD64), FccRII (CD 32), and FcγRIII (CD16). These classes can be further sub-divided into discrete isoforms such as FcγRIIA, FcγRIIB, FcγRIIC, FcγRIIIA and FcγRIIIB that exhibit significant differences in their affinity for individual IgG sub-classes and tissue distribution. One of the difficulties of studying the Fcγ-receptor region on chromosome (1q23-24) is the high level of sequence similarity between each of the Fcγ-receptor genes suggests that the whole Fcγ-receptor gene cluster arose from the duplication of a single ancestral gene. Another complicating factor at this locus is the presence of copy number variation (CNV).

In human patients as well as in experimental animal models, FcγRs have been implicated in immune dysfunction and the development of autoimmunity. The best correlation between impaired FcγRs function and autoimmune pathogenesis is seen in systemic lupus. Various functional variants in FCγR2A, FCγR2B, and FCγR3A have been identified as risk factors for SLE (Nimmerjahn, 2008). These variants might lead to the defective clearance of immune complexes from the circulation therefore will contribute to the deposition in tissues such as the kidney and blood vessels (Lehrnbecher, 1999a; Tsokos, 2001).

FcγRIIA receptor contains ITAM on cell membranes of neutrophils, monocytes, macrophages, dendritic cells and platelets. It is the major receptor for the IgG2 subclass, which is a poor activator of classical complement pathway. It is the only FcR for clearing IgG2-bound immune complexes. The association of FCGR2A alleles with SLE has been studied intensively in several populations (Brown, 2007). Mutations in FCGRs have been shown to alter the function of monocytic cells and B-lymphocytes. For example; the nonsynonymous SNP which result in the substitution of Arginine at amino acid position 131 (R131) of FCGR2A (R131; rs1801274) to Histidine within the ligand binding domain of FcγRIIa diminishes binding to IgG2 results in impaired IgG2-mediated phagocytosis (Parren, 1992a,b; Warmerdam, 1991a,b; Clark, 1991; Salmon, 1996). FcγRIIA R131, might contribute to the risk of proliferative lupus nephritis by activating phagocytes, releasing proinflammatory cytokines and reduced clearance of immune complexes (ICs) (Bredius, 1993; Karassa, 2002). Karassa *et al.* conducted a meta-analysis regarding this polymorphism which included 17 studies, involving a total of 3114 SLE patients and 2580 non-SLE controls of European, African, and Asian descent, demonstrating that the R131 allele was associated with SLE (Karassa, 2002). In other studies conducted in Asians, it has been shown that the FCGRIIA-R131 allele was correlated with certain disease phenotypes. Kobayashi *et al.* studied Japanese SLE patients with or without periodontitis, and found that the R allele was significantly correlated (Kobayashi, 2007). Siriboonrit *et al.* also found in a Japanese cohort that the R allele was significantly increased in patients with lupus nephritis (Siriboonrit, 2003). In various ethnic groups (Europeans, African Americans and Koreans), R131 (rs1801274) showed inconsistent association with susceptibility to SLE, lupus nephritis, or both (Duits, 1995; Yap, 1999; Chen, 2004; Salmon, 1996; Song, 1998). Ethnic differences, disease heterogeneity, genotyping error due to extensive sequence homology among FCGR genes and random fluctuations in small samples might explain these inconsistent associations.

FcγR3IIIA receptor contains ITAM on cell surfaces of natural killer (NK) cells, monocytes, and macrophages. FcγR3A alleles with differential affinity for IgG1 and IgG3 have also been shown to be associated with SLE patients from ethnically diverse groups (Yap, 1999). The nonsynonymous SNP, where valine (V158) of FcγRIIIA changes to phenylalanine (F158) (rs396991) was shown to reduce the IgG1-, IgG3-, and IgG4-binding capacity of the receptor compared to V/V homozygotes. This polymorphism, normally termed FcγRIIIA-176 F/V or FcγRIIIA-158 F/V when excluding the leader sequence, was first reported to be of significant correlation with SLE in the Asian population (Japanese) by Kyogoku et al (Tsuchiya, 2005). Studies in human cohorts have shown that SLE is significantly associated with both alleles, R131 and F158, that encode lower affinity isoforms of FcγRIIA and FcγRIIIA respectively (Lehrnbecher, 1999b). F158 homozygotes bind IgG1- and IgG3-containing ICs less efficiently than V 158 homozygotes, and confers less efficient clearance of ICs than other alleles was associated with SLE susceptibility(Koene, 1998). However, the association between FcγR3A-V/F158 polymorphism and susceptibility to SLE and/or lupus nephritis has been variable in several studies (Tsao, 2004). A meta-analysis of more than 1,000 subjects in each of the three categories (SLE without or without renal involvement, and non-SLE controls) has concluded that the F158 allele confers a 1.2-fold risk for developing lupus nephritis in patients of European, African, and Asian descent but not for SLE susceptibility without renal involvement (Karassa, 2003).

The FcγRIIA-R131 and FcγRIIIA-F158 are often inherited together on the same chromosome as a single-risk haplotype for SLE (Magnusson, 2004). The presence of multiple risk alleles might interact to enhance the risk for SLE (Sullivan, 2003). The relative importance of FcγR2A-H/R131 and FcγR3A-V/F158 to disease progression might depend on the IgG subclass of pathogenic auto antibodies in an individual patient.

A novel polymorphism in FCGR3A, the rs403016 located in the Exon 3 which causes a non-synonymous substitution, the FCGR3A-72R/S, has been found to be associated with SLE in a Chinese SLE cohort, where the R allele contributes to disease susceptibility (Ye, 2006; Pan, 2008).

In a meta-analysis carried out by Lehrnbecher et. al., the development of SLE was significantly associated with the alleles encoding the low affinity isoforms of both FcγRIIA (FcγRIIA-R/R131) and FcγRIIIA (FcγRIIIA-F/F158) (Lehrnbecher, 1999b). More recently, a similar meta-analysis study carried out by Karassa and colleagues found that an FcγRIIA-R/H131 polymorphism represents a significant risk factor for the development of SLE but had no clear effect on susceptibility for lupus nephritis in a large patient cohort (Karassa, 2002).

Lower level evidence exists for a non-synonymous mutation in FcγRIIIA proposed to alter IgG binding affinity, a promoter SNP in FCGR2B that alters transcription factor binding and receptor expression and, in Asian populations, a non-synonymous SNP in exon 6 of FCGR2B suggested to influence B-cell activation (Brown, 2007).

FcγRIIB: FCGR2B receptor is expressed on B cells, dendritic cells, monocytes/macrophages, and mast cells. It contains an ITIM that regulates B-cell survival and proliferation by down-modulating B-cell receptor signaling, and by decreasing antibody-mediated phagocytosis in macrophages (Daeron, 1997).

A nonsynonymous SNP in the transmembrane domain of FcγRIIB (Ile187Thr) that alters the inhibitory function of FcγRIIB on B cells is associated with SLE in Asian populations,(Kyogoku, 2002; Siriboonrit, 2003; Chu, 2004) but not in other populations partly owing to their low allele frequencies (Li, 2003; Kyogoku, 2004; Magnusson, 2004). The FcγR2B encoded by the Thr187 allele results in impaired inhibition of B-cell activation and promotes autoimmunity (Floto, 2005). A functional promoter haplotype (–386G/–120T) of FcγRIIB that confers increased transcription of FcγRIIB has been associated with 1.6-fold risk for SLE in Caucasian Americans (Su, 2004). This haplotype is not in LD with FcγRIIA and FcγRIIIA polymorphisms and is likely to have an independent association with SLE (Kyogoku, 2002).

FcγRIIIB: FCGR3B is expressed solely on neutrophils. It lacks an ITAM domain, so the transmission of intracellular signals is likely to involve cooperation with other transmembrane proteins. Of particular interest are data suggesting that this is achieved through an interaction with complement receptor 3/integrin α_M (Krauss, 1994; Poo, 1995; Stockl, 1995). It is considered low affinity receptor for the Fc region of immunoglobulins gamma. It binds to complexed or aggregated IgG and also monomeric IgG. Contrary to FCγR3A, is not capable to mediate antibody-dependent cytotoxicity and phagocytosis. It may serve as a trap for immune complexes in the peripheral circulation which does not activate neutrophils.

Six SNPS exist in FCGR3B, underlying three different allotypic variants of FCGR3B (NA1, NA2 and SH). The association reported by Hatta *et a.l.*(Hatta, 1999) between the NA2 allotype and SLE in a Japanese population has not been replicated, suggesting that the association between SLE and this genomic region might be influenced by other genetic variations. Both duplication and deficiency of FCGR3B were reported in normal individuals (Clark, 1990; Koene, 1998). The inheritance pattern of FCGR3B in some families affected by SLE has suggested that the copy number variation might be the underlying condition.
The number of copies of FCGR3B in a cell can vary from none to four, with a gene-dose effect that reduced FcγRIIIB copy number being a risk factor for glomerulonephritis in SLE patients. In addition, FCGR3B copy number varies significantly with non-Mendelian inheritance, suggesting that the association of FCGR3B copy number with lupus nephritis is an independent risk factor (Aitman, 2006). Since human FCGR3B is expressed mainly in neutrophils, and it is postulated that SLE patients with low FCGR3B copy number have reduced neutrophil expression, which leads to reduced glomerular clearance of immune complexes, and brings forth susceptibility to SLE and other autoimmune disorders. This observation supports that copy number polymorphism at orthologous regions of diverse genomes is associated with immunologically related disease. It also suggests that genome plasticity, manifested by gene duplication/deletion and copy number polymorphism, is a common cause of genetically complex phenotypes. Fc receptor-like genes (FCRLs): FCLs clustered at 1q21–22 encode proteins that are structurally homologous classical FCGRs. To enhance our understanding of the functional roles of *Fcγ* receptors in SLE, an integrated approach to simultaneously assess CNVs, allotypic variants, SNPs and the functional diversity of these receptors in large-scale case–control studies including multiple ethnic populations is needed to dissect the relative contribution of various variants in this complex FCGR locus to SLE.

2.2 Protein tyrosine phosphatase non-receptor 22 (PTPN22) (1p13)

PTPN22 is a negative regulator for T-cell signal transduction in cellular immunity. It is considered to be the strongest common genetic risk factor for human autoimmunity besides the major histocompatibility complex (MHC) and as an important candidate gene in SLE. A number of candidate gene studies found (SNP rs2476601) R620W polymorphism in the proximal protein-rich SH3-binding domain (+1858T/C), to be associated with the increased risk of SLE (Orozco, 2005). This has been confirmed in a meta-analysis (Lea, 2011) and SLE GWA analysis. This polymorphism was found to be associated with several autoimmune diseases in Caucasians, including T1D, autoimmune thyroid disease, RA and SLE, but not with multiple sclerosis (MS). SNP rs2476601 is not polymorphic in Koreans and Japanese and almost absent in African populations (Gregersen, 2006) while it is more common in northern Europeans (8–15%) compared with southern Europeans (2–10%) (Gregersen, 2009). Suggesting the presence of genetic heterogeneity across various ethnicities.
The lymphoid tyrosine phosphatase protein (LYP), which is encoded by *PTPN22*, is known to regulate immunological synapse formation. LYP is involved in the down-regulation of T-cell activation through its interaction with a negative regulator of TCR signaling C-terminal Src tyrosine kinase (Csk); this interaction is prevented by the arginine to tryptophan amino acid substitution consequent upon the associated mutation rs2476601 R620W (C1858T) (Begovich, 2004; Bottini, 2004).
One would expect this R620W substitution to result in increased T-cell signaling and activation; however, experimental evidence suggests the opposite with TCR signaling

actually reduced in cells carrying the tryptophan variant protein (Vang, 2005). A number of explanations have been proposed including an effect of the mutation on the tyrosine phosphatase activity of LYP, or an effect on the binding of other ligands or the conformation of LYP in response to these ligands (Vang, 2008). At a cellular level the mechanism by which reduced T-cell activation may actually increase the potential for autoimmunity remains a matter for speculation, although the suppression of regulatory T-cells is a possibility (Vang, 2008). A connection between PtPn22 and the type I IFN pathway has been suggested on the basis of elevated serum IFN-α activity and decreased tumor necrosis factor (TNF) levels in patients with SLE carrying the rs2476601 risk allele (Kariuki, 2008). By contrast, another *PTPN22* polymorphism, the loss-of-function mutation Arg263Gln in the catalytic domain (R263Q), leads to reduced phosphatase activity of PtPn22, and, therefore, increases the threshold for TCR signaling has been associated with protection against SLE in European-derived populations (Orru, 2009).

2.3 Interleukin 10 (IL 10) 1q32.1

IL-10 is an important immunoregulatory cytokine in man with both immunosuppressive and immunostimulatory properties (Mosmann, 1994). It is characterized with anti-inflammatory and stimulatory activities, and plays a critical role in the regulation of cellular and humoral immune responses. IL-10 is also involved in the pathology of human autoimmune disease (Llorente, 1994; Cash, 1995; Perez, 1995), particularly in the dysregulation of B-cell function in systemic lupus erythematosus leading to autoantibody production (Itoh, 1995; Llorente, 1995). In addition, its ability to induce T-cell anergy (Luscher, 1994) and inhibit major histocompatibility complex class-I expression (Matsuda, 1994) may be important in its apparent contribution to tumor-related immunosuppression (Kim, 1995; Suzuki, 1995; Fortis, 1996).

It has been known that IL10 production is under strong genetic influence (Westendorp, 1997). Two CA-repeat microsatellites, IL10R (-4 kb) (GeneBank accession number AF295024) and IL10G (-1.1 kb) (GeneBank accession number X78437), and single nucleotide polymorphisms (SNPs) were reported in IL10 promoter that has potential association with IL10 production. These SNPs are located at positions -A3575T, -A2849G, -A2763C, -A1082G, -C819T, and -A592C from the transcription start site. It has been known that -A1082G, -C819T, and -A592C combined to form three haplotypes; GCC, ACC, and ATA linked with different IL10 expression level (Crawley, 1999).

IL-10 has been associated in the pathogenesis of SLE; Increased *IL10* production by peripheral blood B cells and monocytes from patients with SLE is known to correlate with disease activity (Hagiwara, 1996), increased IL-10 productions promotes B-cell hyperactivity and autoantibody production (Llorente, 1995). The association between IL10 promoter haplotypes (defined by three SNPs in the *IL10* promoter region -627C→A, -854C→T and -1117G→A. These single base-pair substitutions produce three different haplotypes, GCC, ACC and ATA,) (Turner, 1997; Eskdale, 1997a) and SLE has been have been reported in European, Hispanic American and Asian populations (Eskdale, 1997b; Mehrian, 1998; Chong, 2004). A large-scale replication study in populations from the USA and Sweden has confirmed *IL10* as a SLE susceptibility locus (Gateva, 2009). However, they were found to have significant association with lupus nephritis.

Levels of IL-10 secretion have been correlated to specific IL10 promoter polymorphisms; a study has shown that the SNP haplotypes in the distal promoter of IL-10 correlate with different IL-10 production phenotype in normal individuals, and high IL-10 haplotype is associated with SLE in African-Americans, which may be a part of their genetic susceptibility to SLE. A meta-analysis of 15 IL-10 studies has shown that the G11 allele is associated with SLE in whole studied populations, and among the promoter SNPs, −A1082G polymorphism, which is found in Asian population only, was also associated with SLE (Nath, 2005). Based on these analyses, IL-10 polymorphisms confer SLE risk in an ethnicity-specific manner (Gateva, 2009; Eskdale, 1997; Mehrian, 1998; Chong, 2004).

2.4 Complement receptor 1 (CR1, CD35), (1q32)

Genome scans have shown linkage (lod score >1.0) at chromosome 1q32, which contains complement components, like complement receptor 1 (**CR1**), complement receptor 2 (CR2), and C4b-binding protein (C4BP) genes and IL10 family members; IL10, IL19, IL20, and IL24, which play a significant role in the pathogenesis of SLE (Johanneson, 2002; Tsao, 1999). The C3b/C4b complement receptor (Gene ID: 1378) (CR1, CD35) is a polymorphic transmembrane single chain glycoprotein expressed on red cell surface binds to C3b and C4b and clears circulating C3- and C4-bearing immune complexes containing (Dykman, 1984).

Functional and structural polymorphisms of CR1 have been reported. The functional polymorphism determines the quantitative expression of CR1 on erythrocytes, i.e. HH, HL, and LL (H = allele correlated with high expression, L = low) (Wilson, 1986). The structural polymorphism exists in its molecular size (Dykman, 1983). The extracellular portion of the CR1 molecule consists of three to five groups of seven short consensus repeats termed long homologous repeats (LHR). The most frequent type of CR1 (F or A) is comprised of four extracellular LHRs and expresses one binding site for C4b and two binding sites for C3b (Wong, 1983). The S (or B) variant of CR1 is characterized by additional C3b binding site on a fifth LHR (Wong, 1989). A meta-analysis for the CR1 functional polymorphisms in SLE shows no significant association of CR1 L allele, L/L genotype, and L/L+L/H genotypes with SLE. However, the same meta-analysis of CR1 structural polymorphisms suggested an association of CR1 S (structural variant of CR1) to be associated with SLE in Caucasians (Nath, 2005).

2.5 Tumor necrosis factor (ligand) SuperFamily, member 4(TNFSF4), 1q25

TNFSF4 (also known as OX40L; 1q25) encodes a cytokine that is expressed on CD40-stimulated B cells, activated antigen-presenting cells (APCs) and vascular endothelial cells. Also its unique receptor, TNFRSF4 (also known as OX40; 1p36), is primarily expressed on activated CD4+ T cells. Their interaction induces the production of CD28-independent co-stimulatory signals to activate CD4+ T cells (Baum, 1994). OX40L-mediated signaling inhibits the generation and function of IL-10-producing CD4+ type 1 regulatory T cells, but induces B-cell activation and differentiation, as well as IL-17 production in vitro (Ito, 2006a; Li, 2008).

These two tumor necrosis factor (TNF) superfamily members (OX40L and OX40) located within proximal intervals showing genetic linkage with SLE (Cunninghame, 2008; Chang, 2009; delGado-Vega, 2009).TNFSF4 has been identified as a susceptibility gene for SLE in multiple studies. Protective and risk haplotypes at TNFSF4 were identified in a study of two cohorts from Minnesota and UK, a haplotype in the upstream region of TNFSF4, marked by SNPs rs844644 and rs2205960, has been shown to correlate with increased cell surface TNFSF4 expression and TNFSF4 transcript and to be associated with SLE (Graham, 2008).

Associations between some *TNFSF4*-tagging SNPs and an increased risk for SLE have been confirmed in GWAS in Chinese populations and in a European replication study; these results were also replicated in four independent SLE datasets from Germany, Italy, Spain and argentine. It has not been fully established how TNFRSF4/ TNFSF4 interactions influence T-cell subset profiles. Most evidence suggests a bias towards a Th2 pattern of cytokine release, although there is also evidence for a down-regulation of regulatory T-cell subsets (Ito, 2006b; Lane, 2000). There is also good evidence that signaling through TNFSF4 can induce B-cell activation and differentiation (Stuber, 1995&1996). TNFRSF4/ TNFSF4 signaling is therefore bi-directional, and the precise immunological consequences of this complex pathway are yet to be clarified. Further studies are needed to localize causal variants and to understand how these polymorphisms affect the pathogenesis of SLE.

2.6 C-reactive protein (CRP), 1q23.2

CRP is a sensitive marker of inflammation. The genes for CRP (CRP) map to 1q23.2 within an interval linked with SLE in multiple populations. It is hypothesized that polymorphism of CRP gene contributes to susceptibility to systemic lupus erythematosus (SLE).

Basal levels of CRP were influenced independently by two polymorphisms at the CRP locus, CRP 2 and CRP 4. Furthermore, the latter polymorphism was linked/associated with SLE and antinuclear autoantibody production. Thus, the polymorphism associated with reduced basal CRP was also associated with the development of SLE.

CRP is normally involved in phagocytosis of apoptotic debris and immune complexes in innate immune response. Defective clearance of products of apoptosis may be the source of autoantigens in SLE, and such phenomenon may also be enhanced by FcγR2A polymorphisms, with FcγR2 receptor being the main receptor for CRP (Bharadwaj, 1999).

During the active phase of SLE, despite the presence of marked tissue inflammation, CRP levels are abnormally low due to reduced synthesis (Russell, 2004). Family-based studies of association and linkage have identified the minor allele of rs1205 in the 3'UTR SNP of CRP to be associated with SLE and antinuclear antibody production (Russell, 2004), and the number of CA repeats correlated with disease risk in a Spanish cohort (Russell, 2004). Also, a single dose of CRP has recently shown to reverse lupus nephritis and nephrotoxic nephritis in mice, suggesting the acute-phase response of CRP may hinder tissue inflammation and damage (Rodriguez, 2005). These results are promising, and future investigation of this gene will not only allow better understanding of the genetic influence of CRP but also its pathophysiology and possible therapeutic options.

Two of several polymorphisms in the CRP gene, designated CRP2 (G/C) and CRP4 (G/A) have been demonstrated to have an impact on baseline serum concentration of CRP, with the C- and A-alleles being associated with lower concentrations (Russell, 2004). Furthermore, the CRP4 A-allele was shown to confer increased susceptibility to SLE in 586 families (P=0.006) (Russell, 2004). The A allele at *CRP* 4 had a relatively high frequency in European and Asian-Indian populations (~0.3) and was present in Afro-Caribbean families too, but at a lower frequency (0.14).

2.7 Poly(ADP-ribose) polymerase (PARP), (1q41–42)

PARP is an enzyme (PARP-1 EC 2.4.2.30) is induced by DNA strand breaks caused by several agents and utilizes NAD to form polyADPR, bound to acceptor proteins. It is responsible for DNA repair, proliferation, stress response, apoptosis, and genomic stability (Oliver, 1999). The involvement of PARP-1 in autoimmune diseases has been suggested especially in systemic lupus erythematosus (SLE) due to the decreased levels of activity and mRNA in SLE patients (Haug 1994). Autoantibodies to PARP are frequently found in patients affected with autoimmune diseases, some of which may prevent caspase-3-mediated PARP cleavage during apoptosis, resulting in the accumulation of autoimmune cells (Decker, 2000). On chromosome 1q41–q42 a 15-cM region has been linked with susceptibility to SLE (Tsao, 1997), this linkage has been confirmed in several independent studies. In a family-based TDT analysis, PARP alleles had skewed transmission to affected offspring, but this finding is not consistent in other multi-ethnic studies (Tsao, 1999).

A polymorphic CA tandem repeat within the PARP promoter region suggested to affect transcription activity has been associated with SLE in some but not other similar studies (Oei, 2001). A study investigated the association of PARP promoter CA tandem repeats polymorphisms with SLE susceptibility in Taiwan. Nine alleles ranging from 12 to 20 repeats were disclosed. No statistically significant association with SLE susceptibility was found in this population however; PARP microsatellite polymorphisms demonstrate associations with clinical subphenotypes such as discoid rash and arthritis, anti-cardiolipin IgG and anti-ds-DNA antibody production. These indicate that PARP CA repeats may play a key role in lupus pathogenesis involving DNA repair of cell damage and consequent autoantibody production. Tsao *et al* demonstrated a skewed transmission of PARP alleles in a family study with the PARP CA8 allele as susceptible and the PARP CA14 allele as a protector of lupus transmission (Tsao, 1999).

In a Korean study, PARP polymorphisms could not prove any statistically significant association with the risk of SLE was observed, however, they found that two single-nucleotide polymorphisms (SNPs -1963A/G and +28077G/A) were significantly associated with an increased risk of nephritis, and one non-synonymous variant [+40329T/C (V762A)] was also significantly associated with an increased risk of arthritis, while the -1963A/G polymorphism showed a protective effect on arthritis in Korean SLE patients (Hur, 2006).

2.8 Toll-like receptor 5 (TLR5), 1q41–q42

At least 10 different *TLR* have been cloned from the human genome to date. Toll-like receptors (TLR) are type I transmembrane proteins contain an extracellular leucine-rich region involved in pathogen recognition and a conserved intracellular Toll/IL-1 receptor domain that activates a signaling pathway. Stimulation of the TLR pathway ends in NF-κB activation and transcription of immune response genes, such as cytokines and chemokines. TLRs play an important role in the activation and regulation of both adaptive and innate immunity. They are considered as excellent candidate genes for genetic susceptibility studies for autoimmune diseases. TLR5 is a critical regulator of inflammatory pathways and maps to chromosome 1q41. Activation of TLR5 triggers production of proinflammatory cytokines, such as IL-6, which, in turn, can stimulate B cells to proliferate, differentiate, and secrete antibodies. Dysregulation of this process may lead to excessive production of cytokines as well as autoantibodies (Dean, 2000).

It was hypothesized that the stop codon variant C1174T (rs5744168) (Arginine to a stop codon at position 392 (R392X) in TLR5, is associated with susceptibility to SLE. This hypothesis was tested by using a TDT in a Caucasian SLE cohort and found that the TLR5 stop codon polymorphism, but not other TLR5 alleles, is associated with protection from developing SLE as subjects with 1174T produced less proinflammatory cytokines (IL-6, TNF-α, and IL-1β) (Hawn, 2003; Hawn, 2005). In addition the same group found that this association was most pronounced in individuals who are seronegative for anti-dsDNA autoantibodies (Tsao, 1999; Hawn, 2005). $TLR5^{R392X}$ may provide protection from SLE by decreasing production of proinflammatory cytokines during infection with flagellated bacteria, which may influence formation of the adaptive immune response. These results suggest a role for the innate immune response in the development of SLE that involves flagellated bacterial infections.

3. Chromosome 2

Locus 2q32- q37 encodes the Programmed cell death 1 gene (PDCD1), Cytotoxic T-lymphocyte associated protein 4 (CTLA4) and STAT4 transcription factor. All were proven to be associated to susceptibility to SLE.

3.1 Programmed cell death 1 gene (PDCD1/ CD279) (2q37)

PDCD1 codes for an immunoreceptor, PD-1, member of the CD28/CTLA4/ICOS co-stimulatory receptor family that bears an inhibitory immunoreceptor tyrosine-based motif (ITIM). It is expressed on activated T- and B-cell surfaces to regulate their peripheral tolerance (Agata 1996; Finger, 1997). PDCD1 is upregulated in T cells following activation, and inhibits TCR signaling and T/B cell survival. It is considered a strong candidate for SLE association.

The human *PDCD1* has an intron enhancer which contains binding sites for other transcription factors that are involved in lymphocyte development and T cell differentiation. PDCD single nucleotide polymorphism (SNP) (PD1.3A, the minor A allele of 7146 G/A) in this intron enhancer alters a binding site for the runt-related transcription factor (RUNX1). The PDCD1 enhancer has a very high GC content (from 50 to 75%). The A allele of the PDCD1 enhancer SNP changes a potential methylation site from CpG to CpA that is surrounded by many other potential methylation sites. Methylation is a known mechanism of regulation of gene activity (Avni, 2000). Whether methylation is involved in the regulation of PDCD1 is under investigation. Changes in methylation can condition the developmental stage of PDCD1 expression.

SNP 7146 G/A was shown to be association with SLE susceptibility and its contribution to SLE development was confirmed in Europeans and Mexicans by inducing lymphocytic hyperactivity in these patients (Prokunina, 2002). PDCD-1 polymorphisms may be a shared genetic factor for multiple autoimmune diseases in humans, and the cellular function leading to disease onset awaits further investigation. PDCD1 7209 CT or 7209 TT genotype exhibited 3.28-fold increased risk of SLE in the Polish and Taiwanese populations (Mostowska, 2008).

The most logical explanation of the mechanism of disease susceptibility for PDCD1 was suggested by Alarcón-Riquelme M *et al* (Alarcón-Riquelme, 2003); The stated: "So what effects could the aberrant function or expression of PDCD1 have in early lymphocyte differentiation that may lead to autoimmune disease, in particular SLE? It mainly depends on at what stage of differentiation does the RUNX1–PDCD1 interaction take place whether it occurs before clonal receptor rearrangements or after. As PDCD1 seems to act during positive selection in the thymus, at least in the mouse, this leads us to suggest that the human mutation may be promoting positive selection of early autoreactive progenitors, leading to an increased "susceptibility" to expand autoreactive T or B cells after antigenic stimuli, however the amount of information to date on PDCD1 in lymphocyte development and its regulation is still an open question".

3.2 Cytotoxic T-lymphocyteassociated protein 4 (CTLA4), (2q33)

CTLA4 is a structural homologue of CD28. It is a negative costimulatory molecule that inhibits T cell activation, and may help to limit T cell responses under conditions of inflammation and prevents autoimmune diseases by promoting anergy. It competes with the binding of CD28 on antigen presenting cells (APCs), and transduces inhibitory signals by activation of serine/threonine phosphatases. Genetic variability in CTLA4 has been implicated in the development of several autoimmune diseases including SLE (Matsushita, 1999). SLE patients have increased levels of soluble CTLA-4. A single nuclear polymorphism (SNP) CT60A/G within the 3′UTR of CTLA4 decreased the production of a spliced variant with inhibitory activity, which indicates the importance of CTLA-4 in providing protection against autoimmunity (Ueda, 2003).

SLE in Caucasians, CTLA-4 polymorphisms of its promoter and exon-1 regions was found to be associated to SLE. Later, in a Chinese cohort, the CTLA-4 promoter (-1722 T/C) polymorphism showed positive evidence (Liu, 2001 & Xu, 2004). However, several genetic studies investigating CTLA-4 polymorphisms and SLE have been negative. Among the positive studies, different mutations were identified within the CTLA4 promoter (−1722T/C, −1661A/G, −319C/T) and exon 1 (+49G/A) in various ethnic groups (Lee, 2005). More work is needed to delineate the genetic relationship between CTLA-4 and SLE.

3.3 Signal transducer and activator of transcription 4 protein (STAT4), (2q32)

STAT4 play key roles in the interferon and Th1 signaling pathway through mediating responses to IL-12 in lymphocytes, and regulates T helper cell differentiation. STAT4 also is known to mediate signals induced by immunologically relevant cytokines including, like IRF5, the Type 1 IFNs (Darnell, 1994 & Watford, 2004). In response to these cytokines, STAT4 activation plays an important role in directing a Th1 T-cell response, and mediates the production of Th1-type cytokines such as IFN-α (Morinobu, 2002; Nguyen, 2002; Nishikomori, 2002). In addition, STAT4 signaling also mediates type 1 IFN signaling in antigen-presenting cells, and may be necessary for the production of IFN-α by these cells (Frucht, 2003 & Fukao, 2001).

STAT4 variation and SLE risk was initially reported in 2007 from a case–control association study (Remmers, 2007). This was subsequently confirmed in both GWA studies. Three SNPs in STAT4, rs7574865, rs11889341, and rs10168266, were then shown to be in significant association with SLE in a Japanese population, with the rs7574865 T allele, in the third intron of STAT4, showing the strongest significance. Interestingly, this rs7574865 risk variant is associated with a more severe SLE phenotype that is characterized by disease onset at a young age (<30 years), a high frequency of nephritis, the presence of antibodies towards double stranded DNA, (Taylor, 2008; Kawasaki, 2008; Sigurdsson, 2008) and an increased sensitivity to IFN-α signaling in peripheral blood mononuclear cells (Kariuki, 2009). In a meta-analysis including Europeans and Asian patients of SLE and RA, the rs7574865 T allele was found to be consistently associated with both diseases (Ji, 2010). Possible functional relevance of risk STAT4 variant has recently strongly suggested by in vivo experiment in SLE patients, in which risk variant of STAT4 (T allele; rs7574865) was simultaneously associated with both lower serum IFN-a activity and greater IFN-α induced gene expression in PBMC in SLE patients.

A risk haplotype (spanning 73 kb from the third intron to the seventeenth exon of STAT4) common to European, Americans, Koreans and Hispanic Americans was also identified

(Namjou, 2009). Functionally, either type I IFN or interleukin (IL)-12 induces phosphorylation of STAT4, which has a signal transduction role in these pathways. Individuals carrying one or more risk alleles of both IRF5 and STAT4 have an increased risk for SLE, suggesting a genetic interaction between these two genes (Sigurdsson, 2008).
The important roles of STAT4 in both innate immunity and Th1 immune response, recent enormous body of evidence of consistent association of STAT4 with SLE in multiple racial groups indicates that a risk variant or a certain risk haplotype of STAT4 has a crucial role in SLE pathogenesis that has yet to be completely determined and could provide new therapeutic targets for SLE and the other autoimmune diseases in future.

4. Chromosome 3

4.1 Phox homology (PX) domain Kinase (PXK), (3p14.3)

PXK is of unknown function. PXK domain containing serine/threonine kinase and act as modulator of Na, K-ATPase enzymatic and ion pump activities (Mao, 2005). It was identified as a novel candidate gene for systemic lupus erythematosus (SLE) from genome-wide association studies (GWAS) in Caucasians (Suarez-Gestal, 2009). The association of PXK rs6445975 with SLE observed in Caucasians was not replication study in Hong Kong Chinese and Koreans (Kim, 2011; Yu, 2011; Yang, 2009). It is possible that PXK has different genetic contribution on SLE between Caucasians and Asians and that the gene is associated with disease subphenotypes rather than with overall susceptibility.

5. Chromosome 4

5.1 BANK, BLK and LYN

All three of these genes play a critical role in controlling the activation of B cells following signaling through the B-Cell Receptor (BCR). Following ligand binding and BCR aggregation, an early intracellular event is the recruitment and activation of Src-family protein tyrosine kinases, including BLK and LYN, which mediate further intracellular signaling. The exact role of these kinases in determining cellular events has yet to be determined with certainty.

5.2 B-cell scaffold protein with ankyrin repeats (BANK1), (4q24)

BANK1 is a B-cell scaffold protein that is tyrosine phosphorylated through the B-cell receptor (BCR) upon B-cell activation, which in turn associates with the tyrosine kinase *Lyn* (Src family of tyrosine kinase) and the calcium channel *IP3R* which results in calcium ion release from the stores of the endoplasmic reticulum (Yokoyama, 2002 & Kozyrev, 2008). *BANK1* is thought to alter B cell activation to increase SLE risk. Polymorphisms in *BANK1* may cause B-cell hyper-responsiveness.
GWAS in European-derived populations have identified associations of *BANK1* and *LYN* with susceptibility to SLE (Kozyrev, 2008 & Guo, 2009). For BANK1 three functional variants with either a non-synonymous SNP (rs10516487; Arg61His), a branch point-site SNP (rs17266594; located in an intron) or a SNP in the ankyrin domain (rs3733197; Ala383Thr) might contribute to the sustained activation of B-cell receptors and the subsequent B-cell hyperactivity that is commonly observed in SLE (Kozyrev, 2008). However, the best functional evidence was found for rs17266594, which altered a branch point upstream of exon 2, resulting in the generation of a novel short isoform, but little

quantitative difference in *BANK1* expression overall. With the exception of the rs10516487 SNP of *BANK1*, which showed a weak association with SLE in an Asian GWAS, the remaining SNPS of *BANK1* have not been confirmed in either Chinese or Asian GWAS, partly owing to the low frequencies of the SNPS in these populations (Chang, 2009).

6. Chromosome 5

6.1 TNIP1 (Tumor necrosis factor α-induced protein 3 (TNFAIP3) interacting protein 1), also known as ABIN (A20-binding inhibitor of NF-κB)-1, (5q32-q33.1)

TNIP1 expression is induced by NF-κB, and in turn, overexpression of TNIP1 inhibits NF-κB activation by TNF (Verstrepen, 2009). TNIP1 was shown to inhibit TNF-induced apoptosis independently of A20 (Oshima, 2009). Two recent GWAS revealed association of TNIP1 intronic SNPs rs7708392 and rs10036748, which are in strong linkage disequilibrium (LD) with SLE in the Caucasian (European-American and Swedish) and Chinese Han populations, respectively (Han, 2009 & Gateva, 2009). Association of TNIP1 with SLE was also confirmed in a Japanese population.

To date, at least 11 splice variants of *TNIP1*have been identified (Verstrepen, 2009). Presence of alternative exon 1A and 1B, as well as splice variants lacking exon 2, has been described. Because rs7708392 is located between exon 1B and exon 2, it is possible that this SNP may influence the usage of the splicing isoform. It is also possible that other causative SNPs in tight LD with rs7708392 may exist. Such a possibility would be addressed by resequencing the entire *TNIP1* gene. *TNIP1* is a shared SLE susceptibility gene in the Caucasian and Asian populations, but the genetic contribution appeared to be greater in the Asians because of the higher risk allele frequency in the population.

7. Chromosome 6

7.1 Major Histocompatibility Complex (MHC), (6p21.31)

A body of evidence has been collected to establish the pivotal role of major histocompatibility complex (MHC) in immune tolerance. The classical MHC locus (6p21.3) 3.6Mb contains at least 250 expressed genes. This locus is divided into the Class I and II regions that encode the antigen-presenting HLA proteins and Class III MHC that contains 58 genes, located between Class I and II regions, only some its genes are of potential immunological interest (e.g. TNF-α and TNF-β, C4A, C4B and C2) and others which have poorly defined function. There is particularly strong linkage disequilibrium between genetic markers in this region which is strongly association with SLE in all GWA studies. It is therefore difficult to establish whether any associated variant is functional or simply observed due to linkage disequilibrium with functional polymorphisms elsewhere. It was as early as 1971 that Grumet *et al.* reported possible relationship between the HLA genes and SLE (Grumet, 1971). MHC alleles on 6p11–21 have shown the most significant association. Although the genetic structure of the MHC makes it a particularly challenging region to study, significant progress has been made over the last year.

The Class II HLA genes are of particular importance, which encode antigen-presenting molecules that play a pivotal role in T-cell immunity. Most evidence has highlighted the DR loci, which are one of the Class II HLA gene complexes. The HLA-DRB1 gene is of particular importance in SLE. For the HLA-DRB1 gene, the serotype of DR2 holds the strongest evidence of disease association. Three class-II-containing-SLE-risk haplotypes (DRB1*1501

(DR2)/DQB1*0602, DRB1*0301) (DR3)/DQB1*0201, and DRB1*0801 (DR8)/DQB1*0402) are consistently associated with SLE in Caucasian populations by family-based TDT (van der Linden, 2001).
Within the MHC class III region, there are genes that encode TNF-α and -β, lymphotoxin-β, complement components C2 and C4, and heat shock protein 70 (Hsp70). In particular, TNFs, C2, and C4 have been implicated in SLE susceptibility. TNF-α is a multifunctional proinflammatory cytokine involved in regulating a wide spectrum of biological processes including cell proliferation, differentiation, and apoptosis, while TNF-β mediates a variety of inflammatory, immunostimulatory, and antiviral responses. Polymorphisms in these genes have been implicated in SLE susceptibility (Pan 2011 & Bettinotti, 1993).
Complement component genes within the MHC class III region include C2, C4A, C4B, and factor B. These genes are closely linked and are usually inherited as a group known as complotype. Deficiencies in complement pathway genes C2, C4, C1q and C3 appear to cause SLE in some people (Kallel-Sellami, 2008). Polymorphisms in C2, C4A and C4B are in linkage disequilibrium with HLA-B and HLA-DR alleles (Alper, 2007) and may predispose to SLE. Also the complete deficiencies of the early components are highly associated with human SLE (Yu, 2007). A homozygous deficiency in one of the early complement components, including C1q, C1r, C1s and C4 in the classical activation pathway, alone can be strong enough to cause the disease, a situation similar to a single gene defect in an autosomal recessive disease. Respectively, 93% and 78% of patients with complete C1q and C4 deficiencies eventually develop SLE or a lupus-like disease (Yu, 2007 & Botto, 2002). In addition, the concordance rates for siblings with homozygous deficiency of C1q or C4 to develop SLE are 90% and 80%, respectively, which are even higher than the rate in monozygotic twins (26–60%) with other genetic defects (Tsao, 2008). Complete deficiency of complement C4 is among the strongest genetic risk factors for human systemic lupus erythematosus (SLE). Further work will be required to determine the effect arising from C4A. C4 is the most polymorphic protein of the complement system. It is encoded by two genes, C4A and C4B, which have minor sequence differences. The resulting proteins have different functional characteristics, with C4A better able to bind immune complexes (Schifferli, 1986). The C4 genes are inherited in a discrete 'RCCX module', which contains one C4 gene (either C4A or C4B) along with three neighboring genes (RP, CYP21 and TNX) (Yang, 1999). The Class III MHC carries between one and four copies of this module; hence each diploid genome has between two and eight C4 genes, which may be either C4A or C4B (Yang, 2007). Carrying less than two copies of C4A has been identified as a risk factor for SLE (Yang, 2007).
The common European haplotype AH8.1 carries multiple variants that have been associated with SLE including DRB1*0301 (DR3), the TNF -308A allele and the C4A complement null allele. Many studies were unable to break down this haplotype below a 1Mb interval covering most of the Class II and II regions (Alper, 2007).

7.2 PR domain containing 1, with ZNF domain - APG5 autophagy 5-like (PRDM1-ATG5 region), (6q21)

PRDM1 acts as a repressor of beta-interferon gene expression. The protein binds specifically to the PRDI (positive regulatory domain I element) of the beta-IFN gene promoter. While, the ATG5 candidate gene function is still obscure and needed to be determined however, both known to play important roles in immunity. Genome-wide association studies suggested the PRDM1-ATG5 gene region as a systemic lupus erythematosus (SLE)-

associated locus both in Caucasian and Asian populations, presumably through upregulating gene expression (Zhou, 2011; Harley, 2008; Gateva, 2009; Han, 2009).
Significant positive correlations with ATG5 expression were identified, suggesting ATG5 as a candidate gene in the region (Harley, 2008). Later GWAS from a Chinese population denied the association between polymorphisms in *ATG5* and SLE, but replicated the association between the intergenic region of *PRDM1-ATG5* (rs548234 and rs6568431) and SLE ((Han, 2009). At the same time, from Caucasian replication data, both *PRDM1* (rs6568431) and *ATG5* (rs2245214) were suggested as candidate genes, because rs6568431 was more close to *PRDM1* and rs6568431 has an r^2 of less than 0.1 with rs2245214. Meta-analysis consolidated the association between rs548234 and SLE ($p=1.28\times10^{-16}$).

7.3 Tumor necrotic factor α-induced protein 3 (TNFAIP3), 6q23

The gene product of *TNFAIP3* is a zinc-finger A20 protein, a ubiquitin-modifying enzyme, which is essential for proteasome degradation and termination of proinflammatory responses mediated by nuclear factor kappa B, thereby preventing inflammation. In humans, genetic surveys have suggested a role for *TNFAIP3* in susceptibility to complex genetic autoimmune disorders, including systemic lupus erythematosus (SLE) (Graham, 2008; Musone, 2008; Bates, 2005; Han, 2009).
Genetic association between variants in *TNFAIP3* and SLE suggest that alterations in activity and/or expression of *TNFAIP3* influence SLE pathophysiology (Graham, 2008; Musone, 2008; Bates, 2005; Han, 2009). Independent genetic associations of SLE and *TNFAIP3* in European-ancestry (EA) subjects have been localized to a region 185 kb upstream of *TNFAIP3* that was first identified with rheumatoid arthritis (Plenge, 2007; Thomson, 2007; Plenge, 2007), a region 249 kb downstream of *TNFAIP3* and a 109 kb haplotype spans the *TNFAIP3* coding region (Musone, 2008; Bates, 2005; Han, 2009) that includes a suggested causal coding variant in exon 3 (rs2230926 T>G; F127C) that reduces the ability of A20 to attenuate NF-κB signaling (Musone, 2008).
Evidence for association with SLE was observed also for a variant within *TNFAIP3* (rs5029939, GWAS *P* value = 2.55×10^{-8}) and two flanking SNPs (rs10499197, GWAS *P* value = 2.11×10^{-6}; rs7749323, GWAS *P* value = 9.63×10^{-7}) in strong LD with rs5029939 (r2>0.95). A SNP located ~185 kb upstream of *TNFAIP3* reported to be associated with risk for RA (204,206) (rs6920220) demonstrated modest association in the SLE GWAS dataset (GWAS P value = 0.01)
By fine mapping and genomic resequencing in ethnically diverse populations Adrianto I *et al*, fully characterized the *TNFAIP3* risk haplotype and isolated a novel TT>A polymorphic dinucleotide (deletion T followed by a T to A transversion) associated with SLE in subjects of European ($P = 1.58 \times 10^{-8}$) and Korean ($P = 8.33 \times 10^{-10}$) ancestry (Adrianto, 2011). This variant, located in a region of high conservation and regulatory potential, bound a nuclear protein complex comprised of NF-κB subunits with reduced avidity. Furthermore, compared with the non-risk haplotype, the haplotype carrying this variant resulted in reduced *TNFAIP3* mRNA and A20 protein expression. These results establish this TT>A variant as the most likely functional polymorphism responsible for the association between *TNFAIP3* and SLE (Adrianto, 2011).
One hundred and twenty seven (127) SNPs in the region of *TNFAIP3* on 6q23 and 347 ancestry informative markers (AIMs) in five diverse ethnic populations were analyzed by Adrianto I *et al*, They discovered a peak associations in European and Asian populations

were seen at markers rs6932056 and rs4896303 in 38 kb and 30 kb downstream of *TNFAIP3*, respectively (Adrianto, 2011).

8. Chromosome 7

8.1 Interferon regulatory factor 5 gene (IRF5), 7q32

IRF5 is one of the key genes of the interferon (IFN)-α pathway. IRF5 is a transcription factor that is responsible for the innate immune response during viral infection. IRF5 is important for trans-activation of type 1 IFN and IFN-responsive genes and for the production of pro-inflammatory cytokines interleukins such as; IL-6, IL-12, and tumor necrosis factor-α (TNF)] after toll like receptor (TLR) signaling induced by immune complexes containing self-antigens and nucleic acids (Takaoka, 2005). *IRF5* is one of the most strongly and consistently SLE-associated loci outside the MHC region in various ethnic groups and was detected using both candidate gene and GWAS approaches (Lee, 2009). Interest in type 1 (IFN-α and -β) IFN pathways was stimulated by the discovery that there is a general up-regulation IFN-inducible genes in SLE (Baechler, 2003 & Bennett, 2003). The best current genetic model proposes an SLE risk haplotype carrying multiple functional SNPs. Several SNPs in IRF5 (rs2004640, rs752637, rs729302, rs10954213etc.) were first found to be associated with SLE in Caucasians (Niewold, 2008; Kim, 2009).

In vitro functional evidence exists for at least two of these polymorphisms at SNP (rs2004640) creates a novel splice site in exon1B allowing the expression of a novel IRF5 isoform (Graham, 2006 & Sigurdsson, 2005) while the second polymorphism (rs10954213) located in the 3′ UTR creates a functional polyadenylation site and hence a shorter and more stable gene transcript (Cunninghame, 2007). To our knowledge, the most consistent evidence of association for this gene with SLE, across different populations including, was observed in the rs2004640 T allele. A meta-analysis has been conducted to study the association of the rs2004640 T allele with SLE; it included 12 studies in Europeans and Asians, it has been concluded that this polymorphism is associated with SLE susceptibility across different ethnic groups (Lee, 2009). In addition, the gene has a polymorphic 30 bp indel (insertion/deletion) in exon 6, which contributes to the diversity in the isoform pattern of IRF5, and a 5 bp indel near the 5'UTR upstream of exon 1A (Sigurdsson, 2008 & Dideberg, 2007).

To understand how IRF5 variants may predispose to SLE we need to understand the physiological role of the Type 1 IFN pathways. The majority of cells produce Type 1 IFNs as part of their early response to viral infection. Particularly large amounts are produced by plasmacytoid dendritic cells, perhaps stimulated by the recognition of viral RNA and DNA through TLR7 and TLR9. In SLE, it is possible that this is also triggered in response to inadequately cleared nucleic acid antigens released from apoptotic cells (Ronnblom, 2002). Type 1 IFNs exert a multitude of downstream effects on the immune system. Perhaps critically, they stimulate Th1 pathways and sustain activated T cells, while also lowering the threshold for B-cell activation through the B-cell receptor (BCR) and promoting B-cell survival and differentiation (Ronnblom, 2002; Braun, 2002; Le Bon, 2001; Marrack, 1999). It can therefore be seen that genetic variants that prolong or alter the actions of IRF5 could result in a prolonged proinflammatory response, and potentially break immunological tolerance. Interestingly, IRF5 signaling has also been shown to play a role in the regulation of cell cycle and apoptosis raising the possibility that susceptibility variants of IRF5 exert their effects at multiple levels (Barnes, 2003).

8.2 Ikaros zinc finger 1(IKZF), 7p12.2

IKZF1 encodes a lymphoid restricted zinc finger transcription factor named Ikaros, which is critically important for the normal development of all lymphoid cells. It regulates lymphocyte differentiation and proliferation (Georgopoulos, 1994), as well as self-tolerance through regulation of B-cell receptor signaling (Wojcik, 2007). Data derived from both GWAS and large replication studies identified *IKZF1* as a novel SLE susceptibility locus in Chinese and European-derived populations (Han, 2009). Yap et al. reported that IKZF1 was involved in the regulation of STAT4 in human T cells, which suggested that STAT4 and IKZF1 might cooperate with each other and play roles in the development of SLE (Yap, 2005). Hu W. *et al,* demonstrated that *IKZF1* mRNA expression levels in PBMCs from patients with SLE were significantly lower than those in healthy controls (Hu, 2011).
Association of SLE and disease phenotype with IKZF1 was studied in Chinese Han origin SLE patients were the allele frequency of rs4917014 (IKZF1) was significantly different in two subphenotypes: renal nephritis (p=0.02) and malar rash (p=0.00038) (He, 2010).

9. Chromosome 8

Several studies have revealed association of SLE susceptibility to different genes within a 700 kb region of locus 8p23.1 (Hom, 2008; Graham, 2008; Harley, 2008). This region contains several candidate genes, including BLK, XKR6, FAM167A/C8orf13 and C8orf12, these genes were in significant linkage disequilibrium (LD), making it difficult to determine whether the different reports are detecting the same association signal. Budarf ML *et al.* found significant association to both the BLK (rs2618476) and XKR6 (rs6985109) genes (Budarf, 2011). Although these two SNPS are separated by 620 kb, there is relatively strong correlation between them (r^2=0.39), allowing the possibility that they may represent the same signal. Here in we will review the evidence of association of both genes BLK, XKR6 with susceptibility to SLE (Budarf, 2011).

9.1 B lymphoid tyrosine kinase (BLK), 8p23.1

BLK encodes a nonreceptor tyrosine-kinase of the src family of proto-oncogenes, which mediates intracellular signaling and influences cell proliferation and differentiation. The human BLK gene was mapped to chromosome 8 at p23.1, and is expressed only in B lymphocytes (Drebin, 1995). The protein has a role in B-cell receptor signaling, B-cell development and tolerance of B cells (Reth, 1997). B cell receptor (BCR) signaling requires a tight regulation of several protein tyrosine kinases and phosphatases, and associated co-receptors. Break of the balance between positive and negative signaling molecules likely modifies the BCR signaling thresholds. Such alterations, together with other factors, may contribute to the disruption of selftolerance in SLE.
BLK has apparently become one of the most important and consistent non-MHC gene for SLE and the other autoimmune diseases across multiple ethnic groups and is one of three key genes (BLK, LYN and BANK) involved in BCR signaling found to be strongly associated with SLE proves the importance of this pathway in disease pathogenesis. B-lymphoid tyrosine kinase (BLK) was one of the top hit in more than one GWA analyses, while LYN was associated with high significance in the International Consortium for Systemic Lupus Erythematosus (SLEGEN) study only. BLK has been implicated in the pathogenesis of SLE and has been investigated in numerous ethnically diverse studies.
GWAS in European-derived populations identified a SNP (rs13277113; located in the promoter region of BLK, maps to the intergenic region between *FAM167A*/C8orf13 and

BLK), of which allele A is associated with reduced expression of *BLK* but increased expression of *FAM167A* (previously referred to as C8orf13) in patients with SLE (Ito, 2010). Another *BLK* SNP (rs2248932), located 43 kb downstream of rs13277113, is also associated with SLE where the risk C allele of rs2248932 was associated with the lower levels of BLK mRNA expression (Zhang, 2010).

Both SNPs have subsequently been confirmed as SLE-associated in Asian populations (Zhang, 2010 & Ito, 2009). Genotyping SNP rs2248932 in SLE patients of Chinese Han confirmed that SNP rs2248932 in BLK gene was significantly associated with SLE ($P = 1.41 \times 10^{-8}$). The association of BLK in Chinese SLE patients was consistent with a dominant model. In contrast to the Caucasian, this risk allele was the major allele in the Chinese Han; the risk allele frequency was higher in Chinese Han than in Caucasian. No association was found between this SNP and any subphenotype of SLE. Fan *et al* performed a meta-analysis to test the association of two SNPs rs13277113 and rs2248932. A significant associations of rs13277113 and SLE were observed for dominant model (AA + AG vs. GG, OR: 1.518), and recessive model (AA vs. AG + GG, OR: 1.553); so were rs2248932 and SLE for dominant model (TT + TC vs. CC, OR: 1.34), and recessive model (TT vs. TC + CC, OR: 1.34) (Fan, 2010).

9.2 X Kell blood group precursor-related family, member 6 (XKR6), 8p23.1

XKR6, a member of a novel family of PDZCBM containing proteins sharing homology with the *C. elegans* gene *ced-8*, which has been implicated in regulating the timing of apoptosis (Giallourakis, 2006). *XKR6* contains an intronic microRNA, hsa-miR-598, which is highly expressed in human peripheral blood mononuclear cells, especially activated B-cells (Lawrie, 2008). Dissecting the relative contribution of XKR6 to SLE risk is likely to be a complicated undertaking, especially given that a polymorphic inversion under apparent selection pressure on 8p23 encompasses the *XKR6, C8orf12, C8orf13,* and *BLK* genes, all of which have been implicated in SLE risk in GWAS studies (Deng, 2008).

9.3 Yamaguchi sarcoma viral (v-yes-1) related oncogene homolog' LYN, 8q12.1

LYN is a Src-tyosine kinase involved in B cell activation by phosphorylating the ITAM domain of the BCR-associated Ig α/β signaling molecules, in turn recruiting and activating the tyrosine kinase SYK, which initiates multiple activating signals. LYN also mediates inhibitory signals by phosphorylating inhibitory receptors such as CD22 and FcγRIIb and may therefore have a critical role as a modulator of B-cell activation thresholds. In the Genome wide association studies (GWAS) of SLE, three B cell signaling molecules *BLK, LYN* and *BANK1* (Hom, 2008; Kozyrev, 2008) were found to be associated with SLE. The best characterized functionally is LYN among the other two kinases *(BANK, BLK)* shown to be associated with SLE. These data suggest that aberrant regulation of B cell signaling may be one mechanism for generating hyper-responsive B cells, which might lead to aberrant B cell development, selection and ultimately influence the production of autoantibodies. Expression of Lyn is significantly decreased in both resting and BCR stimulated peripheral blood B cells from two-thirds of SLE patients compared to controls (Liossis, 2001). Further, statistically significant alterations at the transcriptional level were confirmed by a 2.5-fold decrease in Lyn mRNA in SLE patients compared to healthy individuals. Another group analyzed the level and subcellular distribution of Lyn in SLE

B cells and found that slightly more than half of the SLE patients analyzed had reduced levels of Lyn protein, which was subsequently determined to be due to increased ubiquitination of the protein. Functional differences in LYN ubiquitination have been also associated with SLE risk (Flores-Borja, 2005).

Two SNPs, rs7829816 and rs2667978, showed significant association in some of the cohorts tested, but failed to consistently replicate in all cohorts (Harley, 2008). Lu R. *et al* has performed one of the largest studies to examine the possible genetic association of *LYN* with SLE in multiple large populations of different ancestries (European-derived, African American and Korean). Their study has replicated a previously observed association with rs7829816 (Harley, 2008), however, data from Lu R. *et al* study suggested that this association is not a dominant lupus effect. The strongest and most consistent association found in this study was at rs6983130, which is within the first intron at the 5′ end near the primary transcription initiation site. This SNP showed the strongest association in the European-American female population. A strong gender influence was found with this SNP when analyzing only female subjects. Rs6983130 also showed associations with autoantibodies which is strongly associated with the development of SLE, specifically anti-dsDNA, anti-chromatin, anti-52 kDa Ro and anti-Sm.

10. Chromosome 10

10.1 Mannose-Binding Lectin (MBL), (10q11.2-21)

MBL is very similar to C1q in its structure and function. It is an important element of the innate immune system. MBL comprises a trimer of three identical polypeptides, and several trimmers further combine to form a bouquet-like structure (Holmskov, 1994). MBL recognizes carbohydrate patterns, found on the surface of a large number of pathogenic micro-organisms, including bacteria, viruses, protozoa and fungi and initiates the lectin pathway for opsonization and clearance of pathogens in an antibody-independent manner.

MBL gene comprising four exons and there is only one single functional gene. The normal structural MBL alleles is named A, while the common designation for the 3 variant structural allele B (Gly54Asp), C (Gly57Glu) and D (Arg52Cys) are O. MBL expression is influenced by polymorphic sites in the upstream part of the MBL gene nucleotides substitutions at positions -550, -221 and +4. Absent or low levels of serum MBL is a result of these polymorphisms and might be associated with the development of SLE (Takahashi, 2005 & Pradhan, 2010). Case-control genetic studies of MBL polymorphism were performed in various Ethnic groups. MBL genotyping in SLE confirmed that the MBL functional variants are associated with SLE (Ramasawmy, 2008). Serum MBL levels fluctuate during the course of SLE disease activity and MBL genotypes have been found to be useful in assessing the risk of infection during immunosuppressive treatment the majority of the SLE patients receive.

Two possible explanations for associations between MBL deficiency and occurrence of SLE were proposed (Korb, 1997): (a) MBL can bind to and initiate uptake of apoptotic cells into macrophages (Ogden, 2001 & Okada, 2002), and abnormal clearance of apoptotic cells caused by MBL deficiency may result in overexpression of autoantigens; (b) viral infection is believed to be one of the causes of SLE (Okada, 2002), and MBL deficiency may lead to more frequent infections.

11. Chromosome 11

11.1 Interferon regulatory factor 5 /PHD and RING-finger domains 1(IRF7/ PHRF1) locus, 11p15.5

IRF7 is a transcription factor that can induce transcription of IFN*a* and in turn IFN*a*-induced genes downstream of endosomal TLRs, similar to IRF5 (Barnes, 2004). A SNP near IRF7 was found to be associated with SLE susceptibility in the International Consortium for SLE Genetics (SLEGEN) genome-wide association study (Harley, 2008). The associated SNP (rs4963128) was located 23 kb telomeric to IRF7 in a gene of unknown function named PHD and RING-finger domains 1 (PHRF1; also known as KIAA1542 or CTD-binding SR-like protein rA9). This SNP was in high linkage disequilibrium ($r^2 = 0.94$) with the rs702966 SNP in IRF7 (Harley, 2008). The PHRF1 gene contains PHD-finger and RING-finger domains, and has not been functionally characterized to date. PHD and RING-finger domains both chelate zinc ions, and PHD domains are frequently found in proteins which mediate protein–protein interactions in the cell nucleus (Bienz, 2006).

There is a hypothesizes that the SLE-associated variant discovered in the IRF7/PHRF1 locus in the SLEGEN study (International Consortium for Systemic Lupus Erythematosus Genetics, 2008) could be due to a polymorphism in IRF7 that predisposes to increased IFN*a* production. Then, Salloum R. *et al* have proven this hypothesis by analyzing serum IFN*a* in SLE patients as a quantitative trait to determine associations with haplotype-tagging SNPs in the IRF7/PHRF1 locus (Salloum, 2009). In a joint analysis of European American and Hispanic American subjects, the rs702966 C allele was associated with the presence of anti–double-stranded DNA (anti-dsDNA) antibodies (P=0.0069). The rs702966 CC genotype was only associated with higher serum levels of IFN*a* in European American and Hispanic American patients with anti-dsDNA antibodies (joint analysis $P = 4.1 \times 10^{-5}$) (International Consortium for Systemic Lupus Erythematosus Genetics, 2008). However, the rs702966 C allele was not associated with anti-dsDNA in the African American subjects, and no other significant associations were seen in this group. In African American patients, the rs4963128 T allele downstream of IRF7 was associated with the presence of anti-Sm antibodies ($P = 0.0017$), where subjects with the rs4963128 CT and TT genotypes had higher IFN*a* levels than those with the CC genotype ($P = 0.0012$). The striking differences observed within the African American cohort separated by the presence or absence of anti-Sm antibodies suggest 2 independent patterns of association with IRF7/PHRF1 variants, which cannot be explained by European admixture at the locus. It is possible that the rs4963128 T allele marks a particular element in African-derived chromosomes that associates with anti-Sm antibodies and is not present in the other ancestral backgrounds (Salloum, 2009). Salloum R. *et al* hypothesized that the rs702966 C allele and elements in linkage with it may function similarly across all ancestral backgrounds, although the effect of the anti-Sm–rs4963128 T allele interaction on serum levels of IFN*a* in African Americans is independent of the effect at the rs702966 C allele (Salloum, 2009).

12. Chromosome 16

12.1 *Integrin αM* (ITGAM), 16p11.2

ITGAM is a single-pass type I membrane protein predominantly expressed primarily on neutrophils, macrophages and dendritic cells that is involved in various adhesive interactions to stimulated endothelium, and also in the phagocytosis of complement coated particles. Together with integrin chain β2, *ITGAM* forms a functionally active heterodimer, the integrin αMβ2 molecule to form the cell surface receptor, known as complement receptor 3 (CR3) or Mac-1, can bind a variety of ligands including intercellular adhesion molecule 1 (ICAM-1), the C3bi fragment of activated complement C3, fibrinogen, and factor X. *ITGAM* is perhaps more familiarly known as CD11b or CR3, and it thereby takes part in the uptake of complement-coated particles and the clearance of immune complexes.

The identification of ITGAM as a major susceptibility gene was perhaps the greatest surprise of the GWA analyses because it has been subject to expression studies in the past with little convincing evidence for a role in SLE (Harley, 2008 & Hom, 2008). A non-synonymous SNP in ITGAM, rs1143679, functional mutation results in an Arg77His (R77H), was first associated in European and African descendants SLE patients, where the G allele contributes to disease susceptibility (Nath, 2008 & Han, 2009). This amino acid does not lie within any known ligand binding site, but may alter the confirmation of the I/A domain to which many ligands do bind. This variant could therefore influence leucocyte trafficking mediated via ICAM-1, or equally it could influence the CR3-mediated uptake of apoptotic cells or immune complexes. Functional data is awaited with interest. However, the consistent association of rs1143679 was not replicated in Asian population (Korean and Japanese) because this SNP was monomorphic for 'G' allele (Han, 2009). This result suggests that the genetic association of ITGAM with SLE is unlikely in Asians. However, another group studied Chinese SLE patients living in Hong Kong and found that rs1143679 was associated with SLE, and another related SNP in the gene, rs1143683, was also identified (Yang, 2009). Therefore, it needs to be confirmed in larger number of SLE case-controls in Korean and Japanese populations.

12.2 Deoxyribonuclease DNase I, 16p13.3

DNase I may be the most important nuclease for the removal of DNA from nuclear antigens. Several lines of evidence suggest that defects in DNase I activity play a role in SLE pathogenesis. Studies in SLE patients and in mouse models support the involvement of *DNase I* among the genes involved in the clearance of apoptotic cells. The first evidence was reported by Chitrabamrung *et al.* (Chitrabamrung, 1981) more than two decades ago. These authors found decreased DNaseI activity in patients with SLE. It has been shown that a *DNaseI* knockout mouse develops a lupus-like syndrome (Napirei, 2000) and a nonsense mutation on the DNASEI gene leading to a non-functional protein has been identified in two Japanese girls with SLE. These girls had very low DNaseI activity and high titers of anti-nucleosome and anti-double-stranded DNA (dsDNA) antibodies. Subsequent analysis of several series of SLE patients from different populations showed that this mutation is extremely rare. Bodan˜o A *et al.*, have described two Spanish SLE patients with very low serum DNase I activity harboring three new mutations in the DNASEI coding sequence that account for the reduced enzymatic activity (Bodan˜ o, 2004). The frequency of these new mutations was below 1% both in SLE patients and in the population. Bodan˜o A. *et al.* also found other DNASEI single-nucleotide polymorphisms (SNPs) but there was no evidence suggesting a functional role for them. These studies support the involvement of DNase I in the pathogenesis of SLE.

In a Korean SLE population, 16 SNPs from the DNaseI were studied using a case-control approach. In parallel, common autoantibodies were also examined for the same population. None of the SNPs were in significant association with SLE, however, a non-synonymous SNP in exon 8, namely rs1053874 (which was also known as +2373A/G, and which causes Gln244Arg substitution), was significantly associated with an increased risk of the production of anti-RNP and anti-dsDNA (Shin, 2004). However, the same SNP (+2373A/G) has shown association between the GG allele and SLE susceptibility in Spanish population, but no association with the majority of antinuclear antibodies (anti-dsDNA, anti-ssDNA and anti-RNP) and no effect on DNase I activity (Bodaño , 2006). This discrepancy could be related to heterogeneity between the populations.

13. Chromosome 17

13.1 Monocyte chemo-attractant protein 1 (MCP1), 17q11.2-12

MCP-1, currently also designated CCL2, encodes a β-chemokine that recruits monocyte, eosinophils, and memory T cells to inflammatory sites, to regulate adhesion molecule expression and T-cell functions in acute and possibly chronic inflammation (Charo, 2004). Evidence in human and animal studies suggests a significant role of MCP-1 in the progression of glomerular and tubulointerstitial injuries and glomerulonephriti in patients with SLE (Stahl, 1993; Rovin, 1996; Saitoh, 1998; Rovin 1998). In particular, MCP-1 has been shown to be pathogenic for kidney injury in murine lupus nephritis (Shimizu, 2004), and reported to be involved in glomerulonephritis in SLE patients, in which elevation of serum MCP-1 correlates with disease activity (Tesar, 1998). An increased urine MCP-1 (uMCP-1) level was detected in SLE patients during active renal disease (Rovin, 2005).

SNP (rs1024611) -2518A/G and G/G in MCP1 promoter region may modulate the levels of MCP-1 expression and increased susceptibility to SLE and lupus nephritis in patients from North America (Tucci, 2004). However, the Involvement of the MCP-1 –2518 A>G promoter polymorphism in SLE development and its contribution to some clinical manifestations of SLE remains controversial (Tucci, 2004; Aguilar, 2001; Hwang, 2002; Kim, 2002; Brown, 2007; Liao, 2004; Ye, 2005). In a Spanish study for example, −2518G polymorphism is noted to be associated with cutaneous vasculitis but not SLE or lupus nephritis as genotyping of −2518A/G polymorphism shows no difference in allelic or genotype frequencies in SLE patient and healthy controls (Aguilar, 2001). Further investigation is needed to delineate if ethnic heterogeneity contributes to this gene polymorphism and SLE susceptibility.

14. Chromosome 19

14.1 Tyrosine kinase 2 (TYK2), 19p13.2

TYK2 is part of the Janus kinase that binds to the interferon (IFN)-α receptor (IFNAR), on the cell surface of IFN-producing cells. Binding of IFN-α to its receptor, leads to the phosphorylation and therefore activation of TYK2 (Richter, 1998). Active TYK2 then phosphorylates IFNAR to allow binding of STAT3 and STAT5 (David, 2002) which leads to expression of IFN-α. Deficiency of *TYK2* leads to defects of multiple cytokine pathways, including type I interferon, IL-6, IL-10, IL-12, and IL-23, and to impaired T-helper type 1 differentiation and accelerated T helper type 2 differentiation (Minegishi, 2006). More research needed to clarify which of these pathways is critically affected by the *TYK2* risk allele.

TYK2 gene has been linked to the formation of anti-dsDNA antibodies of Caucasian SLE patients (Namjou, 2002). TYK2 rs2304256 was associated with increased risk of discoid lupus erythematosus (P=0.012). In a joint linkage and association study of 44 SNPs in 13 genes from type I IFN pathway in the Scandinavian population, TYK2 and interferon regulatory factor 5 (IRF5) genes displayed strong association with SLE susceptibility (Sigurdsson, 2005).

The most remarkable result from this study has probably been the association signal observed with the rs2304256 nonsynonymous SNP of TYK2 (OR = 0.79) because this has been a controversial SLE genetic factor. The rs2304256 SNP introduces a valine to phenylalanine change in the Janus homology domain 4 of *TYK2* whose functional relevance has not yet been tested. This nonsynonymous SNP showed the strongest association among the 11 TYK2 SNPs studied in Scandinavian families (Sigurdsson, 2005), but was not associated in a study of UK families (Cunninghame, 2007). This latter study, however, found association with another TYK2 SNP (rs12720270) that was not associated in the Scandinavian study. Finally, the International Consortium for Systemic Lupus Erythematosus Genetics (SLEGEN) GWA study excluded association with the rs12720270 SNP (the rs2304256 SNP was not included in the GWA panels)(International Consortium for Systemic Lupus Erythematosus Genetics, 2008).

TYK2 single nucleotide polymorphisms (SNPs), rs2304256, rs12720270 and rs280519, were genotyped in the Japanese population by Kyogoku C *et. al.* in a case-control association study. Linkage disequilibrium (LD) among TYK2 SNPs was examined and no association was revealed with SLE therefore it was concluded that TYK2 is not a genetic risk factor for SLE in a Japanese population (Kyogoku, 2009).

15. Chromosome X

15.1 Interleukin-1 receptor-associated kinase 1/Methyl-CpG-binding Protein 2 locus (IRAK1/MECP2), Xq28

IRAK1, a serine–threonine protein kinase, regulates multiple pathways in both innate and adaptive immune responses by linking several immune-receptor- complexes to TNF receptor-associated factor 6 in mouse models of lupus, *Irak1* is shown to regulate nuclear factor κB (NFκB) in TCR signaling and Toll/interleukin-1 receptor (TLR) activation, as well as the induction of IFN-α and IFN-γ, (Jacob, 2009) implicating IRAK1 in SLE. In a study of four different ethnic groups, multiple SNPs within *IRAK1* were associated with both adult-onset and childhood-onset SLE (Jacob, 2009). The identified polymorphism C203S in IRAK1 is not in any known functional domain, therefore it was suggested that the association may actually be with its neighbor, methyl-CpG-binding protein 2 (*MECP2*).

MECP2 is an X-linked gene located in a region of LD with *IRAK1*, encoding a protein that represses transcription from methylated promoters, has also been associated with lupus. Polymorphisms in *MECP2* may have relevance to the epigenetic DNA methylation changes found in lupus and discussed below. There is evidence for altered methylation in SLE, (Webb, 2009) as well as differential expression of potentially methylated genes, (Pan, 2009) although, as with *IRAK1*, a contributing causative SNP is not immediately obvious. Indeed, it is possible that both of these strong candidates contribute to the effect.

A large replication study in a European-derived population confirmed the importance of this region (*IRAK1–MECP2*) to SLE. The location of *IRAK1* and *MECP2* on the X chromosome raises the possibility that gender bias of SLE might, in part, be attributed to sex chromosome genes. Further work is required to identify the causal variants (Sestak, 2011).

15.2 Toll-like receptor (TLR7), Xp22.2

TLR7, the protein encoded by this gene is a member of the Toll-like receptor (TLR) family which is single transmembrane cell-surface receptors expressed on many types of cells including macrophages and dendritic cells, plays a fundamental role in pathogen recognition and activation of innate immunity. TLRs generally exist as homodimers. They are highly conserved from Drosophila to humans and share structural and functional similarities. TLR are activated by molecules associated with biological threat and are highly specific towards evolutionary conserved entities on microbes, such as bacterial cell-surface lipopolysaccharides, flagella and unmethylated CpG islands.

Activation of toll-like receptors initiates downstream signaling cascades, initially via the adapter molecules MyD88, Trap, Trif and Tram, leading to NF-kappa-B activation, cytokine secretion and the inflammatory response, regulate intracellular kinases and gene expression. The signaling cascade coupled to toll-like receptor activation is very similar to that of interleukin-1 receptor (IL-1R) activation. It has been suggested that some toll-like receptors may have endogenous ligands, such as Hsp60 and fibrinogen, and this has promoted speculation that endogenous toll-like receptor activators may have a pathological role in autoimmune disease. TLRs play an important role in the pathogenesis of SLE (Vollmer, 2005 & Christensen, 2006). The role of nucleic acid binding TLR7 has become quite apparent in both SLE animal models and human patients. This receptor promotes autoantibodies and cytokines responsible for chronic inflammation (Christensen, 2007 & Savarese, 2008). A recent fine mapping of the 23-kb TLR7 region using 11 SNPs in 1434 SLE cases of Eastern Asian descent versus 1591 controls showed the association of two TLR7 SNPs with SLE (rs5935436 in the promoter, $p=1.8x10^{-3}$; rs3853839 in the 3'-UTR, $p=6.7x10^{-4}$) (in press).

16. Epigenetics involvement in the pathology of SLE

The controversy, we came cross in the previous section, in the association of immunologically related genes with susceptibility to SLE and the incomplete concordance in monozygotic twins affected with SLE, while they carry the same SLE susceptibility genes, are clear indications that genetics is not the only factor that influences susceptibility to SLE. This means that some non-genetic factors can modify gene expression through epigenetic mechanisms, potentially contributing to SLE. The field of epigenetics is rapidly growing especially in studying autoimmune diseases. Epigenetics is the study of heritable modifications in gene function that alter the phenotype without modifying the genetic sequence, these modifications result in the activation or complete/partial gene silencing (Hirst, 2009). It is becoming clear that epigenetic modifications contribute to a variety of pathogenetic processes in which environmental and genetic factors are involved. Much of the variability in severity, organ involvement, and response to therapy among patients with systemic lupus erythematosus (SLE) is blamed on differences in gene expression. That, in turn, is due to epigenetic mechanisms, one of the "master regulators" of gene expression.

Accumulating epidemiological, clinical, and experimental evidence supports the conclusion of the critical role of epigenetic factors in immune programming. Compelling evidence has been gathered supports a role for epigenetic alterations in the pathogenesis of SLE. For example, inhibiting DNA methylation in normal $CD4^{+}$ T cells induces autoreactivity, and these autoreactive cells promote autoantibody production. Furthermore, transferring hypomethylated T cells into syngeneic mice causes a lupus-like disease (Richardson, 1990 & Yung 1997). Understanding this mechanism provides the basis for clarifying how the complex interactions of the genome and epigenome shape immune responses and maintain immune tolerance to self-antigens.

In this section we will discus, in brief, some of the epigenetics mechanisms that are involved in the SLE pathogenesis. These mechanisms play an essential role in gene regulation

Gene	locus	function	P-values	ORs
PTPN22	1p13	T-cell signaling	$<1x10^{-5}$ - $5.2x10^{-6}$	1.49-1.53
FCGR2A	1q21-23	Immune complex clearance Fc Receptor	0.0016 - $6.78x10^{-7}$	1.30-1.35
FCGR3B	1q23.3	Immune complex clearance Fc Receptor	$2.7x10^{-8}$	2.21c
FcGR3A	1q23.3	Immune complex clearance Fc Receptor		1.6
CRP	1q23.2	sensitive marker of inflammation	$6.4x10^{-7}$	
TNFSF4	1q25.1	T-cell signaling	over: $1.91x10^{-6}$	over: 1.63 (T/U) and 1.28b
NMNAT2	1q25.3	Catalyzes the formation of NAD(+)from nicotinamide mononucleotide (NMN) and ATP.	$1x10^{-10}$	1.18
IL10*	1q31–q32	1q24	4.0×10 −8	1.2
TLR5	1q41-q42	innate immunity		
STAT4	2q33	TLR–IFN signaling	$2.8x10^{-9}$ - $8.96x10^{-14}$	1.53-1.50
PDCD1 (CD279)	2q37	pro-B-cells differentiation		1.2
CTLA4 (CD152)	2q33.2	transmits an inhibitory signal to T cells		
PXK	3p14.3	Bind and modulates both Na, K-ATPase enzymatic and ion pump activities	$7.10x10^{-9}$	1.25
BANK1	4q24	B-cell signaling	$3.7x10^{-7}$	1.38
TNIP1	5q33	TNF–NFκB signaling		1.3
The MHC	6p21.3	T-cell signaling	$2.71x10^{-21}$- $1.7x10^{-52}$	2.01-2.36
ATG5	6q21		$1.36x10^{-7}$	1.19
PRDM1	6q21	B-cell signaling	1.74×10 −8	1.3
TNFAIP3	6q23	TNF–NFκB signaling	$2.9x10^{-12}$	1.7
IRF5	7q32	TLR–IFN signaling	$1.65x10^{-11}$ - $3.61x10^{-19}$	1.54-1.72
ICA1	7p21.3		$1.90x10^{-7}$	1.32
IKZF1	7p12	B-cell signaling		1.4
BLK	8p23.1	T-cell signaling	$1x10^{-10}$ -$7x10^{-10}$	1.22-1.39
XKR6	8p23.1		$2.51x10^{-11}$	1.23
LYN	8q12.1		$5.4x10^{-9}$	1.30
C8orf12	8p23.1	miscRNA gene	$4.00x10^{-10}$	1.22
BLK-FAM167A -XKR6 locus	8p23.1	B-cell signaling	$1.7x10^{-8}$	1.2-1.6
MBL	10q11.2-21	element of the innate immune system		
KIAA1542 (near IRF7)	11p15.5	Interferon and TLR7/9 Signaling	$3.00x10^{-10}$	1.28
ITGAM	16p11.2	Neutrophil activity	$3x10^{-11}$ - $1.61x10^{-23}$	1.33-1.62

CD226	18q22.3	member of the Ig-superfamily		
TYK2	19p13.2	Janus kinases (JAKs) protein interferon signaling pathway		
UBE2L3	22q11.2	encodes a member of the E2 ubiquitin-conjugating enzyme	7.53×10^{-8}	1.22
SCUBE1	22q13.2	adhesive molecule	1.21×10^{-7}	1.28
MECP2	Xq28	Chromosomal protein that binds to methylated DNA	1.2×10^{-8}	1.39
IRAK1	Xq28	responsible for IL1-induced upregulation of the transcription factor NF-kappa B		
TLR7	Xp22.2	innate immunity		

Table 1. Top SLE candidate genes categorized by chromosomal location.

through covalent modifications of DNA and histones, and determine regional chromatin structure with consequences on gene expression. We will also discuss the involvement of MicroRNAs (miRNAs) as an epigenetic factor involved in the pathology of SLE.

16.1 Histone covalent modification

The basic chromatin subunit is the nucleosome, which consists of DNA wrapped twice around a histone core. Nucleosomes are then organized into higher order structures forming chromatin fibers (Felsenfeld 2003). Chromatin in its native form is tightly compacted and inaccessible to transcription factors and the transcription initiation machinery. However, histone "tails" protrude from the nucleosome, and are covalently modified by *acetylation, methylation, phosphorylation, ubiquitination, and SUMOylation* (SUMO (small ubiquitin-related modifier) (Felsenfeld 2003). These modifications serve as signals, referred to as the "histone code", that initiate a number of processes including the localized remodeling of chromatin from a compact, transcriptionally silent configuration to a more open structure accessible to the transcription initiation machinery.

16.2 DNA methylation and autoimmunity

DNA methylation refers to the methylation of cytosines in CpG pairs (cytosine and guanine residues separated by a phosphate, which links the two nucleosides together in DNA). Most CpG pairs in the mammalian genome are methylated, with some unmethylated pairs found in the regulatory elements of active genes. Most unmethylated CpGs are found in GC-rich sequences, termed CpG islands. CpG islands contain multiple binding sites for transcription factors, and serve as promoters for the associated gene. Methylation of these promoters can lead to gene silencing where transcriptionally active chromatin is characterized by unmethylated DNA. Convincing evidence indicates that DNA can be actively demethylated and therefore affect gene expresssion. For example, several CpG pairs in the *IL-2* promoter demethylate within 20 minutes of T-cell stimulation, prior to initiation of DNA synthesis (Bruniquel, 2003).

DNA methylation is catalyzed by the enzyme DNA methyltransferases (DNMTs) while and histone acetylation is controlled by histone acetylases (HATs) and deacetylases (HDACs). It is hypothesized that the processes of DNA methylation and histone deacetylation work together through the formation of DNMT/HDAC transcriptional repressor complexes that work in silencing gene expression through establishing a repressive chromatin environment

(Cameron, 1999). However, DNMTs and HDACs lack DNA-binding domains, and are therefore dependent on transcription factors (TFs) for their recruitment to DNA. Zhao M *et al.* set out a study to uncover mechanisms underlying the hypomethylation and hyperacetylation of genes involved in lupus autoimmunity by investigating the involvement of specific TFs. They assessed the activities of 225 TFs in CD4$^+$ T cells from SLE patients relative to healthy controls using a newly developed screening method (Qiao, 2008), and found that the activity of regulatory factor X 1 (RFX1) is significantly downregulated in SLE CD4$^+$ T cells (Zhao, 2010). Follow-up analyses confirmed the result of Zhao M *et al.* study and further revealed that both the expression and activity of RFX1 protein are reduced in SLE CD4$^+$ T cells. Zhao M *et al* (Zhao, 2010) also provided evidence indicating that RFX1 recruits the co-repressors HDAC1 and DNMT1 to the promoter region of CD11a and CD70, thus regulating their expression in CD4$^+$ T cells. Taken together, our findings indicate that reduction of RFX1 plays an important role in inducing autoreactivity and autoantibody overstimulation in SLE.

In addition, DNA hypomethylation appears to induce CD4$^+$ T cell autoreactivity and the inhibition of DNA methylation with 5-azacytidine caused CD4+ T-cell autoreactivity. This lupus-like autoimmunity correlated with overexpression of ITGAL (CD11a) and TNFSF7 (CD70) (Lu, 2002 & 2005). CD11a and CD70 overexpression in these CD4$^+$ T cells is associated with hypomethylation of their respective promoters (Lu, 2002 & 2005). CD11a is the alpha chain of the heterodimeric integrin lymphocyte function-associated antigen-1 (LFA-1) (CD11a/CD18) (ITGAL/Integrin beta-2). Overexpressing LFA-1 by transfection caused an identical autoreactivity (Yung, 1996).LFA-1 plays a central role in adhesive interactions between T cells and other immune system cells including macrophages, dendritic cells and B cells. This protein is also essential for the recruitment of leukocytes into sites of inflammation, antigen-specific T cell activation, helping B cell, as well as alloreactive, cytotoxic T cell and natural killer responses (Shimaoka & Springer, 2003). LFA-1 deficient lupus mice have significantly increased survival, decreased anti-DNA autoantibody formation, and reduced glomerulonephritis (Kevil, 2004). CD70 is expressed on activated T cells and increases pokeweed mitogen (PWM)-stimulated immunoglobulin (Ig) G synthesis, indicating B cell costimulatory functions (Kobata, 1995). Demethylated, autoreactive CD4+ T cells overstimulate antibody production by B cells and kill macrophages (Richardson, 2007), relaeasing apoptotic nuclear material that stimulates lupus-like autoantibodies (Denny, 2006). T-cell hypomethylation correlates with disease activity in SLE, suggesting that DNA hypomethylation may be a key player in the pathogenesis of the disease (Corvetta, 1991).

Furthermore, CD4+ lymphocytes undergo global histone H3 and H4 deacetylation and consequent skewed gene expression. Although multiple lines of evidence highlight the contribution of epigenetic alterations to the pathogenesis of lupus in genetically predisposed individuals, many questions remain to be answered. Attaining a deeper understanding of these matters will create opportunities in the promising area of epigenetic treatments.

16.3 MicroRNAs (miRNAs) and autoimmunity

MicroRNAs (miRNAs) are newly discovered, small (about 23-nucleotide), noncoding ribonucleic acids (RNAs) that function in the posttranscriptional regulation of about 30% of mRNAs by binding to their 3′-untranslated region (3′-UTR), thus targeting them for degradation or translational repression. miRNA are known to regulate cellular processes such as apoptosis, cell cycle, differentiation, and immune functions. The powerful gene regulatory role of miRNAs is now well recognized, where the recent discovery of the gene-regulatory role of miRNAs has led to a paradigm shift in the understanding of expression and function of the mammalian genome. The field of miRNA research gained widespread attention with the recognition of aberrant expression and/or function of miRNAs in a broad range of human diseases including autoimmune diseases (Pauley, 2009).

Recent research evidence has emerged showing the critical role of miRNAs not only for the development of the immune system but also for the function of both innate and adaptive arms of the immune system (Taganov, 2007; Xiao, 2009; Gantier, 2007; O'Connell, 2010; Lodish, 2008; Sonkoly, 2008; Baltimore, 2008). Using state of the art quantitative mass spectrometry two investigators measured the response of thousands of proteins after introducing microRNAs into cultured cells and after knockdown mir-223 in mouse neutrophils. Their results are consistent with each other and demonstrate that changes in the level of a single miRNA may have a significant impact on the levels of hundreds to thousands of proteins (Baek, 2008). These important studies are the first to show the impact of microRNAs on the proteome which indicated that for most interactions microRNAs act as rheostats to make fine-scale adjustments to protein output (Baek, 2008 & Selbach, 2008). Tang et al have shown that miR-146 regulates the level of at least TRAF6, IRAK1, STAT-1, and IFN regulatory factor 5 (IRF-5), all of which are important for the IFN pathway (Tang, 2009). The reported reduction of miR-146 in PBMCs from SLE patients (Tang, 2009) will likely affect the levels of these factors significantly and contribute to overexpression of type I IFN and, thus, disease activity.

It is intriguing that independent studies have demonstrated an increased level of miR-146 in RA patients, but a decreased level in SLE patients, as compared with healthy controls. Given that RA and SLE are both systemic rheumatic diseases, one may be surprised by the finding that miR-146 levels are contradictory in these diseases, and yet, it should not be surprising, since this may simply be reflecting a difference in the overall cytokine profiles between the two diseases, with type I IFN playing a dominant role in SLE, whereas TNFα, interleukin-1 (IL-1), and IL-6 are the principle cytokines in RA. In the coming years, one can expect research reports on miRNA expression in many other autoimmune diseases, as well as more-complete profiling data, with disease activity correlations or a lack thereof.

17. References

Adrianto I, Wen F, Templeton A, Wiley G, King JB, Lessard CJ, Bates JS, Hu Y, Kelly JA, Kaufman KM, Guthridge JM, Alarcón-Riquelme ME; BIOLUPUS and GENLES Networks, Anaya JM, Bae SC, Bang SY, Boackle SA, Brown EE, Petri MA, Gallant C, Ramsey-Goldman R, Reveille JD, Vila LM, Criswell LA, Edberg JC, Freedman BI, Gregersen PK, Gilkeson GS, Jacob CO, James JA, Kamen DL, Kimberly RP, Martin J, Merrill JT, Niewold TB, Park SY, Pons-Estel BA, Scofield RH, Stevens AM, Tsao BP, Vyse TJ, Langefeld CD, Harley JB, Moser KL, Webb CF, Humphrey MB, Montgomery CG, Gaffney PM. Association of a functional variant downstream of TNFAIP3 with systemic lupus erythematosus. Nat Genet. 2011;43(3):253-8.

Aguilar F., Gonz´alez-Escribano MF, ´anchez-Rom´an JS, and N´u˜nez-Rold´an A. "MCP-1 promoter polymorphism in Spanish patients with systemic lupus erythematosus," Tissue Antigens, vol. 58, no. 5, (2001) pp. 335–338.

Aitman TJ, Dong R, Vyse TJ et al. Copy number polymorphism in Fcgr3 predisposes to glomerulonephritis in rats and humans. Nature 2006;439:851–855

Alarcón-Riquelme ME, Prokunina L. Finding genes for SLE: complex interactions and complex populations. J Autoimmun. 2003;21(2):117-20.

Alper CA, Awdeh Z, Raum D, Yunis EJ. Complement genes of the major histocompatibility complex (complotypes), extended haplotypes and disease markers. Biochem Soc Symp. 1986;51:19-28.

Arbuckle MR, McClain MT, Rubertone MV et al. Development of autoantibodies before the clinical onset of systemic lupus erythematosus. N Engl J Med 2003;349:1526–33.

Arnett FC, Edworthy SM, Bloch DA et al. The American Rheumatism Association 1987 revised criteria for the classification of rheumatoid arthritis. Arthritis Rheum 1988;31:315–24.

Baechler EC, Batliwalla FM, Karypis G et al. Interferon-inducible gene expression signature in peripheral blood cells of patients with severe lupus. Proc Natl Acad Sci USA 2003;100:2610–5.

Baek D, Villen J, Shin C, Camargo FD, Gygi SP, Bartel DP. The impact of microRNAs on protein output. Nature 2008;455:64–71.

Baltimore D, Boldin MP, O'Connell RM, Rao DS, Taganov KD. microRNAs: new regulators of immune cell development and function. Nat Immunol 2008;9:839–45.

Barnes BJ, Kellum MJ, Pinder KE, Frisancho JA, Pitha PM. Interferon regulatory factor 5, a novel mediator of cell cycle arrest and cell death. Cancer Res 2003;63:6424–31.

Barnes BJ, Richards J, Mancl M, Hanash S, Beretta L, Pitha PM. Global and distinct targets of IRF-5 and IRF-7 during innate response to viral infection. J Biol Chem 2004;279:45194–207.

Bates JS, et al. Meta-analysis and imputation identifies a 109 kb risk haplotype spanning TNFAIP3 associated with lupus nephritis and hematologic manifestations. Genes Immun. 2009; 10:470–7.

Baum PR, Gayle III RB, Ramsdell F, Srinivasan S, Sorensen RA, Watson ML et al. Molecular characterization of murine and human OX40/OX40 ligand systems: identification of a human OX40 ligand as the HTLV-1-regulated protein gp34. EMBO J 1994; 13: 3992–4001.

Begovich AB, Carlton VE, Honigberg LA et al. A missense single-nucleotide polymorphism in a gene encoding a protein tyrosine phosphatase (PTPN22) is associated with rheumatoid arthritis. Am J Hum Genet 2004;75:330–7.

Bennett L, Palucka AK, Arce E et al. Interferon and granulopoiesis signatures in systemic lupus erythematosus blood. J Exp Med 2003;197:711–23.

Bettinotti MP, Hartung K, Deicher H, Messer G, Keller E, Weiss EH, Albert ED. Polymorphism of the tumor necrosis factor beta gene in systemic lupus erythematosus: TNFB-MHC haplotypes. Immunogenetics. 1993;37(6):449-54.

Bharadwaj D, Stein MP, Volzer M, Mold C, Du Clos TW. The major receptor for C-reactive protein on leukocytes is fcgamma receptor II. J Exp Med 1999;190:585–590

Bienz M. The PHD finger, a nuclear protein-interaction domain. Trends Biochem Sci 2006;31:35–40.

Bodaño A, Amarelo J, Gonza´ lez A, Go´ mez-Reino JJ, Conde C. Novel DNASEI mutations related to systemic lupus erythematosus. Arthritis Rheum 2004;50:4070–73.

Bodaño A, González A, Ferreiros-Vidal I, Balada E, Ordi J, Carreira P, Gómez-Reino JJ, Conde C. Association of a non-synonymous single-nucleotide polymorphism of DNASEI with SLE susceptibility. Rheumatology (Oxford). 2006;45(7):819-23.

Bottini N, Musumeci L, Alonso A et al. A functional variant of lymphoid tyrosine phosphatase is associated with type I diabetes. Nat Genet 2004;36:337–8.

Botto M, Walport MJ. C1q, autoimmunity and apoptosis. Immunobiology 2002;205:395–406.

Braun D, Caramalho I, Demengeot J. IFN-alpha/beta enhances BCR-dependent B cell responses. Int Immunol 2002;14:411–9.

Bredius, RG, de Vries CE, Troelstra A, van Alphen L, Weening RS, van de Winkel JG, Out TA.. Phagocytosis of Staphylococcus aureus and Hemophilus influenzae type B opsonized with polyclonal human IgG1 and IgG2 antibodies. Functional hFcγ RIIa polymorphism to IgG2. J. Immunol. 1993;151, 1463–1472.

Brown EE, Edberg JC, Kimberly RP. Fc receptor genes and the systemic lupus erythematosus diathesis. Autoimmunity 2007;40:567–81.

Brown KS, Nackos E, Morthala S, Jensen LE, Whitehead AS, and Von Feldt JM, "Monocyte chemoattractant protein-1: plasma concentrations and A(−2518)G promoter polymorphism of its gene in systemic lupus erythematosus," Journal of Rheumatology, vol. 34, no. 4, pp. (2007) 740–746.

Bruniquel D and Schwartz RH. Selective, stable demethylation of the interleukin-2 gene enhances transcription by an active process. Nat Immunol 2003;4:235–240.

Budarf ML, Goyette P, Boucher G, Lian J, Graham RR, Claudio JO, Hudson T, Gladman D, Clarke AE, Pope JE, Peschken C, Smith CD, Hanly J, Rich E, Boire G, Barr SG, Zummer M; GenES Investigators, Fortin PR, Wither J, Rioux JD. A targeted association study in systemic lupus erythematosus identifies multiple susceptibility alleles. Genes Immun. 2011;12(1):51-8.

Cameron EE, Bachman KE, Myohanen S, Herman JG and Baylin SB. Synergy of demethylation and histone deacetylase inhibition in the re-expression of genes silenced in cancer, Nat Genet 21 (1999), pp. 103–107.

Cash, J. J., Splawski, J. B., Thomas, R., McFarlin, J. F., Schulze-Koops, H., Davis, L. S., Fujita, K. and Lipsky, P. E. Elevated interleukin-10 levels in patients with rheumatoid arthritis. Arthritis Rheum. 1995;38, 96–104.

Chang YK, Yang W, Zhao M, et al. Association of BANK1 and TNFSF4 with systemic lupus erythematosus in Hong Kong Chinese. Genes Immun. 2009 Jul;10(5):414-20

Chang YK, Yang W, Zhao M, et al. Association of BANK1 and TNFSF4 with systemic lupus erythematosus in Hong Kong Chinese. Genes Immun 2009; 10: 414–420.

Charo IF and Taubman MB, "Chemokines in the pathogenesis of vascular disease," Circulation Research, vol. 95, no. 9, (2004) pp. 858–866,.

Chen JY, Wang CM, Tsao KC, Chow YH, Wu JM, Li CL, Ho HH, Wu YJ, Luo SF.. Fcγ receptor IIa, IIIa, and IIIb polymorphisms of systemic lupus erythematosus in Taiwan. 2004;Ann. Rheum. Dis. 63, 877–880.

Chitrabamrung S, Rubin L, Tan EM. Serum deoxyribonuclease I and clinical activity in systemic lupus erythematosus. Rheumatol Int 1981;1:55–60.

Chong, w. P. et al. Association of interleukin-10 promoter polymorphisms with systemic lupus erythematosus. Genes Immun. 2004;5, 484–492

Chong, w. P. et al. Association of interleukin-10 promoter polymorphisms with systemic lupus erythematosus. Genes Immun. 2004;5, 484–492.

Christensen SR and Shlomchik MJ, "Regulation of lupus-related autoantibody production and clinical disease by Toll-like receptors," Seminars in Immunology, vol. 19, no. 1, (2007) pp.11–23.

Christensen SR, Shupe J, Nickerson K, Kashgarian M, Flavell RA, and Shlomchik MJ. Toll-like receptor 7 and TLR9 dictate autoantibody specificity and have opposing inflammatory and regulatory roles in a murine model of lupus. Immunity 2006;25: 417–428.

Chu ZT, Tsuchiya N, Kyogoku C, Ohashi J, Qian YP, Xu SB, Mao CZ, Chu JY, Tokunaga K. Association of Fcγ receptor IIb polymorphism with susceptibility to systemic lupus erythematosus in Chinese: a common susceptibility gene in the Asian populations. Tissue Antigens 2004;63, 21–27.

Clark MR, Stuart SG, Kimberly RP, Ory PA, Goldstein IM. A single amino acid distinguishes the high-responder from the low-responder form of Fc receptor II on human monocytes. Eur J Immunol 1991;21:1911–6.

Clark, MR., Liu, L., Clarkson, SB., Ory, PA. & Goldstein, IM. An abnormality of the gene that encodes neutrophil Fc receptor III in a patient with systemic lupus erythematosus. J. Clin Invest. 1990;86, 341–346.

Corvetta A, Della Bita R, Luchetti MM, Pomponio G. 5-Methyl-cytosine content of DNA in blood, synovial monnuclear cells and synovial tissue from patients affected by autoimmune rheumatic diseases. J Chromatogr 1991;566:481-91.

Crawley E, Woo P, Isenberg DA. Single nucleotide polymorphic haplotypes of the interleukin-10 5' flanking region are not associated with renal disease or serology in Caucasian patients with systemic lupus erythematosus. Arthritis Rheum. 1999;42(9):2017-8

Cunninghame Graham DS, Akil M, Vyse TJ: Association of polymorphisms across the tyrosine kinase gene, TYK2 in UK SLE families. Rheumatology (Oxford) 2007;46:927-930.

Cunninghame Graham DS, Graham RR, Manku H, et al. Polymorphism at the TNF superfamily gene TNFSF4 confers susceptibility to systemic lupus erythematosus. Nat Genet 2008; 40(1):83-89.

Cunninghame Graham DS, Manku H, Wagner S et al. Association of IRF5 in UK SLE families identifies a variant involved in polyadenylation. Hum Mol Genet 2007;16:579–91.

Daeron M. Fc receptor biology. Annu Rev Immunol 1997;15:203–234

Darnell JE Jr, Kerr IM, Stark GR. Jak-STAT pathways and transcriptional activation in response to IFNs and other extracellular signaling proteins. Science 1994;264:1415–21.

David M. Signal transduction by type I interferons. Biotechniques 2002(Suppl.):58–65.

Dean, G. S., Tyrrell-Price, J., Crawley, E.&Isenberg, D. A. Ann. Rheum. Dis. 2000;59, 243–251.

Deapen D, Escalante A, Weinrib L, Horwitz D, Bachman B, Roy-Burman P, Walker A, Mack TM. A revised estimate of twin concordance in systemic lupus erythematosus. Arthritis Rheum. 1992;35(3):311-8.

Decker P, Isenberg D, Muller S. Inhibition of caspase-3-mediated poly(ADP-ribose) polymerase (PARP) apoptotic cleavage by human PARP autoantibodies and effect on cells undergoing apoptosis. J Biol Chem 2000;275:9043–9046

delGado-Vega AM, Abelson AK, Sanchez E, et al. Replication of the TNFSF4 (OX40L) promoter region association with systemic lupus erythematosus. Genes Immun 2009; 10(3):248-253.

Deng L, Zhang Y, Kang J, Liu T, Zhao H, Gao Y, Li C, Pan H, Tang X, Wang D, Niu T, Yang H, Zeng C.An unusual haplotype polymorphism on human chromosome 8p23 derived from the inversion polymorphism. Hum Mutat 2008;10:1209–16.

Denny MF, Chandaroy P, Killen PD, Caricchio R, Lewis EE, Richardson BC, et al. Accelarated macrophage apoptosis induces autoantibody formation and organ damage in systemic lupus erythematosus. J Immunol 2006;176:2095-104.

Dideberg V, Kristjansdottir G, Milani L, Libioulle C, Sigurdsson S, Louis E, Wiman AC, Vermeire S, Rutgeerts P, Belaiche J, Franchimont D, Van Gossum A, Bours V, Syvänen AC. An insertion-deletion polymorphism in the interferon regulatory Factor 5 (IRF5) gene confers risk of inflammatory bowel diseases. Hum Mol Genet. 2007;16(24):3008-16.

Drebin JA, Hartzell SW, Griffin C, Campbell MJ, Niederhuber JE. Molecular cloning and chromosomal localization of the human homologue of a B-lymphocyte specific protein tyrosine kinase (blk). Oncogene 1995;10(3):477–486

Duits A, Bootsma H, Derksen RH, Spronk PE, Kater L, Kallenberg CG, Capel PJ, Westerdaal NA, Spierenburg GT, Gmelig-Meyling FH. Skewed distribution of IgG Fc receptor IIa (CD32) polymorphism is associated with renal disease in systemic lupus erythematosus patients. Arthritis Rheum. 1995;38,1832–1836.

Dykman TR, Cole JL, Iida K, Atkinson JP. Polymorphismof human erythrocyte C3b/C4b receptor. Proc Natl Acad Sci USA 1983;80:1698–1702

Dykman TR, Hatch JA, Atkinson JP. Polymorphism of the human C3b/C4b receptor. Identification of a third allele and analysis of receptor phenotypes in families and patients with systemic lupus erythematosus. J Exp Med 1984;159:691–703

Eskdale J, Kube D, Tesch H, Gallagher G. Mapping of the human IL10 gene and further characterization of the 5' Xanking sequence. Immunogenetics 1997a;46:120–128.

Eskdale J., wordsworth, P., Bowman, S., Field, M. Gallagher, G. Association between polymorphisms at the human IL-10 locus and systemic lupus erythematosus. Tissue Antigens 1997b, 49, 635–639.

Fan Y, Tao JH, Zhang LP, Li LH, Ye DQ. Association of BLK (rs13277113, rs2248932) polymorphism with systemic lupus erythematosus: a meta-analysis. Mol Biol Rep. 2010 Dec 9. [Epub ahead of print]

Fanciulli M, Norsworthy PJ, Petretto E et al. FCGR3B copy number variation is associated with susceptibility to systemic, but not organ-specific, autoimmunity. Nat Genet 2007; 39: 721–3.

Felsenfeld G and Groudine M. Controlling the double helix. Nature 2003;421: 448–453.

Firestein GS. Kelley's textbook of rheumatology. Philadelphia (USA): W.B. Saunders Company; 2008. p1233.

Flores-Borja F, Kabouridis PS, Jury EC, Isenberg DA, Mageed RA. Decreased Lyn expression and translocation to lipid raft signaling domains in B lymphocytes from patients with systemic lupus erythematosus. Arthritis Rheum. 2005; 52(12):3955–65.

Floto RA, Clatworthy MR, Heilbronn KR, Rosner DR, MacAry PA, Rankin A, Lehner PJ, Ouwehand WH, Allen JM, Watkins NA, Smith KG. Loss of function of a lupus associated FcγRIIb polymorphism through exclusion from lipid rafts. Nat. Med. 2005;11, 1056–1058.

Fortis C, Foppoli M, Gianotti L, Galli L, Citterio G, Consogno G, Gentilini O. and Braga M. Increased interleukin-10 serum levels in patients with solid tumours. Cancer Lett. 1996;104, 1-5.

Frucht DM, Fukao T, Bogdan C, Schindler H, O'Shea JJ, Koyasu S. IFN-gamma production by antigen-presenting cells: mechanisms emerge. Trends Immunol 2001;22:556-60.

Fukao T, Frucht DM, Yap G, Gadina M, O'Shea JJ, Koyasu S. Inducible expression of Stat4 in dendritic cells and macrophages and its critical role in innate and adaptive immune responses. J Immunol 2001;166:4446-55.

Gantier MP, Sadler AJ, Williams BR. Fine-tuning of the innate immune response by microRNAs. Immunol Cell Biol 2007;85: 458-62.

Gateva V, Sandling JK, Hom G, et al. A large-scale replication study identifiesTNIP1, PRDM1, JAZF1, UHRF1BP1 and IL10 as risk loci for systemic lupus erythematosus. Nat Genet 2009;41 : 1228-33 .

Gateva V, Sandling JK, Hom G, Taylor KE, Chung SA, Sun X, Ortmann W, Kosoy R, Ferreira RC, Nordmark G, Gunnarsson I, Svenungsson E, Padyukov L, Sturfelt G, Jönsen A, Bengtsson AA, Rantapää-Dahlqvist S, Baechler EC, Brown EE, Alarcón GS, Edberg JC, Ramsey-Goldman R, McGwin G Jr, Reveille JD, Vilá LM, Kimberly RP, Manzi S, Petri MA, Lee A, Gregersen PK, et al: A large-scale replication study identifies TNIP1, PRDM1, JAZF1, UHRF1BP1 and IL10 as risk loci for systemic lupus erythematosus. Nat Genet 2009; 41:1228-1233.

Gateva, V. et al. A large-scale replication study identifies TNIP1, PRDM1, JAZF1, UHRF1BP1 and IL10 as risk loci for systemic lupus erythematosus. Nat. Genet. 2009;41, 1228-1233.

Gateva, V. et al. A large-scale replication study identifies TNIP1, PRDM1, JAZF1, UHRF1BP1 and IL10 as risk loci for systemic lupus erythematosus. Nat. Genet. 2009;41, 1228-1233.

Georgopoulos K, Bigby M, Wang JH, Molnar A, Wu P, Winandy S, Sharpe A. The Ikaros gene is required for the development of all lymphoid lineages. Cell 1994;79:143-156.

Giallourakis C, Cao Z, Green T, Wachtel H, Xie X, Lopez-Illasaca M, Daly M, Rioux J, Xavier R. A molecular-properties-based approach to understanding PDZ domain proteins and PDZ ligands. Genome Res 2006;16:1056-72.

Graham DS, Graham RR, Manku H, Wong AK, Whittaker JC, Gaffney PM et al. Polymorphism at the TNF superfamily gene TNFSF4 confers susceptibility to systemic lupus erythematosus. Nat Genet 2008; 40: 83-89.

Graham RR, Cotsapas C, Davies L, Hackett R, Lessard CJ, Leon JM et al. Genetic variants near TNFAIP3 on 6q23 are associated with systemic lupus erythematosus. Nat Genet 2008; 40: 1059-1061.

Graham RR, Hom G, Ortmann W, Behrens TW. Review of recent genome-wide association scans in lupus. J Intern Med 2009; 265:680-688.

Graham RR, Kozyrev SV, Baechler EC et al. A common haplotype of interferon regulatory factor 5 (IRF5) regulates splicing and expression and is associated with increased risk of systemic lupus erythematosus. Nat Genet 2006;38:550-5.

Gregersen PK, and Olsson LM. Recent advances in the genetics of autoimmune disease. Annu. Rev. Immunol. 2009;27, 363-391.

Gregersen, PK., Lee, HS., Batliwalla, F, Begovich, AB. PTPN22: Setting thresholds for autoimmunity. Sem. Immunol. 2006;18, 214–22.

Grumet FC, Coukell A, Bodmer JG, Bodmer WF, McDevitt HO. Histocompatibility (HL-A) antigens associated with systemic lupus erythematosus. A possible genetic predisposition to disease. N Engl J Med 1971; 285: 193–196.

Gualtierotti R, Biggioggero M, Penatti AE, Meroni PLUpdating on the pathogenesis of systemic lupus erythematosus. Autoimmun Rev. 2010;10(1):3-7.

Guo L, Deshmukh H, Lu R, et al. Replication of the BANK1 genetic association with systemic lupus erythematosus in a European-derived population. Genes Immun 2009; 10: 531–538.

Hagiwara E, Gourley M., Lee S, Klinman DK. Disease severity in patients with systemic lupus erythematosus correlates with an increased ratio of interleukin-10: interferon-γ-secreting cells in the peripheral blood. Arthritis Rheum. 39, 379–385 (1996).

Han S, Kim-Howard X, Deshmukh H, et al. Evaluation of imputation-based association in and around the integrin-alpha-M (ITGAM) gene and replication of robust association between a non-synonymous functional variant within ITGAM and systemic lupus erythematosus (SLE). Hum Mol Genet 2009;18: 1171–1180.

Han J, Zheng H, Cui Y, Sun L, Ye D, Hu Z, Xu J, Cai Z, Huang W, Zhao G, Xie H, Fang H, Lu Q, Xu J, Li X, Pan Y, Deng D, Zeng F, Ye Z, Zhang X, Wang Q, Hao F, Ma L, Zuo X, Zhou F, Du W, Cheng Y, Yang J, Shen S, Li J, Sheng Y, Zuo X, Zhu W, Gao F, Zhang P, Guo Q, Li B, Gao M, Xiao F, Quan C, Zhang C, Zhang Z, Zhu K, Li Y, Hu D, Lu W, Huang J, Liu S, Li H, Ren Y, Wang Z, Yang C, Wang P, Zhou W, Lv Y, Zhang A, Zhang S, Lin D, Li Y, Low H, Shen M, Zhai Z, Wang Y, Zhang F, Yang S, Liu J, Zhang X. Genome-wide association study in a Chinese Han population identifies nine new susceptibility loci for systemic lupus erythematosus. Nat Genet. 2009;41(11):1234-7.

Han JW, Zheng HF, Cui Y, Sun LD, Ye DQ, Hu Z, Xu JH, Cai ZM, Huang W, Zhao GP, Xie HF, Fang H, Lu QJ, Xu JH, Li XP, Pan YF, Deng DQ, Zeng FQ, Ye ZZ, Zhang XY, Wang QW, Hao F, Ma L, Zuo XB, Zhou FS, Du WH, Cheng YL, Yang JQ, Shen SK, Li J, et al: Genome-wide association study in a Chinese Han population identifies nine new susceptibility loci for systemic lupus erythematosus. Nat Genet 2009; 41:1234-1237.

Hardy J, Singleton A. Genomewide association studies and human disease. N Engl J Med 2009; 360: 1759–1768.

Harley JB, Alarcon-Riquelme ME, Criswell LA, Jacob CO, Kimberly RP, Moser KL, et al. Genomewide association scan in women with systemic lupus erythematosus identifies susceptibility variants in ITGAM, PXK, KIAA1542 and other loci. Nat Genet 2008;40(2):204–10.

Harley JB, Moser KL, Gaffney PM, Behrens TW. The genetics of human systemic lupus erythematosus. Curr Opin Immunol 1998; 10: 690–6.

Hatta Y, Tsuchiya N, Ohashi J, Matsushita M, Fujiwara K, Hagiwara K, Juji T, Tokunaga K. Association of Fcγ receptor IIIB, but not of Fcγ receptor IIA and IIIA polymorphisms with systemic lupus erythematosus in Japanese. Genes Immun. 1999;1, 53–60.

Haug BL, Lee JS, Sibley JT. Altered poly-(ADP-ribose) metabolism in family members of patients with systemic lupus erythematosus. J Rheumatol 1994;21:851–856

Hawn TR, Wu H, Grossman JM, Hahn BH, Tsao BP, Aderem A. A stop codon polymorphism of Toll-like receptor 5 is associated with resistance to systemic lupus erythematosus. Proc Natl Acad Sci U S A. 2005;102(30):10593-7.

Hawn, T. R., Verbon, A., Lettinga, K. D., Zhao, L. P., Li, S. S., Laws, R. J., Skerrett, S. J., Beutler, B., Schroeder, L., Nachman, A., et al. J. Exp. Med. 2003;198, 1563–1572.

He CF, Liu YS, Cheng YL, Gao JP, Pan TM, Han JW, Quan C, Sun LD, Zheng HF, Zuo XB, Xu SX, Sheng YJ, Yao S, Hu WL, Li Y, Yu ZY, Yin XY, Zhang XJ, Cui Y, Yang S. TNIP1, SLC15A4, ETS1, RasGRP3 and IKZF1 are associated with clinical features of systemic lupus erythematosus in a Chinese Han population. Lupus. 2010;19(10):1181-6.

Hirschhorn JN. Genomewide association studies–illuminating biologic pathways. N Engl J Med 2009;360: 1699–1701.

Hirst M, and Marra MA. 2009. Epigenetics and human disease. Int. J. Biochem Cell Biol. 41: 136–146.

Hochberg, M. C. Updating the American College of Rheumatology revised criteria for the classification of systemic lupus erythematosus. Arthritis Rheum. 1997;40, 1725.

Holmskov U, Malhotra R, Sim RB, Jensenius JC. Collectins: collagenous C-type lectins of the innate immune defense system. Immunol Today. 1994;15:67–74.

Hom G, Graham RR, Modrek B, Taylor KE, Ortmann W, Garnier S et al. Association of systemic lupus erythematosus with C8orf13-BLK and ITGAM-ITGAX. N Engl J Med. 2008 Feb 28;358(9):900-9.

Hu W, Sun L, Gao J, Li Y, Wang P, Cheng Y, Pan T, Han J, Liu Y, Lu W, Zuo X, Sheng Y, Yao S, He C, Yu Z, Yin X, Cui Y, Yang S, Zhang X. Down-regulated expression of IKZF1 mRNA in peripheral blood mononuclear cells from patients with systemic lupus erythematosus. Rheumatol Int. 2011;31(6):819-22.

Hunnangkul S, Nitsch D, Rhodes B et al. Familial clustering of non-nuclear autoantibodies and C3 and C4 complement components in systemic lupus erythematosus. Arthritis Rheum 2008;58:1116–24.

Hur JW, Sung YK, Shin HD, Park BL, Cheong HS, Bae SC. Poly(ADP-ribose) polymerase (PARP) polymorphisms associated with nephritis and arthritis in systemic lupus erythematosus. Rheumatology (Oxford). 2006;45(6):711-7.

Hwang SY, Cho ML, Park B, et al.,"Allelic frequency of the MCP-1 promoter −2518 polymorphism in the Korean population and in Korean patients with rheumatoid arthritis, systemic lupus erythematosus and adult-onset Still's disease," European Journal of Immunogenetics, vol.29, no.5,(2002) pp.413–416.

International Consortium for Systemic Lupus Erythematosus Genetics (SLEGEN), Harley JB, Alarcón-Riquelme ME, Criswell LA, Jacob CO, Kimberly RP, Moser KL, Tsao BP, Vyse TJ, Langefeld CD, Nath SK, Guthridge JM, Cobb BL, Mirel DB, Marion MC, Williams AH, Divers J, Wang W, Frank SG, Namjou B, Gabriel SB, Lee AT, Gregersen PK, Behrens TW, Taylor KE, Fernando M, Zidovetzki R, Gaffney PM, Edberg JC, Rioux JD, Ojwang JO, James JA, Merrill JT, Gilkeson GS, Seldin MF, Yin H, Baechler EC, Li QZ, Wakeland EK, Bruner GR, Kaufman KM, Kelly JA. Genome-wide association scan in women with systemic lupus erythematosus identifies susceptibility variants in ITGAM, PXK, KIAA1542 and other loci. Nat Genet. 2008;40(2):204-10

International Schizophrenia Consortium. Rare chromosomal deletions and duplications increase risk of schizophrenia. Nature 2008; 455: 237–41.

Ito I, Kawaguchi Y, Kawasaki A, Hasegawa M, Ohashi J, Kawamoto M, Fujimoto M, Takehara K, Sato S, Hara M, Tsuchiya N. Association of the FAM167A-BLK region with systemic sclerosis. Arthritis Rheum. 2010 Mar;62(3):890-5.

Ito T, Wang YH, Duramad O, Hanabuchi S, Perng OA, Gilliet M et al. OX40 ligand shuts down IL-10-producing regulatory T cells. Proc Natl Acad Sci USA 2006a; 103: 13138–13143.

Ito, I. et al. Replication of the association between the C8orf13-BLK region and systemic lupus erythematosus in a Japanese population. Arthritis Rheum. 2009;60, 553–558.

Itoh K, and Hirohata S, The role of IL-10 in human B cell activation, proliferation, and differentiation.J. Immunol. 1995;154, 4341–4350.

Jacob CO, Zhu J, Armstrong DL, Yan M, Han J, *et al.* Identification of IRAK1 as a risk gene with critical role in the pathogenesis of systemic lupus erythematosus. Proc. Natl Acad. Sci. USA 2009;106, 6256–6261.

Ji JD, Lee WJ, Kong KA, et al. Association of STAT4 polymorphism with rheumatoid arthritis and systemic lupus erythematosus:a meta-analysis. Mol Biol Rep 2010; 37(1): 141–7.

Johanneson B, Lima G, von Salome J, Alarcon-Segovia D, Alarcon-Riquelme ME. A major susceptibility locus for systemic lupus erythematosus maps to chromosome 1q31. Am J Hum Genet 2002;71:1060–1071

Jönsen A, Bengtsson AA, Nived O, Truedsson L, Sturfelt G. Gene-environment interactions in the aetiology of systemic lupus erythematosus. Autoimmunity. 2007;40(8):613-7.

Kallel-Sellami M, Laadhar L, Zerzeri Y, Makni S. Complement deficiency and systemic lupus erythematosus: consensus and dilemma. Expert Rev Clin Immunol. 2008;4(5):629-37.

Karassa FB, Trikalinos TA, Ioannidis JP. Role of the Fcgamma receptor IIa polymorphism in susceptibility to systemic lupus erythematosus and lupus nephritis: a meta-analysis. Arthritis Rheum. 2002;46:1563–1571

Karassa FB, Trikalinos TA, Ioannidis JP. The Fc gamma RIIIA-F158 allele is a risk factor for the development of lupus nephritis: a meta-analysis. Kidney Int 2003;63:1475–82

Kariuki, SN. et al. Cutting edge: autoimmune disease risk variant of STAT4 confers increased sensitivity to IFN-α in lupus patients in vivo. J. Immunol. 2009;182, 34–38.

Kariuki, SN, Crow MK, and Niewold TB. The PTPN22 C1858T polymorphism is associated with skewing of cytokine profiles toward high interferon-α activity and low tumor necrosis factor α levels in patients with lupus. Arthritis Rheum. 2008;58, 2818–23.

Kawasaki, A. et al. Role of STAT4 polymorphisms in systemic lupus erythematosus in a Japanese population: a case-control association study of the STAT1–STAT4 region. Arthritis Res Ther. 2008;10(5):R113.

Kelley VR and Rovin BH, "Chemokines: therapeutic targets for autoimmune and inflammatory renal disease," Springer Seminars in Immunopathology, vol. 24, no. 4, (2003) pp. 411–421.

Kevil CG, Hicks MJ, He X, Zhang J, Ballantyne CM and Raman C et al., Loss of LFA-1, but not Mac-1, protects MRL/MpJ-Fas(lpr) mice from autoimmune disease, Am J Pathol 165 (2004), pp. 609–616.

Kim EM, Bang SY, Kim I, Shin HD, Park BL, Lee HS, Bae SC. Different genetic effect of PXK on systemic lupus erythematosus in the Korean population. Rheumatol Int. 2011 Jan 18. [Epub ahead of print]

Kim HL, Lee DS, Yang SH, et al., "The polymorphism of monocyte chemoattractant protein-1 is associated with the renal disease of SLE," American Journal of Kidney Diseases, vol. 40, no. 6, (2002) pp. 1146–1152.

Kim I, Kim YJ, Kim K, et al. Genetic studies of systemic lupus erythematosus in Asia: where are we now? Genes Immun 2009; 10: 421–432.

Kim I, Kim YJ, Kim K, Kang C, Choi CB, Sung YK, Lee HS, Bae SC.. Genetic studies of systemic lupus erythematosus in Asia: where are we now? Genes Immun 2009; 10:421–432.

Kim J, Modlin RL, Moy RL, Dubinett SM, McHugh T, Nickloff BJ and Uyemura K. IL-10 production in cutaneous basal and squamous cell carcinomas. A mechanism for evading the local T cell immune response. J. Immunol. 1995;155, 2240–47.

Kobata T, Jacquot S, Kozlowski S, Agematsu K, Schlossman SF and Morimoto C, CD27–CD70 interactions regulate B-cell activation by T cells, Proc Natl Acad Sci U S A 92 (1995), pp. 11249–11253.

Kobayashi T, Ito S, Yasuda K, Kuroda T, Yamamoto K, Sugita N, Tai H, Narita I, Gejyo F, Yoshie H. The combined genotypes of stimulatory and inhibitory Fc gamma receptors associated with systemic lupus erythematosus and periodontitis in Japanese adults. J Periodontol. 2007;78(3):467-74.

Kochi Y, Suzuki A, Yamada R, Yamamoto K. Genetics of rheumatoid arthritis: underlying evidence of ethnic differences. J Autoimmun 2009; 32: 158–162.

Koene HR, Kleijer M, Roos D, de Hasse M and Von dem Borne AE, FcγRIIIB gene duplication: evidence for presence and expression of three distinct FcγRIIIB genes in NA(1+,2+)SH(+) individuals. Blood 1998;91, 673–679.

Koene, H. R. et al. The FcγRIIIA-158F allele is a risk factor for systemic lupus erythematosus. Arthritis Rheum. 1998;41,1813–1818.

Korb LC, Ahearn JM. C1q binds directly and specifically to surface blebs of apoptotic human keratinocytes: complement deficiency and systemic lupus erythematosus revisited. J Immunol 1997;158:4525–8.

Kozyrev SV, Abelson AK, Wojcik J, Zaghlool A, Reddy MV Linga, Sanchez E, et al. Functional variants in the B-cell gene BANK1 are associated with systemic lupus erythematosus. Nat Genet. 2008;40(2):211–216.

Krauss JC, PooH, Xue W, Mayo-Bond L, Todd RF III, Petty HR. Reconstitution of antibody-dependent phagocytosis in fibroblasts expressing Fc gamma receptor IIIB and the complement receptor type 3. J Immunol 1994;153:1769–77.

Ku CS, Loy EY, Salim A, Pawitan Y, Chia KS. The discovery of human genetic variations and their use as disease markers: past, present and future. J Hum Genet. 2010;55(7):403-15.

Kyogoku C, Dijstelbloem HM, Tsuchiya N, Hatta Y, Kato H, Yamaguchi A, Fukazawa T, Jansen MD, Hashimoto H, van de Winkel JG, Kallenberg CG, Tokunaga K. Fcγ receptor gene polymorphisms in Japanese patients with systemic lupus erythematosus: contribution of FCGR2B to genetic susceptibility. Arthritis Rheum. 2002;46, 1242–1254.

Kyogoku C, Morinobu A, Nishimura K, Sugiyama D, Hashimoto H, Tokano Y, Mimori T, Terao C, Matsuda F, Kuno T, Kumagai S. Lack of association between tyrosine kinase 2 (TYK2) gene polymorphisms and susceptibility to SLE in a Japanese population. Mod Rheumatol. 2009;19(4):401-6.

Kyogoku C., Tsuchiya N., wu H., Tsao BP and Tokunaga K. Association of Fcγ receptor IIA, but not IIB and IIIA, polymorphisms with systemic lupus erythematosus: a family-based association study in Caucasians. Arthritis Rheum. 2004;50, 671–673.

L.R. Finger, J. Pu, R. Wasserman, R. Vibhakar, E. Louie, R.R. Hardy et al. The human PD-1 gene: complete cDNA, genomic organization, and developmentally regulated expression in B cell progenitors. Gene 197 (1997) pp. 177–187.

Lane P. Role of OX40 signals in coordinating CD4T cell selection, migration, and cytokine differentiation in T helper (Th)1 and Th2 cells. J Exp Med 2000;191:201–6.

Lawrie CH, Saunders NJ, Soneji S, Palazzo S, Dunlop HM, Cooper CD, Brown PJ, Troussard X, Mossafa H, Enver T, Pezzella F, Boultwood J, Wainscoat JS, Hatton CS. MicroRNA expression in lymphocyte development and malignancy. Leukemia 2008;22:1440–1446.

Le Bon A, Schiavoni G, D'Agostino G, Gresser I, Belardelli F, Tough DF. Type I interferons potently enhance humoral immunity and can promote isotype switching by stimulating dendritic cells in vivo. Immunity 2001;14:461–70.

Lea WW, Lee YH. The association between the PTPN22 C1858T polymorphism and systemic lupus erythematosus: a meta-analysis update. Lupus. 2011;20(1):51-7.

Lee YH, Harley JB, Nath SK. CTLA-4 polymorphisms and systemic lupus erythematosus (SLE): a meta-analysis. Hum Genet 2005; 116: 361–367.

Lee YH, Song GG. Association between the rs2004640 functional polymorphism of interferon regulatory factor 5 and systemic lupus erythematosus: a meta-analysis. Rheumatol Int 2009; 29:1137–1142.

Lehrnbecher T, Foster CB, Zhu S, et al. (1999a) Variant genotypes of the low-affinity Fcgamma receptors in two control populations and a review of low-affinity Fcgamma receptor polymorphisms in control and disease populations. Blood 94 (12), 4220–32.

Li J, Li L, Shang X, Benson J, Merle Elloso M, Schantz A et al. Negative regulation of IL-17 production by OX40/OX40L interaction. Cell Immunol 2008; 253: 31–37.

Li X, Wu J, Carter RH, Edberg JC, Su K, Cooper GS, Kimberly RP. A novel polymorphism in the Fcγ receptor IIB (CD32B) transmembrane region alters receptor signaling. Arthritis Rheum. 2003;48, 3242–3252.

Liao CH, Yao TC, Chung HT, See LC, Kuo ML and Huang JL. "Polymorphisms in the promoterregion of RANTES and the regulatory region of monocyte chemoattractant protein-1 among Chinese children with systemic lupus erythematosus," Journal of Rheumatology, vol. 31, no. 10, (2004) pp. 2062–2067.

Liossis SN, Solomou EE, Dimopoulos MA, Panayiotidis P, Mavrikakis MM, Sfikakis PP. B-cell kinase lyn deficiency in patients with systemic lupus erythematosus. J Investig Med. 2001; 49(2):157–65.

Liu MF, Wang CR, Lin LC, Wu CR. CTLA-4 gene polymorphism in promoter and exon-1 regions in Chinese patients with systemic lupus erythematosus. Lupus 2001; 10: 647–649.

Llorente L, Zou W, Levy Y, Richaud-Patin Y, Wijdenes Y, Alcocer-Varela J, Morel-Fourrier B, Brouet J., Alarcon-Segovia D, Galanaud P. et al. Role of interleukin 10 in the B lymphocyte hyperactivity and autoantibody production of human systemic lupus erythematosus. J. Exp. Med. 1995;181, 839–844.

Llorente L., Richaud-Patin Y., Fior R., Alcocer-Varela J., Wijdnes J., Morel-Fourrier B., Galanaud P. & Emilie P. In vivo production of interleukin-10 by non-T cells in rheumatoid arthritis, Sjögren's syndrome, and systemic lupus erythematosus. A potential mechanism of B lymphocyte hyperactivity and autoimmunity.Arthritis Rheum. 1994;37, 1647–1655.

Lodish HF, Zhou B, Liu G, Chen CZ. Micromanagement of the immune system by microRNAs. Nat Rev Immunol 2008;8:120–30.

Lopez P, Mozo L, Gutierrez C, Suarez A. Epidemiology of systemic lupus erythematosus in a northern Spanish population: gender and age influence on immunological features. Lupus 2003;12:860-865.

Lu Q, Kaplan M, Ray D, Ray D, Zacharek S and Gutsch D et al., Demethylation of ITGAL (CD11a) regulatory sequences in systemic lupus erythematosus, Arthritis Rheum 46 (2002), pp. 1282–1291.

Lu Q, Wu A and Richardson BC, Demethylation of the same promoter sequence increases CD70 expression in lupus T cells and T cells treated with lupus-inducing drugs, J Immunol 174 (2005), pp. 6212–6219.

Luscher U, Filgueira L, Juretic A, Zuber M, Luscher L, Heberer M and Spagnoli GC. The pattern of cytokine gene expression in freshly excised human metastatic melanoma suggests a state of reversible anergy of tumor-infiltrating lymphocytes.Int. J. Cancer 1994;57, 612–619.

Magnusson V, Johanneson B, Lima G, Odeberg J, Alarcon- Segovia D, Alarcon-Riquelme ME, SLE Genetics Collaboration Group. Both risk alleles for FcgammaRIIA and FcgammaRIIIA are susceptibility factors for SLE: a unifying hypothesis. Genes Immun 2004;5:130–137

Magnusson V, Zunec R, Odeberg J, Sturfelt G, Truedsson L, Gunnarsson I, Alarcón-Riquelme ME.. Polymorphisms of the Fcγ receptor type IIB gene are not associated with systemic lupus erythematosus in the Swedish population. Arthritis Rheum. 2004;50(4):1348-50.

Mao, H., Ferguson, T. S., Cibulsky, S. M., Holmqvist, M., Ding, C., Fei, H., Levitan, I. B. MONaKA, a novel modulator of the plasma membrane Na,K-ATPase. J. Neurosci. 2005;25: 7934-7943.

Marrack P, Kappler J, Mitchell T. Type I interferons keep activated T cells alive. J Exp Med 1999;189:521–30.

Matsuda M, Salazar F, Petersson M, Masucci G, Hansson J, Pisa, Zhang, QC, Masucci MG and Kiessling R. Interleukin 10 pretreatment protects target cells from tumor- and allo-specific cytotoxic T cells and downregulates HLA class I expression.J. Exp. Med. 1994;180, 2371–2376.

Matsushita M, Tsuchiya N, Shiota M, et al. Lack of a strong association of CTLA-4 exon 1 polymorphism with the susceptibility to rheumatoid arthritis and systemic lupus erythematosus in Japanese: an association study using a novel variation screening method. Tissue Antigens 1999; 54: 578–584.

Mehrian, R. et al. Synergistic effect between IL-10 and bcl-2 genotypes in determining susceptibility to SLE. Arthritis Rheum. 1998;41, 596–602.

Minegishi Y, Saito M, Morio T, Watanabe K, Agematsu K, Tsuchiya S, Takada H, Hara T, Kawamura N, Ariga T, Kaneko H, Kondo N, Tsuge I, Yachie A, Sakiyama Y, Iwata T, Bessho F, Ohishi T, Joh K, Imai K, Kogawa K, Shinohara M, Fujieda M, Wakiguchi H, Pasic S, Abinun M, Ochs HD, Renner ED, Jansson A, Belohradsky BH, et al.: Human tyrosine kinase 2 deficiency reveals its requisite roles in multiple cytokine signals involved in innate and acquired immunity. Immunity 2006;25:745-755

Morinobu A, Gadina M, Strober W et al. STAT4 serine phosphorylation is critical for IL-12-induced IFN-gamma production but not for cell proliferation. Proc Natl Acad Sci USA 2002;99:12281–6.

Mosmann, T. R. Properties and functions of interleukin-10. Adv. Immunol. 1994;56, 1–26.

Mostowska M, Wudarski M, Chwalińska-Sadowska H, Jagodziński PP. The programmed cell death 1 gene 7209 C>T polymorphism is associated with the risk of systemic lupus erythematosus in the Polish population. Clin Exp Rheumatol. 2008;26(3):457-60.

Musone SL, et al. Multiple polymorphisms in the TNFAIP3 region are independently associated with systemic lupus erythematosus. Nat Genet. 2008; 40:1062–4

Namjou B, Nath SK, Kilpatrick J et al. Genome scan stratified by the presence of anti-double-stranded DNA (dsDNA) autoantibody in pedigrees multiplex for systemic lupus erythematosus (SLE) establishes linkages at 19p13.2 (SLED1) and 18q21.1 (SLED2). Genes Immun 2002;3(Suppl 1):S35–S41

Namjou B, Sestak AL, Armstrong DL, et al. High-density genotyping of STAT4 reveals multiple haplotypic associations with systemic lupus erythematosus in different racial groups. Arthritis Rheum 2009; 60: 1085–1095.

Napirei M, Karsunky H, Zevnik B, Stephan H, Mannherz HG, Mo'ro'y T. Features of systemic lupus erythematosus in Dnase 1-deficient mice. Nature Genet 2000;25:177–81.

Nath SK, Han S, Kim-Howard X, et al. A nonsynonymous functional variant in integrin-alpha(M) (encoded by ITGAM) is associated with systemic lupus erythematosus. Nat Genet 2008; 40:152–154.

Nath SK, Harley JB, Lee YH. Polymorphisms of complement receptor 1 and interleukin-10 genes and systemic lupus erythematosus: a meta-analysis. Hum Genet 2005;118(2):225–234

Nguyen KB, Watford WT, Salomon R et al. Critical role for STAT4 activation by type 1 interferons in the interferon-gamma response to viral infection. Science 2002;297:2063–6.

Niewold TB, Kelly JA, Flesch MH, Espinoza LR, Harley JB, Crow MK. Association of the IRF5 risk haplotype with high serum interferon-alpha activity in systemic lupus erythematosus patients. Arthritis Rheum. 2008;58(8):2481-7.

Nimmerjahn F, Ravetch J Fcgamma receptors as regulators of immune responses. Nat Rev Immunol. 2008;8(1):34-47.

Nishikomori R, Usui T, Wu CY, Morinobu A, O'Shea JJ, Strober W. Activated STAT4 has an essential role in Th1 differentiation and proliferation that is independent of its role in the maintenance of IL-12R beta 2 chain expression and signaling. J Immunol 2002;169:4388–98.

O. Avni and A. Rao, T cell differentiation: a mechanistic view. Curr Opin Immunol 12 (2000), pp. 654–659.

O'Connell RM, Rao DS, Chaudhuri AA, Baltimore D. Physiological and pathological roles for microRNAs in the immune system. Nat Rev Immunol 2010;10:111–22.

Oei SL, Shi Y. Poly(ADP-ribosyl)ation of transcription factor Yin Yang 1 under conditions of DNA damage. Biochem Biophys Res Commun 2001;285:27–31

Ogden CA, deCathelineau A, Hoffmann PR, Bratton D, Ghebrehiwet B, Fadok VA, et al. C1q and mannose binding lectin engagement of cell surface calreticulin and CD91 initiates macropinocytosis and uptake of apoptotic cells. J Exp Med 2001;194:781–95.

Okada M, Ogasawara H, Kaneko H, Hishikawa T, Sekigawa I, Hashimoto H, et al. Role of DNA methylation in transcription of human endogenous retrovirus in the pathogenesis of systemic lupus erythematosus. J Rheumatol 2002;29:1678–82.

Oliver FJ, Menissier-de Murcia J, de Murcia G. Poly(ADPribose) polymerase in the cellular response to DNA damage, apoptosis, and disease. Am J Hum Genet 1999;64:1282–1288

Orozco G, Sánchez E, González-Gay MA, López-Nevot MA, Torres B, Cáliz R, Ortego-Centeno N, Jiménez-Alonso J, Pascual-Salcedo D, Balsa A, de Pablo R, Nuñez-Roldan A, González-Escribano MF, Martín J. Association of a functional single-nucleotide polymorphism of PTPN22, encoding lymphoid protein phosphatase, with rheumatoid arthritis and systemic lupus erythematosus. Arthritis Rheum. 2005;52(1):219-24.

Orru V, Tsai SJ, Rueda B, Fiorillo E, Stanford SM, Dasgupta J. A loss-of-function variant of PTPN22 is associated with reduced risk of systemic lupus erythematosus. Hum. Mol. Genet. 2009;18, 569–579.

Oshima S, Turer EE, Callahan JA, Chai S, Advincula R, Barrera J, Shifrin N, Lee B, Benedict Yen TS, Woo T, Malynn BA, Ma A: ABIN-1 is a ubiquitin sensor that restricts cell death and sustains embryonic development. Nature 2009; 457:906-909.

Pan F, Tang X, Zhang K, Li X, Xu J, Chen H, Ye DQ. Genetic susceptibility and haplotype analysis between Fcgamma receptor IIB and IIIA gene with systemic lupus erythematosus in Chinese population. Lupus. 2008;17(8):733-8.

Pan HF, Leng RX, Wang C, Qin WZ, Chen LL, Zha ZQ, Tao JH, Ye DQ. Association of TNF-α promoter-308 A/G polymorphism with susceptibility to systemic lupus erythematosus: a meta-analysis. Rheumatol Int. 2011 Apr 16 [Epub ahead of print].

Pan Y, Sawalha AH. Epigenetic regulation and the pathogenesis of systemic lupus erythematosus. Transl Res 2009;153:4–10 .

Parren PW, Warmerdam PA, Boeije LC, et al. On the interaction of IgG subclasses with the low affinity Fc gamma RIIa (CD32) on human monocytes, neutrophils, and platelets. Analysis of a functional polymorphism to human IgG2. J Clin Invest 1992a;90 (4), 1537–46.

Parren PW, PA, Boeije LC, Capel PJ, van de Winkel JG, Aarden LA. Characterization of IgG FcR-mediated proliferation of human T cells induced by mouse and human anti-

CD3 monoclonal antibodies. Identification of a functional polymorphism to human IgG2 anti-CD3. J Immunol 1992b;148 (3), 695–701.

Pauley KM, Cha S, Chan EK. microRNA in autoimmunity and autoimmune diseases. J Autoimmun 2009;32:189–94.

Perez, L., Orte, J. and Brieva, J. A. Terminal differentiation of spontaneous rheumatoid factor-secreting B cells from rheumatoid arthritis patients depends on endogenous interleukin-10. Arthritis Rheum. 1995;38, 1771–1776.

Plenge RM, et al. Two independent alleles at 6q23 associated with risk of rheumatoid arthritis. Nat Genet. 2007; 39:1477–82.

Plenge RM. Recent progress in rheumatoid arthritis genetics: one step towards improved patient care. Curr Opin Rheumatol 2009; 21:262–271.

Poo H, Krauss JC, Mayo-Bond L, Todd RF III, Petty HR. Interaction of Fc gamma receptor type IIIB with complement receptor type 3 in fibroblast transfectants: evidence from lateral diffusion and resonance energy transfer studies. J Mol Biol 1995;247:597–603.

Pradhan V, Surve P, Ghosh K.Mannose binding lectin (MBL) in autoimmunity and its role in systemic lupus erythematosus (SLE). J Assoc Physicians India. 2010;58:688-90.

Prokunina L, Castillejo-López C, Oberg F, Gunnarsson I, Berg L, Magnusson V, Brookes AJ, Tentler D, Kristjansdóttir H, Gröndal G, Bolstad AI, Svenungsson E, Lundberg I, Sturfelt G, Jönssen A, Truedsson L, Lima G, Alcocer-Varela J, Jonsson R, Gyllensten UB, Harley JB, Alarcón-Segovia D, Steinsson K, Alarcón-Riquelme ME. A regulatory polymorphism in PDCD1 is associated with susceptibility to systemic lupus erythematosus in humans. Nat Genet. 2002;32(4):666-9.

Qiao JY, Shao W, Wei HJ, Sun YM, Zhao YC and Xing WL et al., Novel high-throughput profiling of human transcription factors and its use for systematic pathway mapping, J Proteome Res 7 (2008), pp. 2769–2779.

Ramasawmy R, Spina GS, Fae KC, Pereira AC, Nisihara R, Reason IJM, Grinberg M, Tarasoutchi F, Kalil J, and Guilherme L. Association of Mannose-Binding Lectin Gene Polymorphism but Not of Mannose Binding Serine Protease 2 with Chronic Severe Aortic Regurgitation of Rheumatic Etiology. Clin and vacc Immunol 2008;932-936.

Ramos PS, Kelly JA, Gray-McGuire C et al. Familial aggregation and linkage analysis of autoantibody traits in pedigrees multiplex for systemic lupus erythematosus. Genes Immun 2006;7:417–32.

Remmers EF, Plenge RM, Lee AT et al. STAT4 and the risk of rheumatoid arthritis and systemic lupus erythematosus. N Engl J Med 2007;357:977–86.

Reth, M. & wienands, J. Initiation and processing of signals from the B cell antigen receptor. Annu Rev. Immunol. 1997;15, 453–479.

Richardson B. Primer: epigenetics of autoimmunity. Nat Clin Pract Rheumatol 2007;3:521-7.

Richardson BC, Liebling MR and Hudson JL, $CD4^{+}$ cells treated with DNA methylation inhibitors induce autologous B cell differentiation, Clin Immunol Immunopathol 55 (1990), pp. 368–381.

Richter MF, Dumenil G, Uze G, Fellous M, Pellegrini S. Specific contribution of Tyk2 JH regions to the binding and the expression of the interferon alpha/beta receptor component IFNAR1. J Biol Chem 1998;273:24723–9.

Rodriguez W, Mold C, Kataranovski M, Hutt J, Marnell LL, Du Clos TW. Reversal of ongoing proteinuria in autoimmune mice by treatment with C-reactive protein. Arthritis Rheum 2005;52:642–650

Ronnblom L. Alm GV. Systemic lupus erythematosus and the type I interferon system. Arthritis Res Ther 2003;5:68–75.

Rovin BH and Phan LT, "Chemotactic factors and renal inflammation," American Journal of Kidney Diseases, vol. 31, no. 6, pp. 1065–1084, 1998.

Rovin BH, Doe N, and Tan LC, "Monocyte chemoattractant protein-1 levels in patients with glomerular disease," American Journal of Kidney Diseases, vol.27,no.5,(1996) pp. 640–646.

Rovin BH, Song H, Birmingham DJ, Hebert LA, Yu CY, Nagaraja HN: Urine chemokines as biomarkers of human systemic lupus erythematosus activity. J Am Soc Nephrol 2005;16(2):467-473.

Russell AI, Cunninghame Graham DS, Shepherd C, Roberton CA, Whittaker J, Meeks J, Powell RJ, Isenberg DA, Walport MJ, Vyse TJ. Polymorphism at the C-reactive protein locus influences gene expression and predisposes to systemic lupus erythematosus. Hum Mol Genet. 2004; 1;13(1):137-47.

Saitoh A, Suzuki Y, Takeda M, Kubota K, Itoh K, and Tomino Y, "Urinary levels of monocyte chemoattractant protein (MCP)-1 and disease activity in patients with IgA nephropathy," Journal of Clinical Laboratory Analysis, vol. 12, no. 1, (1998) pp. 1–5.

Salloum R, Franek B, Kariuki S, Utset T, Niewold T. Genetic Variation at the IRF7/KIAA1542 Locus is Associated with Autoantibody Profile and Serum Interferon Alpha Levels in Lupus Patients Clinical Immunology (2009), 131, Supplement, pg. S54-S54

Salmon JE, Millard S, Schachter LA, Arnett FC, Ginzler EM, Gourley MF, Ramsey-Goldman R, Peterson MG, Kimberly RP. Fcγ RIIA alleles are heritable risk factors for lupus nephritis in African Americans. J. Clin. Invest. 1996;97, 1348-1354.

Savarese E, Steinberg C, Pawar RD. et al., "Requirement of Toll-like receptor 7 for pristane-induced production of autoantibodies and development of murine lupus nephritis," Arthritis and Rheumatism, vol. 58, no. 4, (2008) pp. 1107–1115.

Schifferli JA, Steiger G, Paccaud JP, Sjoholm AG, Hauptmann G. Difference in the biological properties of the two forms of the fourth component of human complement (C4). Clin Exp Immunol 1986;63:473–7.

Sebat J, Lakshmi B, Malhotra D et al. Strong association of de novo copy number mutations with autism. Science 2007; 316: 445–9.

Selbach M, Schwanhausser B, Thierfelder N, Fang Z, Khanin R, Rajewsky N. Widespread changes in protein synthesis induced by microRNAs. Nature 2008;455:58–63.

Sestak AL, Fürnrohr BG, Harley JB, Merrill JT, Namjou B. The genetics of systemic lupus erythematosus and implications for targeted therapy. Ann Rheum Dis. 2011;70 Suppl 1:I37-43.

Shimaoka M and Springer TA. Therapeutic antagonists and conformational regulation of integrin function, Nat Rev Drug Discov 2 (2003), pp. 703–716.

Shimizu S, Nakashima H, Masutani K, et al. Anti-monocyte chemoattractant protein-1 gene therapy attenuates nephritis in MRL/lpr mice. Rheumatology (Oxford). 2004;43(9):1121-8.

Shin HD, Park BL, Kim LH, Lee HS, Kim TY, Bae SC. Common DNase I polymorphism associated with autoantibody production among systemic lupus erythematosus patients. Hum Mol Genet 2004;13:2343–50.

Sigurdsson S, Göring HH, Kristjansdottir G, Milani L, Nordmark G, Sandling JK, Eloranta ML, Feng D, Sangster-Guity N, Gunnarsson I, Svenungsson E, Sturfelt G, Jönsen A, Truedsson L, Barnes BJ, Alm G, Rönnblom L, Syvänen AC. Comprehensive evaluation of the genetic variants of interferon regulatory factor 5 (IRF5) reveals a novel 5 bp length polymorphism as strong risk factor for systemic lupus erythematosus. Hum Mol Genet. 2008;17(6):872-81.

Sigurdsson S, Nordmark G, Göring HH, Lindroos K, Wiman AC, Sturfelt G, Jönsen A, Rantapää-Dahlqvist S, Möller B, Kere J, Koskenmies S, Widén E, Eloranta ML, Julkunen H, Kristjansdottir H, Steinsson K, Alm G, Rönnblom L, Syvänen AC: Polymorphisms in the tyrosine kinase 2 and interferon regulatory factor 5 genes are associated with systemic lupus erythematosus. Am J Hum Genet 2005;76:528-537.

Sigurdsson, S. et al. A risk haplotype of STAT4 for systemic lupus erythematosus is overexpressed, correlates with anti-dsDNA and shows additive effects with two risk alleles of IRF5. Hum. Mol. Genet. 2008;17, 2868–2876.

Siriboonrit U, Tsuchiya N, Sirikong M, Kyogoku C, Bejrachandra S, Suthipinittharm P, Luangtrakool K, Srinak D, Thongpradit R, Fujiwara K, Chandanayingyong D, Tokunaga K. Association of Fcgamma receptor IIb and IIIb polymorphisms with susceptibility to systemic lupus erythematosus in Thais. Tissue Antigens. 2003;61(5):374-83.

Song Y, Han CW, Kang SW, Baek HJ, Lee EB, Shin CH, Hahn BH, Tsao BP. Abnormal distribution of Fcγ receptor type IIa polymorphisms in Korean patients with systemic lupus erythematous. Arthritis Rheum. 1998;41(3):421-6.

Sonkoly E, Stahle M, Pivarcsi A. microRNAs and immunity: novel players in the regulation of normal immune function and inflammation. Semin Cancer Biol 2008;18:131–40.

Stahl RA, Thaiss F, Disser M, Helmchen U, Hora K, and Schl¨ondorff D, "Increased expression of monocyte chemoattractant protein-1 in anti-thymocyte antibodyinduced glomerulonephriti," Kidney International, vol. 44, no. 5, (1993) pp. 1036–1047,.

Stockl J, Majdic O, Pickl WF et al. Granulocyte activation via a binding site near the C-terminal region of complement receptor type 3 alpha-chain (CD11b) potentially involved in intramembrane complex formation with glycosylphosphatidylinositolanchored Fc gamma RIIIB (CD16) molecules. J Immunol 1995;154:5452–63.

Stuber E, Neurath M, Calderhead D, Fell HP, Strober W. Cross-linking of OX40 ligand, a member of the TNF/NGF cytokine family, induces proliferation and differentiation in murine splenic B cells. Immunity 1995;2:507–21.

Stuber E, Strober W. The T cell-B cell interaction via OX40-OX40L is necessary for the T cell-dependent humoral immune response. J Exp Med 1996;183:979–89.

Su K, Wu J, Edberg JC et al. A promoter haplotype of the immunoreceptor tyrosine-based inhibitory motif-bearing FcgammaRIIb alters receptor expression and associates with autoimmunity. I. Regulatory FCGR2B polymorphisms and their association with systemic lupus erythematosus. J Immunol 2004;172:7186–7191

Suarez-Gestal M, Calaza M, Endreffy E, Pullmann R, Ordi-Ros J, Sebastiani GD, Ruzickova S, Jose Santos M, Papasteriades C, Marchini M, Skopouli FN, Suarez A, Blanco FJ, D'Alfonso S, Bijl M, Carreira P, Witte T, Migliaresi S, Gomez-Reino JJ, Gonzalez A. Replication of recently identified systemic lupus erythematosus genetic associations: a case-control study.European Consortium of SLE DNA Collections. Arthritis Res Ther. 2009;11(3): R69.

Sullivan, K. E. et al. Analysis of polymorphisms affecting immune complex handling in systemic lupus erythematosus. Rheumatology (Oxford) 2003;42, 446–452 ().

Suzuki T, Tahara H, Narula S, Moore KW, Robbins PD and Lotze MT. Viral interleukin 10 (IL-10), the human herpes virus 4 cellular IL-10 homologue, induces local anergy to allogeneic and syngeneic tumors. J. Exp. Med. 1995;182, 447–486.

Taganov KD, Boldin MP, Baltimore D. microRNAs and immunity:tiny players in a big field. Immunity 2007;26:133–7.

Takahashi R, Tsutsumi A, Ohtani K, Muraki Y, Goto D, Matsumoto I, Wakamiya N, Sumida T Association of mannose binding lectin (MBL) gene polymorphism and serum MBL concentration with characteristics and progression of systemic lupus erythematosus Ann Rheum Dis 2005;64:311–314

Takaoka A, Yanai H, Kondo S et al. Integral role of IRF-5 in the gene induction programme activated by Toll-like receptors. Nature 2005;434:243–249

Tan, E. M. Cohen AS, Fries JF, Masi AT, McShane DJ, Rothfield NF, Schaller JG, Talal N, Winchester RJ. The 1982 revised criteria for the classification of systemic lupus erythematosus. Arthritis Rheum. 1982;25,1271–1277.

Tang Y, Luo X, Cui H, Ni X, Yuan M, Guo Y, et al. MicroRNA-146a contributes to abnormal activation of the type I interferon pathway in human lupus by targeting the key signaling proteins. Arthritis Rheum 2009;60:1065–75.

Taylor, K. E. et al. Specificity of the STAT4 genetic association for severe disease manifestations of systemic lupus erythematosus. PLoS Genet. 2008;4(5):e1000084.

Tesar V, Masek Z, Rychlik I, et al. Cytokines and adhesion molecules in renal vasculitis and lupus nephritis. Nephrol Dial Transplant. 1998;13(7):1662-7.

Thomson W, et al. Rheumatoid arthritis association at 6q23. Nat Genet. 2007; 39:1431-3.

Tian C, Gregersen PK, Seldin MF. Accounting for ancestry: population substructure and genome-wide association studies. Hum Mol Genet 2008;17: R143–R150.

Tsao BP, Cantor RM, Grossman JM et al. PARP alleles within the linked chromosomal region are associated with systemic lupus erythematosus. J Clin Invest 1999;103:1135–1140

Tsao BP, Cantor RM, Grossman JM, Shen N, Teophilov NT, Wallace DJ, Arnett FC, Hartung K, Goldstein R, Kalunian KC, Hahn BH, Rotter JI. PARP alleles within the linked chromosomal region are associated with systemic lupus erythematosus. J Clin Invest 1999;103:1135–1140

Tsao BP, Cantor RM, Kalunian KC et al. Evidence for linkage of a candidate chromosome 1 region to human systemic lupus erythematosus. J Clin Invest 1997;99:725–731.

Tsao BP. Genetic susceptibility to lupus nephritis Lupus 1998;7, 585-590

Tsao BP. Lupus susceptibility genes on human chromosome 1. Int Rev Immunol. 2000;19(4-5):319-34.

Tsao BP. Update on human systemic lupus erythematosus genetics. Curr Opin Rheumatol 2004;16:513–521

Tsao, BP.; Wu, H. The genetics of human lupus. In: Wallace, LC.; Hahn, BH., editors. Dubois' Lupus Erythematosus. Vol. Seventh ed.. Philadeiphia: Lippincott Williams & Wilkins; 2008. p. 54-81.

Tsokos GC (2001; Dec) Systemic lupus erythematosus. A disease with a complex pathogenesis. Lancet 358 (Suppl),S65.

Tsuchiya N, Kyogoku C. Role of Fc gamma receptor IIb polymorphism in the genetic background of systemic lupus erythematosus: insights from Asia. Autoimmunity. 2005;38(5):347-52.

Tucci M, Barnes E.V, Sobel ES, et al., "Strong association of a functional polymorphism in the monocyte chemoattractant protein 1 promoter gene with lupus nephritis," Arthritis and Rheumatism, vol. 50, no. 6, (2004) pp. 1842–1849,.

Turner DM, Williams DM, Sankaran D, Lazarus M, Sinnott PJ, Hutchinson IV. An investigation of polymorphism in the interleukin-10 gene promoter. Eur J Immunogenet 1997;24:1–8

Ueda H, Howson JM, Esposito L et al. Association of the T-cell regulatory gene CTLA4 with susceptibility to autoimmune disease. Nature 2003;423:506–511

van der Linden MW, van der Slik AR, Zanelli E et al. Six microsatellite markers on the short arm of chromosome 6 in relation to HLA-DR3 and TNF-308A in systemic lupus erythematosus. Genes Immun 2001;2:373–380

Vang T, Congia M, Macis MD et al. Autoimmune-associated lymphoid tyrosine phosphatase is a gain-of-function variant. Nat Genet 2005;37:1317–9.

Vang T, Miletic AV, Arimura Y, Tautz L, Rickert RC, Mustelin T. Protein tyrosine phosphatases in autoimmunity. Annu Rev Immunol 2008;26:29–55.

Verstrepen L, Carpentier I, Verhelst K, Beyaert R: ABINs: A20 binding inhibitors of NF-_B and apoptosis signaling. Biochem Pharmacol 2009, 78:105-114.

Vollmer J, Tluk S, Schmitz C, Hamm S, Jurk M, Forsbach A, Akira S, Kelly KM, Reeves WH, Bauer S, and Krieg AM. Immune stimulation mediated by autoantigen binding sites within small nuclear RNAs involves Toll-like receptors 7 and 8. J. Exp. Med. 2005;202: 1575–1585.

Warmerdam PA, van de Winkel JG, Vlug A, Westerdaal NA, Capel PJ. A single amino acid in the second Ig-like domain of the human Fc gamma receptor II is critical for human IgG2 binding. J Immunol 1991;147 (4),n1338–43.

Watford WT, Hissong BD, Bream JH, Kanno Y, Muul L, O'Shea JJ. Signaling by IL-12 and IL-23 and the immunoregulatory roles of STAT4. Immunol Rev 2004;202:139–56.

Webb R, Wren JD, Jeffries M, *et al.* Variants within MECP2, a key transcription regulator, are associated with increased susceptibility to lupus and differential gene expression in patients with systemic lupus erythematosus. Arthritis Rheum 2009; 60: 1076 - 84 .

Westendorp RG, Langermans JA, Huizinga TW, Verweij CL, Sturk A. Genetic influence on cytokine production in meningococcal disease. Lancet. 1997;349(9069):1912-3.

Wilson JG, Murphy EE, Wong WW, Klickstein LB, Weis JH, Fearon DT. Identification of a restriction fragment length polymorphism by a CR1 cDNA that correlates with the number of CR1 on erythrocytes. J Exp Med. 1986 Jul 1;164(1):50-9.

Wojcik H, GriYths E, Staggs S, Hagman J, Winandy S. Expression of a non-DNA-binding Ikaros isoform exclusively in B cells leads to autoimmunity but not leukemogenesis. Eur J Immunol 2007;37:1022–1032.

Wong WW, Cahill JM, Rosen MD, Kennedy CA, Bonaccio ET, Morris MJ, Wilson JG, Klickstein LB, Fearon DT. Structure of the human CR1 gene. Molecular basis of the structural and quantitative polymorphisms and identification of a new CR1-like allele. J Exp Med 1989;169:847–863

Wong WW, Wilson JG, Fearon DT. Genetic regulation of a structural polymorphism of human C3b receptor. J Clin Invest 1983;72:685–693

Wu J et al. OR A novel polymorphism of FcγRIIIa (CD16) alters receptor function and predisposes to autoimmune disease. J Clin Invest 1997; 100: 1059-1070.

Xiao C, Rajewsky K. microRNA control in the immune system:basic principles. Cell 2009;136:26–36.

Xu AP, Yin PD, Su XY. [Association of CTLA-4 promoter -1722 polymorphism with systemic lupus erythematosus in Chinese]. Di Yi Jun Yi Da Xue Xue Bao 2004; 24: 1107–1112.

Y. Agata, A. Kawasaki, H. Nishimura, Y. Ishida, T. Tsubata, H. Yagita et al., Expression of the PD-1 antigen on the surface of stimulated mouse T and B lymphocytes. Int Immunol 8 (1996) pp. 765–772.

Yang W, Ng P, Zhao M, Hirankarn N, Lau CS, Mok CC, Chan TM, Wong RW, Lee KW, Mok MY, Wong SN, Avihingsanon Y, Lee TL, Ho MH, Lee PP, Wong WH, Lau YL. Population differences in SLE susceptibility genes: STAT4 and BLK, but not PXK, are associated with systemic lupus erythematosus in Hong Kong Chinese. Genes Immun. 2009;10(3):219-26.

Yang W, Zhao M, Hirankarn N, et al. ITGAM is associated with disease susceptibility and renal nephritis of systemic lupus erythematosus in Hong Kong Chinese and Thai. Hum Mol Genet 2009;18:2063–2070.

Yang Y, Chung EK, Wu YL et al. Gene copy-number variation and associated polymorphisms of complement component C4 in human systemic lupus erythematosus (SLE): low copy number is a risk factor for and high copy number is a protective factor against SLE susceptibility in European Americans. Am J Hum Genet 2007; 80: 1037–54.

Yang Z, Mendoza AR, Welch TR, Zipf WB, Yu CY. Modular variations of HLA class III genes for serine/threonine kinase RP, complement C4, steroid 21-hydroxylase CYP21 and tenascin TNX (RCCX): a mechanism for gene deletions and disease associations. J Biol Chem 1999;274:12147–12156.

Yang, W. Yang W, Ng P, Zhao M, Hirankarn N, Lau CS, Mok CC, Chan TM, Wong RW, Lee KW, Mok MY, Wong SN, Avihingsanon Y, Lee TL, Ho MH, Lee PP, Wong WH, Lau YL. Population differences in SLE susceptibility genes: STAT4 and BLK, but not PXK, are associated with systemic lupus erythematosus in Hong Kong Chinese. Genes Immun. 2009;10, 219–226.

Yap SN, Phipps ME, Manivasagar M, Tan SY and Bosco JJ. Human Fcγ receptor IIA (FcγRIIA) genotyping and association with systemic lupus erythematosus (SLE) in Chinese and Malays in Malaysia. 1999;Lupus 8, 305–310.

Yap WH, Yeoh E, Tay A, Brenner S, Venkatesh B. STAT4 is a target of the hematopoietic zinc-finger transcription factor Ikaros in T cells. FEBS Lett 2005; 579: 4470–4478.

Ye D, Pan F, Zhang K, Li X, Xu J, Hao J. A novel single-nucleotide polymorphism of the Fcgamma receptor IIIa gene is associated with genetic susceptibility to systemic lupus erythematosus in Chinese populations: a family-based association study. Clin Exp Dermatol. 2006;31(4):553-7.

Ye DQ, Hu YS, Li XP, et al., "The correlation between monocytes chemoattractant protein-1 and the arthritis of sytemic lupus erythematosus among Chinese," Archives of Dermatological Research, vol. 296, no. 8, (2005) pp. 366–371.

Yokoyama K, Su Ih IH, Tezuka T, Yasuda T, Mikoshiba K, Tarakhovsky A et al. BANK regulates BCR-induced calcium mobilization by promoting tyrosine phosphorylation of IP(3) receptor. EMBO J 2002; 21: 83–92.

Yu B, Shao Y, Li P, Zhang J, Zhong Q, Yang H, Hu X, Chen B, Peng X, Wu Q, Chen Y, Guan M, Wan J, Zhang W.Copy number variations of the human histamine H4 receptor gene are associated with systemic lupus erythematosus. Br J Dermatol. 2010;163(5):935-40.

Yu B, Wu Q, Chen Y, Li P, Shao Y, Zhang J, Zhong Q, Peng X, Yang H, Hu X, Chen B, Guan M, Zhang W, Wan J. Polymorphisms of PXK are associated with autoantibody production, but not disease risk, of systemic lupus erythematosus in Chinese mainland population. Lupus. 2011;20(1):23-7

Yu, CY.; Hauptmann, G.; Yang, Y.; Wu, YL.; Birmingham, DJ.; Rovin, BH., et al. Complement deficiencies in human systemic lupus erythematosus (SLE) and SLE nephritis: epidemiology and pathogenesis. In: Tsokos, GC., editor. Systemic Lupus Erythematosus: A Companion to Rheumatology. Philadelphia: Elsevier; 2007. p. 203-213.

Yung R, Chang S, Hemati N, Johnson K and Richardson B, Mechanisms of drug-induced lupus. IV. Comparison of procainamide and hydralazine with analogs in vitro and in vivo, Arthritis Rheum 40 (1997), pp. 1436–1443.

Yung R, Powers D, Johnson K, Ameto E, Carr D, Laing T, et al. Mechanisms of drug-induced lupus II. T cells overexpressing lymphocyte functionassociated antigen 1 become autoreactive and cause a lupus-like disease in systemic mice. J Clin Invest 1996;97:2866-71.

Zhang Z, Zhu KJ, Xu Q, Zhang XJ, Sun LD, Zheng HF, Han JW, Quan C, Zhang SQ, Cai LQ, Xu SX, Zuo XB, Cheng H, Yang S. The association of the BLK gene with SLE was replicated in Chinese Han. Arch Dermatol Res. 2010;302(8):619-24.

Zhao M, Sun Y, Gao F, Wu X, Tang J, Yin H, Luo Y, Richardson B, Lu Q. Epigenetics and SLE: RFX1 downregulation causes CD11a and CD70 overexpression by altering epigenetic modifications in lupus CD4+ T cells. J Autoimmun. 2010;35(1):58-69.

Zhou XJ, Lu XL, Lv JC, Yang HZ, Qin LX, Zhao MH, Su Y, Li ZG, Zhang H. Genetic association of PRDM1-ATG5 intergenic region and autophagy with systemic lupus erythematosus in a Chinese population. Ann Rheum Dis. 2011;70(7):1330-7.

2

Cytokines and Systemic Lupus Erythematosus

Jose Miguel Urra[1] and Miguel De La Torre[2]
[1]*Immunology Service, General Hospital Ciudad Real, Ciudad Real*
[2]*Nephrology Service, Cabueñes Hospital, Asturias*
Spain

1. Introduction

Systemic lupus erythematosus (SLE) is a multisystem autoimmune disease characterized by the production of numerous autoantibodies that typically involves multiple organ systems. As opposed to lupus in animal models, SLE in humans is heterogeneous and affects different individuals with a wide range of disease courses and manifestations. The pathogenesis is still unclear, a myriad of innate and adaptative immune system aberrations in SLE have been identified as major contributors of the disease.

Cytokines are a diverse group of soluble proteins and peptides, produced and released by immune system cells , that act as humoral regulators and modulate the functional activities of individual cells and tissues, playing a pivotal role in the differentiation, maturation, and activation of various immune and no immune cells. Cytokine dysregulation is likely to play a role in the loss of immune tolerance that leads to SLE, and in the damage resulting from the disease. Many of the genes that are associated with risk for lupus are cytokines, regulators of cytokines, or downstream members of cytokine pathways.

Multiple cytokines have been implicated in the disease activity or organ involvement in SLE. Among these, IL-6, Interferon (IFN), B-lymphocyte stimulator (BlyS), IL-10, IL-17 is thought to play an important role in the creation of the characteristic milieu in SLE, which promotes B-cell survival and autoantibody production. On the other hand, also cytokines like IL-10, IL1, TNF-α , IFN, are important in development of the autoimmune injury in renal and central nervous system, the most frequently observed causes of death in patients with SLE. Moreover, recent studies strongly suggest that the cytokines, at least in part, would be implicated in the pathogenesis of accelerated atherosclerosis associated with SLE.

The knowledge of cytokines not only provides new insight into pathogenesis of SLE, but also it has allowed the development of clinical applications such as monitoring of disease and as potential therapeutic targets with the use of several biologic agents, targeting different cytokines or their receptors. Consequently, many trials of anticytokine therapies for SLE are underway.

The focus of the present chapter is to summarize the cytokines which have significant implications in the pathogenesis of SLE, the potential clinical and therapeutic use will be reviewed.

2. SLE gender susceptibility and cytokines

One feature of lupus, which also occurs with other autoimmune diseases, is the influence of gender on disease susceptibility. In fact 90% of people affected by lupus are women (Masi &

Kaslow 1978). Immunological, epidemiological and clinical evidence suggest that female sex hormones play an important role in the etiology and pathophysiology of chronic immune diseases. Abundant studies have suggested that gender differences in susceptibility to SLE are mediated by sex hormones (Rider & Abdou 2001, Cohen-Solal et al 2006, Zandman et al 2007) .The high female prevalence is most marked after puberty: while the pre-puberty female to male ratio is 3 : 1, this increases to 10 : 1 during the childbearing years and decreases again to 8 : 1 after menopause (Lahita et al 1999a). Pregnancy is frequently associated with activity and flares of the disease in SLE patients (Lahita 1999a). Also there is an increased risk of developing SLE in postmenopausal women who received estrogen hormone replacement therapy (Buyon et al 2007) and increased the risk of flares in postmenopausal patients (Straub 2007). Together these considerations indicate that estrogen may be proposed as candidates to explain the sexual dimorphism of SLE. Cytokines are intimately involved with sex hormones, as they regulate the level of sex hormones both systemically and locally, especially in the reproductive organs. The interactions between cytokines and estrogens affect important cellular activities as proliferation and apoptosis (Lahita 1999b).

Estrogens exert their effects by activation of intracellular receptors, the estrogen receptor alpha (ERα) and beta (ERβ) (Green et al 1986). In addition to its intracellular receptors have also been reported membrane receptors that correspond to full-length isoforms of both ERα and ERβ with extracellular functionality (Pedram et al 2006). Both receptors have been identified in the membrane of thymocytes and have a great importance in the proper development of the thymus (Stimson & Hunter 1980). Thus it seems that estrogen receptors influence the adequate development of T lymphocytes. It is well known that low doses of estrogen promote enhanced Th1 responses and increased cell-mediated immunity, while high doses of estrogen lead instead to increased Th2 responses and antibodies production (Maret et al 2003, Bao et al 2002). This effect of estrogens seems to be achieved through direct alteration in the Th cytokine profile from a proinflammatory (IL-2, IFN-γ) to an humoral direction (IL-4, IL-5, IL-9, IL-13). Besides the effect of estrogen on the profile of cytokines released by T cells, estrogen also increases the release of IL-1, IL-6 and TNF by monocytes/macrophages (Kramer et al 2004). SLE patients show immune-related disorders mediated through estrogens. In vitro peripheral blood mononuclear cells in SLE patients show an increase in anti-dsDNA and IL-10 in response to estrogen, and in vivo there are clear differences in hormonal and cytokine levels in SLE *vs* control pregnancies (Doria et al 2004). Although there is much indirect evidence for estrogen involvement in the lupus disease process, the direct role of estrogen/estrogen-receptor mediated pathways in regulating cytokine production in SLE patients has not as yet been clearly defined. The first evidence for a molecular marker of estrogen action in SLE was the estrogen dependent changes in lupus T-cells calcineurin that could alter cytokine regulation (Rider et al 1998). Calcineurin is the target of a class of drugs called calcineurin inhibitors, which includes cyclosporine, pimecrolimus and tacrolimus. Calcineurin induces different transcription factors as NFATs that are important in the transcription of cytokine genes. A recent study demonstrate that blocking estrogens receptor in vivo in SLE pre- menopausal women they reduced the expression of calcineurin in peripheral T cells (Abdou et al 2008). Another possible mechanism of the role of estrogen in gender susceptibility in lupus is the altered expression of its receptors. Peripheral cells of SLE patients showed increased expression of ERα mRNA and decreased expression of ERβ (Iinui et al 2007). ERs are overexpressed in CD4+ and CD8+ cells while is decreased in B cells. The decline in ERβ expression inversely correlated with SLEDAI score. In conclusion, estrogen and its ability to influence on the profiles of cytokines release and immune system regulation is a very powerful factor in the gender susceptibility described in lupus.

3. Cytokines involved in SLE

3.1 Th1/Th2 balance in SLE

The Th1/Th2 balance hypothesis emerge from observations in mice of two subtypes of CD4 T-helper cells differing in cytokine secretion patterns and other functions (Mosmann et al 1986). The concept subsequently was applied to human immunity (Mosmann et al 1989). Th1 cells release significantly INFγ and IL2, and through these mediators Th1- polarized responses are highly protective against infections especially the intracellular pathogens, because of the ability of Th1-type cytokines to activate phagocytes and enhance the cellular response. In contrast Th2 cells release mainly IL4, IL5 IL9 and IL13 and induce the *in situ* survival of eosinophils (through IL-5), promote the production by B lymphocytes of high amounts of antibodies, including IgE (through IL-4 and IL-13), as well as the growth and degranulation of mast cells and basophiles (through IL-4 and IL- 9). (figure 1)

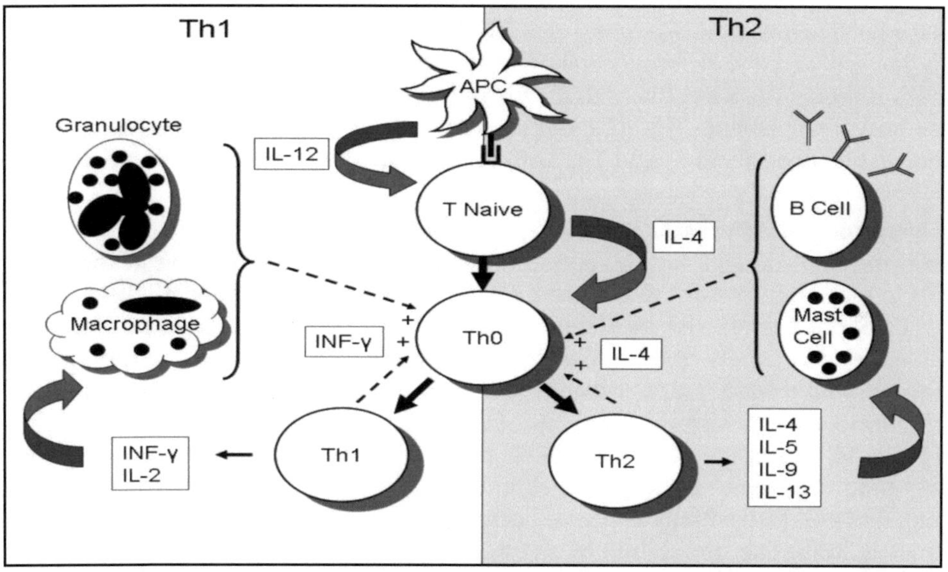

Fig. 1. Diagrammatic representation of the differentiation into Th1 or Th2 cells from naive cells.

Antigen-presenting cells interact with undifferentiated cells secreting specific cytokines that induce differentiation toward Th1 or Th2 cells. INFγ released by Th1 cells and IL4 produced by Th2 cells act as their own growth factors and cross-regulate the other differentiation.
Two features define the Th1/Th2 balance, first each cell subset produced cytokines that served as their own growth factor (autocrine effect) and second the two subsets released cytokines to cross regulate each other's development. Polarization to a subtype or another depends largely on the APC and experience on the antigen. This process is directed by the microenvironment of cytokines resulting in the antigen presentation of APC to T naive cells. A Th1/Th2 imbalance with excess of Th1 predominance appears in organ specific

inflammatory diseases as arthritis, multiple sclerosis and type 1 diabetes, and instead a predominance of Th2 response has been described in allergy and systemic autoimmune diseases (Abbas et al 1996).

The roles of Th1 and Th2 cytokines in the pathogenesis of SLE are controversial. In patients with SLE, Th2 cytokines are increased (Ogawa et al 1992), whereas Th1 cytokines are decreased (Klinman & Steinberg 1995). Thus, SLE was initially considered to be a Th2 predominant disease. However different results contradict this hypothesis like that IFNγ levels in the sera of patients with SLE are significantly elevated and that there is a correlation between the severity of SLE and the amount of IFNγ secreted (Al-Janadi et al 1993). All these findings suggest that the Th1 and Th2 responses are both important in the pathogenesis of lupus associated tissue injury. SLE is a disease involving a wide spectrum of cytokines. SLE patients with arthritis have higher IFNγ levels than the other patients, and conversely, patients with serositis or CNS involvement have higher IL-4 levels (Chang et al 2002). Furthermore SLE patients with nephritis have higher Th1 cytokines in serum and urine than non-nephritis patients (Chang et al 2006). Still more a significant difference in the Th1/Th2 balance in peripheral blood exists between WHO class IV and V lupus nephritis. Th1 cells are predominant in class IV but not in class V (Akahoshi et al 1999). In class V, the number of infiltrating cells was reduced, with a large percentage of CD4 T cells producing IL4 in the peripheral blood (Masutani et al 2001).

SLE is known to be a heterogeneous disease in which a wide range of cytokines are involved, it seems the most likely that Th1 or Th2 dominance depends on the stage of the disease and involvement. The Th2 response would be related to the development and production of autoantibodies, and Th1 with immune-mediated inflammatory activity.

3.2 B-lymphocytic Stimulator (BLyS)

BlyS a member of theTNF family, is also known as the B cell–activating factor(BAFF) and appears to play an important role in the differentiation and survival of B cells (Mackay et al 2002). BlyS can be released in a soluble form or can be expressed as a transmembrane protein on a wide variety of cell types, including monocytes, activated neutrophils, T cells, and DCs and its release is upregulated by IFN-γ, IL-10, G-CSF and CD40L (Nardelli et al 2001, Moore et al 1999, Litinskiy et al 2002, Harigay et al 2008).

BLyS binds to 3 receptors, BAFF-R (BAFF receptor), TACI (transmembrane activator and calcium modulator and cyclophylin ligand anteractor), and BCMA (B-cell maturation antigen), that are differentially expressed during B cell ontogeny (Bossen & Schneider 2006, Bossen et al 2008). The stimulation of all three receptors promotes B-cell differentiation and proliferation. BLyS is the sole ligand for BAFF-R, whereas TACI and BCMA each can bind either BLyS or another TNF family ligand known as a proliferation-inducing ligand (APRIL) (Bossen et al 2008).

After maturation in the bone marrow, newly formed B cells migrate to the secondary lymphoid organs (spleen and lymph nodes). These B cells do not possess all the characteristics of fully mature B cells, and they are referred to as transitional B cells. This transitional stage is an elastic checkpoint where thresholds for negative selection are homeostatically adjusted by free BLyS concentration. At this point an upregulation of BLyS expression can result in the rescue of self-reactive B cells from elimination. This effect explains, at least in part, the greatly increased levels of autoantibody production and associated autoimmune manifestations observed in transgenic mice that overexpress BlyS (Cancro et al 2009, MacKay et al 2007, Zheng et al 2005, Miller et al 2006, Thien et al 2004)

Elevated BLyS serum levels are often observed in SLE patients and correlate with disease activity (Petri et al 2008). Experiments in mice, have been demonstrated causality between BLyS over expression and development of SLE , on the other hand, also had been documented the amelioration of clinical disease in SLE mice following treatment with BlyS antagonist (Mackay et al 1999, Petri et al 2008, Jacob et al 2006)
The primary source of BlyS secretion in SLE remains speculative, a secretion by DCs (dendritic cells), a profoundly dysregulated IFNs in SLE or an increased levels of BLyS resulting from the presentation of self antigens (derived of an defective clearance of apoptotic bodies) to innate immune cells (which express BLyS upon antigenic stimulation) are potentially mechanisms implicated (Cancro et al 2009).
Because BLyS may figure prominently in the development of SLE and it could be a valid target for SLE, therapy with BLyS antagonists have been developed. Belimumab, a fully human monoclonal Ab (IgG1) that binds soluble BLyS and inhibits its binding to TACI, BCMA, and BR3, and Atacicept (TACI-Ig) a soluble, recombinant fusion protein of the human IgG1 Fc and the extracellular domain of the TACI receptor that binds BLyS and APRIL, have been tested in clinical trials. Results from phase III trials have demonstrated the safety profile and efficacy of belimumab in controlling SLE in a broad range of patients (Navarra et al 2011).

3.3 Interferon-α

Interferon alpha (INF-α) is produced mainly by plasmocytoid dendritic cells (PDC) in response to viral infection. INF-α is not one protein, but rather a family of highly related proteins encoded on the short arm of chromosome 9, and called type I INFs. Studies in which cellular mRNAs are screened against thousands of gene sequences have demonstrated that in SLE patients the INF-α induced genes are the most overexpresed of all those assayed (Baechler et al 2003). Evidence of the effect of INF-α in SLE comes from observations on the therapeutic administration of IFN-α in various types of malignancies and hepatitis C infection. Case reports emerged describing the development of lupus associated autoantibodies and even clinical lupus (Niewold & Swedler 2005). Discontinuation of IFN-*a* typically resulted in remission of SLE symptoms, supporting a causal relationship with IFN-*a*. Only a minority of patients treated with IFN-*a* develop SLE (<1% of patients) , these data support the idea that IFN-*a* can be sufficient to induce SLE in some genetically designed individuals. In addition, SLE patients commonly harbor anti INF-α autoantibodies. Anti INF-α antibodies-positive patients have lower levels of serum type I IFN bioactivity and evidence for reduced downstream IFN-pathway and disease activity.
A very strong correlation is consistently observed between the presence of SLE-associated autoantibodies that recognize nucleic acid structures or RNA-containing protein, such as anti-Ro, anti-La, anti-Sm, anti-RNP, and anti-dsDNA and high production of INF-α (Kirou et al 2005). Also lupus patients with high serum IFN*a* had a significantly higher prevalence of cutaneous and renal disease in most studies (Dall'era et al 2005). It is interesting that both of these clinical manifestations share an association with a particular serology (rash with anti-Ro and nephritis with anti-dsDNA).
The principal mechanism through which INF-α is produced in SLE is through Toll-like receptors (TLR). TLR receptors is a family of receptors present in a variety of cells and that recognize characteristics ligand present in pathogens. Some TLR recognize RNA and DNA sequences of single or double chain. A quality of many cases of lupus is the production of

autoantibodies against RNA or DNA containing protein complexes such as Sm, RNP, Ro, and La. Autoantibodies specific for these lupus-associated riboproteins can bind with antigens derived from apoptotic cells. The RNA/DNA found in these complexes are capable of promoting the production of IFN-*α* through the stimulation of TLR. Because some TLR is located in the endosomes, RNA or DNA containing complexes must access the interior of the cell before they are able to act as activators. The Fc portions of the immune complexes are recognized and internalized by cells with Fc receptors in their surface, providing a route of entry for RNA or DNA to reach TLR, resulting in interferon alpha production (Figure 2). This process is especially well established in PDCs on TLR7 and TLR9 (Båve et al 2003).

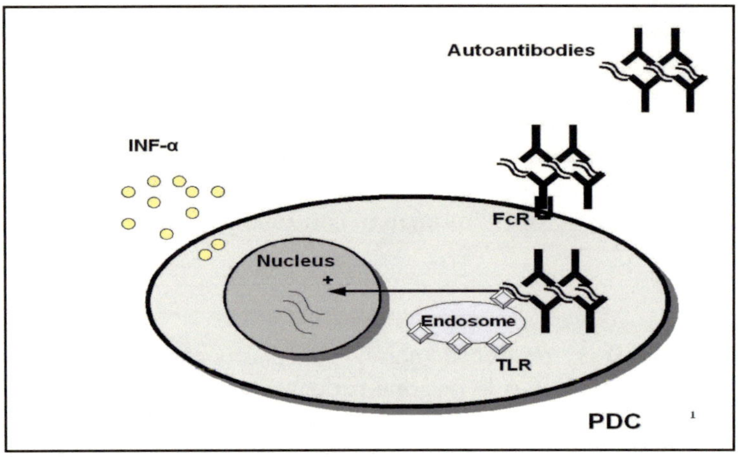

Fig. 2. Induction of INF-α in lupus. RNA/DNA containing immunecomplexes access the interior of the cell through recognition of Fc portion by Fc receptors in PDC membrane. Inside cell the RNA/DNA specific ligand are recognized by Toll-like receptors (TLR). TLR depending signals reach to the cell nucleus and induces transcription of IFN genes.

INF-α generate an effective antigen-presenting cells state by mediating maturation of dendritic cells. Thus INF-α prime the immune system for augmented sensitivity to subsequent stimuli. The activate antigen presenting cell state may also be characterized by an augmented capacity to generate a peripheral T-cell repertoire enriched in autoreactive cells. Dendritic cells are primary activators of T-cells and affect both tolerance and activation, depending of the state of dendritic cells. Dendritic cells from lupus patients are able to present self-antigens to T-cells in a stimulatory rather than regulatory manner, a process which is INF-α dependent (Blanco et al 2001). Moreover PDCs significantly enhance autoreactive B cell proliferation, autoantibody production, and survival in response to TLR activation (Ding et al 2009). Recently it has been reported that activation of the IFN signaling pathway may be linked to the risk of atherosclerosis by affecting plaque formation in patients with SLE (Li et al 2011).

In conclusion, in SLE patients, some autoantibodies are able to induce the production of INF-α. INF-α enhances the autoimmunity and immune response.

3.4 Tumor necrosis factor-α (TNF-α)

TNF-α is a pleiotropic cytokine produced by a variety of cell types including monocytes, lymphocytes and non immunological cell types in response to inflammation, infection and other environmental challenges. There are controversial results about the role of TNF in mice lupus strains. In NZB/W stain diminished production of TNF-α has been reported demonstrating the protective effect of TNF-α (Jacob & McDevitt 1988). In other strains of murine lupus an increased production of TNF-α has been described. In addition, TNF-α concentration correlates with the severity of the illness and anti-TNF therapy is profitable (Boswell et al 1988). Overall, these results show a duality in the role of TNF in lupus, one beneficial and one detrimental.

TNF-α contributes to avoiding the development of autoimmunity and autoantibody production. When introducing inhibitory TNF-α therapies in patients with diseases such as arthritis, spondyloarthropathies or Crohn disease shows the appearance of antinuclear antibodies and anti-ds DNA antibodies (De Ricke et al 2003, Garcia-Planella et al 2003). Normally these antibodies are not pathological, but in a few patients autoantibodies are associated with a SLE-like activity. TNF-α blocker induced lupus is usually benign and the symptoms resolve after TNF blockade stopped (Ramos-Casal et al 2007). It should be noted that these patients do not have the genetic background that makes them susceptible to SLE developing. When using anti-TNF therapy in SLE patients it has been found an elevation of antinuclear and anticardiolipin antibodies in most patients (Aringer et al 2007). This elevation was transient and did not produce complement consumption or lupus flare.

On the other hand numerous studies have shown that TNF blockade in SLE patients suffering from arthritis, nephritis and skin lesions were clinically effective in open clinic trials (Aringer et al 2004, Hayat el al 2007). It has found expression of TNF-α in inflamed tissue biopsies in patients with lupus, which does not occur in healthy individuals (Herrera-Esparza et al 1998), and TNF-α expression is associated with high histological disease activity (Zha et al 2009).

TNF-α performs two major functions: one as an immunoregulatory cytokine and the other as a potent mediator of inflammation. Among the immunoregulatory functions TNF-α induces the release of antiapoptotic molecules, TNF blockade may lead to increased apoptosis (Aringer et al 2007). The resulting increase in apoptotic material could explain why the emerging antibodies appear to exclusively target nuclear antigens and phospholipids, both of which are expressed on apoptotic bodies (Utz et al 1997). In addition, TNF blockade hampers the elimination of autoimmune B lymphocytes by cytotoxic T cells (Via et al 2001). All together could explain the pathways to increased lupus autoantibodies under TNF-α blockade.

The immunecomplexes generated by autoantibodies are deposited in tissues and organs. The deposit of immunecomplexes mediated inflammatory process triggered largely by TNF-α. The expression of TNF-α activates the local inflammation and tissue damage. TNF-*a* is the most important proinflammatory cytokine and a harbinger of tissue destruction, and it is at the top of a pro-inflammatory "cascade" leading to tissue damage. In contrast to the complex role of TNF-*a* in apoptosis and in immune regulation, its powerful proinflammatory effects are unequivocal. At the tissue level, TNF blockade induces remission of inflammation and hence tissue recovery. Anyway in the use of anti-TNF therapy is important to note the dual activity of this cytokine.

3.5 IL-6

IL6 is a pleiotropic cytokine, structurally, it shares homology with other cytokines: oncostatin M, IL11, leukaemia inhibitory factor, ciliary neurotrophic factor and cardiotrophin (Hirano, 1998). It was known initially as B-cell stimulatory factor 2 because it stimulates B cell growth and maturation to antibody-producing plasma cells. It is produced by a wide range of cell types including, monocytes, T cells, fibroblasts, synoviocytes and endothelial cells. IL-6 beyond his capacity of B cell activation and promotion of Ig production, play an important role in governing inflammation process (Ishihara et al., 2002).

IL-6 responses are transmitted through gp130, which serves as the universal signal-transducing receptor subunit for all IL-6-related cytokines. Although this classically occurs through IL-6 binding to its membrane-bound receptor (IL-6R), it is clear that a soluble form of the cognate IL-6 receptor (sIL-6R) affords IL-6 with an alternative mechanism of gp130 activation. This additional mode of cell activation is termed IL-6 trans-signaling and results from formation of a sIL-6R_IL-6 complex, which can directly bind cellular gp130. Because gp130 is ubiquitously expressed within tissue, trans-signaling provides IL-6 with the capacity to activate cells that would not intrinsically respond to IL-6 itself (Hibi et al., 1990; Hirano et al., 1994; McLoughlin et al., 2005). Therefore, IL-6 and gp130 signaling plays a critical role in the inflammatory process and tissue injury (Nechemia-Arbely et al., 2008).

An association between IL-6 and progression of lupus has been published for several murine models of SLE. The direct role of IL-6 in controlling autoantibody production has been demonstrated in the pristane induced model of lupus (Richards et al., 1998). On the other hand the administration of recombinant IL-6 to female NZB/W mice exacerbates the progression of glomerulonephritis (Ryffel et al., 1994). Anti IL-6 monoclonal antibody given in MRL lpr lupus prone mice, has been shown to cause a decrease in renal damage and a temporary reduction in levels of anti-dsDNA antibody production (Kiberd 1993).

Elevated levels of IL-6 have been found in the serum and in the urine of active SLE patients (Chun et al., 2007; Grondal et al., 2000; Horii et al., 1993). Raised expression of gp130, has been found in patients with active SLE, while an important reduction in the gp130 expression on B lymphocytes was observed when the activity of the disease had disappeared after readjusting its immunosuppressive treatment (De La Torre et al., 2009). Therefore, monitoring the frequency of gp130, could provide a useful tool in the diagnosis and monitoring of disease activity in patients with lupus.

Beyond the ability of IL-6 to stimulate B-lymphocyte differentiation into immunoglobulin secreting cells, IL-6 in concert with TGF-B is a critical cofactor for Th17 development, whereas the absence of IL-6 induces Foxp3, thereby specifying Treg development (Weaver et al., 2006). The two T-cell subsets play prominent roles in immune functions: Th17 cell is a key player in the pathogenesis of autoimmune diseases and protection against bacterial infections, while Treg functions to restrain excessive effector T-cell responses (Kimura et al., 2010).

Factors leading to the constitutive expression of IL-6 in SLE have not been elucidated yet, they may involve other regulator cytokines, like IL-10, or may be due, at least in part, to genetic differences (Linker et al., 1999; Tackey et al., 2004).

Recently, tocilizumab, a humanized monoclonal antibody against the α-chain of the IL-6 receptor, which prevents the binding of IL-6 to membrane bound and soluble IL-6 receptor, has been tested in SLE patients, with promising results (Illei et al., 2010).

3.6 IL-2

The cytokine IL-2 is a multifactorial cytokine. It was initially identified as a potent T cell growth factor, however, more recent data strongly indicate that IL-2 is essential for immune tolerance (Humrich et al., 2010). IL-2 constitutes a key element in the maintenance of the homeostasis between a proliferative immune response and the induction of tolerance, which supports the involvement of this cytokine in diverse autoimmunity disorders, such as SLE (Sharma et al., 2011). Predominantly produced by activated CD4+ and CD8+ T cells, IL-2 exerts its functions trough the interaction with its receptor (IL-2R) (Kammer, 2005).

It has been reported that production of IL-2 is decreased in patients with SLE (Sharma et al., 2011). Transcriptional regulators responsible for the transcription or suppression of IL-2 production are imbalanced in SLE T cells and this explains the reduced IL-2 levels found in SLE patients (Solomou et al., 2001). The decreased production of IL-2 in SLE patients most likely contributes to various immune defects such as decreased Treg production, decreased activation-induced cell death (AICD), and potentially decreased cytotoxic T lymphocytes (Lieberman & Tsokos 2010).

IL-2 signals are critical for the outcome of a CD8+ T cell response. Recently it was discovered that a strong IL-2 signal promotes the progressive acquisition of effector T cell functions (such as perforin and granzyme B expression, the hallmarks of CD8+ T cell cytotoxicity) but decreases the capacity to generate cells with memory features. By contrast, in conditions of weak IL-2 signaling, T cells fail to acquire the full program of effectors differentiation.(Pipkin et al., 2010)

IL-2 module activation-induced cell death (AICD). The activation of AICD is a mechanism of self tolerance in which apoptosis of autoreactive lymphocytes is induced after repeated stimulation. The deficiency in activation induced cell death might be related to the persistence of autoreactive T cell clones that eventually may lead to the activation of B cell subsets, with the subsequent production of autoantibodies and the development of autoimmune disorders (Gómez-Martín et al., 2009).

IL-2 is also required for the expansion and conversion of $CD4^{+}foxp3^{-}T$ cells into $CD4^{+}$ $foxp3^{+}$ cells or regulatory T cells (Treg) (Setoguchi et al., 2005; Zheng et al., 2007;). Tregs cells, are necessary for maintaining tolerance to self antigens and they are able to do is by suppressing self-reactive T cells (Buckner , 2010). It has been well recognized that a decline in Tregs as a critical event in the development of systemic autoimmunity both mice and SLE patients (Valencia et al., 2007; Suzuki et al., 1995). On the other hand, recently IL-2 signaling has been shown to play a role in inhibiting the development of Th17 cells (Tato et al., 2007; Ma et al., 2010). Thus, the effects of IL-2 on Treg and Th17 cells may serve to promote auto-reactivity while at the same time inhibiting a counter regulatory response (discussed later).

3.7 IL-17

Interleukin 17 (IL-17) is a proinflammatory cytokine that is involved in defending the host against extracellular, some intracellular pathogens and fungi (Bettelli et al., 2008; Khader et al., 2010). IL-17 promote inflammation on several levels, as their receptors are expressed on both hematopoietic cells and non hematopoietic cells. Il-17 exerts its effects through the recruitment of monocytes and neutrophils by increasing the local production of chemokines. IL-17 can also stimulate B-cell antibody production (Hsu et al., 2008; Mitsdoerffer et al., 2010).

Recent studies have reported that production of IL-17 is abnormally high in patients with SLE. Its levels are increased in SLE sera and correlate with SLE disease activity. Moreover, the frequency of IL-17-producing T cells is increased in the peripheral blood of patients with SLE (Crispín & Toscos, 2010; Shah et al., 2010). Recent evidence indicates that a significant fraction of the IL-17 produced in SLE derives from Th17 cells and $CD3^{+}CD4^{-}CD8^{-}$ (double negative or DN) T cells (Nalbandian et al., 2009).

The identification of Th17-lineage-specific transcription factors, established Th17 cells as an independent T-cell subset. Differentiation of naïve T cells into Th17 cells depends on TGF-β and IL-6, being IL-23 essential for expansion and maintenance of pathogenic Th17 cells (Jäger & Kuchroo, 2010). Interestingly, the participation of TGF-β in the differentiation of Th17 cells places the Th17 lineage in close relationship with $CD4^{+}CD25^{+}Foxp3^{+}$ regulatory T cells (Tregs), as TGF-β also induces differentiation of naive T cells into $Foxp3^{+}$ Tregs in the peripheral immune compartment (Korn et al., 2009).

In light of this knowledge, now is the general notion that there is a reciprocal relationship between pro-inflammatory IL-17-producing Th17 cells and protective $Foxp3^{+}$ Tregs. The presence of pro-inflammatory cytokines like IL-6, which is induced during infection, inflammation or injury, inhibited the induction of $Foxp3^{+}$ Tregs and simultaneously promoted Th17-cell differentiation (Bettelli et al., 2006). On the other hand, tolerance induction was associated with decreased IL-6 production and increased TGF-β production that paralleled a reduction in the fraction of IL-17-producing T cells and a reciprocal increase in regulatory T cells (Kang et al., 2007). Therefore, some authors support the notion that therapeutic intervention in SLE should focus on therapeutic agents that can regulate the immune balance between Th17 and Treg cells rather than on those that exclusively regulate Th17 cells or a specific cytokine (Yang et al., 2011).

3.8 IL-10

Interleukin (IL)-10 is one of the most important cytokine with anti-inflammatory properties. Today it its known that the ability to synthesize IL-10 is not limited to certain T cells subsets, but is characteristic of almost all leukocytes. Very important sources in vivo appear to be mainly monocytes and macrophages as well as Th cells (Sabat et al., 2010).

IL-10 is a potent inhibitor of antigen presentation. The other profound effect of IL-10 is to inhibit the production of proinflammatory cytokines and mediators from macrophages and DCs. The major inflammatory cytokines, IL-1, IL-6, IL-12, and tumor necrosis factor (TNF), are all dramatically repressed following exposure to IL-10. On the other hand, IL-10 can costimulate B-cell activation, prolong B-cell survival, and contribute to class switching in B cells (Mosser & Zhang, 2008).

Multiple studies have reported high levels of IL-10 in SLE patients and in murine models of lupus, and this increase correlated with disease activity (Capper et al., 2004; Hagiwara et al., 1996; Houssiau et al., 1995; Park et al., 1998). However, the specificity of these findings is unclear. A recent study that investigated the role of IL-10 in a novel congenic model of lupus, B6.Sle1.Sle2.Sle3 (B6.TC) showed, that although B6.TC mice produced higher IL-10 levels that nonautoimmune control mice, an overexpression of IL-10 decreased T-cell activation, auto-antibody production and autoimmune pathogenesis (Blenman et al., 2006). Interestingly, other study has recently been shown that the presence of immune complexes and IFNα a cytokine implicated in the pathogenesis of SLE, decreases the capacity of IL-10 to suppress inflammation, limiting therefore the anti-inflammatory effect of this cytokine (Yuan et al., 2011). These results reinforce the notion that IL-10 exerts multiple functions and we must be cautious in equating high levels of IL-10 and increased pathogenesis in systemic autoimmunity (Blenman et al., 2006).

4. Cytokines in organ damage

4.1 Cutaneous lupus and cytokines

Cutaneous lupus erythematosus represents an autoimmune disease characterized by photosensitivity, apoptosis of keratinocytes and an inflammatory infiltrate in superficial and/or deep compartments of the skin. Skin disease is the second most common manifestation in SLE patients. Although clearly there is a link between the skin and systemic manifestations of SLE, often the skin may flare independently or patients may have SLE without skin disease. Treatments also may improve the skin, systemic disease, or both, suggesting that there are differences pathogenetically between skin and systemic findings in cutaneous lupus.

UV-irradiation is a well-known trigger of apoptosis in keratinocytes and there is accumulating evidence that abnormalities in the generation and clearance of apoptotic material is an important source of antigens in autoimmune diseases (Caricchio et al 2003). Phototesting studies suggest that both UVB and UVA are potentially pathogenic wavelengths, although it is clear that UVA induction requires higher doses of light relative to UVB. UV light can induce the binding of autoantibodies to selected nuclear antigens located on blebs or apoptotic bodies of skin. It has been suggested that these bleb-associated antigens may then be phagocyted, packaged, and presented to lymphocytes, thereby stimulating autoimmune responses (Casciola-Rosen & Rosen 1997). The high presence of anti-Ro antibodies in cutaneous involvement in lupus might be explained because anti-Ro antibodies might interfere with protection from UV damage as genetic knock-out of 60kD Ro resulted in an SLE-like illness in multiple strains of mice that were susceptible to UV damage (Xue et al 2003).

Exposure of keratinocytes to UVB results in the synthesis of many pro-inflammatory cytokines, including tumor necrosis factor-a (TNF-α) interleukin-1α (IL-1α), IL-6, IL-8, and IL-10 (Brink et al 2000). TNF-α is not only involved in the mediation of local inflammatory reactions within the epidermis, but may also enter the circulation and cause systemic effects. There is an association of subacute cutaneous LE with the extended HLA haplotype DRB1*03-B*08. Contained within this haplotype is the TNF2 allele, a TNFα promoter polymorphism, associated with increased TNFα production (Werth et al 2000).

UV induced injury trigger the initial chemokine production and release results in a first wave of skin-homing memory T cells and plasmacytoid dendritic cells (PDCs) via chemokine driven pathways. DNA, RNA, and immune complexes, present in skin containing apoptotic material, can serve as IFN-alpha inducers in PDCs . There is a higher frequency of PDCs in skin compared to the blood of patients with SLE, suggesting that PDCs migrate from the circulation into the skin. Under normal conditions PDCs are not able to respond to self nucleic acids, but in lupus PDCs became activated to produce INF-α by self nucleic acids in complex with autoantibodies to DNA or nucleoproteins. These immuno-complexes trigger innate activation of PDC through TLR7 and 9 and lead to sustained production of INF-α (show Figure 2) that may induce an unabated maturation of dendritic cells and the activation of autoreactive T cells. Enhanced type I IFN signaling promotes Th1-biased inflammation in cutaneous lupus. IFN-α can amplify cutaneous inflammation via the induction of chemokines that recruit potentially auto-reactive T cells into the skin. For example, IFN-α induces the production of chemokines, CXCL9, CXCL10, and CXCL11, which recruit chemokine receptor CXCR3 expressing lymphocytes, including Th1 cells and CD8+ T cells, from peripheral blood into inflamed skin (Wenzel et al 2005). Large numbers of CXCR3+ lymphocytes are detected in cutaneous lupus skin lesions. The majority of these infiltrating cells are memory T CD4+ lymphocytes. Among memory T cell subsets, CXCR3 is predominantly expressed on the surface of IFN-γ-producing Th1 cells, generating a proinflammatory effector response (Meller et al 2005). Hence, UV-irradiation may induce chemokine production and release, subsequently recruiting a first wave of skin-homing memory T cells and PDCs to sites of UV-injury which produce cytokine-mediated inflammation and tissue damage.

4.2 Neuropsychiatric SLE

Neuropsychiatric systemic lupus erythematosus (NPSLE) involves neurological manifestations seen in the central, peripheral, and autonomic nervous systems as well as psychiatric disorders in patients with SLE in which other causes have been excluded. NPSLE may occur at any time during the course of the disease, and symptoms are extremely diverse, ranging from depression, psychosis, and seizures to stroke (Committee on Neuropsychiatric Lupus Nomenclature 1999). Though the pathophysiology of NPSLE has not yet been elucidated, two mechanisms of damage, specifically those produced by autoantibodies, and inflammatory mediators, are implicated in NPSLE. The most common neuropathologic features are multifocal microinfarcts many of them due to the effect of anti-cardiolipin antibodies (Hanlyet al 1992).

Cytokines and chemokines have been implicated in the pathophysiology of NPSLE. Of the different cytokines studied, interleukin-6 (IL-6) has been shown to have the strongest positive association with NPSLE (Fragoso-Loyo et al 2007). IL-6 is a cytokine with high proinflammatory activity. IL-6 level in the CSF of NPSLE was reported to be elevated without damage of the blood-brain barrier, demonstrating an intrathecal synthesis of IL-6. In addition, the expression of IL-6 mRNA was elevated in the hippocampus and cerebral cortex, suggesting that IL-6 expression was increased within the entire CNS of NPSLE (Hirohata & Hayakawa 1999). Furthermore, when IL-6 activity was followed throughout symptom remission, they noted a decrease in CSF IL-6 activity measured indirectly, but not in serum IL-6 activity (Hirohata & Miyamoto 1990). A recent study has shown that the sensitivity and specificity of CSF IL-6 for diagnosis of lupus psychosis was 87.5% and 92.3%, respectively, indicating that CSF IL-6 might be an effective marker for the diagnosis of lupus psychosis (Hirohata et al 2009). Although some cytokines are important biomarkers of NPSLE, the mechanism for the elevated levels of cytokines is thus far unknown. Immune complexes in SLE can stimulate IFN-*α* and there is strong evidence in humans and in mice that IFN-*α* can cause neuropsychiatric manifestations. It has recently described using a bioassay containing plasmacytoid dendritic cells, that NPSLE CSF induced significantly higher IFN-*α* compared with CSF from patients with multiple sclerosis or other autoimmune disease controls. NPSLE CSF was 800-fold more potent at inducing IFN-*α* compared with paired serum, due to inhibitors present in serum (Santer et al 2009). Further immunological studies are expected to show how autoantibodies in SLE patients work to promote the cytokine storm associated with the pathophysiology of NPSLE.

4.3 Cytokines role in lupus nephropathy

Renal involvement in SLE is present in over 50% of patient with active SLE and remains a major cause of end-stage renal disease and it is associated with a greater than four-fold increase in mortality in recent series (Bernatsky et al., 2006; Boumpas et al., 1995). The pathologic manifestations of lupus nephritis (LN) are extremely diverse and may affect any or all renal compartments. The complexity of renal manifestations can be most easily approached using the World Health Organization Classification revised and updated in 2004 (Weening et al., 2004).

The picture of cytokines present in LN is already complex and no single-cell population or cytokine has been decisively identified as a key mediator. Elevated circulating levels and/or tissue mRNA transcripts for several cytokines are reported in lupus patients and mice. On the other hand, the data regarding the relative importance of Th1-type versus Th2-type cytokines are inconsistent (Foster, 2005; Theofilopoulos et al., 2001).

The development of laser-manipulated micro dissection (LMD) from clinical biopsy specimens, together with messenger RNA (mRNA) expression analysis in the targeted glomeruli or specific regions of interest, using real-time quantitative PCR, has allowed to explore the single-cell cytokine profile of the samples from the LN patients. Interestingly a recent study, using LMD and PCR analysis of renal biopsy samples from LN patients has showed a negative correlation between the level of IL-2 and renal damage while a positive correlation between IL-17 and renal damage was evidenced. Indicating that IL-2 and IL-17 play opposite roles in SLE development, suggesting that IL-2 may play a role in protecting against SLE development, while IL-17 might have a reverse effect (Wang et al., 2010). On the other hand, recent studies have highlighted the potential importance of the Th17 immune response in renal inflammatory disease. These include the identification and characterization of IL-17-producing T cells in nephritic kidneys of mice and humans, as well as evidence for the contribution of IL-17 and the IL-23/Th17 axis to renal tissue injury in LN (Turner et al., 2010; Zhang et al., 2009).

5. Conclusions

This chapter has focused in the new insights about the role of cytokine in the pathogenesis of Systemic Lupus Erythematosus. The imbalance in the levels of cytokines and their receptors found in SLE is clearly crucial to the development of the pathology of the disease. The cytokines are actively involved in both favoring the production of auto-antibodies as generating inflammation in affected tissues. Interactions between the cytokine milieus are complex and the attenuation of one cytokine would need to be approached with caution, considering effects on the cytokine network as a whole. There are still many facets of immunopathology of SLE elicited by cytokines to be elucidated. A more in-depth understanding of these cytokines may be of clinical significance in the context of devising biomarkers or therapeutic agents. Cytokine therapy, is highly probable that, in the future will take a relevant place in the therapeutic armamentarium of autoimmune disorders.

6. Acknowledgements

We thank Dr. Luis Caminal, Autoimmune Diseases Unit, Hospital Universitario Central de Asturias, sincerely for suggestions.

7. References

Abbas AK, Murphy KM, & Sher A. (1996). Functional diversity of helper T lymphocytes. *Nature* Vol 383 No 6603 (Oct 1996) pp 787-793. ISSN 0028-0836.

Abdou NI. Rider V. Greenwell C. Li X., & Kimler BF.(2008) Fulvestrant (Faslodex), an estrogen selective receptor downregulator, in therapy of women with systemic lupus erythematosus. Clinical, serologic, bone density, and T cell activation marker studies: a double-blind placebo-controlled trial. *The Journal of Rheumatology* Vol 35 No 5 (May 2008) pp 797-803.ISSN 0315-162X.

Akahoshi M, Nakashima H, Tanaka Y, Kohsaka T, Nagano S, Ohgami E, Arinobu Y, Yamaoka K, Niiro H, Shinozaki M, Hirakata H, Horiuchi T, Otsuka T, & Niho Y. (1999) Th1/Th2 balance of peripheral T helper cells in systemic lupus erythematosus. *Arthritis and Rheumatism* Vol 42 No 8 (Aug 1999) pp 1644–8. ISSN 0004-3591.

Al-Janadi M, Al-Balla S, Al-Dalaan A, & Raziudin S. (1993). Cytokine profile in systemic lupus erythematosus, rheumatoid arthritis and other rheumatic disease. *Journal of Clinical Immunology* Vol 13 No1 (Jan 1993) pp 58–67. ISSN 0271-9142.

Aringer M, Graninger WB, Steiner G, & Smolen JS. (2004). Safety and efficacy of tumor necrosis factor alpha blockade in systemic lupus erythematosus: an open-label study. *Arthritis and Rheumatism* Vol 50 No 10 (Oct 2004) pp 3161-3169. ISSN 0004-3591.

Aringer M, Steiner G, Graninger WB, Höfler E, Steiner CW, & Smolen JS. (2007). Effects of short-term infliximab therapy on autoantibodies in systemic lupus erythematosus. *Arthritis and Rheumatism* Vol 56 No 1 (Jan 2007) pp 274-279. ISSN 0004-3591.

Baechler EC, Batliwalla FM, Karypis G, Gaffney PM, Ortmann WA, Espe KJ, Shark KB, Grande WJ, Hughes KM, Kapur V, Gregersen PK, & Behrens TW. (2003). Interferon inducible gene expresion signature in peripheral blood cells of patients with severe Lupus. *Proceedings of the National Academy of Sciences of the United States of America* Vol 100 No 5 (Mar 2003) pp 2610-2615. ISSN 0027-8424.

Bao M. Yang Y. Jun HS, &. Yoon JW. (2002) Molecular mechanisms for gender differences in susceptibility to T cellmediated autoimmune diabetes in nonobese diabetic mice. *Journal of Immunology* Vol 168 No10 (May 15 2002) pp 5369-5375 ISSN 0022-1767.

Båve U, Magnusson M, Eloranta ML, Perers A, Alm GV, & Rönnblom L. (2003) FcγRIIa is expressed on natural IFN-α- producing cells (plasmacytoid dendritic c ells) and is required for the IFN-α production induced by apoptotic cells combined with Lupus IgG. *Journal of Immunology* Vol 171 No 6 (Sept 2003) pp 3296–3302. ISSN 0022-1767.

Bernatsky,S.;Boivin, JF; Joseph, L.; Manzi, S.; Ginzle,r E.; Gladman, DD.; Urowitz, M.; Fortín, PR.; Petri, M.; Barr, S.; Gordon, C.; Bae, SC.; Isenberg, D.; Zoma, A.; Aranow, C.; Dooley, MA.; Nived .; Sturfelt, G.; Steinsson, K.; Alarcón, G.; Senécal, JL.; Zummer, M.; Hanly, J.; Ensworth. S.; Pope, J.; Edworthy, S.; Rahman, A.; Sibley, J.; El-Gabalawy, H.; McCarthy, T.; St Pierre, Y.; Clarke, A. & Ramsey-Goldman, R. (2006) . Mortality in systemic lupus erythematosus. *Arthritis and Rheumatism* Vol. 54, No. 8, (Aug 2006), pp. 2550–2557 ISSN 0004-3591.

Bettelli, E; Oukka, M.; Kuchroo, VK. & Korn, T. (2009). IL-17 and Th17 Cells. *Annual reviews of Immunology*. Vol. 27 (2009), pp. 485-517. ISSN 0732-0582.

Bettelli, E.; Korn, T.; Oukka, M. & Kuchroo, VK. (2008) Induction and effector functions of T(H)17 cells. *Nature* Vol. 453, (Jun 2008), pp. 1051-7. ISSN 0028-0836.

Bettelli, E.; Carrier, Y.; Gao, W.; Korn, T.; Strom, TB.; Oukka, M.; Weiner, HL. & Kuchroo, VK. (2006). Reciprocal developmental pathways for the generation of pathogenic effector TH17 and regulatory T cells. *Nature* Vol. 441, (May 2006), pp. 235-8. ISSN 0028-0836.

Blanco P, Palucka AK, Gill M, Pascual V, & Banchereau J.(2001). Induction of dendritic cell diferentiation by INF-α in systemic lupus erythemotosus. *Science* Vol 294 No 5546 (Nov 2001) pp 1540-1543. ISSN 0193-4511.

Blenman, KR.; Duan, B.: Xu, Z.; Wan, S.; Atkinson, MA.; Flotte, TR.; Croker, BP. & Morel,L. (2006). IL-10 regulation of lupus in the NZM2410 murine model. *Laboratory Investigations*. Vol 86, No 11, (Nov 2006), pp. 1136-48 ISSN 0023-6837

Bossen C.; Cachero TG.; Tardivel A.; Ingold K.; Willen L.; Dobles M.; Scott ML.; Maquelin A.; Belnoue E.; Siegrist CA.; Chevrier S.; Acha-Orbea H.; Leung H.; Mackay F.; Tschopp J & Schneider P. (2008). TACI, unlike BAFF-R, is solely activated by oligomeric BAFF and APRIL to support survival of activated B cells and plasmablasts, *Blood* Vol 111 No 3 (Feb 2008), pp. 1004–1012 ISSN 0006-4971.

Bossen C, & Schneider P.(2006). BAFF.; APRIL and their receptors: structure, function and signaling. *Seminars in Immunology*. Vol 18 No 5 (Oct 2006) pp:263–75, ISSN 1044-5323.

Boswell JM; Yui MA, Burt DW, & Kelley VE. (1988). Increased tumor necrosis factor and IL-1 beta gene expression in the kidneys of mice with lupus nephritis. *Journal of Immunology* Vol 14 No9 (Nov 1988) pp 3050-3054. ISSN 0022-1767.

Boumpas, DT.; Auston, HA.; Fessler, BJ.; Balow, JE.; Klippel, JH. & Lockshin, MD. (1995). Systemic lupus erythematosus: Emerging concepts. Part I. Renal neuropsychiatric, cardiovascular pulmonary and hematologic disease. *Annals of Internal Medicine* Vol. 122, No.12, (Jun 1995), pp. 940-950. ISSN 0003-4819.

Brink N, Szamel M, Young AR, Wittern KP, & Bergemann J. (2000). Comparative quantification of IL-1beta, IL-10, IL-10r, TNFalpha and IL-7 mRNA levels in UV-irradiated human skin in vivo. *Inflammation Research* Vol 49 No 6 (Jun 2000) pp 290-296. ISSN 1023-3830.

Buckner, JH. (2010). Mechanisms of impaired regulation by CD4(+)CD25(+)FOXP3(+) regulatory T cells in human autoimmune diseases. *Nature Reviews of Immunology*. Vol. 10, No.12,(Dec 2010), pp. 849-59. ISSN 1474-1733.

Buyon JP, Petri MA, Kim MY, Kalunian KC, Grossman J, Hahn BH, Merrill JT, Sammaritano L, Lockshin M, Alarcón GS, Manzi S, Belmont HM, Askanase AD, Sigler L, Dooley MA, Von Feldt J, McCune WJ, Friedman A, Wachs J, Cronin M, Hearth-Holmes M, Tan M, & Licciardi F. (2007)The effect of combined estrogen and progesterone hormone replacement therapy on disease activity in systemic lupus erythematosus: a randomized trial. *Annals of Internal Medicine* Vol 142 No 21 (Jun 2005) pp 953–62. ISSN 0003-4819.

Cancro MP.; D'Cruz DP & Khamashta MA. (2009). The role of B lymphocyte stimulator(BLyS) in systemic lupus erythematosus. *Journal of Clinical Investigations*. Vol 119. No 5 (May 2009), pp. 1066-73 ISSN 0021-9738.

Capper, ER.; Maskill, JK.; Gordon, C. & Blakemore, AI. (2004). Interleukin (IL)-10, IL-1ra and IL-12 profiles in active and quiescent systemic lupus erythematosus: could longitudinal studies reveal patient subgroups of differing pathology?.*Clinical and Experimental Immunology*. Vol 138, No 2 (Nov 2004), pp. 348-56, ISSN 0009-9104.

Caricchio R, McPhie L, & Cohen PL. (2003). Ultraviolet B radiation-induced cell death: critical role of ultraviolet dose in inflammation and lupus autoantigen redistribution. *Journal of Immunology* Vol 171 No 11 (Dec 2003) pp 5778–86.ISSN 0022-1767.

Casciola-Rosen L, & Rosen A. (1997). Ultraviolet light-induced keratinocyte apoptosis: A potential mechanism for the induction of skin lesions and autoantibody production in LE. *Lupus*. Vol 6 No 2 pp 175-80. ISSN 0961-2033.

Chan R.W.-Y., Lai F.M.-M., Li E.K.-M., Tam L.-S., Chow K.-M., Li P.K.-T., & Szeto C.. (2006). Imbalance of Th1/Th2 transcription factors in patients with lupus nephritis.

Rheumatology (Oxford, England) Vol 45 No 8 (Aug 2006) pp 951-957. ISSN 1462-0324.

Chang DM, Su WL, & Chu SJ. (2002)The expression and significance of intracellular T helper cytokines in systemic lupus erythematosus. *Immunological Investigations* Vol 31 No 1 (Febr 2002) pp 1-12. ISSN 0882-0139.

Chun, H.Y.; Chung, J.W.; Kim, H.A.; Yun, J.M.; Jeon, J.Y.; Ye, Y.M.; Kim, S.H., Park, H.S. & Suh, C.H.J. (2007). Cytokine IL-6 and IL-10 as biomarkers in systemic lupus erythematosus. *Clinical. Immunology*. Vol. 27, No. 5, (Sep 2007), pp. 461-466. ISSN 0271-9142.

Cohen-Solal JF, Jeganathan V, Grimaldi CM, Peeva E, & Diamond B (2006) Sex hormones and SLE: influencing the fate of auto reactive B cells. *Current topics in microbiology and immunology* Vol 305 No 1 pp 67–88. ISSN 0070-217X

Committee on Neuropsychiatric Lupus Nomenclature.(1999). The American College of Rheumatology nomenclature and case definitions for neuropsychiatric lupus syndromes. *Arthritis and Rheumatism.* Vol 42 No 4 (Apr 1999) pp 599–608.ISSN 0004-3591.

Crispín, JC. & Tsokos, GC. (2010). IL-17 in systemic lupus erythematosus. *Journal of Biomedicine and Biotechnology.* (Apr 2010): 943254. ISSN 1110-7243.

Dall'era MC, Cardarelli PM, Preston BT, Witte A, & Davis JC Jr. (2005). Type I interferon correlates with serological and clinical manifestations of SLE *Annals of the rheumatic diseases* Vol. 64, no. 12 (Dec 2005) pp. 1692–1697.ISSN 0003-4967.

De La Torre, M.; Urra, J.M. & Blanco, J. (2009). Raised expression of cytokine receptor gp130 subunit on peripheral lymphocytes of patients with active lupus. A useful tool for monitoring the disease activity?. *Lupus* Vol. 18, No 3, (Mar 2009), pp. 216- 222. ISSN 0961-2033.

De Rycke L, Kruithof E, Van Damme N, Hoffman IE, Van den Bossche N, Van den Bosch F, Veys EM, & De Keyser F. (2003) Antinuclear antibodies following infliximab treatment in patients with rheumatoid arthritis or spondylarthropathy. *Arthritis and Rheumatism* Vol 48: No 4 (Apr 2003) pp 1015-1023.ISSN 0004-3591.

Ding C, Cai Y, Marroquin J, Ildstad ST, & Yan J.(2009). Plasmacytoid Dendritic Cells Regulate Autoreactive B Cell Activation via Soluble Factors and in a Cell-to-Cell Contact Manner. *Journal of Immunology* Vol 183 No 11 (Dec 1 2009) pp 7140-7149. ISSN 0022-1767.

Doria A, Ghirardello A, Iaccarino L, Zampieri S, Punzi L, Tarricone E, Ruffatti A, Sulli A, Sarzi-Puttini PC, Gambari PF, & Cutolo M.(2004)Pregnancy, cytokines and disease activity in systemic lupus erythematosus. *Arthritis and Rheumatism* Vol 51 No 6 (Dec 15 2004) pp 989–95. ISSN 0004-3591.

Foster, MH. (1999). Relevance of systemic lupus erythematosus nephritis animal models to human disease. *Seminars in Nephrology.* Vol 19, No 1 (Jan 1999), pp.12-24. ISSN 0270-9295.

Fragoso-Loyo H, Richaud-Patin Y, Orozco-Narváez A, Dávila-Maldonado L, Atisha-Fregoso Y, Llorente L, & Sánchez-Guerrero J. (2007). Interleukin-6 and chemokines in the neuropsychiatric manifestations of systemic lupus erythematosus. *Arthritis and Rheumatism.* Vol 56 No 4 (Apr 2007) pp 1242–50. ISSN 0004-3591.

Garcia-Planella E, Domènech E, Esteve-Comas M, Bernal I, Cabré E, Boix J, & Gassull MA. (2003). Development of antinuclear antibodies and its clinical impact in patients with Crohn's disease treated with chimeric monoclonal anti-TNFalpha antibodies (infliximab). *European journal of gastroenterology & hepatology* Vol 15 No 4 (Apr 2003 pp 351-354. ISSN 0954-691X .

Gómez-Martín, D.; Díaz-Zamudio, M.; Crispín, JC. & Alcocer-Varela, J. (2009) Interleukin 2 and systemic lupus erythematosus: beyond the transcriptional regulatory net abnormalities. *Autoimmunity reviews*. Vol.9, No. 1 (Sep 2009), pp. 34-9. ISSN 1568-9972.

Green GL. Gilna P. Waterfield M. Baker A. Hort Y. & Shine J. (1986). Sequence and expression of human estrogen receptor complementary DNA. *Science* Vol 231 No 4742 (Mar 1986) pp 1150-1154. ISSN 0193-4511.

Grondal, G.; Gunnarsson, I.; Ronnelid, J.; Rogberg, S.; Klareskog, L. & Lundberg, I. (2000). Cytokine production,serum levels and disease activity in systemic lupus erythematosus *Clinical and Experimental Rheumatology* Vol. 18, No. 5, (Sep-Oct 2000, pp. 565-570. ISSN 0392-856X.

Hagiwara, E.; Gourley, MF.; Lee, S. & Klinman, DK. (1996). Disease severity in patients with systemic lupus erythematosus correlates with an increased ratio of interleukin-10:Interferon- gamma-secreting cells in the peripheral blood. *Arthritis and Rheumatism* Vol. 39, No 3 (Mar 1996), pp.379-385, ISSN 0004-3591 .

Hanly JG, Walsh NM, &bSangalang V. (1992). Brain pathology in systemic lupus erythematosus. *Journal of Rheumatolology* Vol 19 No (May 1992) pp 732–41.ISSN 0315-162X .

Harigai M.; Kawamoto M.; Hara M.; Kubota T.; Kamatani N & Miyasaka N.(2008) Excessive production of IFN-γ in patients with systemic lupus erythematosus and its contribution to induction of B lymphocyte stimulator/B cell-activating factor/TNF ligand superfamily-13B. *Journal of Immunology*. Vol 181:. No. 3 (Aug 2008), pp. 2211–2219, ISSN 0022-1767 .

Hayat SJ, Uppal SS, Narayanan Nampoory MR, Johny KV, Gupta R, & Al-Oun M. (2007). Safety and efficacy of infliximab in a patient with active WHO class IV lupus nephritis. *Clinical Rheumatology* Vol 26 No 6 (Jun 2007) pp 973-975. ISSN 0770-3198.

Herrera-Esparza R, Barbosa-Cisneros O, Villalobos-Hurtado R, & Avalos-Díaz E. (1998). Renal expression of IL-6 and TNFα genes in lupus nephritis *Lupus* Vol 7 No 3 (Mar 1998) pp 154–158. ISSN 0961-2033.

Hibi,M.;Murakami,M.; Saito, M.; Hirano, T.; Taga, T. & Kishimoto, T. (1990). Molecular cloning and expression of an IL-6 signal transducer, gp130. *Cell* Vol. 63. No. 6, (Dec 1990), pp. 1149-1157. ISSN 0092-8674.

Hirano, T. (1998). Interleukin 6 and its receptor: ten years later. *International reviews of Immunology* Vol. 16, (1998), pp. 249–284 ISSN 0883-0185.

Hirano, T.; Matsuda, T. & Nakajima, K. (1994). Signal transduction through gp-130 is shared among the receptor for the interleukin-6 related cytokine subfamily. *Stem Cells* Vol. 12, No. 3 (May 1994), pp. 262–277. ISSN 1066-5099.

Hirohata S, Kanai Y, Mitsuo A, Tokano Y, & Hashimoto H; NPSLE Research Subcommittee. (2009). Accuracy of cerebrospinal fluid IL-6 testing for diagnosis of lupus psychosis. A multicenter retrospective study. *Clinical Rheumatology* Vol 28 No 11 (Nov 2009) pp 1319-23. ISSN 0770-3198.

Hirohata S, & Hayakawa K. (1999). Enhanced interleukin-6 messenger RNA expression by neuronal cells in a patient with neuropsychiatric systemic lupus erythematosus. *Arthritis and Rheumatism* Vol 42 No 12 (Dec 1999) pp 2729–30. ISSN 0004-3591.

Hirohata S,& Miyamoto T. (1990). Elevated levels of interleukin-6 in cerebrospinal fluid from patients with systemic lupus erythematosus and central nervous system involvement. *Arthritis and Rheumatism.* Vol 33 No 5 (May 1990) pp 644–9. ISSN 0004-3591.

Horii, Y.; Iwano, M.; Hirata, E.; Shiiki, H.; Fujii, Y.; Dohi, K. & Ishikawa, H. (1993). Role of interleukin-6 in the progression of mesiangial proliferative glomerulonephritis. *Kidney International Suppl* Vol. 39, (Jan1993), pp. S71-5 ISSN 0098-6577.

Houssiau, FA.; Lefebvre, C.; Vanden Berghe, M.; Lambert, M.; Devogelaer,JP. & Renauld, JC. (1995). Serum interleukin 10 titers in systemic lupus erythematosus reflect disease activity. *Lupus*, Vol.4, No 5, (Oct 1995), pp. 393-5, ISSN 0961-2033

Hsu, HC.; Yang, P.; Wang, J.; Wu, Q.; Myers, R.; Chen, J.; Yi, J.; Guentert, T.; Tousson, A.; Stanus, AL.; Le, TV.; Lorenz, RG.; Xu, H.; Kolls, JK.; Carter, RH.; Chaplin, DD.; Williams, RW. & Mountz, JD. (2008). Interleukin 17-producing T helper cells and interleukin 17 orchestrate autoreactive germinal center development in autoimmune BXD2 mice. *Nature Immunology.* 2008 Vol. 9, No 2, pp. 166-75. ISSN 1529- 2908.

Humrich, JY.; Morbach, H.; Undeutsch, R.; Enghard, P.; Rosenberger, S.; Weigert. O.; Kloke, L.; Heimann, J.; Gaber, T.; Brandenburg, S.; Scheffold, A.; Huehn, J.; Radbruch, A.; Burmester, GR. & Riemekasten, G. (2010) Homeostatic imbalance of regulatory and effector T cells due to IL-2 deprivation amplifies murine lupus. *Proc Natl Acad Sci U S A.* Vol. 107, No. 1 (Jan 2010), pp. 204-9. ISSN 0027-8424.

Iinui A, Ogasawara H, Naito T, Sekigawa I, Takasaki Y, Hayashida Y, Takamori K, & Ogawa H. (2007) Estrogen receptor expression by peripheral blood mononuclear cells of patients with systemic lupus erythematosus. *Clinical Rheumatology* Vol 26 No 10 (Oct 2007) pp 1675-1678. ISSN 0770-3198.

Ishihara, K. & Hirano, T. (2002). IL-6 in autoimmune disease and chronic inflammatory proliferative disease. *Cytokine & Growth Factor Reviews.* 2002 Vol. 13, (Aug-Oct 2002), pp. 357-68. ISSN 1359-6101.

Jacob CO, & McDevitt HO. (1988). Tumour necrosis factor-alpha in murine autoimmune lupus' nephritis. *Nature* Vol 331:No 6154 (Jan 28, 1988) pp 356-358. ISSN 0028-0836.

Jacob CO.; Pricop L.; Putterman C.; Koss MN.; Liu Y.; Kollaros M.; Bixler SA.;Ambrose CM.; Scott ML & Stohl W. (2006). Paucity of clinical disease despite serological autoimmunity and kidney pathology in lupus-prone New Zealand Mixed 2328 mice defi cient in BAFF. *Journal of Immunology* Vol 177 No 4 (Aug 2006), pp. 2671-2680, ISNN 0022-1767.

Jäger, A. & Kuchroo, VK. (2010). Effector and regulatory T-cell subsets in autoimmunity and tissue inflammation. *Scandinavian Journal of Immunology.* Vol. 72, No 3, (Sep 2010), pp. 173-84. ISSN 0300-9475.

Kammer, GM. (2005) Altered regulation of IL-2 production in systemic lupus erythematosus: an evolving paradigm. *Journal of Clinical Investigations.* 2005 Vol 115, No. 4, pp. 836-40. ISSN 0021-9738.

Kang, HK.; Liu, M. & Datta SK. (2007). Low-dose peptide tolerance therapy of lupus generates plasmacytoid dendritic cells that cause expansion of autoantigen-specific regulatory T cells and contraction of inflammatory Th17 cells. *Journal of Immunology* Vol. 178, No. 2 (Jun2007), pp. 7849-58. ISSN 0022-1767.

Khader, SA. & Gopal, R. (2010). IL-17 in protective immunity to intracellular pathogens. *Virulence*. Vol. 1 No.5 (Sep-Oct 2010), pp. 423-7. ISSN 2150-5594.

Kiberd, BA. (1993). Interleukin-6 receptor blockage ameliorates murine lupus nephritis. *Journal of American Society of Nephrology* Vol. 4, No. 1, (Jul 1993), pp. 58–61 ISSN 1046-6673.

Kirou KA, Lee C, George S, Louca K, Peterson MG, & Crow MK. (2005). Activation of the interferon-α pathway identifies a subgroup of systemic lupus erythematosus patients with distinct serologic features and active disease. *Arthritis and Rheumatism* Vol 52 No 5 (May 2005) pp 1491–1503. ISSN 0004-3591.

Klinman DM, & Steinberg AD. (1995). Inquiry into murine and human lupus. *Immunological reviews* Vol 144 No (Apr 1995) pp 157–93. ISSN 0277-9366.

Kramer PR. Kramer SF., & Guan G. (2004)17 β-estradiol regulates cytokine release through modulation of CD16 expression in monocytes and monocyte-derived macrophages. *Arthritis and rheumatism* Vol 50 No 6 (Jun 2004) pp 328-337. ISSN 0004-3591.

Lahita RG. (1999) The role of sex hormones in systemic lupus erythematosus. *Current opinion in rheumatology*. Vol 11 No 5 (Sept 1999) pp 352–356. ISSN 1040-8711.

Lahita RG.(1999) Emerging concepts for sexual predilection in the disease systemic lupus erythematosus. *Annals of the New York Academy of Sciences* Vol 876: No (Jun 1999) pp 64–70. ISSN 0077-8923.

Laurence, A.; Tato, CM.; Davidson, TS.; Kanno, Y.; Chen, Z.; Yao, Z.; Blank, RB.; Meylan, F.; Siegel, R.; Hennighausen, L.; Shevach, EM. & O'shea, JJ. (2007) Interleukin-2 signaling via STAT5 constrains T helper 17 cell generation. *Immunity* Vol. 26, No. 3, (Mar 2007), pp. 371-381 ISSN 1074-7613.

Li J, Fu Q, Cui H, Qu B, Pan W, Shen N, & Bao C. (2011). Interferon-α priming promotes lipid uptake and macrophage-derived foam cell formation: A novel link between interferon-α and atherosclerosis in lupus. *Arthritis and Rheumatism*. Vol 63 No 2 (Feb 2011) pp 492-502. ISSN 0004-3591.

Lieberman, LA. & Tsokos, GC. (2010). The IL-2 defect in systemic lupus erythematosus disease has an expansive effect on host immunity. *Journal of Biomedicine and Biotechnology*. (Jun 2010) ISSN 1110-7243.

Litinskiy MB.; Nardelli B.; Hilbert DM.; He B.; Schaffer A.; Casali P. & Cerutti A. (2002). DCs induce CD40-independent immunoglobulin class switchingthrough BLyS and APRIL. *Nature Immunology*. Vol 3, No 9 (Sep 2002), pp. 822-829, ISSN 1529-2908.

Ma, J.; Yu, J.; Tao, X.; Cai, L.; Wang, J. & Zheng, SG. (2010). The imbalance between regulatory and IL-17-secreting CD4+ T cells in lupus patients. *Clinical Rheumatology*. Vol. 29, No. 11, (Nov 2010), pp. 1251-8. ISSN 0770-3198.

Mackay F.; Silveira PA & Brink R. (2007). B cells and the BAFF/APRIL axis: fast-forward on autoimmunity and signaling. *Current Opinion in Immunology*.Vol 19 No 3 (Jun 2007), pp. 327-36. ISSN 0952-7915.

Mackay F, & Browning.JL. (2002). BAFF: a fundamental survival factor for B cells. *Nature. Reviews. Immunology*. vol 2: No.7 (Jul 2002), pp.465–475, ISSN 1474-1733.

Mackay F.; Woodcock SA.; Lawton P.; Ambrose C.; Baetscher M.; Schneider P.; Tschopp J & Browning JL (1999). Mice transgenic for BAFF develop lymphocytic disorders along with autoimmune manifestations. *The Journal of Experimental Medicine* Vol 190 No 11 (Dec 1999), pp. 1697-1710, ISSN 0022-1007.

Maret A, Coudert JD, Garidou L, Foucras G, Gourdy P, Krust A, Dupont S, Chambon P, Druet P, Bayard F, & Guéry JC. (2003) Estradiol enhances primary antigen-specific CD4 T cell responses and Th1 development in vivo. Essential role of estrogen receptor-α expression in hematopoietic cells. *European journal of immunology* Vol 33 No 2 (Feb 2003) pp 512- 521. ISSN 0014-2980.

Masi AT, & Kaslow RA. (1978). Sex effects in systemic Lupus Erithematosus: A clue to pathogenesis. *Arthritis and Rheumathism* . Vol 21 No 4 (May 1978) pp 480-484. ISSN 0004-3591.

Masutani K, Akahoshi M, Tsuruya K, Tokumoto M, Ninomiya T, Kohsaka T, Fukuda K, Kanai H, Nakashima H, Otsuka T, & Hirakata H. (2001) Predominance of Th1 immune response in diffuse proliferative lupus nephritis. *Arthritis and rheumatism* Vol 44 No 9 (Sept 2001) pp 2097–106. ISSN 0004-3591.

McLoughlin, RM.; Jenkins, BJ.; Grail, D.; Williams, AS.; Fielding, CA.; Parker ,CR.; Ernst, M.; Topley, N. & Jones, SA. (2005). IL-6 trans-signaling via STAT3 directs T cell infiltration in acute inflammation *Proc Natl Acad Sci U S A*. Vol. 102, No 27, (Jul 2005), pp. 9589-94. ISSN 0027-8424.

Meller S, Winterberg F, Gilliet M, Müller A, Lauceviciute I, Rieker J, Neumann NJ, Kubitza R, Gombert M, Bünemann E, Wiesner U, Franken-Kunkel P, Kanzler H, Dieu-Nosjean MC, Amara A, Ruzicka T, Lehmann P, Zlotnik A, & Homey B. (2005). Ultraviolet radiation-induced injury, chemokines, and leukocyte recruitment: an amplification cycle triggering cutaneous lupus erythematosus. *Arthritis and Rheumatism* Vol 52 No 5 (May 2005) pp 1504-16. ISSN 0004-3591.

Miller JP.; Stadanlick JE & Cancro MP. (2006).Space, selection, and surveillance: setting boundaries with BLyS. *Journal of Immunology* Vol 176 No 11 (Jun 2006,) pp. 6405-10, ISNN 0022-1767.

Mitsdoerffer, M.; Lee, Y.; Jäger, A.; Kim, HJ.; Korn, T.; Kolls, JK.; Cantor, H.; Bettelli, E. & Kuchroo, VK. (2010). Proinflammatory T helper type 17 cells are effective B-cell helpers. *Proc Natl Acad Sci U S A*. Vol. 107, No. 32, (Aug 2010), pp.14292-7 ISSN 0027-8424.

Moore PA.; Belvedere O.; Orr A.; Pieri K.; LaFleur DW.; Feng P.; Soppet D.; Charters M.;Gentz R.; Parmelee D.; Li Y.; Galperina O.; Giri J.; Roschke V.; Nardelli B.; Carrell J.; Sosnovtseva S.; Greenfield W.; Ruben SM.; Olsen HS.;Fikes J, & Hilbert M. (1999.) BlyS: member of the tumor necrosis factor family and B lymphocyte stimulator, *Science*, Vol 285(5425). No 9 (Jul1999), pp. 260-263, ISSN 0193-4511.

Mosmann TR, & Coffman RL. (1989). TH1 and TH2 cells: different patterns of lymphokine secretion lead to different functional properties. *Annual reviews of immunology* Vol 7 pp 145-173. ISSN 0732-0582.

Mosmann TR, Cherwinski H, Bond MW, Giedlin MA, & Coffman RL. (1986). Two types of murine helper T cell clone. I. Definition according to profiles of lymphokine activities and secreted proteins. *Journal of Immunology* Vol 136 No 7 (Apr 1 1986) pp 2348-2357.ISSN 0022-1767.

Mosser, DM. & Zhang, X. (2008). Interleukin-10: new perspectives on an old cytokine. *Immunology reviews*. Vol. 226 (Dec 2008), pp. 205-18 ISSN:0105-2896.

Nalbandian, A.; Crispín, JC. & Tsokos, GC. (2009). Interleukin-17 and systemic lupus erythematosus: current concepts. *Clinical and Experimental Immunology*. Vol. 157, No 2, (Aug 2009), pp. 209-15. ISSN 0009-9104.

Nardelli B.; Belvedere O.; Roschke V.; Moore PA.; Olsen HS.; Migone TS.; Sosnovtseva S.; Carrell JA.; Feng P.; Giri JG & Hilbert DM.(2001). Synthesis and release of B-lymphocyte stimulator from myeloid cells. *Blood*. Vol 97. No 1(Jan 2001), pp. 98-204,ISSN 0006-4971.

Navarra SV.; Guzmán RM.; Gallacher AE.; Hall S.; Levy RA.; Jimenez RE.; Li EK.; Thomas M.; Kim HY.; León MG.; Tanasescu C.; Nasonov E.; Lan JL.; Pineda L.; Zhong ZJ.; Freimuth W & Petri MA; BLISS-52 Study Group. (2011). Efficacy and safety of belimumab in patients with active systemic lupus erythematosus: a randomised, placebo-controlled, phase 3 trial. *Lancet* Vol 26 No 377(Feb 2011), pp. 721-31, ISSN 0140-6736.

Nechemia-Arbely, Y.; Barkan, D.; Pizov, G.; Shriki, A.; Rose-John, S.; Galun, E. &, Axelrod, JH. (2008). IL-6/IL-6R axis plays a critical role in acute kidney injury. *Journal of American Society of Nephrology*. Vol.19, No. 6, (Jun 2008), pp.1106-15 ISSN 1046-6673.

Niewold TB, & Swedler WI.(2005) Systemic lupus erythematosus arising during interferon-alpha therapy for cryoglobulinemic vasculitis associated with hepatitis C. *Clinical Rheumatology*. Vol 24 No 2 (Ap 2005) pp 178–181. ISSN 0770-3198.

Ogawa N, Itoh M, & Goto Y. (1992). Abnormal production of B cell growth factor in patients with systemic lupus erythematosus. *Clinical and experimental immunology* Vol 89 No 1 (Jul 1992) pp 26–31. ISSN 0009-9104.

Park, YB.; Lee. SK; Kim, DS.; Lee, J.; Lee, CH. & Song, CH. (1998). Elevated interleukin-10 levels correlated with disease activity in systemic lupus erythematosus. *Clinical and experimental Rheumatology*, Vol. 16, No 3, (May-Jun 1998), pp. 283-8, ISSN 0392-856X.

Pedram A. Razandi M. & Levin R. (2006) Nature of functional estrogens receptors at the plasma membrane. *Molecular Endocrinology (Baltimore, Md.)*. Vol 20 No 9 (Sept 2006): pp 1996-2009. ISSN 0888-8809.

Petri M.; Stohl W.; Chatham W.; McCune WJ.; Chevrier M.; Ryel J.; Recta V.; Zhong J. & Freimuth W (2008). Association of plasma B lymphocyte stimulator levels and disease activity in systemic lupus erythematosus. *Arthritis and Rheumatism* Vol 58 No 8 (Aug 2008), pp 2453-2459, ISSN 0004-3591.

Pipkin, ME.; Sacks, JA.; Cruz-Guilloty, F.; Lichtenheld, MG.; Bevan, MJ. & Rao, A. (2010) Interleukin-2 and inflammation induce distinct transcriptional programs that promote the differentiation of effector cytolytic T cells. *Immunity*. Vol. 32, No 1 (Jan 2010), pp. 79-90. ISSN 1074-7613.

Ramanujam M.; Wang X.; Huang W.; Liu Z.; Schiffer L.; Tao H.; Frank D.; Rice J.; Diamond B.; Yu KO.; Porcelli S & Davidson. (2006). A.Similarities and differences between selective and nonselective BAFF blockade in murine SLE. *Journal of Clinical Investigations*, Vol 116 No 3 (Mar2006), pp. 724-734, ISSN 0021-9738.

Ramos-Casals M, Brito-Zerón P, Muñoz S, Soria N, Galiana D, Bertolaccini L, Cuadrado MJ,& Khamashta MA . (2007). Autoimmune diseases induced by TNF-tageted therapies: analysis of 233 cases. *Medicine (Baltimore)* Vol 86 No 4 (Jul 2007) pp 242-251. ISSN 0025-7974.

Richards, HB.; Satoh, M.; Shaw, M.; Libert, C.; Poli, V. & Reeves, WH. (1998). Interleukin 6 dependence of anti-DNA antibody production: evidence for two pathways of autoantibody formation in pristane-induced lupus. *The Journal of Experimental Medicine* Vol. 188, No. 5, (Sep 1998), pp. 985–990 ISSN 0022-1007.

Rider V, & Abdou NI. (2001). Gender differences in autoimmunity: molecular basis for estrogen effects in systemic lupus erythematosus. *International immunopharmacology.* Vol 1 No 6 (Jun 2001) pp 1009–1024. ISSN 1567-5769.

Rider V. Foster RT. Evans M. Suenaga R. & Abdou NI.(1998) Gender differences in autoimmune diseases: estrogen increases calcineurin expression in systemic lupus erythematosus. *Clinical immunology and immunopathology* Vol 82 No 2 (Nov 1998) pp 258-262.ISSN 0090-1229.

Ryffel, B.; Car, BD.; Gunn, H.; Roman, D.; Hiestand, P. & Mihatsch ,MJ. (1994). Interleukin-6 exacerbates glomerulonephritis in (NZB × NZW)F1 mice. *American Journal of Pathology* Vol. 144, No. 5, (May 1994), pp. 927-937 ISSN 0002-9440.

Sabat, R.; Grütz, G.; Warszawska, K.; Kirsch, S; Witte, E.; Wolf, K. & Geginat, J. (2010).Biology of interleukin-10. Cytokine& *Growth Factor reviews.* Vol. 21, No 5 (Oct 2010), pp.331-44, ISSN 1359-6101.

Santer DM, Yoshio T, Minota S, Möller T, & Elkon KB.(2009) Potent induction of IFN-alpha and chemokines by autoantibodies in the cerebrospinal fluid of patients with neuropsychiatric lupus. *Journal of Immunology.* Vol 182 No 2 (Jan 12, 2009) pp 1192–1201.ISSN 0022-1767.

Setoguchi, R.; Hori, S.; Takahashi, T. & Sakaguchi, S. (2005). Homeostatic maintenance of natural Foxp3+ CD25+CD4+ regulatory T cells by interleukin 2 and induction of autoimmune disease by IL-2 neutralization. *Journal of Experimental Medicine* Vol. 201, No. 5, (Mar 2005), pp.723–735 ISSN 0022-1007.

Shah, K.; Lee, WW.; Lee, SH.; Kim, SH.; Kang, SW.; Craft, J. & Kang, I. (2010). Dysregulated balance of Th17 and Th1 cells in systemic lupus erythematosus. *Arthritis Research and Therapy.* Vol. 12, No. 2, (2010); R53, ISSN 1478-6354.

Sharma, R.; Fu, SM. & Ju, ST. (2011) IL-2: a two-faced master regulator of autoimmunity. *Journal of Autoimmunity.* Vol. 36, N0 2, (Mar 2011), pp 91-7. ISSN 0896-8411.

Solomou, EE.; Juang, YT.; Gourley, MF.;Kammer, GM. & and Tsokos, GC. (2001).Molecular basis of deficient IL-2 production in T cells from patients with systemic lupus erythematosus. *Journal of Immunology,* Vol. 166, No. 6, (Mar 2001), pp. 4216–4222. ISSN0022-1767.

Stimson WH. & Hunter IC.(1980) Oesrtrogen induced immunoregulation mediated through the thymus. *Journal of clinical & laboratory immunology* Vol 4 No 1 (Jul 1980) pp 27-33. ISSN 0141-2760.

Straub RH. (2007) The complex role of estrogens in inflammation. *Endocrine Reviews* Vol 28 No 5 (Aug 2007) pp 521-574. ISSN 0163-769X.

Suzuki, H.; Kündig, TM.; Furlonge,r C.; Wakeham, A.; Timms, E.; Matsuyama, T.: Schmits, R.; Simard, JJ.; Ohashi, PS. & Griesser, H. (1995) Deregulated T cell activation and autoimmunity in mice lacking interleukin-2 receptor beta. *Science* Vol. 268, (Jun 1995), pp. 1472–1476. ISSN 0036-8075.

Theofilopoulos, AN.; Koundouris, S.; Kono, DH. & Lawson, BR.. (2001) The role of IFN-gamma in systemic lupus erythematosus: a challenge to the Th1/Th2 paradigm in autoimmunity. *Arthritis Research* Vol. 3, No 3, (Feb 2001), pp. 136-41 ISSN 1465-9905.

Thien M.; Phan TG.; Gardam S.; Amesbury M.; Basten A.; Mackay F, & Brink R. (2004). Excess BAFF rescues self-reactive B cells from peripheral deletion and allows them to enter forbidden follicular and marginal zone niches. *Immunity* Vol 20 No 6 (Jun 2004), pp. 785-798, ISSN 1074-7613.

Turner, JE.; Paust, HJ; Steinmetz, OM. & Panzer, U. (2010). The Th17 immune response in renal inflammation. *Kidney International*. Vol. 77, No 12, (Jun 2010), pp. 1070-5. ISSN 0085-2538.

Utz PJ, Hottelet M, Schur PH, & Anderson P. (1997). Proteins phosphorylated during stress-induced apoptosis are common targets for autoantibody production in patients with systemic lupus erythematosus. *Journal of Experimental Medicine* Vol 185 No 3 (Mar 1997) pp 843-854. ISSN 0022-1007.

Valencia, X.; Yarboro C.; Illei, G. & P. E. Lipsky, PE. (2007) Deficient CD4+CD25high T regulatory cell function in patients with active systemic lupus erythematosus., *Journal of Immunology* Vol. 178, No. 4, (2007), pp. 2579-2588 ISSN 0022-1767.

Via CS, Shustov A, Rus V, Lang T, Nguyen P, & Finkelman FD. (2001) In vivo neutralization of TNF-alpha promotes humoral autoimmunity by preventing the induction of CTL. *Journal of Immunology* Vol 167 No 12 (Dec 15 2001) pp 6821-6826. ISSN 0022-1767.

Wang, Y.; Ito, S.; Chino, Y.; Goto, D.; Matsumoto, I.; Murata, H.; Tsutsumi, A.; Hayashi, T.; Uchida, K.; Usui, J.; Yamagata, K. & Sumida, T. (2010) Laser microdissection-based analysis of cytokine balance in the kidneys of patients with lupus nephritis. *Clinical and Experimental Immunology*. Vol. 159, No 1, (Jan 2010), pp.1-10 ISSN 0009-9104.

Weening JJ.; D'Agati, VD.; Schwartz, MM.; Seshan, SV.; Alpers, CE.; Appel, GB., Balow,JE.; Bruijn ,JA.; Cook, T.; Ferrario, F.; Fogo, AB.; Ginzler, EM.; Hebert, L.; Hill, G.; Hill, P.; Jennette, JC.; Kong, NC.; Lesavre, P.; Lockshin, M.; Looi, LM.; Makino, H.; Moura, LA. & Nagata, M. (2004).The classification of glomerulonephritis in systemic lupus erythematosus revisited. *Journal of American Society of Nephrology*. Vol. 15, No 2, (Feb 2004), pp. 241-50. ISSN 1046-6673.

Wenzel J, Uerlich M, Wörrenkämper E, Freutel S, Bieber T, & Tüting T. (2005). Scarring skin lesions of discoid lupus erythematosus are characterized by high numbers of skin-homing cytotoxic lymphocytes associated with strong expression of the type I interferon-induced protein MxA. The *British journal of dermatology*. Vol 153 No 5 (Nov 2005) pp 1011-5. ISSN 0007-0963.

Werth VP, Zhang W, Dortzbach K, & Sullivan K. (2000). Association of a promoter polymorphism of TNFalpha with subacute cutaneous lupus erythematosus and distinct photoregulation f transcription. *The Journal of investigative dermatology* Vol 115 No 4 (Oct 2000) pp 726-30.ISSN 0022-202X.

Xue D, Shi H, Smith JD, Chen X, Noe DA, Cedervall T, Yang DD, Eynon E, Brash DE, Kashgarian M, Flavell RA, & Wolin SL. (2003). A lupus-like syndrome develops in mice lacking the Ro 60-kDa protein, a major lupus autoantigen. *Proceedings of the National Academy of Sciences of the United States of America.* Vol 100 No 13 (Jun 24, 2003) pp 7503-8. ISSN 0027-8424.

Yang, J.; Yang, X.; Zou, H.; Chu, Y. & Li, M. (2011). Recovery of the immune balance between Th17 and regulatory T cells as a treatment for systemic lupus erythematosus. *Rheumatology (Oxford)* (Apr 2011) ISSN 1462-0324.

Yuan, W.; DiMartino, SJ.; Redecha, PB.; Ivashkiv, LB. & Salmon, JE. (2011). Systemic lupus erythematosus monocytes are less responsive to interleukin-10 in the presence of immune complexes. *Arthritis and Rheumatism.* (Jan 2011), Vol.63, No 1, pp. 212-8. ISSN 0004-3591.

Zandman-Goddard G, Peeva E, & Shoenfeld Y (2007) Gender and autoimmunity. *Autoimmunity reviews* Vol 6 No 6 (Jun 2006) pp 366–372. ISSN 1568-9972.

Zhang, Z.; Kyttaris, VC. & Tsokos, GC. (2009). The role of IL-23/IL-17 axis in lupus nephritis. *Journal of Immunology.* Vol 183, No. 5, (Sep 2009), pp. 3160-9. ISSN 0022-1767.

Zheng Y.; Gallucci S.; Gaughan JP.; Gross JA & Monestier M.(2005) A role for B cell-activating factor of the TNF family in chemically induced autoimmunity. *Journal of Immunology* Vol 175 No 5 (Nov 2005), pp. 6163-8, ISNN 0022-1767.

Zheng, SG.; Wang, J.; Wang, P.; Gray, JD. & Horwitz, DA. (2007). IL-2 is essential for TGF-β to convert naïve CD4+CD25− cells to CD25+Foxp3+ regulatory T cells and for expansion of these cells. *Journal of Immunology* Vol. 178, No. 4 (Feb 2007), pp. 2018–2027 ISSN 0022-1767.

Zhu L, Yang X, Ji Y, Chen W, Guan W, Zhou SF, & Yu X. (2009). Up-regulated renal expression of TNF-α signalling adapter proteins in lupus glomerulonephritis. *Lupus*, Vol 18 No 2 (Feb 2009) pp 116–127. ISSN 0961-2033.

3

Interferon and Apoptosis in Systemic Lupus Erythematosus

Daniel N. Clark and Brian D. Poole
Brigham Young University
USA

1. Introduction

Systemic lupus erythematosus (SLE) is generally diagnosed long after the disease begins. This means that the cause of the disease is hard to find, buried in the past. In the search for the elusive causal agents for SLE, one candidate is the immune signaling molecule, interferon (IFN). Interferon is a secreted signaling protein, or cytokine, which is expressed at higher levels in SLE patients and has been associated with incidence and severity of the disease.

A combination of environmental triggers and genetic susceptibility combine to initiate SLE. Although there are many etiological components, they usually converge on a heightened state of activation for the immune system, with resultant increases in interferon production and interferon signaling. That is to say that interferon could be thought of as either a causative agent, a result of the disease, or both.

This chapter will discuss the basics of interferon function and how de-regulation of apoptosis can lead to interferon production due to immune complexes. We will then discuss how the functioning of the immune system changes in someone with SLE, the genes which are associated with risk for SLE, and clinical manifestations of interferon in SLE.

2. How interferon works in the context of SLE

Interferon is a signaling protein which is secreted to activate neighboring cells in response to viruses or other infections. It is a cytokine, or immune signaling molecule which allows communication between cells. When a cell is infected with a virus, interferon is produced and secreted as a warning to other cells to prepare for an infection. Interferons alpha (IFNα) and beta (IFNβ) are the type I interferons, and interferon gamma (IFNγ) is the type II interferon. Most of the cells in the human body have receptors for type I IFN, whereas certain immune cells express the receptor for type II IFN (Su, et al., 2004). The proteins are made by many different cells, but generally speaking, IFNα is of leukocyte origin, IFNβ is of fibroblast origin, and IFNγ is made by lymphocytes (Lucero, et al., 1982). Other less studied interferons also exist, and interferons are conserved among many species. This chapter will talk mostly about type I interferons, which are IFNα and IFNβ.

The main purpose of interferon is to shut down a cell before a virus can take it over, although it has many other jobs (Niewold, et al., 2010). Interferon signaling leads to increased apoptosis, which is a normal response to control viral spread or to decrease the size of a tumor (Takaoka, et al., 2003). If one cell can undergo apoptosis before a virus can replicate and infect other cells, the infection is halted (Luker, et al., 2005).

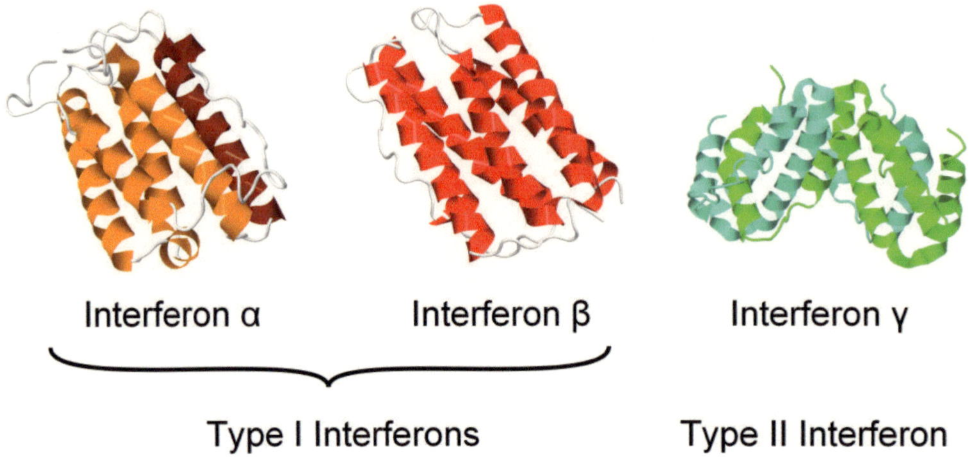

Fig. 1. Interferon protein structures. Interferons alpha and beta, the type I interferons, have a common structure composed mainly of five alpha helices (shown are IFNα2a and IFNβ1 based on PDB files 1itf and 1au1, respectively). Although the monomers of each are very similar in structure, the functional form of both is a dimer, and the two dimerize differently, IFNα2a along homologous surfaces and IFNβ1 on opposing sides of the protein (Karpusas, et al., 1997). IFNγ is show in its dimerized form, with the two colors representing two intertwined monomers (based on PDB file 1hig). Not shown to scale; figures drawn with Jmol (Jmol, 2011).

Interferon can be produced in response to infection, other cytokines, mitogens and several signaling pathways. Once produced it is secreted where it can be recognized by other cells, which is called paracrine signaling, or by the cell which produced it, called autocrine signaling. One type of cell, the plasmacytoid dendritic cell (pDC) is a natural IFN producer, and is able to make very large amounts of IFNα (Ronnblom & Alm, 2001).

When interferon ligates an interferon receptor, signaling pathways are activated. Interferon causes an increase in the expression of both major histocompatibility complexes (MHCI and MHCII) for presentation of viral peptides to T cells, which can then lead to activation of other cells in order to kill infected cells, and remove them (Fruh & Yang, 1999). Interferon also increases intracellular levels of protein kinase R (PKR) which recognizes viral nucleic acids and activates RNase L to degrade viral RNAs. PKR also slows protein synthesis by inactivating translational initiation factors, so that viral proteins synthesis is slowed (Pindel & Sadler, 2011). p53 is also activated, which is pro-apoptotic (Takaoka, 2003). Interferons activate immune cells, especially natural killer cells and macrophages (Murray, 1988). This activation cascade is normally "turned off" after an infection is cleared to prevent damage to uninfected cells. However this activation state is not reduced to the normal levels in individuals with SLE, where a higher level of interferon is present (T. Kim, et al., 1987; Ytterberg & Schnitzer, 1982). This higher amount of interferon is also measurable by an increase in the expression of interferon-stimulated genes seen in lupus patients, called the interferon response signature (Baechler, et al., 2003; Bennett, et al., 2003; Feng, et al., 2006).

This means that IFN is turned on and that it is actively affecting how other cells are functioning.

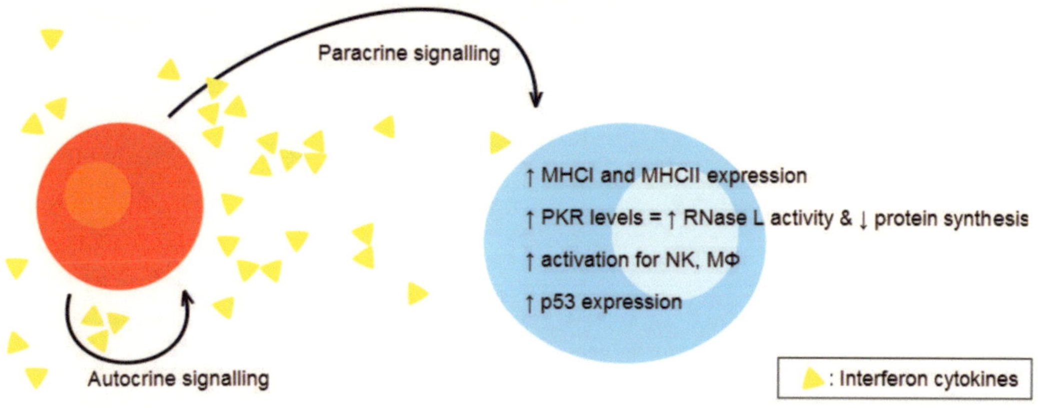

Fig. 2. Cell to cell IFN signaling and its effects. One cell produces interferon and either another cell (paracrine signaling) or the same cell (autocrine signaling) receives the signal. ↑: an increase, ↓: a decrease, MHC: major histocompatibility complex, PKR: protein kinase R, NK: natural killer cell, MΦ: macrophage

As a general feature of autoimmune diseases such as SLE, the immune system is in an "always on" state, which can lead to a breach in the body's natural tolerance to self. Once this self tolerance is lost, autoimmune disease can result. In addressing why the immune system generates an attack against one's own body, the over activation of the immune system, including the overproduction of interferon in SLE patients is a part of this picture.

3. Interferon leads to apoptosis, and the SLE-apoptosis connection

One effect of interferon production is the release of autoantigens due to increased cell death. This release is normally controlled by a process called efferocytosis, or apoptotic cell removal, where cell debris are processed by immune cells or neighboring cells which remove them by phagocytosis. Defects in apoptotic pathways have been noted in individuals with SLE (Gaipl, et al., 2006). Examples of why this occurs have been studied. For example, in SLE patients there is an overexpression of both soluble and membrane-bound Fas. Fas is a receptor which when ligated signals to a cell to undergo apoptosis. The levels of Fas also correlate with the amount of apoptotic lymphocytes and disease activity of SLE (Li, et al., 2009; Sahebari, et al., 2010). Mouse models of lupus commonly have genetic variations in apoptotic pathways such the Fas/Fas L pathway and interferon pathways.

Mouse as well as human SLE patients make antibodies to self antigens. This is likely because of over-exposure of potential autoantigens to the immune system. This could be due to an increased amount of apoptosis, or a decrease in the rate of clearance of apoptotic debris. Apoptosis, which can be induced by interferon, is also part of the natural cycle of cellular growth and death. Cells undergoing apoptosis are recognized as dead by other cells, so that they are cleared (Munoz, et al., 2010).

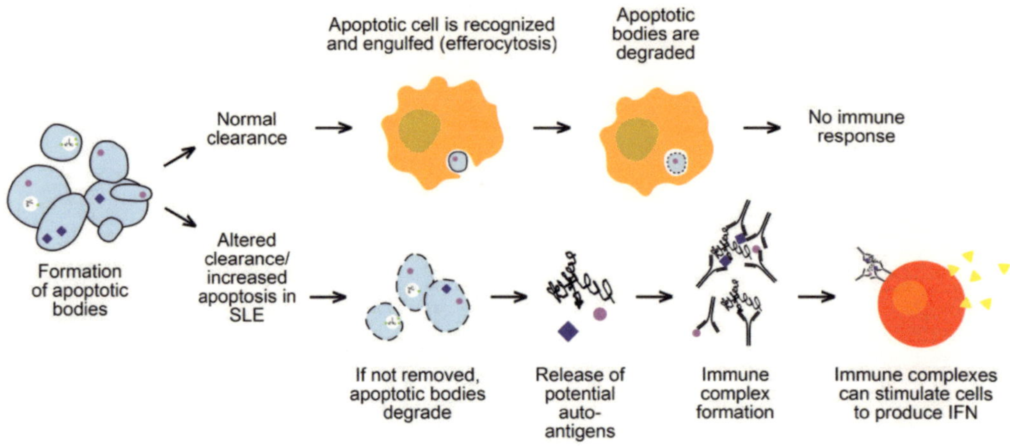

Fig. 3. Production of interferon can begin with defects in apoptosis. This can be due to either an increase in apoptosis or a decrease in clearance of apoptotic debris. If contents are released, they can form immune complexes with autoantibodies. These immune complexes can cause cells to produce interferon. Manipulating this pathway is also a common characteristic of mouse models of lupus.

3.1 Mouse models allow the study of IFN and apoptosis pathways

Mouse models have been very useful in understanding the etiology and pathogenesis of lupus. Two approaches to experimental mice have been used to generate information about the role of interferon in lupus. In the first approach, interferon-related genes are knocked out and the resulting effects on lupus are studied. For the second, established lupus mouse models are studied on a molecular level for differences in interferon pathways or interferon-related effects. These two approaches often overlap, as in cases where interferon-related genes are knocked out in lupus-prone mice. Several established lupus mouse models include the MRL/lpr mice, NZW/NZB, and others. These are mice that spontaneously develop lupus, and several of them have been investigated to understand the role of interferon in their pathogenesis. Although a complete description of the mouse models for lupus is beyond the scope of this or any one publication, a few illustrative examples represent the power of these model systems.

One mouse model that is especially relevant for the study of interferon in lupus is the BXSB/MpJ (BXSB) or Yaa mouse. These mice spontaneously develop lupus-like disease in a sex-linked fashion because of a duplication of the Toll-like receptor 7 (TLR7) gene on the Y chromosome (Izui, et al., 1994). TLR7 is responsible for inducing interferon in response to viral infection or autoantibody production.

Another interesting mouse for the study of interferon is the NZB/NZW mouse. These mice spontaneously develop a lupus-like autoimmune disease. They have been used to investigate the role of several interferon-related molecules and cells. For example, treating these mice with interferon accelerates disease in a T-cell like manner (Z. Liu, et al., 2010; Mathian, et al., 2005), while knocking out or inhibiting interferon-related genes slows or eliminates the development of lupus-like symptoms (Jorgensen, et al., 2007; Sharma, et al., 2005). These mice have been used to clarify the interactions between sex hormones and interferon in lupus etiology (Bynote, et al., 2008; Panchanathan, et al., 2009; Panchanathan, et al., 2010), and they serve as an excellent all-around model for spontaneous development of lupus.

The role of several interferon-related molecules has been examined using a combination of mouse models. As an example, consider the gene interferon regulatory factor five (IRF5). This gene is an interferon-regulating gene which will be described in section 5.2 below. It was discovered that knockout of IRF5 prevents or inhibits the development of lupus in MRL/lpr mice, $Fc\gamma^{-/-}$ Yaa mice, and pristine-injected mice (Richez, et al., 2010; Savitsky, et al., 2010; Tada, et al., 2011).

Mouse models for lupus represent a powerful and flexible mechanism for investigating the role of multiple aspects of lupus. However, it must be remembered that the mutations or disease manifestations in these mice are not necessarily related to those seen in human lupus, and therefore the results observed must be interpreted with caution.

4. A cycle of autoantibody production

When it comes to SLE we may think of interferon production as a cycle, which begins when an environmental trigger, such as a viral infection, UV light damage or medical treatment activates the immune system to produce interferon.

Normally B cells which produce antibodies to self-antigens undergo negative selection, where they receive signals to die off or become inactivated if they make antibody against a self-antigen. This self-tolerance is breached in SLE (Cancro, et al., 2009), and the self-antigens released from damaged or apoptotic cells during or after initial triggering events become the targets of autoantibodies. When autoantibodies are produced, they are made by B cells as well as plasma cells, which are a mature differentiated form of B cells.

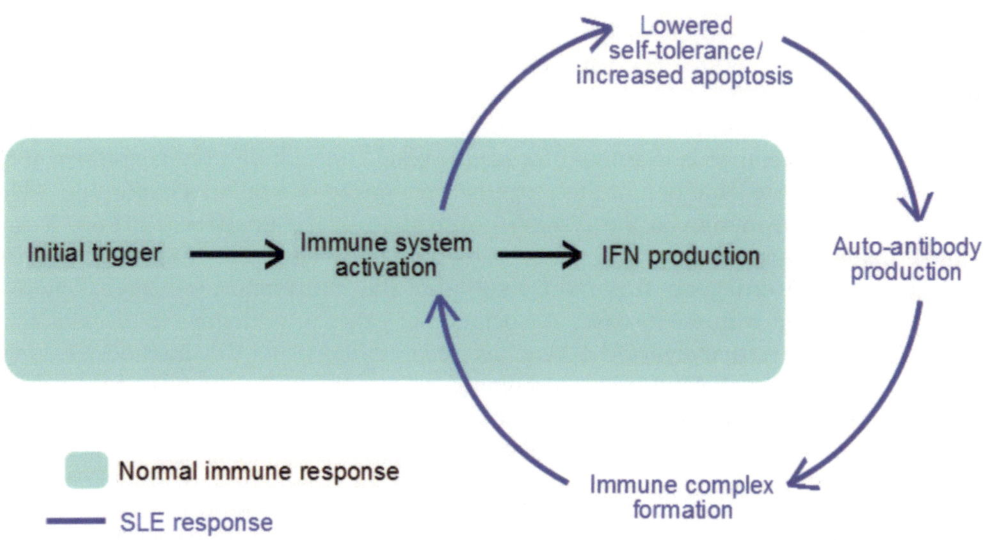

Fig. 4. The altered immune response in SLE generates a cycle. In blue is a cycle which exists in SLE, amplifying the amount of IFN present. This cycle needs a trigger, but once it begins, it can leave the immune system in an "always on" state.

Autoantibodies lead to the production of interferon by forming immune complexes which are immunostimulatory (Ronnblom, et al., 2011). Immune complexes are composed of aggregates of antibody and antigen molecules which are processed by the body. These immune complexes are a main source of SLE pathology, as they obstruct small passages in areas of the body such as the kidneys and joints (Crispin, et al., 2010).

Immune complexes may include the common SLE autoantigens such as RNA-containing protein complexes like Sm, RNPs, Ro, and La. Having a combination of both nucleic acids and protein complexed with antibody means many pathways can be turned on. For example, antibody can stimulate an immune cell through an Fc receptor, nucleic acids can stimulate cells through Toll-like receptors (TLRs), and proteins can be recognized by other antibodies.

Immune cells are activated by immune complexes and the cycle continues. Interferon production is instigated by immune cells which recognize part of the complex, be it the antibody, the antigen, or other associated molecules.

5. SLE genetic risk screens identify genes in interferon signaling pathways

We have looked at the disease state of SLE, and how the immune system functions improperly to instigate disease. Things begin when an environmental trigger works on the genetic background of varying degrees of susceptibility. Genetic susceptibility is thought to account for at least 20% of the risk for SLE (Deapen, et al., 1992). To find the actual genes involved, studies are performed to determine the linkage or association of a variation in the genome to a particular disease.

One important method is called a genome wide association study (GWAS). These GWA studies genotype thousands of individuals, grouped into SLE patients and non-patients comparing them at thousands of single nucleotide polymorphisms (SNPs). These studies reveal the genomic regions which contain disease-associated genes, because the variations are more common in people with the disease. Individual genes or gene pathways are pinpointed, and can ultimately lead to treatment strategies. Many genes have been identified that contain SNPs which confer risk to SLE.

These studies are especially useful for diseases with unknown or complex genetic components. The genome is examined for sets of single nucleotide polymorphisms (SNPs). When sets of SNPs are usually inherited together in a group it is called a haplotype. When a haplotype is more common in the disease group than in the unaffected group, it can be assumed that it is associated with the disease. Although specific genes are sometimes found which may predict a disease, it is more likely that the information will reveal molecular pathways associated with the disease. Association of genes or pathways to diseases such as heart disease, asthma, diabetes and others have been found using this method (Stranger, et al., 2011). The amount of effect is measured as an odds ratio (OR), which is a measure of the strength of association of the disease with a haplotype. A median OR value is around 1.3, with some genes having much higher association ORs. For example, one of the lupus-associated haplotypes TREX1, has a published OR of 25 (Lee-Kirsch, et al., 2007). In such cases, the genetic risk is almost certainly associated with the disease.

An important caveat to these tests is that they answer the question, "What?" but not the question, "How?" That is, they identify genetic loci which confer risk to SLE, but then further studies are needed to show what functional changes affect people with a risk haplotype. For most of the genes, we do not know what functional role they play. However it is promising to note that the genes are within certain pathways, some of which are already associated with lupus.

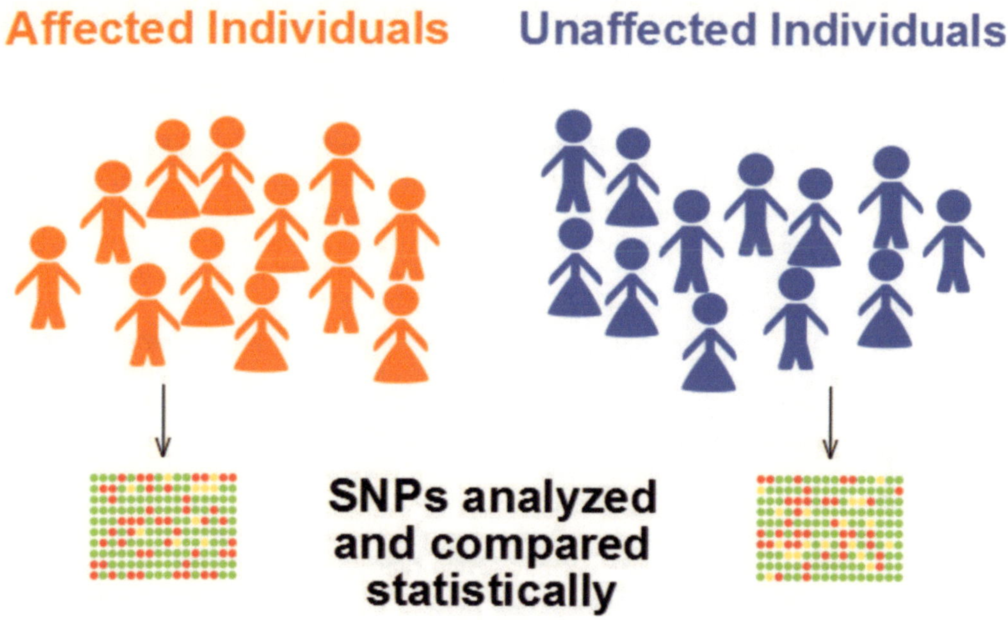

Fig. 5. Genome wide association studies (GWAS). Genome-wide association studies aim to discover the genetic risk component of a disease by finding differences in a group with the disease compared to a group of unaffected control individuals.

Several review articles have reviewed the findings of many lupus GWAS with varying degrees of certainty (R.R. Graham, et al., 2009; I.T.W. Harley, et al., 2009; Moser, et al., 2009; Rhodes & Vyse, 2008; Sebastiani & Galeazzi, 2009). In some cases the indicated susceptibility genes are common in many ethnicities and populations, while others are specific to certain groups. The statistical significance of many of these genes is well established, while others are novel and need to be replicated by other groups. An important finding is that most of the genes that have been identified in GWA studies can be grouped into several functional pathways. We will focus on the genes in the IFN pathway and the pathways involving clearing of apoptotic cells and immune complexes.

5.1 Interferon production pathways

Intracellular signaling pathways which control interferon production include the production of type I interferons by interferon regulatory factors (IRFs), and the production of type II interferon by STAT4. IRFs are activated by TLRs, which are extracellular or endosomal pattern recognition molecules. TLRs 7, 8, and 9 recognize nucleic acids and are endosomal. Maintaining these TLRs in the endosome instead of the cell surface is an important barrier to too frequent TLR activation. Once the nucleic acids are brought into the cells through endocytosis, the TLRs become activated to turn on IRFs. TLR 8 and TLR 9 have both been identified as lupus risk genes (Armstrong, et al., 2009; Xu, et al., 2009).

TLRs begin a signaling cascade through a MyD88 signaling complex. MyD88 activates another confirmed locus of SLE risk, the gene which encodes IL1 receptor-associated kinase 1

(IRAK1). In Sle1 and Sle3 mouse models of lupus, IRAK deficiency eliminated most lupus symptoms (Jacob, et al., 2009), which highlights the importance of IRAK1. Since this gene is on the X chromosome, it could help explain why lupus is more common among women. The MyD88 complex can be affected by osteopontin (OPN). It regulates IFNα production in plasmacytoid dendritic cells, which are the body's main IFNα producer cell (Cao & Liu, 2006). The lupus-risk variant of OPN was tied to high IFNα levels in certain lupus patients (Kariuki, et al., 2009b).

Two interacting proteins involved in inflammation, TNFα-induced protein 3 (TNFAIP3) and TNFAIP3-interacting protein 1 (TNIP1), are also lupus risk loci (Gateva, et al., 2009; Musone, et al., 2008). TNFAIP3 encodes the protein A20, which abrogates NFκB after an inflammatory response, and lupus-risk variants of this gene are associated with blood and kidney manifestations (Bates, et al., 2009). TNIP1 interacts with TNFAIP3 as well as affecting several other signal transduction pathways.

Interferon regulatory factors are activated next, downstream of TLRs; they are transcription factors which travel to the nucleus to bind DNA to initiate transcription. IRF5 binds to a sequence-specific region of DNA to induce IFN production. It has been confirmed as a risk factor for SLE in among several ethnicities (Kawasaki, et al., 2008; Kelly, et al., 2008; Lee & Song, 2009; Reddy, et al., 2007; Shimane, et al., 2009). There are three main genetic variants within IRF5, one copy number variant with either two or four copies of a 30-bp sequence, and two SNPs (R.R. Graham, et al., 2007b). The rs2004640 SNP changes the first exon, although this exon does not encode protein. The other SNP, rs10954213, creates an early polyadenylation sequence, which yields shorter more stable mRNA (D.S.C. Graham, et al., 2007a). Work has shown that these variants increase the amount of IFN in the presence of SLE autoantibodies (Niewold, et al., 2008; Salloum, et al., 2009).

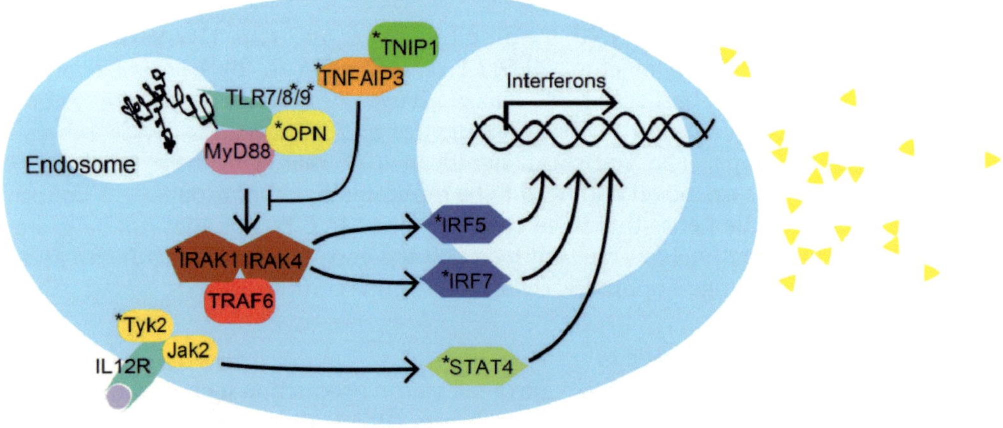

Fig. 6. Interferon production pathways are affected by lupus-risk genes. The * represents genes which have been identified as having risk for lupus. The endosomal TLRs (7, 8, and 9) can bind to autoantigenic nucleic acids and signal through a MyD88 complex which can be affected by association with osteopontin (OPN). If it is not blocked by TNFAIP3, this activates an IRAK signaling complex to phosphorylate the IRF5 and IRF7 transcription factors to produce type I IFN. IL-12 or IL-23 signal through Tyk2/Jak2 to activate the STAT4 transcription factor to produce type II IFN, commonly in T helper cells (Watford, et al., 2004).

IRF7 is associated with SLE risk by its proximity to SNPs in the IRF7/KIAA1542 locus (J.B. Harley, et al., 2008; Suarez-Gestal, et al., 2009). IRF7 SNPs have been shown to lead to increased IFNα levels and alter of which autoantibodies are made (Salloum, et al., 2009).

Signal transducer and activator of transcription 4 (STAT4) is also associated with risk for SLE. It is a transcription factor which activates genes in proliferation, differentiation and apoptosis pathways. Two STAT4 SNPs have been examined, rs7574865 increases sensitivity to IFNα (Kariuki, et al., 2009a), and rs3821236 causes STAT4 to be transcribed at higher levels and is additive with IRF5 risk loci so that when both are present, the risk to SLE is multiplied (Abelson, et al., 2009; Sigurdsson, et al., 2008).

5.2 Genes associated with apoptosis and immune complexes

Another set of risk genes can be placed into a functional group of apoptosis-associated genes. As we read earlier in the chapter, defects in apoptosis can lead to the presence of potential autoantigens. For example, a cell undergoes apoptosis and instead of being cleared by other cells, its contents are released. The cellular contents can contain things like nucleic acids, RNA binding proteins, and others which are common lupus autoantigens. If antibodies bind to these antigens, a complex of multiple antibodies and multiple antigens can aggregate. The resultant immune complexes can be broken down through reactions with complement components, which are commonly found at low levels in SLE patients (C.C. Liu & Ahearn, 2009). If they are not broken down, they reach areas such as the kidneys or joints, which can be damaged by these immune complexes. This is how organ damage usually occurs in lupus patients.

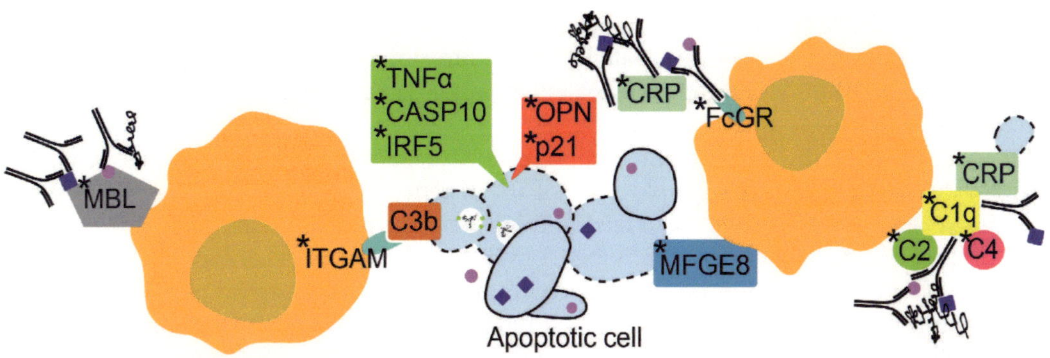

Fig. 7. Genes associated with risk for lupus in the apoptosis pathway. The * represents genes which have been identified as having risk for lupus. TNFα, CASP10 and IRF5 are pro-apoptotic whereas OPN and p21 are anti-apoptotic. These genes all have a role in how much apoptosis is occurring. Once apoptosis has transpired, the cell must be cleared. Parts of apoptotic cells or immune complexes can be recognized by other cells to facilitate their removal. This is aided by recognition molecules such as the complement components shown here.

The problem of creating autoantibodies could stem from too much apoptosis or too little clearance of apoptotic debris. Genes identified in GWA studies that could alter the amount of apoptosis include TNFα, caspase 10, IRF5, osteopontin and p21.

TNFα was identified as a risk factor for lupus in certain ethnicities (Jimenez-Morales, et al., 2009; Lin, et al., 2009). TNFα is a cytokine which is produced and secreted to signal to other cells and is found at high levels in the serum of lupus patients (Davas, et al., 1999; Emilie, et al., 1996; Sabry, et al., 2006). Part of its function is to induce apoptosis—when a cell binds TNFα, it activates the caspase cascade. Caspases are proteases which are activated under certain conditions and are a hallmark of apoptosis. They cleave other caspases as well, and the combined proteolytic activity of several different activated caspases breaks down cellular components as the cell prepares to die. Caspase 10 is part of this cascade and is another lupus susceptibility gene (Armstrong, et al., 2009). Caspase 8, is activated by TNF signaling, and cleaves caspase 10, which then cleaves caspases 3 and 7. IRF5, as well as being a transcription factor which helps produce IFN, is also a tumor suppressor gene which is commonly inactivated in cancers. This is because of IRF5's pro-apoptotic function.

Osteopontin (OPN) and p21 are also lupus risk genes, both anti-apoptotic. OPN promotes proliferation, as well as prevention of death under apoptotic stimuli (Standal, et al., 2004). A mimic of p21 was used in the treatment of murine lupus in the NZB/NZW mouse, and it was found to dramatically reduce the disease (Goulvestre, et al., 2005).

So, there are genes which dysregulate the amount of apoptosis, and they are associated with risk for lupus. But this is only half of the picture; the other part is the clearance of apoptotic cells or immune complexes. Several SLE susceptibility genes in this pathway have been identified as well. Active SLE can be assessed when low levels of complement proteins are found in circulation. Complement can function against microbes during an infection, but can also help to degrade immune complexes. Once attached, they can help cells recognize and degrade them. Other proteins function to bind apoptotic cells or immune complexes to facilitate their uptake by other cells.

Integrin αM (ITGAM) has been convincingly associated to SLE (Nath, et al., 2008). Risk variants of ITGAM have been associated with certain clinical manifestations of lupus (Kim-Howard, et al., 2010). It is a cell receptor which binds to OPN or to complement C3b. C3b binds to apoptotic cells or immune complexes.

SLE association with complement components C1q, C2, C4a and C4b have large OR values, meaning that the risk haplotypes of these genes are causing a large effect. When C1q is expressed at low levels it can lead to lupus, and it was shown to increase the amount the of IFN produced due to immune complexes (Lood, et al., 2009). Complement components function by binding immune complexes by the Fc region of antibody or by binding to other parts of apoptotic cells, which can opsonize them for easier uptake by other cells. Cells can then remove the immune complex or apoptotic debris by endocytosis. Receptors for the Fc region of antibody have also been implicated in SLE risk (Lee-Kirsch, et al., 2007). These receptors can bind to antibody within an immune complex.

Other proteins such as milk fat globule EGF factor 8 (MFG-E8) and C-reactive protein (CRP) can bind to apoptotic cells by recognizing phospholipids on their membranes. MFG-E8 binds to phosphatidylserine, an "eat me" signal which is expressed on apoptotic cells. The MFG-E8 knockout mouse gets SLE because of failure to remove apoptotic cells (Yamaguchi, et al., 2010). CRP binds to phosphocholine, which is present on dying or damaged cells. Both MFG-E8 and CRP are lupus risk genes (Batuca & Alves, 2009; Hu, et al., 2009; H.A. Kim, et al., 2009). Low mannose-binding lectin (MBL) levels can lead to higher levels of apoptosis is this lupus-risk associated gene (Pradhan, et al., 2010).

The number of genes associated with risk for SLE will likely increase, though we have an interesting pool of genes already that point to certain pathways associated with the disease. The interferon and apoptosis pathways are certainly important in SLE etiopathogenesis.

6. Clinical component of interferon and SLE

Many researchers have sought to determine if higher levels of IFN, which is common in lupus patients, is a cause of lupus or an effect of lupus. An interesting occurrence can happen when someone undergoes treatment with IFNα. The presence of increased levels of IFN leads to lupus or a lupus-like syndrome (Gota & Calabrese, 2003; Ioannou & Isenberg, 2000; Niewold & Swedler, 2005). Because the lupus symptoms usually disappear after IFN treatment ends, this connection suggests that IFN may be more of a cause than an effect. In a small number of cases, some patients also develop SLE as a result of these IFN treatments. Furthermore, within a family, the levels of interferon among all members correlate, suggesting that this is a heritable trait (Niewold, et al., 2007). That is, even the siblings of a lupus patient with high IFN levels are more likely to have higher IFN levels. This also supports a causal role for IFN.

Clinically, disease activity can be measured and correlated to other observations to determine the cause of the different levels of activity. One item linked to SLE activity is interferon, where higher levels of IFN in the serum correlated with more severe disease in most cases (Bauer, et al., 2009; Dall'Era, et al., 2005; Feng, et al., 2006; Landolt-Marticorena, et al., 2009; Petri, et al., 2009; Zhuang, et al., 2005).

Common autoantibodies also correlate with IFN levels. A very strong correlation is consistently observed between IFNα levels and the presence of antibodies to common SLE autoantigens like Ro, La, Sm, RNP, and dsDNA (Kirou, et al., 2005).

Another set of findings has to do with properties of main producer of IFNα, the plasmacytoid dendritic cells (pDCs). High numbers of IFN-producing pDCs have been observed in lupus skin lesions (Blomberg, et al., 2001; Farkas, et al., 2001). Since the cells are present at the scene of the crime, the increased interferon could have to do with the pathology in these cases.

At the time of writing, two clinical drug trials for SLE are being conducted, Sifalimumab is in Phase II, and Rontalizumab is in Phase I. Both are antibodies, designed to block interferon alpha signaling by binding it to prevent its recognition by neighboring cells (Clinical Trials, 2011). If these drugs are found to be effective, it will show that IFN plays a critical role in the pathogenesis of lupus. In addition, the United States Food and Drug Administration recently approved an antibody to B lymphocyte stimulator (BLyS) to treat SLE called Belimumab (Sanz, et al., 2011). This should help control the selective apoptosis and autoantibody production to some degree.

7. Conclusions

Several themes have been examined in this chapter. Specifically that the production of interferon is tied to lupus and that apoptosis, clearance of apoptotic cells, and the formation of immune complexes are events that can augment the production of interferon. Exciting findings about the actual genetic causes of SLE are being examined which will lead to better treatments for this complex disease. Although most of the data discussed in this chapter are inferential, there is a large body of evidence in support of the hypothesis that increased interferon signaling promotes an autoimmune state in those genetically prone to SLE.

8. References

Abelson, A.K.; Delgado-Vega, A.M.; Kozyrev, S.V.; Sanchez, E.; Velazquez-Cruz, R.; Eriksson, N.; Wojcik, J.; Reddy, M.; Lima, G.; D'Alfonso, S.; Migliaresi, S.; Baca, V.; Orozco, L.; Witte, T.; Ortego-Centeno, N.; Abderrahim, H.; Pons-Estel, B.A.; Gutierrez, C.; Suarez, A.; Gonzalez-Escribano, M.F.; Martin, J.; Alarcon-Riquelme, M.E. & Grp, A. (2009). STAT4 associates with systemic lupus erythematosus through two independent effects that correlate with gene expression and act additively with IRF5 to increase risk. *Annals of the Rheumatic Diseases*, 68 pp. 1746-1753

Armstrong, D.L.; Reiff, A.; Myones, B.L.; Quismorio, F.P.; Klein-Gitelman, M.; McCurdy, D.; Wagner-Weiner, L.; Silverman, E.; Ojwang, J.O.; Kaufman, K.M.; Kelly, J.A.; Merrill, J.T.; Harley, J.B.; Bae, S.C.; Vyse, T.J.; Gilkeson, G.S.; Gaffney, P.M.; Moser, K.L.; Putterman, C.; Edberg, J.C.; Brown, E.E.; Ziegler, J.; Langefeld, C.D.; Zidovetzki, R. & Jacob, C.O. (2009). Identification of new SLE-associated genes with a two-step Bayesian study design. *Genes and Immunity*, 10 pp. 446-456

Baechler, E.C.; Batliwalla, F.M.; Karypis, G.; Gaffney, P.M.; Ortmann, W.A.; Espe, K.J.; Shark, K.B.; Grande, W.J.; Hughes, K.M.; Kapur, V.; Gregersen, P.K. & Behrens, T.W. (2003). Interferon-inducible gene expression signature in peripheral blood cells of patients with severe lupus. *Proceedings of the National Academy of Sciences of the United States of America*, 100 pp. 2610-2615

Bates, J.S.; Lessard, C.J.; Leon, J.M.; Nguyen, T.; Battiest, L.J.; Rodgers, J.; Kaufman, K.M.; James, J.A.; Gilkeson, G.S.; Kelly, J.A.; Humphrey, M.B.; Harley, J.B.; Gray-McGuire, C.; Moser, K.L. & Gaffney, P.M. (2009). Meta-analysis and imputation identifies a 109 kb risk haplotype spanning TNFAIP3 associated with lupus nephritis and hematologic manifestations. *Genes and Immunity*, 10 pp. 470-477

Batuca, J. & Alves, J.D. (2009). C-reactive protein in systemic lupus erythematosus. *Autoimmunity*, 42 pp. 282-285

Bauer, J.W.; Petri, M.; Batliwalla, F.M.; Koeuth, T.; Wilson, J.; Slattery, C.; Panoskaltsis-Mortari, A.; Gregersen, P.K.; Behrens, T.W. & Baechler, E.C. (2009). Interferon-Regulated Chemokines as Biomarkers of Systemic Lupus Erythematosus Disease Activity A Validation Study. *Arthritis and Rheumatism*, 60 pp. 3098-3107

Bennett, L.; Palucka, A.K.; Arce, E.; Cantrell, V.; Borvak, J.; Banchereau, J. & Pascual, V. (2003). Interferon and granulopoiesis signatures in systemic lupus erythematosus blood. *Journal of Experimental Medicine*, 197 pp. 711-723

Blomberg, S.; Eloranta, M.L.; Cederblad, B.; Nordlind, K.; Alm, G.V. & Ronnblom, L. (2001). Presence of cutaneous interferon-alpha producing cells in patients with systemic lupus erythematosus. *Lupus*, 10 pp. 484-490

Bynote, K.K.; Hackenberg, J.M.; Korach, K.S.; Lubahn, D.B.; Lane, P.H. & Gould, K.A. (2008). Estrogen receptor-alpha deficiency attenuates autoimmune disease in (NZB x NZW)F1 mice. *Genes Immun*, 9 pp. 137-152

Cancro, M.P.; D'Cruz, D.P. & Khamashta, M.A. (2009). The role of B lymphocyte stimulator (BLyS) in systemic lupus erythematosus. *Journal of Clinical Investigation*, 119 pp. 1066-1073

Cao, W. & Liu, Y.J. (2006). Opn: key regulator of pDC interferon production. *Nature Immunology*, 7 pp. 441-443

ClinicalTrials.gov. (2011) http://www.clinicaltrials.gov

Crispin, J.C.; Liossis, S.N.C.; Kis-Toth, K.; Lieberman, L.A.; Kyttaris, V.C.; Juang, Y.T. & Tsokos, G.C. Pathogenesis of human systemic lupus erythematosus: recent advances. *Trends in Molecular Medicine*, 16 pp. 47-57

Dall'Era, M.C.; Cardarelli, P.M.; Preston, B.T.; Witte, A. & Davis, J.C. (2005). Type I interferon correlates with serological and clinical manifestations of SLE. *Annals of the Rheumatic Diseases*, 64 pp. 1692-1697

Davas, E.M.; Tsirogianni, A.; Kappou, I.; Karamitsos, D.; Economidou, I. & Dantis, P.C. (1999). Serum IL-6, TNF alpha, p55 srTNF alpha, p75 srTNF alpha, srIL-2 alpha levels and disease acitivity in systemic lupus erythematosus. *Clinical Rheumatology*, 18 pp. 17-22

Deapen, D.; Escalante, A.; Weinrib, L.; Horwitz, D.; Bachman, B.; Royburman, P.; Walker, A. & Mack, T.M. (1992). A revised estimate of twin concordance in systemic lupus erythematosus. *Arthritis and Rheumatism*, 35 pp. 311-318

Emilie, D.; Llorente, L. & Galanaud, P. (1996). Cytokines and systemic lupus erythematosus. *Annales De Medecine Interne*, 147 pp. 480-484

Farkas, L.; Beiske, K.; Lund-Johansen, F.; Brandtzaeg, P. & Jahnsen, F.L. (2001). Plasmacytoid dendritic cells (natural interferon-alpha/beta-producing cells) accumulate in cutaneous lupus erythematosus lesions. *American Journal of Pathology*, 159 pp. 237-243

Feng, X.B.; Wu, H.; Grossman, J.M.; Hanvivadhanakul, P.; FitzGerald, J.D.; Park, G.S.; Dong, X.; Chen, W.L.; Kim, M.H.; Weng, H.H.; Furst, D.E.; Gorn, A.; McMahon, M.; Taylor, M.; Brahn, E.; Hahn, B.H. & Tsao, B.P. (2006). Association of increased interferon-inducible gene expression with disease activity and lupus nephritis in patients with systemic lupus erythematosus. *Arthritis and Rheumatism*, 54 pp. 2951-2962

Fruh, K. & Yang, Y. (1999). Antigen presentation by MHC class I and its regulation by interferon gamma. *Current Opinion in Immunology*, 11 pp. 76-81

Gaipl, U.S.; Sheriff, A.; Franz, S.; Munoz, L.E.; Voll, R.E.; Kalden, J.R. & Herrmann, M. (2006). Inefficient clearance of dying cells and autoreactivity. *Current Concepts in Autoimmunity and Chronic Inflamation*, 305 pp. 161-176

Gateva, V.; Sandling, J.K.; Hom, G.; Taylor, K.E.; Chung, S.A.; Sun, X.; Ortmann, W.; Kosoy, R.; Ferreira, R.C.; Nordmark, G.; Gunnarsson, I.; Svenungsson, E.; Padyukov, L.; Sturfelt, G.; Jonsen, A.; Bengtsson, A.A.; Rantapaa-Dahlqvist, S.; Baechler, E.C.; Brown, E.E.; Alarcon, G.S.; Edberg, J.C.; Ramsey-Goldman, R.; McGwin, G.; Reveille, J.D.; Vila, L.M.; Kimberly, R.P.; Manzi, S.; Petri, M.A.; Lee, A.; Gregersen, P.K.; Seldin, M.F.; Ronnblom, L.; Criswell, L.A.; Syvanen, A.C.; Behrens, T.W. & Graham, R.R. (2009). A large-scale replication study identifies TNIP1, PRDM1, JAZF1, UHRF1BP1 and IL10 as risk loci for systemic lupus erythematosus. *Nature Genetics*, 41 pp. 1228-U1293

Gota, C. & Calabrese, L. (2003). Induction of clinical autoimmune disease by therapeutic interferon-alpha. *Autoimmunity*, 36 pp. 511-518

Goulvestre, C.; Chereau, C.; Nicco, C.; Mouthon, L.; Weill, B. & Batteux, F. (2005). A mimic of p21(WAF1)/(CIP1) ameliorates murine lupus. *Journal of Immunology,* 175 pp. 6959-6967

Graham, D.S.C.; Manku, H.; Wagner, S.; Reid, J.; Timms, K.; Gutin, A.; Lanchbury, J.S. & Vyse, T.J. (2007a). Association of IRF5 in UK SLE families identifies a variant involved in polyadenylation. *Human Molecular Genetics,* 16 pp. 579-591

Graham, R.R.; Hom, G.; Ortmann, W. & Behrens, T.W. (2009). Review of recent genome-wide association scans in lupus. *Journal of Internal Medicine,* 265 pp. 680-688

Graham, R.R.; Kyogoku, C.; Sigurdsson, S.; Vlasova, I.A.; Davies, L.R.; Baechler, E.C.; Plenge, R.M.; Koeuth, T.; Ortmann, W.A.; Hom, G.; Bauer, J.W.; Gillett, C.; Burtt, N.; Cunninghame Graham, D.S.; Onofrio, R.; Petri, M.; Gunnarsson, I.; Svenungsson, E.; Ronnblom, L.; Nordmark, G.; Gregersen, P.K.; Moser, K.; Gaffney, P.M.; Criswell, L.A.; Vyse, T.J.; Syvanen, A.C.; Bohjanen, P.R.; Daly, M.J.; Behrens, T.W. & Altshuler, D. (2007b). Three functional variants of IFN regulatory factor 5 (IRF5) define risk and protective haplotypes for human lupus. *Proc Natl Acad Sci U S A,* 104 pp. 6758-6763

Harley, I.T.W.; Kaufman, K.M.; Langefeld, C.D.; Harley, J.B. & Kelly, J.A. (2009). Genetic susceptibility to SLE: new insights from fine mapping and genome-wide association studies. *Nature Reviews Genetics,* 10 pp. 285-290

Harley, J.B.; Alarcon-Riquelme, M.E.; Criswell, L.A.; Jacob, C.O.; Kimberly, R.P.; Moser, K.L.; Tsao, B.P.; Vyse, T.J.; Langefeld, C.D. & Int Consortium Systemic Lupus, E. (2008). Genome-wide association scan in women with systemic lupus erythematosus identifies susceptibility variants in ITGAM, PXK, KIAA1542 and other loci. *Nature Genetics,* 40 pp. 204-210

Hu, C.Y.; Wu, C.S.; Tsai, H.F.; Chang, S.K.; Tsai, W.I. & Hsu, P.N. (2009). Genetic polymorphism in milk fat globule-EGF factor 8 (MFG-E8) is associated with systemic lupus erythematosus in human. *Lupus,* 18 pp. 676-681

Ioannou, Y. & Isenberg, D.A. (2000). Current evidence for the induction of autoimmune rheumatic manifestations by cytokine therapy. *Arthritis and Rheumatism,* 43 pp. 1431-1442

Izui, S.; Merino, R.; Fossati, L. & Iwamoto, M. (1994). The role of the Yaa gene in lupus syndrome. *Int Rev Immunol,* 11 pp. 211-230

Jacob, C.O.; Zhu, J.K.; Armstrong, D.L.; Yan, M.; Han, J.; Zhou, X.J.; Thomas, J.A.; Reiff, A.; Myones, B.L.; Ojwang, J.O.; Kaufman, K.M.; Klein-Gitelman, M.; McCurdy, D.; Wagner-Weiner, L.; Silverman, E.; Ziegler, J.; Kelly, J.A.; Merrill, J.T.; Harley, J.B.; Ramsey-Goldman, R.; Vila, L.M.; Bae, S.C.; Vyse, T.J.; Gilkeson, G.S.; Gaffney, P.M.; Moser, K.L.; Langefeld, C.D.; Zidovetzki, R. & Mohan, C. (2009). Identification of IRAK1 as a risk gene with critical role in the pathogenesis of systemic lupus erythematosus. *Proceedings of the National Academy of Sciences of the United States of America,* 106 pp. 6256-6261

Jimenez-Morales, S.; Velazquez-Cruz, R.; Ramirez-Bello, J.; Bonilla-Gonzalez, E.; Romero-Hidalgo, S.; Escamilla-Guerrero, G.; Cuevas, F.; Espinosa-Rosales, F.; Martinez-Aguilar, N.E.; Gomez-Vera, J.; Baca, V. & Orozco, L. (2009). Tumor necrosis factor-alpha is a common genetic risk factor for asthma, juvenile rheumatoid arthritis, and systemic lupus erythematosus in a Mexican pediatric population. *Human Immunology*, 70 pp. 251-256

Jmol: an open-source Java viewer for chemical structures in 3D. http://www.jmol.org

Jorgensen, T.N.; Roper, E.; Thurman, J.M.; Marrack, P. & Kotzin, B.L. (2007). Type I interferon signaling is involved in the spontaneous development of lupus-like disease in B6.Nba2 and (B6.Nba2 x NZW)F(1) mice. *Genes Immun*, 8 pp. 653-662

Kariuki, S.N.; Kirou, K.A.; MacDermott, E.J.; Barillas-Arias, L.; Crow, M.K. & Niewold, T.B. (2009a). Cutting Edge: Autoimmune Disease Risk Variant of STAT4 Confers increased Sensitivity to IFN-alpha in Lupus Patients In Vivo. *Journal of Immunology*, 182 pp. 34-38

Kariuki, S.N.; Moore, J.G.; Kirou, K.A.; Crow, M.K.; Utset, T.O. & Niewold, T.B. (2009b). Age- and gender-specific modulation of serum osteopontin and interferon-alpha by osteopontin genotype in systemic lupus erythematosus. *Genes and Immunity*, 10 pp. 487-494

Karpusas, M.; Nolte, M.; Benton, C.B.; Meier, W.; Lipscomb, W.N. & Goelz, S. (1997). The crystal structure of human interferon beta at 2.2-angstrom resolution. *Proceedings of the National Academy of Sciences of the United States of America*, 94 pp. 11813-11818

Kawasaki, A.; Kyogoku, C.; Ohashi, J.; Miyashita, R.; Hikami, K.; Kusaoi, M.; Tokunaga, K.; Takasaki, Y.; Hashimoto, H.; Behrens, T.W. & Tsuchiya, N. (2008). Association of IRF5 polymorphisms with systemic lupus erythematosus in a Japanese population: support for a crucial role of intron 1 polymorphisms. *Arthritis Rheum*, 58 pp. 826-834

Kelly, J.A.; Kelley, J.M.; Kaufman, K.M.; Kilpatrick, J.; Bruner, G.R.; Merrill, J.T.; James, J.A.; Frank, S.G.; Reams, E.; Brown, E.E.; Gibson, A.W.; Marion, M.C.; Langefeld, C.D.; Li, Q.Z.; Karp, D.R.; Wakeland, E.K.; Petri, M.; Ramsey-Goldman, R.; Reveille, J.D.; Vila, L.M.; Alarcon, G.S.; Kimberly, R.P.; Harley, J.B. & Edberg, J.C. (2008). Interferon regulatory factor-5 is genetically associated with systemic lupus erythematosus in African Americans. *Genes Immun*, 9 pp. 187-194

Kim-Howard, X.; Maiti, A.K.; Anaya, J.M.; Bruner, G.R.; Brown, E.; Merrill, J.T.; Edberg, J.C.; Petri, M.A.; Reveille, J.D.; Ramsey-Goldman, R.; Alarcon, G.S.; Vyse, T.J.; Gilkeson, G.; Kimberly, R.P.; James, J.A.; Guthridge, J.M.; Harley, J.B. & Nath, S.K. ITGAM coding variant (rs1143679) influences the risk of renal disease, discoid rash and immunological manifestations in patients with systemic lupus erythematosus with European ancestry. *Annals of the Rheumatic Diseases*, 69 pp. 1329-1332

Kim, H.A.; Chun, H.Y.; Kim, S.H.; Park, H.S. & Suh, C.H. (2009). C-Reactive Protein Gene Polymorphisms in Disease Susceptibility and Clinical Manifestations of Korean Systemic Lupus Erythematosus. *Journal of Rheumatology*, 36 pp. 2238-2243

Kim, T.; Kanayama, Y.; Negoro, N.; Okamura, M.; Takeda, T. & Inoue, T. (1987). Serum levels of interferons in patients with systemic lupus-erythematosus. *Clinical and Experimental Immunology*, 70 pp. 562-569

Kirou, K.A.; Lee, C.; George, S.; Louca, K.; Peterson, M.G.E. & Crow, M.K. (2005). Activation of the interferon-alpha pathway identifies a subgroup of systemic lupus erythematosus patients with distinct serologic features and active disease. *Arthritis and Rheumatism*, 52 pp. 1491-1503

Landolt-Marticorena, C.; Bonventi, G.; Lubovich, A.; Ferguson, C.; Unnithan, T.; Su, J.; Gladman, D.D.; Urowitz, M.; Fortin, P.R. & Wither, J. (2009). Lack of association between the interferon-alpha signature and longitudinal changes in disease activity in systemic lupus erythematosus. *Annals of the Rheumatic Diseases*, 68 pp. 1440-1446

Lee-Kirsch, M.A.; Gong, M.; Chowdhury, D.; Senenko, L.; Engel, K.; Lee, Y.A.; de Silva, U.; Bailey, S.L.; Witte, T.; Vyse, T.J.; Kere, J.; Pfeiffer, C.; Harvey, S.; Wong, A.; Koskenmies, S.; Hummel, O.; Rohde, K.; Schmidt, R.E.; Dominiczak, A.F.; Gahr, M.; Hollis, T.; Perrino, F.W.; Lieberman, J. & Hubner, N. (2007). Mutations in the gene encoding the 3 '-5 ' DNA exonuclease TREX1 are associated with systemic lupus erythematosus. *Nature Genetics*, 39 pp. 1065-1067

Lee, Y.H. & Song, G.G. (2009). Association between the rs2004640 functional polymorphism of interferon regulatory factor 5 and systemic lupus erythematosus: a meta-analysis. *Rheumatology International*, 29 pp. 1137-1142

Li, L.H.; Li, W.X.; Wu, O.; Zhang, G.Q.; Pan, H.F.; Li, X.P.; Xu, J.H.; Dai, H. & Ye, D.Q. (2009). Fas expression on peripheral blood lymphocytes in systemic lupus erythematosus: relation to the organ damage and lymphocytes apoptosis. *Molecular Biology Reports*, 36 pp. 2047-2052

Lin, Y.J.; Chen, R.H.; Wan, L.; Sheu, J.J.C.; Huang, C.M.; Lin, C.W.; Chen, S.Y.; Lai, C.H.; Lan, Y.C.; Hsueh, K.C.; Tsai, C.H.; Lin, T.H.; Huang, Y.M.; Chao, K.; Chen, D.Y. & Tsai, F.J. (2009). Association of TNF-alpha gene polymorphisms with systemic lupus erythematosus in Taiwanese patients. *Lupus*, 18 pp. 974-979

Liu, C.C. & Ahearn, J.M. (2009). The search for lupus biomarkers. *Best Practice & Research in Clinical Rheumatology*, 23 pp. 507-523

Liu, Z.; Bethunaickan, R.; Huang, W.; Lodhi, U.; Solano, I.; Madaio, M.P. & Davidson, A. (2011). Interferon-alpha accelerates murine systemic lupus erythematosus in a T cell-dependent manner. *Arthritis Rheum*, 63 pp. 219-229

Lood, C.; Gullstrand, B.; Truedsson, L.; Olin, A.I.; Alm, G.V.; Ronnblom, L.; Sturfelt, G.; Eloranta, M.L. & Bengtsson, A.A. (2009). C1q Inhibits Immune Complex-Induced Interferon-alpha Production in Plasmacytoid Dendritic Cells A Novel Link Between C1q Deficiency and Systemic Lupus Erythematosus Pathogenesis. *Arthritis and Rheumatism*, 60 pp. 3081-3090

Lucero, M.A.; Magdelenat, H.; Fridman, W.H.; Pouillart, P.; Billardon, C.; Billiau, A.; Cantell, K. & Falcoff, E. (1982). Comparison of effects of leukocyte and fibroblast interferon on immunological parameters in cancer-patients. *European Journal of Cancer & Clinical Oncology*, 18 pp. 243-251

Luker, K.E.; Hutchens, M.; Schultz, T.; Pekosz, A. & Luker, G.D. (2005). Bioluminescence imaging of vaccinia virus: Effects of interferon on viral replication and spread. *Virology*, 341 pp. 284-300

Mathian, A.; Weinberg, A.; Gallegos, M.; Banchereau, J. & Koutouzov, S. (2005). IFN-alpha induces early lethal lupus in preautoimmune (New Zealand Black x New Zealand White) F1 but not in BALB/c mice. *J Immunol*, 174 pp. 2499-2506

Moser, K.L.; Kelly, J.A.; Lessard, C.J. & Harley, J.B. (2009). Recent insights into the genetic basis of systemic lupus erythematosus. *Genes and Immunity*, 10 pp. 373-379

Munoz, L.E.; Lauber, K.; Schiller, M.; Manfredi, A.A. & Herrmann, M. (2010). The role of defective clearance of apoptotic cells in systemic autoimmunity. *Nature Reviews Rheumatology*, 6 pp. 280-289

Murray, H.W. (1988). Interferon-gamma, the activated macrophage, and host defense against microbial challenge. *Annals of Internal Medicine*, 108 pp. 595-608

Musone, S.L.; Taylor, K.E.; Lu, T.T.; Nititham, J.; Ferreira, R.C.; Ortmann, W.; Shifrin, N.; Petri, M.A.; Kamboh, M.I.; Manzi, S.; Seldin, M.F.; Gregersen, P.K.; Behrens, T.W.; Ma, A.; Kwok, P.Y. & Criswell, L.A. (2008). Multiple polymorphisms in the TNFAIP3 region are independently associated with systemic lupus erythematosus. *Nature Genetics*, 40 pp. 1062-1064

Nath, S.K.; Han, S.Z.; Kim-Howard, X.; Kelly, J.A.; Viswanathan, P.; Gilkeson, G.S.; Chen, W.; Zhu, C.; McEver, R.P.; Kimberly, R.P.; Alarcon-Riquelme, M.E.; Vyse, T.J.; Li, Q.Z.; Wakeland, E.K.; Merrill, J.T.; James, J.A.; Kaufman, K.M.; Guthridge, J.M. & Harley, J.B. (2008). A nonsynonymous functional variant in integrin-alpha M (encoded by ITGAM) is associated with systemic lupus erythematosus. *Nature Genetics*, 40 pp. 152-154

Niewold, T.B.; Clark, D.N.; Salloum, R. & Poole, B.D. Interferon Alpha in Systemic Lupus Erythematosus. *Journal of Biomedicine and Biotechnology*, pp. 8

Niewold, T.B.; Hua, J.; Lehman, T.J.A.; Harley, J.B. & Crow, M.K. (2007). High serum IFN-alpha activity is a heritable risk factor for systemic lupus erythematosus. *Genes and Immunity*, 8 pp. 492-502

Niewold, T.B.; Kelly, J.A.; Flesch, M.H.; Espinoza, L.R.; Harley, J.B. & Crow, M.K. (2008). Association of the IRF5 risk haplotype with high serum interferon-alpha activity in systemic lupus erythematosus patients. *Arthritis and Rheumatism*, 58 pp. 2481-2487

Niewold, T.B. & Swedler, W.I. (2005). Systemic lupus erythematosus arising during interferon-alpha therapy for cryoglobulinemic vasculitis associated with hepatitis C. *Clinical Rheumatology*, 24 pp. 178-181

Panchanathan, R.; Shen, H.; Bupp, M.G.; Gould, K.A. & Choubey, D. (2009). Female and male sex hormones differentially regulate expression of Ifi202, an interferon-inducible lupus susceptibility gene within the Nba2 interval. *J Immunol*, 183 pp. 7031-7038

Panchanathan, R.; Shen, H.; Zhang, X.; Ho, S.M. & Choubey, D. (2010). Mutually positive regulatory feedback loop between interferons and estrogen receptor-alpha in mice: implications for sex bias in autoimmunity. *PLoS ONE*, 5 pp. e10868

Petri, M.; Singh, S.; Tesfasyone, H.; Dedrick, R.; Fry, K.; Lal, P.G.; Williams, G.; Bauer, J.W.; Gregersen, P.K.; Behrens, T.W. & Baechler, E.C. (2009). Longitudinal expression of type I interferon responsive genes in systemic lupus erythematosus. *Lupus*, 18 pp. 980-989

Pindel, A. & Sadler, A. The Role of Protein Kinase R in the Interferon Response. *Journal of Interferon and Cytokine Research*, 31 pp. 59-70

Pradhan, V.; Surve, P. & Ghosh, K. Mannose binding lectin (MBL) in autoimmunity and its role in systemic lupus erythematosus (SLE). *J Assoc Physicians India*, 58 pp. 688-690

Reddy, M.V.; Velazquez-Cruz, R.; Baca, V.; Lima, G.; Granados, J.; Orozco, L. & Alarcon-Riquelme, M.E. (2007). Genetic association of IRF5 with SLE in Mexicans: higher frequency of the risk haplotype and its homozygozity than Europeans. *Hum Genet*, 121 pp. 721-727

Rhodes, B. & Vyse, T.J. (2008). The genetics of SLE: an update in the light of genome-wide association studies. *Rheumatology*, 47 pp. 1603-1611

Richez, C.; Yasuda, K.; Bonegio, R.G.; Watkins, A.A.; Aprahamian, T.; Busto, P.; Richards, R.J.; Liu, C.L.; Cheung, R.; Utz, P.J.; Marshak-Rothstein, A. & Rifkin, I.R., (2010) IFN regulatory factor 5 is required for disease development in the FcγRIIB$^{-/-}$ Yaa and FcγRIIB$^{-/-}$ mouse models of systemic lupus erythematosus. *J Immunol*, 184 pp. 796-806

Ronnblom, L. & Alm, G.V. (2001). A pivotal role for the natural interferon alpha-producing cells (plasmacytoid dendritic cells) in the pathogenesis of lupus. *Journal of Experimental Medicine*, 194 pp. F59-F63

Ronnblom, L.; Alm, G.V. & Eloranta, M.L. The type I interferon system in the development of lupus. *Seminars in Immunology*, 23 pp. 113-121

Sabry, A.; Sheashaa, H.; El-husseini, A.; Mahmoud, K.; Eldahshan, K.F.; George, S.K.; Abdel-Khalek, E.; El-Shafey, E.M. & Abo-Zenah, H. (2006). Proinflammatory cytokines (TNF-alpha and IL-6) in Egyptian patients with SLE: Its correlation with disease activity. *Cytokine*, 35 pp. 148-153

Sahebari, M.; Hatef, M.R.; Rezaieyazdi, Z.; Abbasi, M.; Abbasi, B. & Mahmoudi, M. Correlation between Serum Levels of Soluble Fas (CD95/Apo-1) with Disease Activity in Systemic Lupus Erythematosus Patients in Khorasan, Iran. *Archives of Iranian Medicine*, 13 pp. 135-142

Salloum, R.; Franek, B.; Kariuki, S.; Utset, T. & Niewold, T. (2009). T.16. Genetic Variation at the IRF7/KIAA1542 Locus is Associated with Autoantibody Profile and Serum Interferon Alpha Levels in Lupus Patients. *Clinical Immunology*, 131 pp. S54-S54

Sanz, I.; Yasothan, U. & Kirkpatrick, P. Belimumab. *Nature Reviews Drug Discovery*, 10 pp. 335-336

Savitsky, D.A.; Yanai, H.; Tamura, T.; Taniguchi, T. & Honda, K. (2010). Contribution of IRF5 in B cells to the development of murine SLE-like disease through its transcriptional control of the IgG2a locus. *Proc Natl Acad Sci U S A*, 107 pp. 10154-10159

Sebastiani, G.D. & Galeazzi, M. (2009). Immunogenetic studies on systemic lupus erythematosus. *Lupus*, 18 pp. 878-883

Sharma, R.P.; He, Q. & Riley, R.T. (2005). Lupus-prone NZBWF1/J mice, defective in cytokine signaling, are resistant to fumonisin hepatotoxicity despite accumulation of liver sphinganine. *Toxicology*, 216 pp. 59-71

Shimane, K.; Kochi, Y.; Yamada, R.; Okada, Y.; Suzuki, A.; Miyatake, A.; Kubo, M.; Nakamura, Y. & Yamamoto, K. (2009). A single nucleotide polymorphism in the IRF5 promoter region is associated with susceptibility to rheumatoid arthritis in the Japanese population. *Annals of the Rheumatic Diseases*, 68 pp. 377-383

Sigurdsson, S.; Nordmark, G.; Garnier, S.; Grundberg, E.; Kwan, T.; Nilsson, O.; Eloranta, M.L.; Gunnarsson, I.; Svenungsson, E.; Sturfelt, G.; Bengtsson, A.A.; Jonsen, A.; Truedsson, L.; Rantapaa-Dahlqvist, S.; Eriksson, C.; Alm, G.; Goring, H.H.H.; Pastinen, T.; Syvanen, A.C. & Ronnblom, L. (2008). A risk haplotype of STAT4 for systemic lupus erythematosus is over-expressed, correlates with anti-dsDNA and shows additive effects with two risk alleles of IRF5. *Human Molecular Genetics*, 17 pp. 2868-2876

Standal, T.; Borset, M. & Sundan, A. (2004). Role of osteopontin in adhesion, migration, cell survival and bone remodeling. *Experimental Oncology*, 26 pp. 179-184

Stranger, B.E.; Stahl, E.A. & Raj, T. Progress and Promise of Genome-Wide Association Studies for Human Complex Trait Genetics. *Genetics*, 187 pp. 367-383

Su, A.I.; Wiltshire, T.; Batalov, S.; Lapp, H.; Ching, K.A.; Block, D.; Zhang, J.; Soden, R.; Hayakawa, M.; Kreiman, G.; Cooke, M.P.; Walker, J.R. & Hogenesch, J.B. (2004). A gene atlas of the mouse and human protein-encoding transcriptomes. *Proceedings of the National Academy of Sciences of the United States of America*, 101 pp. 6062-6067

Suarez-Gestal, M.; Calaza, M.; Endreffy, E.; Pullmann, R.; Ordi-Ros, J.; Sebastiani, G.D.; Ruzickova, S.; Santos, M.J.; Papasteriades, C.; Marchini, M.; Skopouli, F.N.; Suarez, A.; Blanco, F.J.; D'Alfonso, S.; Bijl, M.; Carreira, P.; Witte, T.; Migliaresi, S.; Gomez-Reino, J.J.; Gonzalez, A. & European Consortium, S.D. (2009). Replication of recently identified systemic lupus erythematosus genetic associations: a case-control study. *Arthritis Research & Therapy*, 11 pp.

Tada, Y.; Kondo, S.; Aoki, S.; Koarada, S.; Inoue, H.; Suematsu, R.; Ohta, A.; Mak, T.W. & Nagasawa, K. (2011). Interferon regulatory factor 5 is critical for the development of lupus in MRL/lpr mice. *Arthritis Rheum*, 63 pp. 738-748

Takaoka, A.; Hayakawa, S.; Yanai, H.; Stoiber, D.; Negishi, H.; Kikuchi, H.; Sasaki, S.; Imai, K.; Shibue, T.; Honda, K. & Taniguchi, T. (2003). Integration of interferon-alpha/beta signalling to p53 responses in tumour suppression and antiviral defence. *Nature*, 424 pp. 516-523

Watford, W.T.; Hissong, B.D.; Bream, J.H.; Kanno, Y.; Muul, L. & O'Shea, J.J. (2004). Signaling by IL-12 and IL-23 and the immunoregulatory roles of STAT4. *Immunological Reviews*, 202 pp. 139-156

Xu, C.J.; Zhang, W.H.; Pan, H.F.; Li, X.P.; Xu, J.H. & Ye, D.Q. (2009). Association study of a single nucleotide polymorphism in the exon 2 region of toll-like receptor 9 (TLR9) gene with susceptibility to systemic lupus erythematosus among Chinese. *Molecular Biology Reports*, 36 pp. 2245-2248

Yamaguchi, H.; Fujimoto, T.; Nakamura, S.; Ohmura, K.; Mimori, T.; Matsuda, F. & Nagata, S. Aberrant splicing of the milk fat globule-EGF factor 8 (MFG-E8) gene in human systemic lupus erythematosus. *European Journal of Immunology*, 40 pp. 1778-1785

Ytterberg, S.R. & Schnitzer, T.J. (1982). Serum interferon levels in patients with systemic lupus-erythematosus. *Arthritis and Rheumatism*, 25 pp. 401-406

Zhuang, H.Y.; Narain, S.; Sobel, E.; Lee, P.Y.; Naconales, D.C.; Kelly, K.M.; Richards, H.B.; Segal, M.; Stewart, C.; Satoh, M. & Reeves, W.H. (2005). Association of anti-nucleoprotein autoantibodies with upregulation of Type I interferon-inducible gene transcripts and dendritic cell maturation in systemic lupus erythematosus. *Clinical Immunology*, 117 pp. 238-250

4

Fas Pathway of Cell Death and B Cell Dysregulation in SLE

Roberto Paganelli, Alessia Paganelli and Maria C. Turi
Department of Medicine and Sciences of Aging
University "G. d'Annunzio" of Chieti-Pescara
and Ce.S.I.- U.d'A. Foundation, Chieti scalo (CH)
Italy

1. Introduction

Systemic lupus erythematosus (SLE) is a generalized autoimmune disease affecting several organ systems, characterized by the presence of a vast array of autoantibodies, characteristically directed to nuclear antigens (ANA) (Arbuckle et al, 2003, Hahn, 1998, Rothman and Isenberg, 2008). Systemic lupus erythematosus (SLE) is the second most common human autoimmune disease affecting between 400 and 1000 per million people worldwide (Craft, 2011).

SLE is caused by the breakdown of tolerance to nuclear self-antigens, which leads to activation of autoreactive B cells that produce autoantibodies against self-nucleic acids and associated proteins (Lande et al, 2011). These autoantibodies bind self-nucleic acids released by dying cells, and form immune complexes that are deposited in different parts of the body, leading to detrimental inflammation and tissue damage. A key early event that triggers autoimmunity in SLE is the chronic innate activation of plasmacytoid dendritic cells (pDCs) to secrete type I interferons (IFNs) (Theofilopoulos et al, 2005; Ronnblom et al, 2006; Banchereau and Pascual, 2006). The high levels of type I IFNs induce an unabated differentiation of monocytes into dendritic cells that stimulate autoreactive B and T cells (Blanco et al, 2001), licensing T cells recognize autoantigens and lower the activation threshold of autoreactive B cells (LeBon et al, 2006), thereby promoting autoimmunity in SLE.

Analysis of genes encoding components of the interferon pathway has led to extensive support for an association of polymorphic variants of interferon regulatory factor 5 (*IRF5*) with SLE (Bennett et al, 2003; Crow, 2008; Niewold et al,2007;). Recent genomewide association studies confirm associations of HLA and *STAT4* variants with SLE and also the role of *PTPN22* (International Consortium, 2008; Rieck et al, 2007; Remmers et al, 2007). New reports of genetic SNPs associations include the B-cell-receptor–signaling pathway and the mechanisms of adhesion of inflammatory cells to the vasculature (Hom et al, 2008; Kozyrev et al, 2008).

The heterogeneity of clinical manifestations and the disease's unpredictable course (Tan et al, 1982) characterized by flares and remissions are very likely a reflection of heterogeneity at the origin of disease, with a final common pathway leading to loss of tolerance to nuclear antigens. Impaired clearance of immune complexes and apoptotic material and production of autoantibodies have long been recognized as major pathogenic events (Arbuckle et al, 2003; Rothman and Isenberg, 2008). Apoptotic defects underlie some models of autoimmune diseases, and they have been proposed in the pathogenesis of SLE, a prototypic autoimmune disorder.

SLE disease activity can be difficult to monitor, and flares are unpredictable in both frequency and severity. Certain clinical laboratory tests, including anti-double-stranded DNA antibodies (anti-dsDNA), complement factor levels, and the erythrocyte sedimentation rate (ESR) are often measured as potential indicators of disease activity (Ippolito et al, 2011).

Neutrophils are part of the innate immune response and they have long been suspected to play a role in SLE pathogenesis. Nevertheless, their role has not been elucidated until very recently.

In 1948, Hargraves et al. described mature bone marrow neutrophils containing intracytoplasmic nuclear material in 25 SLE patients at the Mayo Clinic (Hargraves, 1948). This phenomenon, which they called the "LE cell," helped develop the first diagnostic test for this disease (Haserick and Bortz, 1949a). In 1949, Haserick and Bortz found that plasma from 50 to 75% of patients with SLE reproduced the LE cell phenomenon in vitro, with the formation of clumps of neutrophils around amorphous masses of nuclear material (Haserick and Borts, 1949b). Subsequent reports described the LE factor binding to nuclear components, including RNPs and histones. The identification of anti-nuclear antibodies (Baugh et al, 1960; Hahn, 1998) later replaced the LE cell as a diagnostic test, and switched the focus of lupus research from neutrophils to B cells, which now seems to switch back again (see below, NETosis).

2. Types of cell death

In human adults, billions of cells die every day as part of the body's natural processes. Cells that become damaged by microbial infection or mechanical stress also die. The cell death that occurs in the physiological setting is programmed (Nagata et al, 2010).

Four different cell-death processes (apoptosis, cornification, necrosis, and autophagy) have been officially proposed (Kroemer et al., 2009). In apoptosis, the cell and nuclei condense and become fragmented and are engulfed by phagocytes (Kerr et al., 1972). Apoptosis is the major death process, but necrosis and autophagic cell death have also been proposed to play roles in programmed cell death (Kroemer et al., 2009). Dying cells secrete a "find me" signal, and they expose an "eat me" signal on their surface. In response to the "find me" signal, macrophages approach the dead cells; they then recognize the "eat me" signal (Ravichandran and Lorenz, 2007).

The machinery used for the engulfment and degradation of the extruded nuclei appears similar to that used for the removal of apoptotic cells. Mice deficient in the engulfment of apoptotic cells develop SLE-type autoimmune diseases (Hanayama et al., 2004). A defect in the degradation of the chromosomal DNA from engulfed cells in mice activates macrophages, leading to lethal anemia in embryos and chronic arthritis in adults (Kawane et al., 2001; Kawane et al., 2006). These observations indicate that dead cells and the nuclei expelled from erythroid precursor cells need to be swiftly cleared for animals to maintain homeostasis.

2.1 High mobility group box 1 (HMGB1)

In 1999, K.J. Tracey and colleagues discovered that the abundant chromatin-associated protein HMGB1 is secreted by activated macrophages during inflammation, and plays a critical role as a late mediator of lethal endotoxemia and sepsis (Wang et al, 1999). Since this initial report, the cytokine activity of HMGB1 has been confirmed by many groups and HMGB1 has now been proposed to be a crucial mediator in the pathogenesis of many diseases including sepsis, arthritis, and cancer (Erlandsson Harris and Andersson, 2004; Dumitriu et al, 2005; Ulloa and Messmer, 2006).

HMGB1 is an intracellular protein that when present in the extracellular milieu acts as a "necrotic marker" for the immune system. Recent studies indicate that damaged or necrotic cells can release HMGB1 into the extracellular milieu, where it triggers inflammatory responses. In contrast to necrosis, cells undergoing programmed cell death or apoptosis induce negligible inflammation in the surrounding tissue (Yang et al, 2004), which is attributed in part, to the retention of HMGB1 within the apoptotic cells (Kokkola, 2003). Indeed, there are two mechanisms for cells to liberate HMGB1 into the extracellular milieu . The first mechanism is a "passive release" of HMGB1 from damaged or necrotic cells: extracellular HMGB1 acts as an immune-stimulatory signal that indicates the extent of tissue injury (Wang et al, 2004; Yang, 2004), promotes the recruitment of mononuclear cells to clear cellular debris and protects against possible infection that often follows trauma (Carriere et al, 2007). The second mechanism is an "active secretion" of HMGB1 from immune cells to act as a pro-inflammatory cytokine during an immunological challenge.

IL-33, the most recent addition to the IL-1 family, is a potent proinflammatory cytokine that induces production of Th2-associated cytokines IL-4, IL-5, and IL-13, both in vitro and in vivo (Schmitz, 2005). Surprisingly, IL-33 has also been described as an abundant chromatin associated nuclear factor, which associates with mitotic chromosomes in living cells and with interphase chromatin in the nucleus of endothelial cells in vivo (Baekkevold, 2003). IL-33 therefore constitutes a second example of a chromatin associated cytokine (Yamada, 2007).

2.2 NETosis

Neutrophils in circulation are directed by cytokines into infected tissues, where they encounter invading microbes. This encounter leads to the activation of neutrophils and the engulfment of the pathogen into a phagosome. In the phagosome, two events are required for antimicrobial activity. First, the presynthesized subunits of the NADPH oxidase assemble at the phagosomal membrane and transfer electrons to oxygen to form superoxide anions. Second, the granules fuse with the phagosome, discharging antimicrobial peptides and enzymes. Together, they are responsible for microbial killing (Klebanoff, 1999). Patients with mutations in the NADPH oxidase suffer from chronic granulomatous disease (CGD; Heyworth et al., 2003).

Upon activation, neutrophils release extra cellular traps (neutrophil extracellular traps [NETs]; Brinkmann et al., 2004). NETs are composed of chromatin decorated with granular proteins, including LL-37, antibiotic peptides, neutrophil peptides and nuclear proteins, e.g. histones and HMGB1. These structures bind Gram-positive and -negative bacteria. Activated neutrophils initiate a process where first the classical lobulated nuclear morphology and the distinction between eu- and hetero-chromatin are lost. Later, all the internal membranes disappear, allowing NET components to mix. Finally, NETs emerge from the cell as the cytoplasmic membrane is ruptured by a process that is distinct from necrosis or apoptosis. This active process is dependent on the generation of ROS by NADPH oxidase (Fuchs et al., 2007). With the loss of nuclear and granular membranes, the decondensed chromatin comes into direct contact with cytoplasmic and granular

components. 120 min after activation the granular marker neutrophil elastase colocalizes with chromatin. NETs were detected after PMA activation, but not after incubation with Fas antibody (inducing apoptosis) or treatment with *S. aureus* toxins (inducing necrosis).
Together, these data indicate that neither apoptosis nor necrosis lead to NET formation, and that NET-inducing cell death is different from both apoptosis and necrosis by morphological and molecular criteria. A hitherto unknown form of active cell death apparently evolved to allow neutrophils to kill microbes post mortem. In this form of cell death, the potent cationic antimicrobial peptides and proteins of neutrophils are mixed with chromatin and released to form NETs. Interestingly, the generation of ROS by NADPH oxidase is required for efficient phagocytic killing, and ROS act as a second messenger to trigger NET formation (Lande et al, 2011).
Importantly, in this form of cell death DNA fragmentation is not activated, allowing the chromatin to unfold in the extracellular space. NETs can bind and kill microbes by providing a high local concentration of antimicrobial peptides and, at the same time, minimize tissue damage by sequestering the noxious granule enzymes (Fuchs et al, 2007). Therefore, intact nucleosomes decorated with antimicrobial peptides and nuclear proteins may be released in NETosis, whose dysregulation has been postulated to represent a critical event in SLE pathogenesis (Craft, 2011).

3. Cell death as driving force for autoantibodies production

Phagocytes engulf dead cells, which are recognized as dead by virtue of a characteristic "eat me" signal exposed on their surface. Inefficient engulfment of dead cells activates the immune system, causing disease (such as SLE). The molecular details of these processes have been recently superbly reviewed in Cell (Nagata, 2010).
During apoptosis, the asymmetric distribution of phospholipids of the plasma membrane gets lost and phosphatidylserine (PS) is translocated to the outer leaflet of the plasma membrane. There, PS acts as one major "eat me" signal that ensures efficient recognition and uptake of apoptotic cells by phagocytes. PS recognition of activated phagocytes induces the secretion of anti-inflammatory cytokines like interleukin-10 (Fadok, 2001). Accumulation of dead cells containing nuclear autoantigens in sites of immune selection may provide survival signals for autoreactive B-cells.
The production of antibodies against nuclear structures determines the initiation of chronic autoimmunity in systemic lupus erythematosus. Various soluble molecules and biophysical properties of the surface of apoptotic cells play significant roles in the appropriate recognition and further processing of dying and dead cells. High mobility group box 1 (HMGB1), C-reactive protein (CRP), and anti-nuclear autoantibodies may contribute to the etiopathogenesis of the disease (Craft, 2011).

3.1 Autoantibodies in SLE

Patients with SLE have autoantibodies in their sera against nuclear components (anti-ribonucleoprotein and anti-DNA antibodies) and sometimes exhibit circulating DNA or nucleosomes (Rumore and Steinman, 1990). As unengulfed apoptotic cells are present in the germinal centers of the lymph nodes of some SLE patients and macrophages from these patients often show a reduced ability to engulf apoptotic cells, a deficiency in the clearance of apoptotic cells is proposed to be one of the causes of SLE (Gaipl et al., 2006). Apoptotic corps are disposed by phagocytes (Savill, 1994) and show immunosuppressive activity (Voll,

1997) and recently are reported to be conducive to generation of B regulatory cells (see below) (Gray 2007).

There is increasing evidence that in systemic lupus erythematosus, nucleosomes, the basic chromatin component, represent both a driving immunogen and a major in vivo target for antibodies (Casciola-Rosen, 1994; Huggins et al, 1999). Either a disturbed apoptosis or a reduced clearance of apoptotic cells by phagocytes may lead to an increased exposure of apoptotic nucleosomes protected by HMGB1, to the immune system (Urbonaviciute et al., 2008). One possible new source of HMGB1-nucleosome complexes is thought to derive from NETosis (Lande, 2011; Garcia-Romo, 2011).

3.2 The Fas/FasL pathway of apoptosis in SLE

Apoptosis is activated by two pathways, the intrinsic and extrinsic pathways (Ow et al., 2008). Fas ligand (FasL), tumor necrosis factor (TNF), and TRAIL (TNF-related apoptosis-inducing ligand) are type II membrane proteins that can activate the extrinsic death pathway (Krammer, 2000; Nagata, 1997; Strasser et al., 2009). The binding of FasL to its receptor (Fas) induces the formation of the death inducing signaling complex (DISC), consisting of Fas, an adaptor protein (FADD), and procaspase 8. Formation of the DISC leads to the processing and activation of caspase 8. In both the intrinsic and extrinsic pathways, apoptosis is completed by the cleavage of a set of cellular proteins (more than 500 substrates) by effector caspases (caspases 3 and 7) (Lüthi and Martin, 2007; Timmer and Salvesen, 2007).

Fas is a 43 kDa glycoprotein molecule which is involved in inducing apoptosis in both B and T lymphocytes (Singh, 1995). In the murine MRL/lpr/lpr model of systemic lupus erythematosus (SLE), the lymphoproliferation (lpr) mutation results in defective transcription of the gene that codes for the Fas protein. MRL mice which carry the homozygous recessive lpr mutation develop a severe early-onset genetically predetermined autoimmune syndrome. Susceptibility to SLE is found to be associated with many genes (see Table 1), one of which is APO-1/Fas gene, which is present on chromosome 10 in humans (Singh et al, 2009). The APO-1/Fas promoter contains consensus sequences for binding of several transcription factors that affect the intensity of Fas expression in cells. The mutations in the APO-1/Fas promoter are associated with risk and severity in various autoimmune diseases. A decreased rate of apoptosis may possibly be related also to elevated levels of soluble Fas (sFas) which can inhibit Fas mediated apoptosis of lymphocytes (Kruse et al, 2010).

GENETIC	TYPE I IFN *(Irf-5, etc)*	TLRs (7 to 9)	B cell R and activation	Apoptotic control and disposal
FACTORS	Complement factors (classical/alternate)	NETs control	CD4 activation	*ITGAM* *FcGRII*

Table 1. Possible genetic loci controlling SLE predisposition; they include antigen presentation, IFN type-I production by pDCs, activation of autoreactive T and B cells and neutrophils, complement cascade and nucleic acid sensing and antibody signalling.

In overwhelming majority of situations alterations in Fas and FasL expression are viewed in frames of Fas-mediated apoptosis (Tinazzi et al, 2009; Nozawa, 1997). Telegina et al. (2008) tested a possible involvement of Fas-ligand-mediated "reverse signaling" in the pathogenesis of autoimmune diseases such as rheumatoid arthritis (RA) and SLE. The results indicated that high level of sFas in RA patient blood correlates with a high activity of disease; in SLE patients with elevated sFas level there was a correlation between sFas concentration and tissue and organ damage. In serum sFas is present in oligomeric form (Tokano, 1996). Oligomeric sFas demonstrated cytotoxicity in lymphocyte primary culture and in transformed cells, while non-toxic recombinant Fas-ligand partially blocked this effect (Telegina, 2008). Levels of sFas correlated with the percentages of activated B cells defined as CD20(+)CD38(+) cells. Serum levels of sFas correlate with percentages of activated B cells but not with that of activated T cells (Bijl, 1998). There is a significant correlation between serum concentrations of sFas and serum IL-18 in SLE patients (Sahebari, 2010). sFas and TNFα serum levels are increased in SLE patients (Miret et al, 2001). sFas levels seems to be secondary to TNFα action, which is enhanced in inflammatory conditions such as SLE. Bcl-2 antigen expression and IL-10 serum levels are related to the maintenance of SLE activity. These alterations may interfere with the apoptotic process.

3.2.1 Role of Fas/FasL in SLE

Fas ligand (FasL), an apoptosis-inducing member of the TNF cytokine family, and its receptor Fas are critical for the shutdown of chronic immune responses and prevention of autoimmunity. Accordingly, mutations in their genes cause severe lymphadenopathy and autoimmune disease in mice and humans. FasL function is regulated by deposition in the plasma membrane and metalloprotease-mediated shedding. mFasL is essential for cytotoxic activity and constitutes the guardian against lymphadenopathy, autoimmunity and cancer, whereas excess sFasL appears to promote autoimmunity (O'Reilly et al., 2009). Lymphocytes from aged autoimmune MRL/lpr mice overexpress Fas ligand (FasL), and are cytotoxic against Fas+ target cells. This cytotoxic potential is only partly due to FasL, as wild-type MRL+/+ lymphocytes are not able to kill Fas+ targets after induction of FasL (Hadj-Slimane et al, 2004). IFN alpha, which is increased in SLE, induces overexpression of Fas on lymphocyte surface of lpr mice.

In healthy subjects, more memory than naive T lymphocytes undergo TNF alpha-induced apoptosis. By contrast, in patients with SLE, more naive T cells undergo apoptosis with TNFalpha (Habib et al, 2009). Enhanced apoptosis of T cells in SLE seems to be independent of disease activity or medication. Finally, inhibition experiments showed that apoptosis in the presence of TNFalpha was only partly blocked by anti-FasL antibody (Habib, 2009). Another study showed that mFas expression levels were significantly higher among SLE patients than in healthy controls, and the expression levels had a positive correlation with the early apoptosis rate of mononuclear cells in SLE patients (Li et al, 2009).

Data from several studies demonstrate increasing serum concentrations of the soluble molecules sFas and sFasL starting the first days after birth, indicating possibly a gradual decrease of apoptosis in early neonatal life (Telegina, 2009). In our study (Turi et al., 2009) SLE patients with lower ratios of sFas/sFasL in their sera were of younger age, and had a shorter disease duration (as calculated by the time from diagnosis) and also shorter duration of therapy and/or less organ damage. This pointed to the association of the index with age, which resulted to be strongly correlated with this parameter. Therefore the main variable associated with changes of the sFas/sFasL ratio is the age of the subjects.

Neutrophil apoptosis was significantly increased in patients with juvenile-onset SLE as compared with the noninflamed controls (Midgley et al, 2009). Concentrations of TRAIL and FasL were significantly increased in sera from patients with juvenile-onset SLE, but formation of NETs was not assessed in this study. Finally, it has been reported that SLE serum is capable of inducing apoptosis independent of Fas or TNF-R (Bengtsson et al, 2008).

3.3 Type I Interferons and apoptosis

Type I IFN (IFN-I) was firstly described in 1957 as a soluble factor responsible for viral resistance in vitro. IFN-I can be considered a "director" of protective immune responses (Sozzani et al, 2010). The recent finding of the so-called interferon signature in patients suffering from different autoimmune diseases has underlined its possible role in the pathogenesis of these diseases (Obermoser and Pascual, 2010). Type I IFN has immunoregulatory functions by affecting cell proliferation and by inducing antiinflammatory responses (Cantaert et al, 2010).

pDCs, specialized type I IFN producers, significantly enhance autoreactive B cell proliferation, autoantibody production, and survival in response to TLR and BCR stimulation (Thibault, 2009). IFNAR2-/- B cells fail to upregulate nucleic acid-sensing Toll-like receptors TLR7 as well as TLR9 expression in response to IFN-I (Ding et al, 2009). In addition, serum levels of IFN-alpha increase in parallel with the Fas-dependent cytotoxic potential of lymphocytes from MRL/lpr mice as they age (Hadj-Slimane, 2004). MRL/lpr lymphocytes overexpressed mRNA for the IFN-alpha receptor (IFNAR-1 and IFNAR-2) chains of the IFN-I receptor and exhibited high endogenous levels of phosphorylated Stat1. These data suggest that IFN-alpha plays an important role in the SLE-like syndrome occurring in MRL/lpr mice, and link aberrant apoptosis caused by FasL to high levels of IFN-I.

It has been found that type 1 IFNs protect human B cells in culture from spontaneous apoptosis and from apoptosis mediated by anti-CD95 agonist, in a dose- and time-dependant manner (Badr et al, 2010). Such effect on human B cells was totally abrogated by blockade of IFNR1 chain. PI3Kδ, Rho-A, NFκB and Bcl-2/Bcl_{XL} are active downstream of IFN receptors and are the major effectors of IFN-I-rescued B cells from apoptosis. Furthermore, marked reduction in numbers of CD20 positive B cell in both spleen and Peyer's patches was seen in mice treated with anti-IFNR1. Type I IFNs can stimulate B-cell proliferation and differentiation into antibody-secreting plasma cells, and differentiation of immature monocytes into antigen presenting dendritic cells. These dendritic cells can activate autoreactive lymphocytes and promote autoantibody production (Ding, 2009). These functions of type I IFN, coupled with impaired clearance of apoptotic debris in SLE patients, promote formation of immune complexes, which are potent inducers of type I IFN (Craft, 2011). Inappropriate IFN production and/or an inability to dampen IFN responses thus may initiate a positive feedback loop, resulting in perpetuation of the autoimmune response.

4. B cell phenotypes in SLE

4.1 B lymphocytes development

Cells that have recently emerged from the bone marrow and have yet to acquire follicular markers such as IgD and CD23, but that express very low levels of CD21 and invariably express high levels of CD24 and AA4.1, are called T1 or newly formed (NF) B cells (Carsetti, 2004a). These cells do not require BAFF (B cell–activating factor of the TNF family) for their survival (Schneider, 2001), but like all B cells they depend on signals from the BCR for survival (Kraus, 2004; Hardy and Hayakawa, 2001). These cells, after emerging from the marginal sinus, mature and are drawn into follicles following a CXCL13 gradient (Pillai,

2008), initially become transitional follicular B cells, and eventually give rise to at least two lineages of B cells, mature FO B cells and MZ B cells. Transitional follicular B cells can be subdivided into two distinct categories. NF (newly formed)/T1 (transitional stage 1) B cells are believed to differentiate into T2-FP (transitional stage 2-follicular precursors), which may either differentiate into mature FO B cells or sequentially into T2-MZP (transitional stage 2-MZ B cell precursors) or MZ (marginal zone) B cells (Cariappa and Pillai, 2002).

Although MZ B cells are defined primarily on the basis of their anatomical localization (Martin and Kearney, 2002), the surface expression of a number of markers can also be used to characterize these cells. In rodents the only secondary lymphoid organ in which cells bearing surface markers characteristic of MZ B cells are normally found is the spleen. Unlike follicular B cells that express high levels of IgD and CD23, with either high or low levels of IgM, MZ B cells express high levels of IgM and very low levels of IgD and CD23 (Oliver, 1999). They also express higher levels of CD21 (complement receptor type II), CD1d (an MHC class Ib protein linked to the presentation of lipid antigens), CD38 (an ADP-ribosyl cyclase), CD9 (a scavenger receptor family protein), and CD25 (the α chain of the IL-2 receptor) than those on follicular B cells. MZ B cells also express higher levels of B7 proteins than do follicular B cells and overall are described as having an "activated" phenotype (Oliver, 1997).

4.1.1 Transitional B cells

To identify human transitional B cells, two developmentally regulated markers, CD24 and CD38, are used in combination with the B-lineage marker CD19. In the peripheral blood, all cells of the B lineage (CD19pos) coexpress CD24 and CD38, and, conversely, all non-B cells (CD19neg) lack CD24. (Carsetti, 2004b) Three populations of B cells can be discriminated based on the relative distribution of CD24 and CD38. The CD24brightCD38neg population includes 60% of all B cells and only 2% expressed high levels of both CD24 and CD38 (CD24brightCD38bright). To distinguish mature from memory B cells, the expression of CD27 (a marker of memory cells) can be studied in the three populations. Essentially all CD24brightCD38neg cells are memory B cells, and mature B cells correspond to the CD24dullCD38pos population. CD24brightCD38bright cells lack CD27 (Carsetti 2004 a, b). The analysis of IgM and IgD in the CD24brightCD38bright population shows that transitional B cells coexpress IgM and IgD. IL-10 produced by B cells can downregulate autoimmune disease in EAE (Fillatreau et al., 2002), collagen-induced arthritis (Mauri et al., 2003), and inflammatory bowel disease (Mizoguchi et al., 2002). IL-10-deficient (Il10-/-) mice also have enhanced hypersensitivity responses (Berg et al., 1995). Neutralizing IL-10 by monoclonal antibody (mAb) treatment also enhances these responses, whereas systemic IL-10 administration reduces them (Ferguson et al., 1994; Schwarz et al., 1994). IL-10 is secreted by multiple cell types, including T cells, monocytes, macrophages, mast cells, eosinophils, and keratinocytes, and can suppress both Th1 and Th2 polarization (Yanaba, 2008) and inhibit macrophage antigen presentation and proinflammatory cytokine production (Asadullah et al., 2003). Thus, B cells and IL-10 play important inhibitory roles during T cell-mediated inflammatory responses.

4.1.2 Negative regulation by B cells

B cells have been recently shown to negatively regulate autoimmunity and inflammation in numerous mouse models (Bouaziz, 2008). Mizoguchi and Bhan (2006) were the first to use the term 'regulatory B cells' to designate B cells with regulatory properties. Suppressor/regulatory B-cell populations have predominantly been identified using diverse mouse models of autoimmune diseases, suggesting that autoimmunity itself promotes the expansion of these cells as a compensatory mechanism to limit self-directed inflammation.

Immunological tolerance exemplifies the capacity of the immune system to downmodulate host immune responses (Shevach, 2000). Several regulatory T-cell subsets have been identified that contribute to immunological tolerance, including naturally arising CD4+CD25+Forkhead box protein 3 (FoxP3)+ regulatory T cells (Sakaguchi, 2004) and T-regulatory type 1 cells that produce high amounts of interleukin-10 (Groux, 1997). B cells are generally considered to be positive regulators of immune responses.

Whether negative regulation is a general property of B cells induced as a consequence of normal B-cell activation or whether only a specific subset of B cells posses this property has also been unknown. However, it has been recently shown that regulatory B cells are a phenotypically unique (CD1dhi CD5+) and rare subset of B cells in the spleens of naı¨ve wildtype mice that can significantly influence T-cell activation and some inflammatory responses (Yanaba, 2008). This specific subset of regulatory B cells only produces IL-10 and is responsible for most IL-10 production by B cells. Other regulatory B-cell subsets that may also exist (Mauri and Ehrestein, 2008, Bouaziz, 2008).

Stimulation of arthritogenic B cells with an agonistic anti-CD40 and collagen generated a subset of B cells producing IL-10 (Mauri, 2007). Transfer of collagen and anti-CD40-stimulated Bcells to syngeneic immunized mice prevented the induction of arthritis and ameliorated established disease. This suppressive effect was associated with a downregulation of Th1 cytokines and was dependent upon the release of IL-10 because B cells isolated from IL-10- deficient mice stimulated with collagen and anti-CD40 failed to suppress disease (Mauri et al, 2007). The engagement of CD40 on B cells is also a principal requirement for the generation of Bregs in EAE. Additional in vivo results have shown that MZ B cells participate in the suppression of systemic lupus erythematosus (Lenert et al, 2005). After anti-CD40 treatment an increase of IL-10 production and a decrease of IFN-gamma release was observed (Mauri, 2000) so it was suggested that the therapeutic effect observed after administration of anti-CD40, could have been achieved by redirecting pathogenic Th1 type response toward the "protective" Th2 type (Harris et al, 2000). These data show that the dialogue between B and T cells during an (auto)-immune response is not one sided and demonstrate that B cells have a strong impact in conditioning T cell differentiation.

4.2 Breg phenotype(s)

Further phenotypical identification showed that the majority of CD19+CD38hiCD24hi B cells were also IgMhiIgDhiCD5+CD10+CD20+CD27-CD1dhi (Blair et al, 2010). Interestingly, the majority of the CD19+CD5+CD1dhiB cells (71%), previously reported to be regulatory in experimental models of inflammation (Matsushita et al., 2008; Yanaba et al., 2008a), are contained within the CD24hiCD38hi B cell subset. Co-culture of CD4+ T cells with CD19+CD24hiCD38hi B cells significantly suppressed the frequencies of CD4+IFN-γ+ and CD4+TNF-α+ T cells.

The group of Mauri evaluated whether there was a numerical deficit in CD19+CD38hiCD24hi B cells in patients with SLE (Blair et al, 2010). The absolute cell numbers were not statistically different from controls. In contrast, the numbers of both CD19+CD38intCD24int and CD19+CD24hiCD38- B cells were both significantly reduced in

SLE patients. These results suggest that the inability of SLE CD19+CD38hiCD24hi B cells to suppress the expression of proinflammatory cytokines by CD4+ T cells is unlikely to be due to a numerical deficiency. Depleting CD19+ CD38hiCD24hi B cells from PBMCs of healthy donors and SLE patients leads to an increased production of inflammatory cytokines such as IFN gamma and TNF alpha in healthy donors, suggesting an immunoregulatory effect, but this was not observed in SLE patients.

4.3 Other novel B cell subsets

A novel subset of circulating memory B cells with >2-fold higher levels of CD19 [CD19(hi) B cells] correlates with long-term adverse outcomes in SLE (Nicholas et al, 2008). These B cells do not appear anergic, as they exhibit high basal levels of phosphorylated Syk and ERK1/2, signal transduce in response to BCR crosslinking, and can become plasma cells in vitro. Autoreactive anti-Smith (Sm) B cells are enriched within this subset. Quantitative genetic variation in CD19 expression correlates with autoimmunity (Sato et al, 2000). CD19(hi) B cells have elevated CXCR3 levels and chemotax in response to its ligand CXCL9. Thus, CD19(hi) B cells are precursors to anti-self PCs, and identify an SLE patient subset likely to experience poor clinical outcomes (Nicholas, 2008). CD19(hi)CD21(lo/neg) B cells of uncertain origin are expanded also in common variable immunodeficiency patients with autoimmune features (Warnatz et al, 2002).

B cell functions are under the regulation of B cell antigen receptor (BCR)-induced signals and by specialized cell surface coreceptors, or "response regulators", which inform B cells of their microenvironment. These response regulators include CD19 and CD22 (Fujimoto and Sato, 2007). Importantly, this “CD19/CD22 loop" is significantly related to an autoimmune phenotype in mice. Thus, the CD19/CD22 loop may be a potential therapeutic target. Regulatory B cells that produce IL-10 are now recognized as an important component of the immune system .

4.4 Role of TLR 7 and 9

A previously uncharacterized population of B cells has been recently described in aged mice, called Age-associated B cells (ABCs), which express integrin α_X chain CD11c (Rubtsov et al, 2011). This subset is present also in young lupus-prone mice. Upon stimulation, $CD11c^+$ B cells secrete autoantibodies and depletion of these cells *in vivo* leads to reduction of autoreactive antibodies. Toll-like receptor 7 (TLR7) is crucial for development of this B cell population. A similar population of B cells was observed in elderly women with autoimmune disease (Rubtsov et al, 2011). Age-associated mature B cells have been described also by Hao et al (2011): they are refractory to BCR and CD40 stimulation but respond to TLR9 or TLR7 stimulation and divide maximally upon combined BCR and TLR ligation, leading to Ig production and preferential secretion of IL-10. They derive from normal mature B cells but have lost the need of BLyS for survival. Finally, they present antigen effectively and favor polarization to a TH17 profile. It has been reported four years ago (Treml, 2007) that TLR9 stimulates TACI expression in all follicular and marginal zone B cells, but only BLyS enhances survival in TLR stimulated B cells. Following the exit from the bone marrow, peripheral B cells develop through transitional type 1 (T1) and transitional type 2 (T2) B-cell stages. Emerging data suggest that the T2 subset is the immediate precursor of the mature B-cell populations. T2 cells uniquely activate a proliferative, pro-survival, and differentiation program in response to B-cell antigen receptor (BCR) engagement. The type of signal(s) encountered by T2 cells lead to their differential maturation toward the follicular mature versus marginal zone mature B-cell populations (Su et al, 2004).

Among the principal targets of autoantibodies produced in murine SLE are nucleic acid-protein complexes, such as chromatin and ribonucleoproteins, and the envelope glycoprotein gp70 of endogenous retroviruses. The preferential production of these autoantibodies is apparently promoted by the presence of genetic abnormalities leading to defects in the elimination of apoptotic cells and to an enhanced expression of endogenous retroviruses. Moreover, recent studies revealed that the innate receptors TLR7 and TLR9 are critically involved in the activation of dendritic cells and autoreactive B cells through the recognition of endogenous DNA- or RNA-containing antigens and subsequent development of autoimmune responses against nuclear autoantigens (Santiago-Raber et al, 2009). Furthermore, the regulation of autoimmune responses against endogenous retroviral gp70 by TLR7 suggested the implication of endogenous retroviruses in this autoimmune response. Clearly, further elucidation of the precise molecular role of TLR7 and TLR9 in the development of autoimmune responses will help to develop novel therapeutic strategies and targets for SLE (Goeken et al, 2010).

4.5 Relationship of B1 to Breg cells

B1 cells constitute a specialized B cell lineage with remarkable properties that include spontaneous secretion of immunoglobulin, autoreactive repertoire skewing, focused memory characteristics, abnormal receptor signaling, induction of Th17 cell differentiation, and production of immunomodulatory IL-10. A particularly exciting issue is the relationship of B1 cells to regulatory B cells and the extent to which these cell types may be one and the same (Cancro, 2009).

Colonna-Romano et al (2009) describe the IgD^-CD27^- double-negative B cell population which is increased in the elderly. Most of these cells are IgG^+. Evaluation of the telomere length and expression of the ABCB1 transporter and anti-apoptotic molecule, Bcl2, shows that they have the markers of memory B cells. These cells do not act as antigen presenting cells, as indicated by the low levels of CD80 and DR, nor do they express significant levels of the CD40 molecule necessary to interact with T lymphocytes through the ligand, CD154 (Duffau et al, 2010). The authors hypothesize that these expanded cells are late memory or exhausted cells that have down-modulated the expression of CD27.

It is interesting to note that platelets are the main source of circulating CD154, and they can stimulate IFN typeI production from pDCs as well as ligate CD40 on autoreactive B cells (Duffau et al, 2010; Craft, 2011).

5. SLE as the result of defects both in apoptosis control and B cell regulation

Recent data have emerged to support the role of IFN alpha in both control of cell death and regulation of B lymphocyte functions. Two papers (Lande, 2011; Garcia-Romo, 2011) have reported the induction of neutrophil changes due to autoantibodies to DNA or RNA in immune complexes interacting with FcγRIIa as well as TLRs in the presence of inflammatory cytokines and IFN type I, resulting in the formation of NETs which represent a type of cell death with DNA extrusion and release of antimicrobial peptides and cytolytic enzymes that is very effective in defence against bacteria.

5.1 Neutrophils, NETosis and B cells

SLE neutrophils undergo accelerated spontaneous apoptosis in vitro, and SLE sera induce the apoptosis of healthy neutrophils, and nuclear material such as DNA and histones, which comprises the major structural components of NETs, is released in immunogenic form. The inappropriate amplification of this phenomenon in SLE perpetuates B cell stimulation to produce anti-DNA and -RNA antibodies, as well as autoantibodies to antibiotic peptides, and also, via TLR 7 and 9 interactions, IFN alpha production by pDC (Craft, 2011). IFNα in turn primes neutrophils for death with NET formation, which makes more immunogenic DNA and RNA available to the immune system. Both IFN-α and SLE serum up-regulate neutrophil TLR7 expression. In addition, sera from ~40% of SLE patients contain TLR7 ligands in the form of ICs derived from antibodies recognizing small nuclear RNA/RNA binding protein complexes. These ICs have been shown to activate pDCs and induce type I IFN secretion. Anti-RNP antibodies are not efficient activators of pDCs in vitro, however, unless combined with dying cells, which provide the substrate to form ICs that might be internalized via FcγRIIa.

Anti-RNP Ig-induced SLE NETosis requires FcγRIIa and endosomal TLR7 signaling and depends on the formation of ROS. Furthermore, anti-RNP antibodies induce SLE but not healthy neutrophils to secrete high levels of LL37 and HMGB1, two endogenous proteins that contribute to increase the immunogenicity and uptake of mammalian DNA by pDCs. Therefore other sources of immunogenic nuclear material has to be present, and this is provided by increased apoptosis, mostly due to Fas/FasL dysregulation, and inefficient disposal of IC due to complement and reticulo-endothelial defects.

5.2 Fas/FasL dysregulation in SLE

The Fas(CD95) antigen and its ligand (FasL, CD95L) are members of the TNF/TNFR families, expressed on the surface of immune and other cell types. They regulate one important extrinsic apoptotic pathway, by higher or lower expression and by their splice or cleaved soluble variants, sFas and sFasL (Sheriff et al., 2004; Tinazzi et al., 2009). Peripheral T cell apoptosis is upregulated in active SLE, in parallel with high expression of both membrane-bound and soluble Fas (Silvestris et al., 2003; Hao et al., 2006). Previous studies postulated that sFas down-regulates apoptosis in vitro through its blockade of the FasL of cytotoxic cells. This paradox has been examined by Silvestris et al. (2003) and Hao et al. (2006), but it is still unresolved. The situation is even more complex since autoantibodies to FasL have been detected in sera of SLE patients which contribute to inhibit apoptotic cell death of lymphocytes (Suzuki et al., 1998). In our study (Turi et al, 2009) we confirmed that though slightly increased values of both sFas and sFasL are found in SLE patients compared to normal subjects, a very scattered distribution is observed. No definitive answer to the importance of these differences may derive from examining one factor when many contribute to the final effect, so we decided to derive and index from the ratio of the values of sFas to sFasL, which is about 50 in normal controls. This ratio has been found to be lower in younger subjects, being related to age, both in SLE patients and healthy controls. Apoptosis resistance is modulated during aging, and the changes in the sFas/sFasL ratio may be involved in this phenomenon. As clarified by the study by O'Reilly (2009), sFasL does not efficiently mediate Fas-induced apoptosis, therefore its increase in serum equals to an additive anti-apoptotic mechanism in conjunction with elevated sFas circulating levels and autoantibodies to FasL.

6. Conclusion

Systemic lupus erythematosus (SLE) is a chronic autoimmune disease characterized by the production of high-titer IgG autoantibodies directed against nuclear autoantigens. Type I interferon (IFN-I) has been shown to play an important pathogenic role in this disease. Common hypotheses about SLE pathogenesis suggest that environmental triggers, such as infectious agents, operate in the context of both susceptibility genes and epigenetic modifications, resulting in alterations in antigen presentation, lymphoid signaling, apoptosis, and antigen/IC clearance. Decreased numbers of neutrophils, dendritic cells, and lymphocytes are common features of SLE. pDCs accumulate at sites of inflammation such as the skin and the kidney, where they secrete type I interferon (IFN). Upon exposure to SLE serum, healthy monocytes differentiate into mature DCs in an IFN-I–dependent fashion. SLE display a type I IFN signature as measured by peripheral blood mononuclear cell (PBMC) gene expression profiling. The second most prevalent PBMC transcriptional signature corresponds to neutrophil-specific genes, and differential expression of these genes correlates with disease activity. Indeed, polymorphisms in genes expressed by neutrophils, such as ITGAM/CD11b, rank among the highest in the scale of SLE susceptibility. Polymorphisms in genes along the IFN and TLR signaling pathways (that is, IRF5, TLR7, IRAK1, STAT4, etc.) could amplify the response of SLE neutrophils to TLR7 triggering. Polymorphisms affecting thresholds of B cell activation and/or deficient removal of ICs might contribute to prolonged neutrophil exposure to activating ICs. Polymorphisms in FcgRIIa could affect the internalization and/or endosomal trafficking of SLE-specific ICs in neutrophils and pDCs.

Our review has highlighted some recent aspects of the main points relating to these issues, both at the cellular and molecular level, with discussion of the role of NETs formation, TLR 7/9 signaling, apoptosis increased proneness, and the induction both of autoantibodies and IFN-I overproduction. The consequences of these pathogenetic changes are then defined in terms of autoantigens presentation, B lymphocyte dysregulation and IC formation with organ damage. We mainly studied the alterations occurring at quantitative and functional level in the Fas/FasL apoptotic pathway, but also touched upon several other issues such as the relationship of newly identified B cell subsets to autoimmunity, and the role of nuclear cytokines in autoantibody stimulation. We believe that the key aspects of SLE pathogenesis have now been uncovered, and await the composition of their temporal sequence in a unified view of this multifaceted systemic autoimmune disorder.

7. Acknowledgments

Studies reported here have been supported by grants of the Faculty of Medicine of Chieti (60%) for 2009-11 and PRIN 2009 from the Italian Ministry of University (MIUR) to R.P. Studies on B reg have been carried out by M.C.T. as part of a PhD Fellowship at the University of Chieti.

8. Note added in proof

Since completion of this chapter, a review was published in the section of Clinical implications of Basic research of the N Engl J Med (Bosch X (2011). Systemic lupus erythematosus and the neutrophil. N Engl J Med 365;8 (Aug.25) 758-60) discussing the work of Lande and Garcia-Romo reviewed here. No mention of HMGB1 is to be found in the review, however much emphasis was put on antimicrobial peptides (LL-37, which is also implicated in psoriasis) and antagonistic molecules for TLR signalling; the main message was on the new therapeutic aspects and the generalization of these findings (of neutrophil NETosis as pathogenetic mechanism) to vasculitis with ANCA antibodies.

9. References

Arbuckle MR, Mc Clain MT, Rubertone MV, Scofield RH, Dennis GJ, James JA, Harley JB (2003). Development of autoantibodies before the clinical onset of systemic lupus erythematosus. N Engl J Med 349:1526-33.

Asadullah, K., Sterry, W., and Volk, H.D. (2003). Interleukin-10 therapy-review of a new approach. Pharmacol. Rev. 55, 241–269.

Badr G, Saad H, Waly H, Hassan K, Abdel-Tawab H, Alhazza IM, Ahmed EA. (2010). Type I interferon (IFN-alpha/beta) rescues B-lymphocytes from apoptosis via PI3Kdelta/Akt, Rho-A, NFkappaB and Bcl-2/Bcl(XL). Cell Immunol. 263:31-40.

Baekkevold, E.S. et al. (2003) Molecular characterization of NF-HEV, a nuclear factor preferentially expressed in human high endothelial venules. Am. J. Pathol. 163, 69–79

Banchereau J., V. Pascual (2006). Type I interferon in systemic lupus erythematosus and other autoimmune diseases. Immunity 25, 383–392

Baugh C. W., P. M. Kirol, M. V. Sachs, (1960). Demonstration and titration of anti-nuclear antibodies in systemic lupus erythematosus. Can. Med. Assoc. J. 83, 571–580.

Bengtsson AA, Gullstrand B, Truedsson L, Sturfelt G. (2008). SLE serum induces classical caspase-dependent apoptosis independent of death receptors. Clin Immunol. 126:57-66.

Bennett L., A. K. Palucka, E. Arce, V. Cantrell, J. Borvak, J. Banchereau, V. Pascual, (2003). Interferon and granulopoiesis signatures in systemic lupus erythematosus blood. J. Exp. Med. 197, 711–723

Berg, D.J., Leach, M.W., Kuhn, R., Rajewsky, K., Muller, W., Davidson, N.J., and Rennick, D. (1995). Interleukin 10 but not interleukin 4 is a natural suppressant of cutaneous inflammatory responses. J. Exp. Med. 182, 99–108.

Bijl M, van Lopik T, Limburg PC, Spronk PE, Jaegers SM, Aarden LA, Smeenk RJ, Kallenberg GG. (1998). Do elevated levels of serum-soluble fas contribute to the persistence of activated lymphocytes in systemic lupus erythematosus? J Autoimmun. 11:457-63.

Blair PA, Noreña LY, Flores-Borja F, Rawlings DJ, Isenberg DA, Ehrenstein MR, Mauri C. (2010). CD19(+) CD24(hi)CD38(hi) B cells exhibit regulatory capacity in healthy individuals but are functionally impaired in systemic Lupus Erythematosus patients. Immunity. 32:129-40.

Blanco P., A. K. Palucka, M. Gill, V. Pascual, J. Banchereau, (2001). Induction of dendritic cell differentiation by IFN-a in systemic lupus erythematosus. Science 294, 1540–1543

Bouaziz JD, Yanaba K, Tedder TF. (2008) Regulatory B cells as inhibitors of immune responses and inflammation. Immunol Rev. 224:201-14.

Brinkmann, V., U. Reichard, C. Goosmann, B. Fauler, Y. Uhlemann, D.S. Weiss, Y. Weinrauch, and A. Zychlinsky. (2004). Neutrophil extracellular traps kill bacteria. *Science*. 303:1532–1535.

Cancro MP, Y Hao, JL. Scholz, RL. Riley, D Frasca, DK. Dunn-Walters, BB. Blomberg (2009) B cells and aging: molecules and mechanisms. *Trends Immunol.* 30: 313–318.

Cantaert T, Baeten D, Tak PP and van Baarsen LGM. (2010). Type I IFN and TNFα cross-regulation in immune-mediated infl ammatory disease: basic concepts and clinical relevance. Arthr Res Ther 12:219.

Cariappa A, Pillai S. (2002). Antigen dependent B-cell development. *Curr Opin Immunol* 14:241–9.

Carriere, V. et al. (2007) IL-33, the IL-1-like cytokine ligand for ST2 receptor, is a chromatin-associated nuclear factor in vivo. Proc. Natl. Acad. Sci. U. S. A. 104, 282–287.

Carsetti R. (2004a) Characterization of B-cell maturation in the peripheral immune system. Methods Mol Biol. 271:25-35.

Carsetti R, Rosado MM, Wardmann H. (2004b) Peripheral development of B cells in mouse and man. Immunol Rev. 197:179-91.

Casciola-Rosen, L. A., G. Anhalt, and A. Rosen. (1994). Autoantigens targeted in systemic lupus erythematosus are clustered in two populations of surface structures on apoptotic keratinocytes. *J. Exp. Med.* 179: 1317–1330.

Colonna-Romano G, M Bulati, A Aquino, M Pellicanò, S Vitello, D Lio, G Candore and C Caruso (2009). A double-negative (IgD−CD27−) B cell population is increased in the peripheral blood of elderly people. Mech Ageing Dev 130: 681-90.

Craft J (2011). Dissecting the immune cell mayhem that drives lupus pathogenesis. Sci Transl Med 3, 73ps9.

Crow M.K. (2008). Collaboration, Genetic Associations, and Lupus Erythematosus. N Engl J Med 358: 956-61.

Ding C, Cai Y, Marroquin J, Ildstad ST, Yan J. (2009). Plasmacytoid dendritic cells regulate autoreactive B cell activation via soluble factors and in a cell-to-cell contact manner. J Immunol. 183:7140-9.

Duffau P., J. Seneschal, C. Nicco, C. Richez, E. Lazaro, I. Douchet, C. Bordes, J.-F. Viallard, C. Goulvestre, J.-L. Pellegrin, B. Weil, J.-F. Moreau, F. Batteux, P. Blanco (2010). Platelet CD154 potentiates interferon-a secretion by plasmacytoid dendritic cells in systemic lupus erythematosus. Sci. Transl. Med. 2, 47ra63.

Dumitriu, I. E., P. Baruah, A. A. Manfredi, M. E. Bianchi, and P. Rovere-Querini. (2005). HMGB1: guiding immunity from within. *Trends Immunol.* 26: 381–387.

Erlandsson Harris, H., and U. Andersson. (2004). Mini-review: the nuclear protein HMGB1 as a proinflammatory mediator. *Eur. J. Immunol.* 34: 1503–1512.

Fadok, V.A., Bratton, D.L., Guthrie, L., and Henson, P.M. (2001). Differential effects of apoptotic versus lysed cells on macrophage production of cytokines: role of proteases. J. Immunol. *166*, 6847–6854.

Ferguson, T.A., Dube, P., and Griffith, T.S. (1994). Regulation of contact hypersensitivity by interleukin 10. J. Exp. Med. 179, 1597–1604.

Fillatreau, S., Sweenie, C.H., McGeachy, M.J., Gray, D., and Anderton, S.M. (2002). B cells regulate autoimmunity by provision of IL-10. Nat. Immunol. 3, 944–950.

Fuchs TA,U Abed, C Goosmann, R Hurwitz, I Schulze, V Wahn, Y Weinrauch, V Brinkmann, A Zychlinsky (2007) Novel cell death program leads to neutrophil extracellular traps. J Cell Biol 176, 231–241.

Fujimoto M, Sato S. (2007). B cell signaling and autoimmune diseases: CD19/CD22 loop as a B cell signalling device to regulate the balance of autoimmunity. J Dermatol Sci. 46:1-9.

Gaipl, U.S., Kuhn, A., Sheriff, A., Munoz, L.E., Franz, S., Voll, R.E., Kalden, J.R., and Herrmann, M. (2006). Clearance of apoptotic cells in human SLE. Curr. Dir. Autoimmun. *9*, 173–187.

Garcia-Romo G.S., S. Caielli, B. Vega, J. Connolly, F. Allantaz, Z. Xu, M. Punaro, J. Baisch, C.Guiducci, R. L.Coffman, F. J.Barrat, J. Banchereau,V. Pascual, (2011). Netting neutrophils are major inducers of type I IFN production in pediatric systemic lupus erythematosus. Sci. Transl. Med. 3, 73ra20

Goeken JA, T Layer, S Fleenor, M Laccheo and P Lenert (2010) B-cell receptor for antigen modulates B-cell responses to complex TLR9 agonists and antagonists: implications for systemic lupus erythematosus. Lupus 19, 1290–1301.

Gray M, Miles K, Salter D, Gray D, Savill J. (2007). Apoptotic cells protect mice from autoimmune inflammation by the induction of regulatory B cells. Proc Natl Acad Sci USA 104:14080–5

Groux, H., A. O'Garra, M. Bigler, M. Rouleau, S. Antonenko, J. E. de Vries, and M. G. Roncarolo. (1997). A CD4+ T cell subset inhibits antigen-specific T cell responses and prevents colitis. *Nature* 389: 737–742.

Habib HM, Taher TE, Isenberg DA, Mageed RA. (2009). Enhanced propensity of T lymphocytes in patients with systemic lupus erythematosus to apoptosis in the presence of tumour necrosis factor alpha. Scand J Rheumatol. 38:112-20.

Hadj-Slimane R, Chelbi-Alix MK, Tovey MG, Bobé P. (2004). An essential role for IFN-alpha in the overexpression of Fas ligand on MRL/lpr lymphocytes and on their spontaneous Fas-mediated cytotoxic potential. J Interferon Cytokine Res. 24:717-28.

Hahn BH (1998). Antibodies to DNA. N Engl J Med 338:1359-68.

Hanayama, R., Tanaka, M., Miyasaka, K., Aozasa, K., Koike, M., Uchiyama, Y., and Nagata, S. (2004). Autoimmune disease and impaired uptake of apoptotic cells in MFG-E8-deficient mice. Science *304*, 1147–1150.

Hao, J.H., Ye, D.Q., Zhang, G.Q., Liu, H.H., Dai, H., Huang, F., Pan, F.M., Su, H., Dong, M.X., Chen, H., Wang, Q., Zhang, X.J. (2006): Elevated levels of serum soluble Fas are associated with organ and tissue damage in systemic lupus erythematosus among Chinese. Arch. Dermatol. Res. 297, 329-332.

Hao Y, O'Neill PJ, Naradikian MS, Scholz JL, Cancro MP. (2011). A B-cell subset uniquely responsive to innate stimuli accumulates in aged mice. Blood. 118:1294-304

Hardy RR, Hayakawa K. (2001). B cell development pathways. *Annu. Rev. Immunol.* 19:595–621

Hargraves M.M., H. Richmond, R. Morton, (1948). Presentation of two bone marrow elements; the tart cell and the L.E. cell. Mayo Clin. Proc. 23, 25–28

Harris, D.P., L. Haynes, P.C. Sayles, D.K. Duso, S.M. Eaton, N.M. Lepak, L.L. Johnson, S.L. Swain, and F.E. Lund. (2000). Reciprocal regulation of polarized cytokine production by effector B and T cells. *Nat. Immunol.* 1:475–482.

Haserick J.R., D. W. Bortz (1949a). A new diagnostic test for acute disseminated lupus erythematosus. Cleve. Clin. Q. 16, 158–161

Haserick J.R., D. W. Bortz, (1949b). Normal bone marrow inclusion phenomena induced by lupus erythematosus plasma. J. Invest. Dermatol. 13, 47–49.

Heyworth, P.G., A.R. Cross, and J.T. Curnutte. (2003). Chronic granulomatous disease. *Curr. Opin. Immunol.* 15:578–584.

Hom G, Graham RR, Modrek B, et al. (2008) Association of systemic lupus erythematosus with *C8orf13–BLK* and *ITGAM–ITGAX*. N Engl J Med 358: 900–909.

Huggins, M. L., I. Todd, M. A. Cavers, S. R. Pavuluri, P. J. Tighe, and R. J. Powell. (1999). Antibodies from systemic lupus erythematosus (SLE) sera define differential release of autoantigens from cell lines undergoing apoptosis. *Clin. Exp. Immunol.*118: 322–328.

International Consortium for Systemic Lupus Erythematosus Genetics, Harley JB, Alarcon-Riquelme ME, et al. (2008). A genomewide association scan in women with systemic lupus erythematosus identifies risk variants in ITGAM, PXK, KIAA1542 and other loci and confirms multiple loci contributing to disease susceptibility. Nat Genet 40, 204–210

Ippolito A., DJ Wallace, D Gladman, PR Fortin, M Urowitz, V Werth, M Costner, C Gordon, GS Alarcón, R et al. (2011) Autoantibodies in systemic lupus erythematosus: comparison of historical and current assessment of seropositivity. Lupus 20, 250–255.

Kawane, K., Fukuyama, H., Kondoh, G., Takeda, J., Ohsawa, Y., Uchiyama, Y., and Nagata, S. (2001). Requirement of DNase II for definitive erythropoiesis in the mouse fetal liver. Science *292*, 1546–1549.

Kawane, K., Ohtani, M., Miwa, K., Kizawa, T., Kanbara, Y., Yoshioka, Y., Yoshikawa, H., and Nagata, S. (2006). Chronic polyarthritis caused by mammalian DNA that escapes from degradation in macrophages. Nature *443*,998–1002.

Kerr, J.F., Wyllie, A.H., and Currie, A.R. (1972). Apoptosis: a basic biological phenomenon with wide-ranging implications in tissue kinetics. Br. J. Cancer *26*, 239–257.

Klebanoff, S.J. (1999). Oxygen metabolites from phagocytes. *In* J.I. Gallin and R. Snyderman, editors. Infl ammation: Basic Principles and Clinical Correlates. Lippincott Williams & Wilkins, Philadelphia. 721–768

Kokkola R, Li J, Sundberg E, Aveberger AC, Palmblad K, Yang H, et al. (2003) Successful treatment of collagen-induced arthritis in mice and rats by targeting extracellular high mobility group box chromosomal protein 1 activity. Arthritis Rheum 48:2052–8.

Kozyrev SV, Abelson A-K, Wojcik J, et al. (2008) Functional variants in the B cell gene BANK1 are associated with systemic lupus erythematosus. Nat Genet 40: 211–216..

Krammer, P.H. (2000). CD95's deadly mission in the immune system. Nature *407*, 789–795.

Kraus M, Alimzhanov MB, Rajewsky N, Rajewsky K. (2004). Survival of resting mature B lymphocytes depends on BCR signaling via the Igα/β heterodimer. *Cell* 117:787–800

Kroemer, G., Galluzzi, L., Vandenabeele, P., Abrams, J., Alnemri, E.S., Baehrecke, E.H., Blagosklonny, M.V., El-Deiry, W.S., Golstein, P., Green, D.R., et al; Nomenclature Committee on Cell Death 2009. (2009). Classification of cell death: recommendations of the Nomenclature Committee on Cell Death 2009. Cell Death Differ. *16*, 3–11.

Kruse K, Janko C, Urbonaviciute V, Mierke CT, Winkler TH, Voll RE, Schett G, Muñoz LE, Herrmann M. (2010). Inefficient clearance of dying cells in patients with SLE: anti-dsDNA autoantibodies, MFG-E8, HMGB-1 and other players. Apoptosis. 15:1098-113.

Lande R, D. Ganguly, V. Facchinetti, L. Frasca, C. Conrad, J. Gregorio, S. Meller, G. Chamilos, R. Sebasigari, V. Riccieri, R. Bassett, H. Amuro, S. Fukuhara, T. Ito, Y.-J. Liu, M. Gilliet, (2011). Neutrophils activate plasmacytoid dendritic cells by releasing self-DNA-peptide complexes in systemic lupus erythematosus. Sci. Transl. Med. 3, 73ra19

Le Bon A., C. Thompson, E. Kamphuis, V. Durand, C. Rossmann, U. Kalinke, D. F. Tough (2006). Cutting edge: Enhancement of antibody responses through direct stimulation of B and T cells by type I IFN. J. Immunol. 176, 2074–2078.

Lenert, P., R. Brummel, E. H. Field, and R. F. Ashman. (2005). TLR-9 activation of marginal zone B cells in lupus mice regulates immunity through increased IL-10 production. *J. Clin. Immunol.* 25: 29–40.

Li LH, Li WX, Wu O, Zhang GQ, Pan HF, Li XP, Xu JH, Dai H, Ye DQ. (2009). Fas expression on peripheral blood lymphocytes in systemic lupus erythematosus: relation to the organ damage and lymphocytes apoptosis. Mol Biol Rep. 36:2047-52.

Loken MR, Shah VO, Hollander Z, Civin CI. (1988). Flow cytometric analysis of normal B lymphoid development. Pathol Immunopathol Res. 7:357-70.

Lüthi, A.U., and Martin, S.J. (2007). The CASBAH: a searchable database of caspase substrates. Cell Death Differ. *14*, 641–650.

Martin F, Kearney JF. (2002). Marginal zone B cells. *Nat. Rev. Immunol.* 2:323– 35

Mauri, C., L.T. Mars, and M. Londei. (2000). Therapeutic activity of agonistic monoclonal antibodies against CD40 in a chronic autoimmune inflammatory process. *Nat. Med.* 6:673–679.

Mauri, C., Gray, D., Mushtaq, N., and Londei, M. (2003). Prevention of arthritis by interleukin 10-producing B cells. J. Exp. Med. 197, 489–501.

Mauri, C. and Ehrenstein, M.R. (2007) Cells of the synovium in rheumatoid arthritis. B cells. Arthritis Res. Ther. 9, 205-10.

Mauri C, Ehrenstein MR. (2008). The 'short' history of regulatory B cells. Trends Immunol 29:34–40.

Midgley A, McLaren Z, Moots RJ, Edwards SW, Beresford MW. (2009). The role of neutrophil apoptosis in juvenile-onset systemic lupus erythematosus. Arthritis Rheum. 60:2390-401.

Miret C, Font J, Molina R, Garcia-Carrasco M, Filella X, Ramos M, Cervera R, Ballesta A, Ingelmo M. (2001). Relationship of oncogenes (sFas, Bcl-2) and cytokines (IL-10, alfa-TNF) with the activity of systemic lupus erythematosus. Anticancer Res. 21(4B):3053-9.

Mizoguchi, A., Mizoguchi, E., Takedatsu, H., Blumberg, R.S., and Bhan, A.K. (2002). Chronic intestinal inflammatory condition generates IL-10-producing regulatory B cell subset characterized by CD1d upregulation. Immunity 16,219–230.

Mizoguchi A, Bhan AK. (2006). A case for regulatory B cells. J Immunol. 176:705-10.

Moschese V, Orlandi P, Di Matteo G, Chini L, Carsetti R, Di Cesare S, Rossi P. (2004). Insight into B cell development and differentiation. Acta Paediatr Suppl. 93(445):48-51.

Nagata, S. (1997). Apoptosis by death factor. Cell *88*, 355–365.

Nagata S, Hanayama R, Kawane K (2010). Autoimmunity and the clearance of dead cells. Cell 140: 619-630.

Nicholas MW, Dooley MA, Hogan SL, Anolik J, Looney J, Sanz I, Clarke SH. (2008). A novel subset of memory B cells is enriched in autoreactivity and correlates with adverse outcomes in SLE. Clin Immunol. 126:189-201.

Niewold TB, Hua J, Lehman TJ, Harley JB, Crow MK. (2007). High serum IFN-alpha activity is a heritable risk factor for systemic lupus erythematosus. Genes Immun 8:492-502.

Nozawa, K., Kayagaki, N., Tokano, Y., Yagita, H., Okumura, K., Hasimoto, H. (1997): Soluble Fas (APO-1, CD95) and soluble Fas ligand in rheumatic diseases. Arthritis Rheum. 40, 1126-1129.

Obermoser G, Pascual V. (2010). The interferon-alpha signature of systemic lupus erythematosus. Lupus. 19:1012-9.

Oliver AM, Martin F, Gartland GL, Carter RH, Kearney JF. (1997). Marginal zone B cells exhibit unique activation, proliferative and immunoglobulin secretory responses. *Eur. J. Immunol.* 27:2366–74

Oliver AM, Martin F, Kearney JF. (1999). IgMhighCD21high lymphocytes enriched in the splenic marginal zone generate effector cells more rapidly than the bulk of follicular B cells. *J. Immunol.* 162:7198–207

O' Reilly LA, Tai L, Lee L, Kruse EA, Grabow S, Fairlie WD, Haynes NM, Tarlinton DM, Zhang JG, Belz GT, Smyth MJ, Bouillet P, Robb L, Strasser A. (2009). Membrane-bound Fas ligand only is essential for Fas-induced apoptosis. Nature. 461(7264):659-63.

Ow, Y.P., Green, D.R., Hao, Z., and Mak, T.W. (2008). Cytochrome c: functions beyond respiration. Nat. Rev. Mol. Cell Biol. *9*, 532–542.

Pillai, S., A. Cariappa, and S. T. Moran. (2005). Marginal zone B cells. *Annu. Rev.Immunol.* 23: 161–196.

Ravichandran, K.S., and Lorenz, U. (2007). Engulfment of apoptotic cells: signals for a good meal. Nat. Rev. Immunol. *7*, 964–974.

Remmers EF, Plenge RM, Lee AT, et al. (2007). *STAT4* and the risk of rheumatoid arthritis and systemic lupus erythematosus. N Engl J Med 357:977-86.

Rieck M, Arechiga A, Onengut-Gumuscu S, Greenbaum C, Concannon P, Buckner JH. (2007). Genetic variation in PTPN22 corresponds to altered function of T and B lymphocytes. J Immunol 179:4704-10.

Rönnblom L, Eloranta ML, Alm GV. (2006). The type I interferon system in systemic lupus erythematosus. Arthritis Rheum 54:408-20.

Rothman A, Isenberg DA (2008). Systemic lupus erythematosus. N Engl J Med 358:929-39.

Rubtsov A.V. , K Rubtsova, A Fischer, R T. Meehan, J Z. Gillis, JW. Kappler, and P Marrack (2011) TLR7-driven accumulation of a novel CD11c$^+$ B-cell population is important for the development of autoimmunity. Blood. 118(5):1305-15

Rumore, P.M., and Steinman, C.R. (1990). Endogenous circulating DNA in systemic lupus erythematosus. Occurrence as multimeric complexes bound to histone. J. Clin. Invest. *86*, 69–74.

Sahebari M, Rezaieyazdi Z, Nakhjavani MJ, Hatef M, Mahmoudi M, Akhlaghi S. (2010). Correlation between serum concentrations of soluble Fas (CD95/Apo-1) and IL-18 in patients with systemic lupus erythematosus. Rheumatol Int. DOI: 10.1007/s00296-010-1633-9

Sakaguchi, S. (2004). Naturally arising CD4_ regulatory T cells for immunologic self tolerance and negative control of immune responses. *Ann. Rev. Immunol.* 22:531–562.

Salmon JE, Millard S, Schacter LA, et al. (1996). Fc gamma RIIA alleles are heritable risk factors for lupus nephritis in African Americans. J Clin Invest 97:1348-54.

Santiago-Raber M-L, L Baudino and S Izui (2009). Emerging roles of TLR7 and TLR9 in murine SLE. J Autoimmunity 33:231-8.

Sato S, Hasegawa M, Fujimoto M, Tedder TF, Takehara K. (2000). Quantitative genetic variation in CD19 expression correlates with autoimmunity. J Immunol. 165:6635-43.

Savill, J., V. Fadok, P. Henson, and C. Haslett. (1993). Phagocyte recognition of cells undergoing apoptosis. *Immunol. Today* 14: 131–136.

Schmitz J, Owyang A, Oldham E, Song Y, Murphy E, McClanahan TK, Zurawski G, Moshrefi M, Qin J, Li X, Gorman DM, Bazan JF, Kastelein RA. (2005) IL-33, an interleukin-1-like cytokine that signals via the IL-1 receptor-related protein ST2 and induces T helper type 2-associated cytokines. Immunity 23, 479–490

Schneider P, Takatsuka H, Wilson A, Mackay F, Tardivel A, et al. (2001). Maturation of marginal zone and follicular B cells requires B cell activating factor of the tumor necrosis factor family and is independent of B cell maturation antigen. *J.Exp. Med.* 194:1691–97

Sheriff, A., Gaipl, U.S., Voll, R.E., Kalden, J.R., Herrmann, M. (2004): Apoptosis and systemic lupus erythematosus. Rheum. Dis. Clin. North Am. 30, 505-527.

Shevach, E. M. (2000). Regulatory T cells in autoimmunity. *Ann. Rev. Immunol.* 18:423–449.

Sigurdsson S, Göring HH, Kristjansdottir G, et al. (2008). Comprehensive evaluation of the genetic variants of interferon regulatory factor 5 reveals a novel 5bp length polymorphism as strong risk factor for systemic lupus erythematosus. Hum Mol Genet 17:872-81.

Silvestris, F., Grinello, D., Tucci, M., Cafforio, P., Dammacco, F. (2003): Enhancement of T cell apoptosis correlates with increased serum levels of soluble Fas (CD95/Apo-1)in active lupus. Lupus 12, 8-14.

Singh AK. (1995). Lupus in the Fas lane? J R Coll Physicians Lond. 29:475-8.

Singh R, Pradhan V, Patwardhan M, Ghosh K. (2009). APO-1/Fas gene: Structural and functional characteristics in systemic lupus erythematosus and other autoimmune diseases. Indian J Hum Genet. 15:98-102.

Sozzani S, Bosisio D, Scarsi M, Tincani A. (2010). Type I interferons in systemic autoimmunity. Autoimmunity. 43:196-203.

Strasser, A., Jost, P.J., and Nagata, S. (2009). The many roles of FAS receptor signaling in the immune system. Immunity *30*, 180–192.

Su TT, Guo B, Wei B, Braun J, Rawlings DJ. (2004). Signaling in transitional type 2 B cells is critical for peripheral B-cell development. Immunol Rev. 197:161-78.

Suzuki, N., Ichino, M., Mihara, S., Kaneko, S., Sakane, T. (1998): Inhibition of Fas/Fas ligand-mediated apoptotic cell death of lymphocytes in vitro by circulating anti-Fas ligand autoantibodies in patients with systemic lupus erythematosus. Arthritis Rheum. 41, 344-353.

Tan EM, Cohen AS, Fries JF, et al. (1982). The 1982 revised criteria for the classification of systemic lupus erythematosus. Arthritis Rheum 25:1271-7

Telegina E, Reshetnyak T, Moshnikova A, Proussakova O, Zhukova A, Kuznetsova A, Ivanov A, Paltsev M, Beletsky I. (2009). A possible role of Fas-ligand-mediated "reverse signaling" in pathogenesis of rheumatoid arthritis and systemic lupus erythematosus. Immunol Lett. 122:12-7.

Theofilopoulos A,N., R. Baccala, B. Beutler, D. H. Kono (2005). Type I interferons (a/b) in immunity and autoimmunity. Annu. Rev. Immunol. 23, 307–336

Thibault DL, Graham KL, Lee LY, Balboni I, Hertzog PJ, Utz PJ. (2009). Type I interferon receptor controls B-cell expression of nucleic acid-sensing Toll-like receptors and autoantibody production in a murine model of lupus. Arthritis Res Ther. 11:R112.

Timmer, J.C., and Salvesen, G.S. (2007). Caspase substrates. Cell Death Differ. *14*, 66–72.

Tinazzi, E., Puccetti, A., Gerli, R., Rigo, A., Migliorini, P., Simeoni, S., Beri, R., Dolcino, M., Martinelli, N., Corrocher, R., Lunardi, C. (2009): Serum DNase I, soluble Fas/FasL levels and cell surface Fas expression in patients with SLE: a possibile explanation for the lack of efficacy of hrDNase I treatment. Int. Immunol. 21, 237-243.

Tokano, Y., Miyake, S., Kayagaki, N., Nozawa, K., Morimoto, S., Azuma, M., Yagita, H., Takasaki, Y., Okumura, K., Hashimoto, H. (1996): Soluble Fas molecule in the serum of patients with systemic lupus erythematosus. J. Clin. Immunol. 16, 261-265.

Treml LS, Carlesso G, Hoek KL, Stadanlick JE, Kambayashi T, Bram RJ, Cancro MP, Khan WN. (2007). TLR stimulation modifies BLyS receptor expression in follicular and marginal zone B cells. J Immunol. 178:7531-9.

Turi MC, D'Urbano M, Celletti E, Alessandri C, Valesini G, Paganelli R. (2009). Serum Fas/FasL ratio in sistemi lupus erythematosus (SLE) is a function of age. Arch Gerontol Geriatr S1:221-6.

Ulloa L, D Messmer (2006). High-mobility group box 1 (HMGB1) protein: Friend and foe. Cytokine & Growth Factor Reviews 17:189–201

Urbonaviciute V, et al. (2008) Induction of infl amatory and immune responses by HMGB1 nucleosome complexes: implications for the pathogenesis of SLE. J. Exp. Med. 205:3007-3018

Voll , R.E. , M. Herrmann , E.A. Roth , C. Stach , J.R. Kalden , and I. Girkontaite . (1997). Immunosuppressive eff ects of apoptotic cells. *Nature* . 390 : 350 - 351 .

Wang, H., Bloom, O., Zhang, M., Vishnubhakat, J.M.,Ombrellino, M.,Che, J., Frazier, A., Yang, H., Ivanova, S., Borovikova, L., Abraham E, Andersson J, Andersson U, Molina PE, Abumrad NN, Sama A, Tracey KJ (1999). HMG-1 as a late mediator of endotoxin lethality in mice. Science 285:248 –251.

Wang H., H. Yang & K Tracey (2004). Extracellular role of HMGB1 in inflammation and sepsis. Journal of Internal Medicine 255: 320–331

Warnatz K, Wehr C, Dräger R, Schmidt S, Eibel H, Schlesier M, Peter HH. (2002). Expansion of CD19(hi)CD21(lo/neg) B cells in common variable immunodeficiency (CVID) patients with autoimmune cytopenia. Immunobiology. 206:502-13.

Yamada S, Maruyama I (2007). HMGB1, a novel inflammatory cytokine. Clin Chim Acta 375:36–42

Yanaba K, Bouaziz JD, Haas KM, Poe JC, Fujimoto M, Tedder TF. (2008). A regulatory B cell subset with a unique CD1dhiCD5+ phenotype controls T cell-dependent inflammatory responses. Immunity. 28:639-50.

Yang H, Ochani M, Li J, Qiang X, Tanovic M, Harris HE, et al. (2004). Reversing established sepsis with antagonists of endogenous high-mobility group box 1. Proc Natl Acad Sci USA 101:296–301.

5

Regulation of Nucleic Acid Sensing Toll-Like Receptors in Systemic Lupus Erythematosus

Cynthia A. Leifer and James C. Brooks
College of Veterinary Medicine, Cornell University
USA

1. Introduction

Autoimmune disease is an aberrant response of the immune system to self. Unlike the adaptive immune system, the innate immune system is not selected during development and was originally thought to inherently discriminate between host and foreign molecular structures (Janeway, 1989). This is true for many innate immune receptor ligands including lipopolysaccharide, which is only synthesized by Gram-negative bacteria. However, some innate immune receptors detect nucleic acids that are shared between microbes and the host. Immune complexes containing nucleic acids are a hallmark of Systemic Lupus Erythematosus (SLE), and the nucleic acid sensing Toll-like receptors (TLRs) respond to the DNA and RNA within these complexes thereby contributing to disease. Defects in regulation of this class of innate immune receptors likely play a key role in precipitation of disease. Here we review nucleic acid sensing TLRs in SLE and recent advances in our understanding of the regulatory mechanisms governing TLR activity. Since breakdown of regulatory mechanisms controlling response of nucleic acid-sensing TLRs likely contributes to development of SLE, targeting specific proteins in these regulatory pathways has the potential to block nucleic acid-driven autoimmune inflammation.

2. Nucleic acid sensing toll-like receptors in SLE

2.1 Toll-like receptors

Toll-like receptors (TLRs) are a family of innate immune receptors that directly detect molecular structures and initiate signaling. Engagement of TLRs initiates innate immune responses that promote microbial killing and antigen presentation to educate T cells and B cells. At least 10 different TLRs recognize various microbial structures such as lipopeptides (TLR1, TLR2, and TLR6), lipopolysaccharide (TLR4), bacterial flagellin (TLR5), double stranded RNA (dsRNA, TLR3), single stranded RNA (ssRNA, TLR7, TLR8), and single stranded DNA (ssDNA, TLR9) (Takeda, et al. 2003).

TLRs are type 1 transmembrane receptors with C-termini facing the cytoplasm of the cell and ectodomains either at the cell surface or in the lumen of intracellular compartments. The cytoplasmic domain has homology with the IL-1 and IL-18 receptors and has been called the Toll/IL-1-like receptor domain (TIR). The three-dimensional structures of two TLR cytoplasmic TIR domains have been solved and are globular with many surfaces for protein-protein interactions (Xu, et al. 2000). The TIR domain associates with several adapter proteins that initiate signal transduction. These adapters include myeloid differentiation factor 88 (MyD88), and TIR-domain-containing adapter-inducing interferon-β (TRIF, also known as MyD88 adapter-like, MAL), which promote production of proinflammatory cytokines and type I interferons. The ectodomain is composed of a series of leucine rich repeats that form a curved solenoid. Alignment studies predicted a model structure for the ectodomains of TLRs (Bell, et al. 2003), which was supported by crystallographic studies (Bell, et al. 2005; Choe, et al. 2005). TLRs are expressed on a wide variety of cell types including B cells, T cells, dendritic cells, macrophages, and intestinal epithelial cells, although different cell types have unique repertoires of TLR expression (Takeda, et al. 2003). For example, human plasmacytoid dendritic cells express the nucleic acid-sensing TLRs, TLR7 and TLR9. TLR7- and TLR9-dependent responses by both B cells and plasmacytoid dendritic cells have been proposed to contribute to SLE (Marshak-Rothstein, 2006).

2.2 Nucleic acids as TLR ligands

Multiple nucleic acids, including ssRNA, dsRNA, and DNA, induce inflammatory responses. For DNA, the response is dependent on a 5′- cytosine-guanosine-3′ dinucleotide (CpG). The central cytosine must be unmethylated, and is active when surrounded by specific bases, which together form the CpG motif (Krieg, 2002). These CpG motifs are rare in vertebrate DNA due to reduced frequency of the CG dinucleotide (CpG suppression) and increased frequency of cytosine methylation (Cardon, et al. 1994; Klinman, et al. 1996; Krieg, et al. 1995). However, CpG motifs are present and functional in bacterial DNA, in plasmid DNA produced in bacteria, and in synthetic DNA. Variation of sequence and physical structure of synthetic DNAs have resulted in characterization of at least four types of CpG oligodeoxynucleotides each with different activity on cells. Three are stimulatory, and one is inhibitory (Gursel, et al. 2003; Verthelyi, et al. 2001). Inhibitory DNAs do not require a CpG motif and the mechanism of inhibition has not been clearly defined (Gursel, et al. 2003; Krieg, et al. 1998; Lenert, et al. 2003). Type A CpG DNAs (also called D) induce robust type I interferon production, while type B CpG DNAs (also called K) induce B cell proliferation and proinflammatory cytokine production (Verthelyi, et al. 2001). The last class type C CpG DNAs have properties of both type A and type B CpG DNAs and thus induces both types of cellular responses (Vollmer, et al. 2004).

Regardless of their class, CpG DNAs require endocytosis and acidification of endosomes for activity (Figure 1). Blockade of uptake by immobilization of the CpG DNA on beads inhibits the B cell proliferative activity of synthetic CpG DNAs (Manzel & Macfarlane, 1999). Inhibition of endosomal acidification blocks CpG DNA-induced cytokine release by macrophages (Hacker, et al. 1998). Furthermore, cellular activation by CpG DNA initiates on endosomes (Ahmad-Nejad, et al. 2002). Vertebrate DNAs are poorly internalized, which contributes to their poor stimulatory activity. However, vertebrate DNA is stimulatory when in complex with proteins such as high mobility group box 1 (HMGB1), the antimicrobial peptide LL37, or anti-DNA antibodies (Lande, et al. 2007; Leadbetter, et al. 2002; Tian, et al. 2007). Whether the CpG DNA induces proinflammatory cytokines or type I interferon also depends on the endosomal compartment where the DNA is retained (Honda, et al. 2005). Honda and colleagues demonstrated that different types of DNA were trafficked to and retained within different endosomal compartments. For example, the type I interferon inducing CpG DNAs (type A) rapidly co-localized with FITC-dextran, a marker for early endosomes, but failed to co-localize with lysosomal markers. In contrast, rapid localization with lysosomal markers correlated with proinflammatory cytokine production induced by type B CpG DNAs. In another study the outcome of cellular responses to the DNA types could be swapped by changing the physical and chemical properties of the DNA (Guiducci, et al. 2006). Multimerization of type B CpG DNAs, so that their physical structure resembled type A CpG DNAs, caused them to be retained in early endosomes and induce A-type responses. Response of B cells was also dependent on CpG DNA type and delivery mechanism (Avalos, et al. 2009). These studies strongly correlated location of DNA detection with cellular outcome and suggested that manipulation of localization and receptor recognition could change the outcome of cellular response.

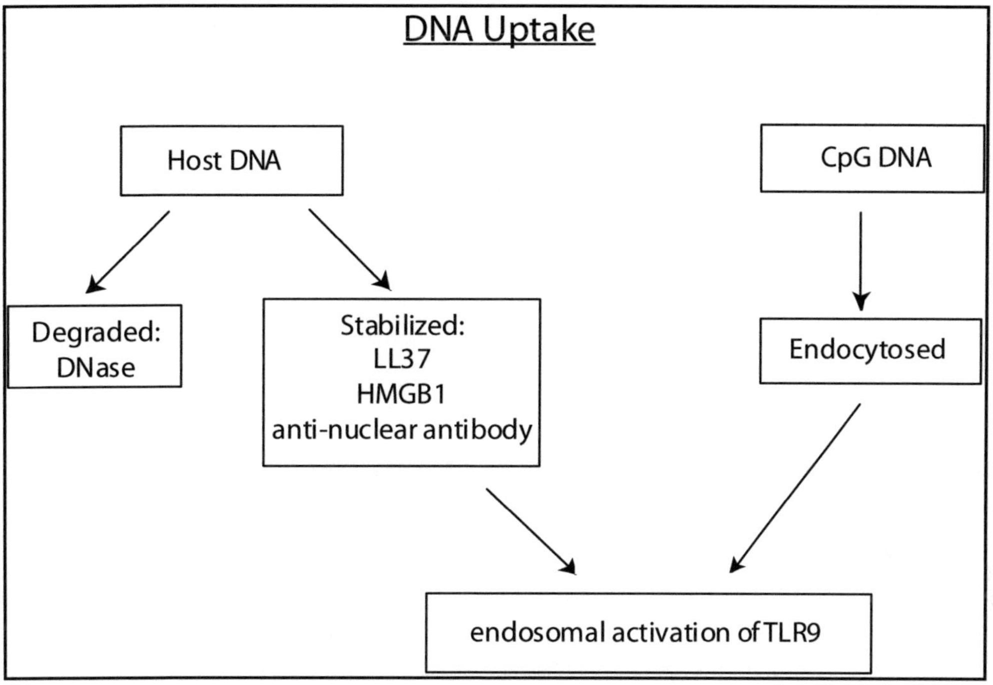

Fig. 1. DNA uptake into the cell. Host DNA is degraded in the extracellular space by DNase and does not normally induce inflammatory responses. However, several host proteins including LL37, HMGB1, and anti-nuclear antibodies stabilize host DNA and facilitate uptake into the endosomal compartment. Endocytosed host DNA activates TLR9. Unlike host DNA, synthetic CpG DNAs, or bacterial DNA, are efficeintly endocytosed and activate TLR9.

At concentrations of CpG DNA used by many investigators, uptake occurs by fluid phase endocytosis. Uptake of CpG DNA reached a plateau at 2 hours, was slowed at low temperature and was inhibited by known endocytosis inhibitors such as sodium azide and cytochalasin B (Yakubov, et al. 1989). Yet, at lower concentrations, uptake was significantly more efficient, which indicated that the CpG DNA was internalized by receptor-mediated endocytosis. Using radiolabeled cells, multiple groups demonstrated specific DNA binding proteins that likely assisted in internalization and trafficking of CpG DNA to the correct endosomal compartment where it encountered TLR9 (Beltinger, et al. 1995; Yakubov, et al. 1989). However, the identity of these receptors remains unknown. During the internalization process, CpG DNA transits though both early and late endosomes, which is important because, as mentioned above, CpG DNAs trigger different cellular outcomes depending on the compartment where signaling initiates.

A hallmark of SLE is elevated serum antibodies to nuclear components, which enhance response to DNA (Leadbetter, et al. 2002). Immune complexes from SLE patient serum were enriched in CG content within the DNA, consistent with increased presence of potential stimulatory motifs (Sano & Morimoto, 1982). Complexes with DNA bound to anti-idiotype B cell receptors (rheumatoid factor) and to Fc receptors to mediate internalization (Boule, et al. 2004; Leadbetter, et al. 2002). By either mechanism the uptake was very efficient and delivered the complexes to the endosomal compartment. Synergistic cytokine production and autoantibody induction by enhanced uptake of DNA-containing immune complexes likely contributes to the induction and propagation of anti-nucleic acid antibody production so frequently observed in SLE.

Internalization of CpG DNA and host DNA is also facilitated by several other host proteins including high mobility group protein 1 (HMGB-1), and the antimicrobial peptide LL37. The cationic antimicrobial peptide LL37 was highly elevated in the skin of patients with psoriases (Lande, et al. 2007). LL37 formed a stable complex with host DNA, and induced a TLR9-dependent, DNase-sensitive, type I interferon response from human plasmacytoid dendritic cells. The nuclear factor HMGB1 is retained within cells under normal conditions, but cell death and inflammation releases HMGB1, which formed a stable complex with host DNA. Association of CpG DNA-A with HMGB1 dramatically enhanced production of type I interferon (Tian, et al. 2007). In fact, HMGB1 was found in immune complexes with host DNA. Altogether, these studies demonstrate that while host DNA alone is not very immunostimulatory, association with a variety of different proteins, present in disease states, promote endosomal uptake where the DNA can associate with TLRs and induce pathologic interferon responses.

2.3 The role of TLRs in B cells and DC in SLE models

Mouse models have provided significant experimental evidence for the importance of TLRs in SLE. Deficiency in UNC93B1, a chaperone-like protein required for endocytic trafficking of nucleic acid-sensing TLRs, results in less severe disease in induced models of SLE in mice (Kono, et al. 2009). Furthermore, UNC93B1 protein is upregulated in SLE (Nakano, et al. 2010), underscoring the importance of TLRs in disease manifestations. The Y-linked autoimmune accelerator (Yaa) mutation, which accelerates and enhances spontaneous disease on the B6/FcRIIB -/- background, is due to TLR7 gene duplication (Pisitkun, et al. 2006), and disease in Fas-deficient MRL/lpr mice is dependent on TLR7 expression (Christensen, et al. 2006). Together these studies show that nucleic acid-sensing TLRs contribute to SLE.

The role for TLR9 in SLE-like disease in mice is less clear. TLR9 deficient mice have reduced anti-DNA antibodies, but enhanced disease (Christensen, et al. 2005). Despite these limitations, much is known about the regulation of TLR9, and TLR9 remains a good model to study the regulation of nucleic acid-sensing TLRs. A specific role for TLR9 in B cell responses to DNA containing immune complexes was supported by studies using a mouse expressing a transgenic "rheumatoid factor" receptor. In vitro stimulation with immune complexes that included DNA, such as anti-nucleosome complexes, induced proliferation of the transgenic B cells, but non-nucleic acid complexes, such as BSA-anti-BSA complexes did not. The response was DNase sensitive and dependent on MyD88 and uptake of the immune complexes into the endosomal compartment (Leadbetter, et al. 2002). Therefore, while TLR9 may not be a major contributor to disease in patients, defects in TLR9 regulation may have very specific functional consequences and a better understanding of the regulatory mechanisms may provide necessary information to therapeutically target TLR9 and other nucleic acid-sensing TLRs.

Patients with SLE have high levels of type I interferons in the blood and their peripheral blood mononuclear cells have a characteristic upregulation of interferon regulated genes (Bennett, et al. 2003). Plasmacytoid dendritic cells circulating in the blood are a major source of type I interferons and were originally called natural interferon producing cells (NIPCs). In humans, this subset of dendritic cells expresses predominantly TLR7 and TLR9 (Hornung, et al. 2002; Krug, et al. 2004). Production of type I interferons by plasmacytoid dendritic cells can be induced by immune complexes produced in abundance in patients with SLE (Ronnblom & Alm, 2001). Dendritic cells have Fc receptors on their cell surface that capture and internalize immune complexes, which induces interferon in a CpG motif- and TLR9-dependent manner (Boule, et al. 2004; Yasuda, et al. 2009). High circulating type I interferon correlates with immune pathology and disease severity in SLE. Therefore, TLR9 contributes to interferon production, and interferon can in turn augment TLR9-dependent responses.

2.4 Nucleic acid-sensing TLRs detection of self-ligands

When the stimulatory activity of CpG DNA was first described, it was thought to represent microbial DNA and that self-DNA was non-stimulatory. This was due to the requirement for the central CG dinucleotide, unmethylation of the C, and for selectivity for surrounding bases. These arguments held for many years, but it was known, even then, that the mammalian genome had the potential to induce TLR9-mediated responses (Ishii, et al. 2001; Yasuda, et al. 2005). Many studies, including the ones reviewed below, have been focussed on understanding what regulates TLR9 mediated responses and why self-DNA is not normally detected. However, recent studies suggest that TLR9 signaling is important for normal responses like wound repair.

Cells go to great lengths to assure DNA is not released into the extracellular milieu when they die by condensing and digesting their DNA during apoptosis. However, necrosis and neutrophil extracellular trap (NET) formation intentionally releases DNA that can induce inflammatory responses (Garcia-Romo, et al. 2011; Lande, et al. 2011; Villanueva, et al. 2011). Interestingly, SLE neutrophils were primed by high type I interferon levels in vivo, and in response to immune complexes, the neutrophils from SLE patients generated NETs that had a high content of DNA, LL37 and HMGB1. These proteins protected the DNA from degradation and facilitated internalization, and thereby increased the inflammatory potential of the host DNA. Therefore, since it is purposefully released under certain conditions, there must be other regulatory mechanisms to avoid response to host DNA. DNase is present in serum and in the extracellular environment and degrades potentially stimulatory host DNA. DNase deficient mice were born healthy but develop lupus like disease around six months of age (Napirei, et al. 2000). Heterozygous mice had increased serum concentrations of anti-nuclear antibodies, and more glomerulonephritis. However, in homozygous DNase deficient mice these SLE parameters were even higher. Mutations in DNase have been identified in SLE patients (Yasutomo, et al. 2001), and together these studies suggest that DNase is an important mechanism to prevent response to host DNA.

Interestingly, recent studies have shown that detection of self-DNA may be a normal biological process, and is, in fact, critical for wound healing (Gregorio, et al. 2010; Sato, et al. 2010). In the absence of TLR9, full thickness biopsy wound healing was delayed, and application of CpG DNA enhanced healing in a TLR9 dependent manner (Sato, et al. 2010). These data suggest that TLR9 plays an important role in wound healing. In a different model, tape stripping-induced epidermal injury induced plasmacytoid dendritic cell and neutrophil infiltration (Guiducci, et al. 2010). This response was accompanied by production of type I interferon, and was dependent on the signaling adapter molecule MyD88. Treatment of wild-type mice with a TLR7-TLR9 inhibitor inhibited the response, implicating these TLRs in the process. In lupus-prone mice, the same tape-stripping procedure led to chronic wounds with a type I interferon signature that resembled SLE skin lesions. Therefore, detection of DNA and RNA by TLR9 and TLR7 is important for normal wound healing. Dysregulation of this pathway in SLE likely contributes to autoimmune inflammation, especially in the skin, and is a potential target for therapeutic intervention.

3. Regulation of TLR9

3.1 Compartmentalization of TLR9

Infectious agents replicate in various locations outside and inside cells. Bacteria and viruses are internalized into endosomes, and some can escape into the cytoplasm. Therefore, positioning of TLRs is important for detecting components of microbes in the varied locations where they can reside. Some TLRs, such as TLR2, TLR4, and TLR5, are expressed at the cell surface to detect ligands expressed on the surface of bacteria (lipopolysaccharide, TLR4; lipopeptides, TLR2; and flagellin, TLR5). However, nucleic acids, such as DNA and RNA, are encapsulated within bacteria and viruses, and are only released upon internalization into endosomes. To accommodate this, nucleic acid sensing TLRs are localized intracellularly. For example, TLR9 is primarily found in the endoplasmic reticulum (ER) of resting cells (Latz, et al. 2004; Leifer, et al. 2004) where it colocalizes with ER, and not endosomal, markers. Since detection of DNA occurs in endosomes, these data suggest that that there is an induced trafficking event that leads to TLR9 entry into this compartment (Leifer, et al. 2004). The unique compartmentalization of nucleic acid-sensing TLRs has been proposed as a major regulatory mechanism to prevent response to host DNA (Barton, et al. 2006). Fusion of the ectodomain of TLR9 with the transmembrane domain and cytoplasmic tail of TLR4 created a protein that localized to the cell surface. This change in localization endowed the TLR9 ectodomain with the ability to respond to host DNA (Barton, et al. 2006). These data support a model where TLR9 is specifically trafficked intracellularly to avoid access to the extracellular milieu, thereby preventing recognition of host DNA.

3.2 Trafficking of TLR9 through the Golgi to localize in the endolysosomes

While TLR9 predominantly resides in the ER it must traffic to the endosomal compartment where it encounters endocytosed CpG DNA (Latz, et al. 2004; Leifer, et al. 2004) (Figure 2). Normally, transmembrane or secreted proteins synthesized in the ER traffic through the Golgi to access the cell surface or intracellular endosomes. However, TLR9 was sensitive to endoglycosidase H (endo H) treatment, which indicated that TLR9 had not reached the

Golgi (Latz, et al. 2004). In 2009 Chockalingam et al., showed that Brefeldin A inhibited TLR9 response to CpG DNA (Chockalingam, et al. 2009). Since Brefeldin A is a small molecule that inhibits transport of proteins from ER to Golgi, TLR9 signaling appeared to be dependent on Golgi trafficking.

When proteins traffic through the Golgi, the high mannose glycans are processed to hybrid forms that are still cleaved by Endo H; therefore, highly specific lectins were used to determine whether TLR9 had glycan modifications indicative of Golgi transit (Chockalingam, et al. 2009). Lectins are plant proteins that selectively recognize carbohydrate structures. For example, *Datura stramonium* (DS) lectin specifically recognizes "Galβ1→4GlcNac" structures present only on proteins that have been processed by Golgi resident enzymes. DS lectin bound to TLR9, which confirmed that TLR9 trafficked through the Golgi during synthesis (Chockalingam, et al. 2009). TLR9 immunoprecipitated from the lysosomal compartment of HEK293 cells also bound DS lectin, and co-immunoprecipitated with the signaling adapter MyD88 (Chockalingam, et al. 2009). These data indicated that lysosomal TLR9 had transited through the Golgi and contributed to signaling.

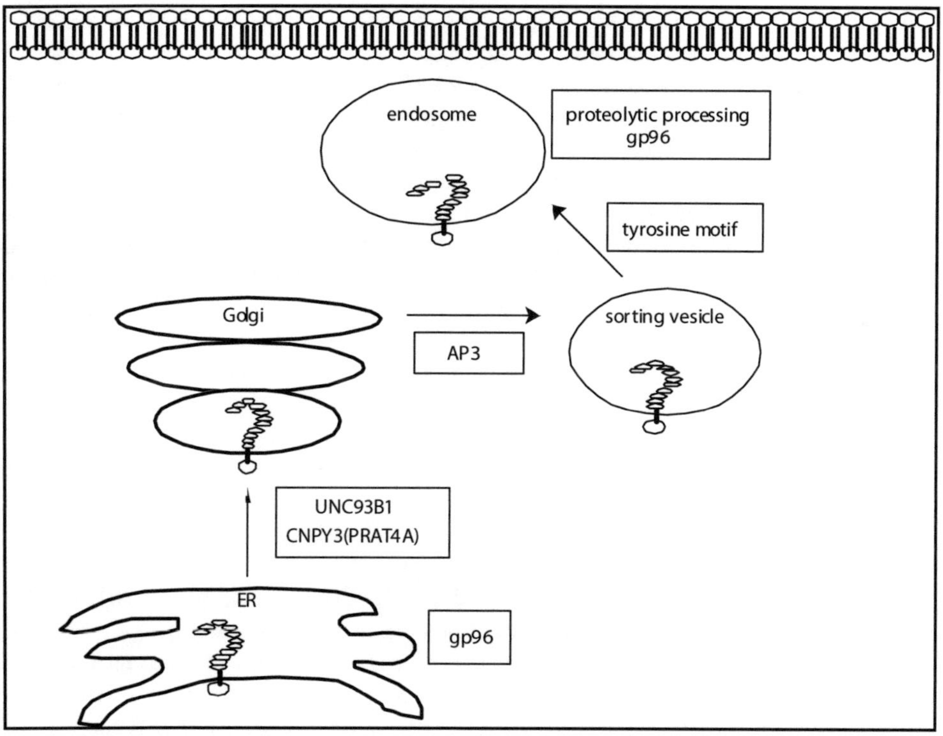

Fig. 2. Regulation of TLR9 trafficking. After synthesis in the ER TLR9 associates with gp96. TLR9 traffics out of the ER to the Golgi in a manner dependent on gp96, PRAT4A, and UNC93B1. TLR9 traffics from the Golgi to a sorting vesicle in an AP3 dependent manner where it is then sorted to the endosomal compartment via a cytoplasmic tyrosine motif. In the endosomal compartment TLR9 is proteolytically processed either active or negative regulatory forms that modulate TLR9 signaling. Lack of gp96 prevents TLR9 proteolytic processing.

3.3 Proteins that regulate intracellular localization and trafficking

Several proteins are critical for TLR9 trafficking both out of the ER and to the endosomal compartment (Figure 2): UNC93B1, adapter protein 3 (AP3), a protein associated with TLR4 (PRAT4A), Slc15a4, and glycoprotein 96 (gp96, also known as glucose regulated protein 94 (gp94). Recessive N-ethyl-N-nitrosourea-induced mutagenesis revealed a mouse line that lacked response to TLR3, TLR7, and TLR9 ligands. These mice had a single point mutation (H412R) in UNC93B1 (Tabeta, et al. 2006). In dendritic cells from these mice, TLR7 and TLR9 did not localize to the endosomal compartment (Kim, et al. 2008). Interestingly, UNC93B1 seems to play opposing roles in regulation of TLR7 and TLR9 (Fukui, et al. 2009). Reconstitution of UNC93B1 deficient cells with UNC93B1 containing a single point mutation (D34A) resulted in hyperresponsivenss to TLR7, yet hyporesponsiveness to TLR9, ligands. Therefore, the role of UNC93B1 in regulation of nucleic acid sensing TLRs is clearly important and interfering with UNC93B1 function has different effects on signaling by different TLRs.

Two ER luminal proteins, gp96 and PRAT4A, are essential for TLR9 exit from the ER. PRAT4A, also known as CNPY3, bound to TLR9, which depended on methionine 145 of PRAT4A (Kiyokawa, et al. 2008). In the absence of PRAT4A, TLR9 did not access endosomes, and PRAT4A deficient cells lacked response through all TLRs, except TLR3 (Takahashi, et al. 2007). The heat shock protein gp96 also bound to TLR9 and was required for B cell and macrophage response to CpG DNA (Randow & Seed, 2001; Yang, et al. 2007). A pre-B cell line with a frame-shift mutation in gp96 was 10,000 times less sensitive to LPS then the non-mutant line, which was due to a lack of TLR4 on the cell surface (Randow & Seed, 2001). This study suggested that gp96 regulated trafficking of TLRs. Further studies using a mouse with macrophage specific knockout of gp96 showed that gp96 is essential for TLR9 trafficking and signaling, and was in fact a chaperone for all TLRs except TLR3 (Liu, et al. 2010; Yang, et al. 2007). In 2011 Liu et al., demonstrated that gp96 and PRAT4A directly interacted to form a multimeric complex with TLR9 (Liu, et al. 2010). Very recent studies using gp96 specific inhibitors have examined the role of gp96 after TLR9 synthesis and trafficking is complete. These studies show that gp96 remains associated with TLR9 in the endosomal compartment and that specific inhibitors block CpG DNA signaling and cause a loss of TLR9 protein (JC Brooks and CA Leifer unpublished observations). This suggests that gp96 has an additional function in regulating the conformational stability of TLR9 in the endosomal compartment.

Cytoplasmic proteins are also important for TLR9 trafficking. Plasmacytoid DCs from adapter protein 3 (AP3) deficient mice failed to induce a type I interferon response after CpG DNA stimulation despite normal IL-12 production (Sasai, et al. 2010). AP3 is a cytosolic protein that associates with endosomes and sorts transmembrane proteins from the endosomal compartment to lysosome-related organelles (Bonifacino & Traub, 2003). In the absence of AP3, TLR9 did not colocalize with markers for lysosome-related organelles (Sasai, et al. 2010). This group suggested that it was these lysosome-related organelles that were critical for induction of type I interferons (Sasai, et al. 2010). However, this conclusion contradicts previously published studies showing that initiation of signaling that results in type I interferon production occurs on early endosomes (Guiducci, et al. 2006; Honda, et al. 2005). In a separate study using the same AP3 deficient mice, both proinflammatory and type I interferon production were lost. Therefore, AP3 is important for TLR9-induced cytokine production, but its exact role in TLR9 biology remains unclear.

Recent data have shown that TLR9 signaling also depends on Slc15a4, a twelve-spanning transmembrane oligopeptide transporter that localizes to the endolysosomal compartment (Blasius, et al. 2010; Yamashita, et al. 1997). Cells from Slc15a4 deficient mice lack response to nucleic acid sensing TLRs (Blasius, et al. 2010). Again, the specific role of Slc15a4 remains unknown, but may involve endolysosomal transport of TLR9 or a TLR9-associated protein required for TLR9 function.

3.4 Specific motifs in TLR9 that regulate localization and trafficking

Localization of TLRs is regulated by sequences in their transmembrane domains and cytoplasmic tails. Fusion of TLR4 to the transmembrane and cytoplasmic tail of various TLRs resulted in distinct localizations of the chimeric proteins (Nishiya & DeFranco, 2004). For example, TLR4 by itself localized to the cell surface, and fusion of TLR4's ectodomain with the transmembrane and cytoplasmic tail of TLR1, TLR2, TLR5, or TLR6 resulted in similar localization. In contrast, when TLR4 was fused to the transmembrane and cytoplasmic tail of any of the nucleic acid-sensing TLRs, the resulting chimeric receptor was not detected at the cell surface. Further studies using different approaches identified different motifs in TLR9 responsible for this localization (Barton, et al. 2006; Leifer, et al. 2006). TLR9's ectodomain fused to TLR4's transmembrane and cytoplasmic domains localized to the cell surface (Barton, et al. 2006). The chimera retained the ability to respond to CpG DNA, yet was resistant to endosomal acidification inhibitors. Interestingly, TLR9 associates with UNC93B1 via the transmembrane domain and this may explain, in part, the requirement for this association in TLR9 signaling.

The cytoplasmic tail of TLR9 also contains a specific localization motif (Leifer, et al. 2006). In this study, the ectodomain of the IL-2 receptor alpha chain, which normally localized to cell surface, was fused to the transmembrane and cytoplasmic tail of different TLRs (Leifer, et al. 2006). A fusion with the TLR4 transmembrane and cytoplasmic tail localized to the cell surface; however, a fusion with the same regions of TLR9 was not. Truncation analysis revealed that deletion of all but four amino acids of the cytoplasmic tail generated a protein that was robustly expressed at the cell surface, ruling out a contribution of the transmembrane domain to intracellular localization. It is unclear why these two studies showed opposite requirements for TLR9 transmembrane domain. Regardless, additional truncations and mapping identified a 14 amino acid motif that was important for TLR9 intracellular localization. Follow-up studies showed that mutation of a critical tyrosine (888) within this motif abolished proinflammatory cytokine production. Interestingly, this mutant maintained normal interferon responses suggesting that this motif was required for trafficking TLR9 to the compartment selectively required for induction of proinflammatory cytokines (A Chockalingam and CA Leifer unpublished observations). It remains to be determined if this motif is necessary for association with AP3 or other regulatory proteins.

3.5 Proteolytic regulation of TLR9

In addition to trafficking to specific endocytic compartments, several recent studies have demonstrated that TLR9 is proteolytically processed in endosomes and that this processing regulates TLR9 function (Chockalingam, et al. 2011; Ewald, et al. 2011; Ewald, et al. 2008; Park, et al. 2008; Sepulveda, et al. 2009). The ectodomain of TLR9 contains 25 leucine rich repeats. The first 14 and the second 15 leucine-rich repeats are interrupted by a region predicted to have very little secondary structure, often referred to as the hinge (Bell, et al.

2003). The first described proteolytic event was mapped to this hinge region through a mass spectrometric approach (Park, et al. 2008). The form of TLR9 generated encompasses one-half of the ectodomain and all of the transmembrane and cytoplasmic tail (Figure 3). This proteolytic event is inhibited by endosomal acidification inhibitors and by broad-spectrum cathepsin inhibitors (Ewald, et al. 2008; Park, et al. 2008). Additional studies with specific cathepsin inhibitors, and in cathepsin deficient mice, did not reveal a unique cathepsin responsible for the cleavage. An independent study, showed an additional proteolytic event (Sepulveda, et al. 2009). While this study did not reveal the precise location of the proteolysis, a specific enzyme, asaparagine endopeptidase was shown to be important. A more recent study suggested that stepwise processing of TLR9 is required to attain fully functional proteolytically processed TLR9 (Ewald, et al. 2011). Interestingly, knockdown of either PRAT4A (CNPY3) or gp96 by shRNA targeting resulted in a loss of proteolytic processing of TLR9, and suggested that these chaperones were required for TLR9 to access endosomes (Liu, et al. 2010).

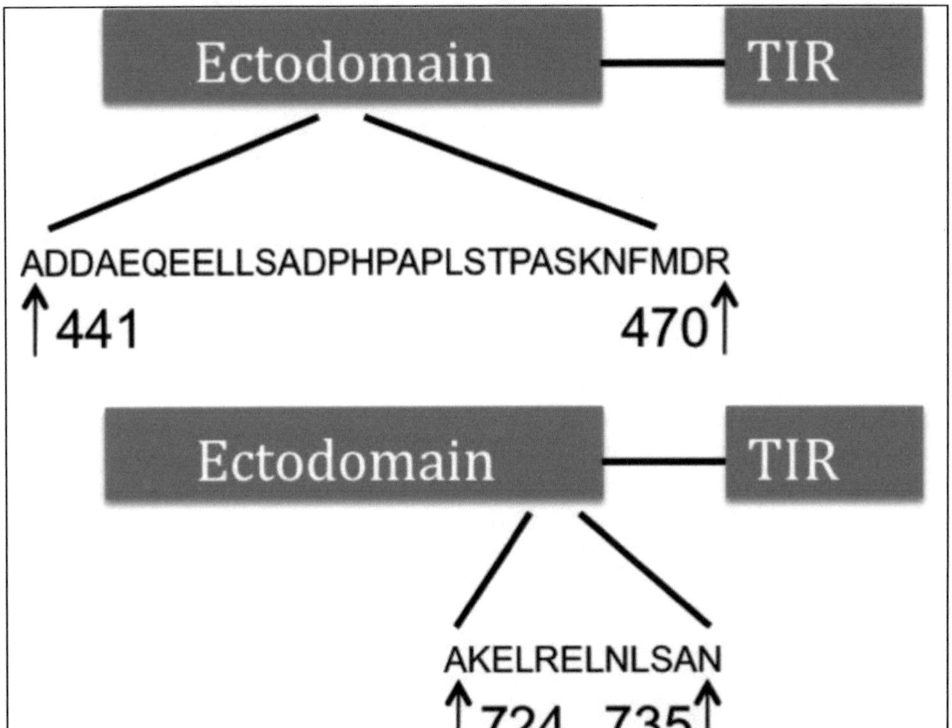

Fig. 3. Proteolytic processing of TLR9. The ectomain of TLR9 is proteolytically processed into two forms. The first form is active and consists of one half of the ectodomain of TLR9 and the transmembrane and cytoplasmic tail (amino acids 471-1032) The second form is a negative regulator of TLR9 signaling and consists of almost the entire ectodomain with no transmembrane or cytoplasmic tail. This form, called soluble TLR9, is released into endosomes, but is not secreted. By binding to internalized DNA, and to full-length TLR9, this form blocks signaling. The relative ratio of these two fragments likely determines the cellular response upon exposure to DNA.

TLR9 is also proteolytically processed at a completely different position to generate a negative regulator of TLR9 signaling (Chockalingam, et al. 2011). This proteolytic event resulted in generation of an intact ectodomain separated from the transmembrane domain and cytoplasmic tail (Figure 2). This soluble form of TLR9 bound to CpG DNA, associated with full length TLR9, and dominant negatively inhibited responses by the full-length receptor (Chockalingam, et al. 2011). In contrast to the other proteolytic cleavage events, generation of soluble TLR9 occurred in cells expressing endogenous TLR9 (Chockalingam, et al. 2011). Soluble TLR9 is likely important in regulating TLR9 responses since intestinal epithelial cells poorly responded to CpG DNA, and abundantly generated soluble TLR9 (Chockalingam, et al. 2011). Therefore, correlative studies on TLR9 in different pathological conditions must account for the complexity of TLR9 post-translational modification.

4. Conclusion

In this review we have highlighted recent studies describing regulatory mechanisms governing nucleic acid-sensing TLRs. While TLRs are critical for host defence against infection, some TLRs recognize ligands shared between infectious agents and the host (Marshak-Rothstein & Rifkin, 2007). Despite complex regulatory mechanisms, these TLRs do contribute to autoimmune disease (Marshak-Rothstein, 2006). Recent studies have revealed multiple post-translational mechanisms that regulate this family of TLRs, and if dysregulated could also contribute to the development of autoimmune disease. By exploiting mechanisms that control nucleic acid sensing TLRs we will relieve TLR-mediate autoimmune inflammation.

Host DNA and RNA are not typically inflammatory since there are several regulatory mechanisms to prevent availability of host DNA. These include preventing its release (apoptosis), and degrading it once it is released (DNase). Association with various host proteins such as HMGB1, LL37, and autoantibodies stabilize host DNA and enhance its uptake where it gains access to intracellular nucleic acid sensing TLRs (Lande, et al. 2007; Leadbetter, et al. 2002; Tian, et al. 2007). When this occurs, especially by anti-nuclear antibodies, host DNA and RNA enhance type I interferon production from dendritic cells and promote proliferation and antibody production from B cells. Defects in expression of the nucleic acid stabilizing proteins changes susceptibility to autoimmunity in mouse models. Development of drugs that block stabilization of DNA by these host proteins, and thereby block proinflammatory or interferon responses, will reduce autoinflammation and offer new ways to treat SLE.

The nucleic acid-sensing TLRs are also carefully regulated to avoid response to host DNA. To avoid detection of host DNAs and RNAs, nucleic acid-sensing TLRs are excluded from the cell surface (Latz, et al. 2004; Leifer, et al. 2004). Several proteins including UNC93B1, and gp96 regulate nucleic acid-sensing TLR access to endosomes (Kim, et al. 2008; Yang, et al. 2007). Specific parts of TLR9 have been found to be important for this regulation and may interact with some of the localization regulators (Barton, et al. 2006; Leifer, et al. 2006). Development of drugs that affect the activity of these proteins would change the intracellular distribution of TLRs, thereby affecting the ability of these receptors to detect and respond to nucleic acids.

Once nucleic acid-sensing TLRs do reach endosomes, they are proteolytically processed (Chockalingam, et al. 2011; Ewald, et al. 2008; Park, et al. 2008), which modifies their function. Cleavage at two different locations within the ectodomain leads to either activation (Ewald, et al. 2008; Park, et al. 2008), or inhibition (Chockalingam, et al. 2011), of TLR9 activity. Specific identification of the enzymes responsible for these proteolytic events will provide new targets for drug development to interfere with TLR signaling and response to host DNA.

When host DNA, or RNA, does activate a TLR, it induces robust inflammation and production of pathologic levels of cytokines such as type I interferon. While several contributing factors to the development of SLE have been found, new data on post-translational regulation of nucleic acid-sensing TLRs show that we still have much to learn. Dysregulation in any of these regulatory proteins will change the intracellular localization of TLR9 and could potentially lead to aberrant response to host nucleic acids. Identifying these regulatory pathways is the first step to understanding how defects in these pathways lead to disease. Specifically targeting these regulatory proteins within these pathways will reduce, or restore, function as necessary to return the regulatory networks to the non-disease state. Therefore, future studies should be focused on improving our understanding of the basic regulatory networks for nucleic acid-sensing TLRs so that we may determine which are defective in SLE. Our hope is that these studies will lead to novel drug development, and improve our repertoire of options to treat autoimmune disease.

5. Acknowledgments

Studies from the Leifer lab described in this review were supported by awards to CAL (NCI K22CA113705, and NIAID AI076588). The authors would like to thank A Chockalingam for helpful suggestions.

6. References

Ahmad-Nejad, P, Hacker, H, Rutz, M, Bauer, S, Vabulas, RM, & Wagner, H. (2002) Bacterial CpG-DNA and lipopolysaccharides activate Toll-like receptors at distinct cellular compartments. European Journal of Immunolology 32:1958-1968.

Avalos, AM, Latz, E, Mousseau, B, Christensen, SR, Shlomchik, MJ, Lund, F, & Marshak-Rothstein, A. (2009) Differential cytokine production and bystander activation of autoreactive B cells in response to CpG-A and CpG-B oligonucleotides. Journal of Immunology 183:6262-6268.

Barton, GM, Kagan, JC, & Medzhitov, R. (2006) Intracellular localization of Toll-like receptor 9 prevents recognition of self DNA but facilitates access to viral DNA. Nature Immunology 7:49-56.

Bell, JK, Botos, I, Hall, PR, Askins, J, Shiloach, J, Segal, DM, & Davies, DR. (2005) The molecular structure of the Toll-like receptor 3 ligand-binding domain. Procedings of the National Academy of Science U S A 102:10976-10980.

Bell, JK, Mullen, GE, Leifer, CA, Mazzoni, A, Davies, DR, & Segal, DM. (2003) Leucine-rich repeats and pathogen recognition in Toll-like receptors. Trendsin Immunol 24:528-533.

Beltinger, C, Saragovi, HU, Smith, RM, LeSauteur, L, Shah, N, DeDionisio, L, Christensen, L, Raible, A, Jarett, L, & Gewirtz, AM. (1995) Binding, uptake, and intracellular trafficking of phosphorothioate-modified oligodeoxynucleotides. Journal of Clinical Investigation 95:1814-1823.

Bennett, L, Palucka, AK, Arce, E, Cantrell, V, Borvak, J, Banchereau, J, & Pascual, V. (2003) Interferon and granulopoiesis signatures in systemic lupus erythematosus blood. Journal of Experimental Medicine 197:711-723.

Blasius, AL, Arnold, CN, Georgel, P, Rutschmann, S, Xia, Y, Lin, P, Ross, C, Li, X, Smart, NG, & Beutler, B. (2010) Slc15a4, AP-3, and hermansky-pudlak syndrome proteins are required for Toll-like receptor signaling in plasmacytoid dendritic cells. Procedings of the National Academy of Science U S A 107:19973-19978.

Bonifacino, JS, & Traub, LM. (2003) Signals for sorting of transmembrane proteins to endosomes and lysosomes. Annual Review of Biochemistry 72:395-447.

Boule, MW, Broughton, C, Mackay, F, Akira, S, Marshak-Rothstein, A, & Rifkin, IR. (2004) Toll-like receptor 9-dependent and -independent dendritic cell activation by chromatin-immunoglobulin G complexes. Journal of Experimental Medicine 199:1631-1640.

Cardon, LR, Burge, C, Clayton, DA, & Karlin, S. (1994) Pervasive CpG suppression in animal mitochondrial genomes. Procedings of the National Academy of Science U S A 91:3799-3803.

Chockalingam, A, Brooks, JC, Cameron, JL, Blum, LK, & Leifer, CA. (2009) TLR9 traffics through the Golgi complex to localize to endolysosomes and respond to CpG DNA. Immunology and Cell Biology 87:209-217.

Chockalingam, A, Cameron, JL, Brooks, JC, & Leifer, CA. (2011) Negative regulation of signaling by a soluble form of Toll-like receptor 9. European Journal of Immunology DOI: 10.1002/eji.201041034

Choe, J, Kelker, MS, & Wilson, IA. (2005) Crystal structure of human Toll-like receptor 3 (TLR3) ectodomain. Science 309:581-585.

Christensen, SR, Kashgarian, M, Alexopoulou, L, Flavell, RA, Akira, S, & Shlomchik, MJ. (2005) Toll-like receptor 9 controls anti-DNA autoantibody production in murine lupus. Journal of Experimental Medicine 202:321-331.

Christensen, SR, Shupe, J, Nickerson, K, Kashgarian, M, Flavell, RA, & Shlomchik, MJ. (2006) Toll-like receptor 7 and TLR9 dictate autoantibody specificity and have opposing inflammatory and regulatory roles in a murine model of lupus. Immunity 25:417-428.

Ewald, SE, Engel, A, Lee, J, Wang, M, Bogyo, M, & Barton, GM. (2011) Nucleic acid recognition by Toll-like receptors is coupled to stepwise processing by cathepsins and asparagine endopeptidase. Journal of Experimental Medicine 208:643-651.

Ewald, SE, Lee, BL, Lau, L, Wickliffe, KE, Shi, GP, Chapman, HA, & Barton, GM. (2008) The ectodomain of Toll-like receptor 9 is cleaved to generate a functional receptor. Nature 456:658-662.

Fukui, R, Saitoh, S, Matsumoto, F, Kozuka-Hata, H, Oyama, M, Tabeta, K, Beutler, B, & Miyake, K. (2009) Unc93B1 biases Toll-like receptor responses to nucleic acid in dendritic cells toward DNA- but against RNA-sensing. Journal of Experimental Medicine 206:1339-1350.

Garcia-Romo, GS, Caielli, S, Vega, B, Connolly, J, Allantaz, F, Xu, Z, Punaro, M, Baisch, J, Guiducci, C, Coffman, RL, Barrat, FJ, Banchereau, J, & Pascual, V. (2011) Netting neutrophils are major inducers of type I IFN production in pediatric Systemic Lupus Erythematosus. Science Translational Medicine 3:73ra20.

Gregorio, J, Meller, S, Conrad, C, Di Nardo, A, Homey, B, Lauerma, A, Arai, N, Gallo, RL, Digiovanni, J, & Gilliet, M. (2010) Plasmacytoid dendritic cells sense skin injury and promote wound healing through type I interferons. Journal of Experimental Medicine 207:2921-2930.

Guiducci, C, Ott, G, Chan, JH, Damon, E, Calacsan, C, Matray, T, Lee, KD, Coffman, RL, & Barrat, FJ. (2006) Properties regulating the nature of the plasmacytoid dendritic cell response to Toll-like receptor 9 activation. Journal of Experimental Medicine 203:1999-2008.

Guiducci, C, Tripodo, C, Gong, M, Sangaletti, S, Colombo, MP, Coffman, RL, & Barrat, FJ. (2010) Autoimmune skin inflammation is dependent on plasmacytoid dendritic cell activation by nucleic acids via TLR7 and TLR9. Journal of Experimental Medicine 207:2931-2942.

Gursel, I, Gursel, M, Yamada, H, Ishii, KJ, Takeshita, F, & Klinman, DM. (2003) Repetitive elements in mammalian telomeres suppress bacterial DNA-induced immune activation. Journal of Immunology 171:1393-1400.

Hacker, H, Mischak, H, Miethke, T, Liptay, S, Schmid, R, Sparwasser, T, Heeg, K, Lipford, GB, & Wagner, H. (1998) CpG-DNA-specific activation of antigen-presenting cells requires stress kinase activity and is preceded by non-specific endocytosis and endosomal maturation. EMBO Journal 17:6230-6240.

Honda, K, Ohba, Y, Yanai, H, Negishi, H, Mizutani, T, Takaoka, A, Taya, C, & Taniguchi, T. (2005) Spatiotemporal regulation of MyD88-IRF-7 signalling for robust type-I interferon induction. Nature 434:1035-1040.

Hornung, V, Rothenfusser, S, Britsch, S, Krug, A, Jahrsdorfer, B, Giese, T, Endres, S, & Hartmann, G. (2002) Quantitative expression of Toll-like receptor 1-10 mRNA in cellular subsets of human peripheral blood mononuclear cells and sensitivity to CpG oligodeoxynucleotides. Journal of Immunology 168:4531-4537.

Ishii, KJ, Suzuki, K, Coban, C, Takeshita, F, Itoh, Y, Matoba, H, Kohn, LD, & Klinman, DM. (2001) Genomic DNA released by dying cells induces the maturation of apcs. Journal of Immunology 167:2602-2607.

Janeway, CA, Jr. (1989) Approaching the asymptote? Evolution and revolution in immunology. Cold Spring Harorb Symposium on Quantative Biology 54 Pt 1:1-13.

Kim, YM, Brinkmann, MM, Paquet, ME, & Ploegh, HL. (2008) UNC93B1 delivers nucleotide-sensing Toll-like receptors to endolysosomes. Nature 452:234-238.

Kiyokawa, T, Akashi-Takamura, S, Shibata, T, Matsumoto, F, Nishitani, C, Kuroki, Y, Seto, Y, & Miyake, K. (2008) A single base mutation in the PRAT4A gene reveals differential interaction of PRAT4A with Toll-like receptors. International Immunology 20:1407-1415.

Klinman, DM, Yi, AK, Beaucage, SL, Conover, J, & Krieg, AM. (1996) CpG motifs present in bacteria DNA rapidly induce lymphocytes to secrete interleukin 6, interleukin 12, and interferon gamma. Proceedings of the National Academy of Science U S A 93:2879-2883.

Kono, DH, Haraldsson, MK, Lawson, BR, Pollard, KM, Koh, YT, Du, X, Arnold, CN, Baccala, R, Silverman, GJ, Beutler, BA, & Theofilopoulos, AN. (2009) Endosomal TLR signaling is required for anti-nucleic acid and rheumatoid factor autoantibodies in lupus. Proceedings of the National Academy of Science U S A 106:12061-12066.

Krieg, AM. (2002) CpG motifs in bacterial DNA and their immune effects. Annual Review of Immunology 20:709-760.

Krieg, AM, Wu, T, Weeratna, R, Efler, SM, Love-Homan, L, Yang, L, Yi, AK, Short, D, & Davis, HL. (1998) Sequence motifs in adenoviral DNA block immune activation by stimulatory CpG motifs. Proceedings of the National Academy of Science U S A 95:12631-12636.

Krieg, AM, Yi, AK, Matson, S, Waldschmidt, TJ, Bishop, GA, Teasdale, R, Koretzky, GA, & Klinman, DM. (1995) CpG motifs in bacterial DNA trigger direct B-cell activation. Nature 374:546-549.

Krug, A, French, AR, Barchet, W, Fischer, JA, Dzionek, A, Pingel, JT, Orihuela, MM, Akira, S, Yokoyama, WM, & Colonna, M. (2004) TLR9-dependent recognition of MCMV by iPC and DC generates coordinated cytokine responses that activate antiviral NK cell function. Immunity 21:107-119.

Lande, R, Ganguly, D, Facchinetti, V, Frasca, L, Conrad, C, Gregorio, J, Meller, S, Chamilos, G, Sebasigari, R, Riccieri, V, Bassett, R, Amuro, H, Fukuhara, S, Ito, T, Liu, YJ, & Gilliet, M. (2011) Neutrophils activate plasmacytoid dendritic cells by releasing self-DNA-peptide complexes in Systemic Lupus Erythematosus. Science Translational Medicine 3:73ra19.

Lande, R, Gregorio, J, Facchinetti, V, Chatterjee, B, Wang, YH, Homey, B, Cao, W, Wang, YH, Su, B, Nestle, FO, Zal, T, Mellman, I, Schroder, JM, Liu, YJ, & Gilliet, M. (2007) Plasmacytoid dendritic cells sense self-DNA coupled with antimicrobial peptide. Nature 449:564-569.

Latz, E, Schoenemeyer, A, Visintin, A, Fitzgerald, KA, Monks, BG, Knetter, CF, Lien, E, Nilsen, NJ, Espevik, T, & Golenbock, DT. (2004) TLR9 signals after translocating from the ER to CpG DNA in the lysosome. Nature Immunology 5:190-198.

Leadbetter, EA, Rifkin, IR, Hohlbaum, AM, Beaudette, BC, Shlomchik, MJ, & Marshak-Rothstein, A. (2002) Chromatin-IgG complexes activate B cells by dual engagement of IgM and Toll-like receptors. Nature 416:603-607.

Leifer, CA, Brooks, JC, Hoelzer, K, Lopez, JL, Kennedy, MN, Mazzoni, A, & Segal, DM. (2006) Cytoplasmic targeting motifs control localization of Toll-like receptor 9. Journal of Biological Chemistry 281:35585-35592.

Leifer, CA, Kennedy, MN, Mazzoni, A, Lee, C, Kruhlak, MJ, & Segal, DM. (2004) TLR9 is localized in the endoplasmic reticulum prior to stimulation. Journal of Immunology 173:1179-1183.

Lenert, P, Rasmussen, W, Ashman, RF, & Ballas, ZK. (2003) Structural characterization of the inhibitory DNA motif for the type A (D)-CpG-induced cytokine secretion and NK-cell lytic activity in mouse spleen cells. DNA Cell Biology 22:621-631.

Liu, B, Yang, Y, Qiu, Z, Staron, M, Hong, F, Li, Y, Wu, S, Hao, B, Bona, R, Han, D, & Li, Z. (2010) Folding of Toll-like receptors by the hsp90 paralogue gp96 requires a substrate-specific cochaperone. Nature Communications 1:79.

Manzel, L, & Macfarlane, DE. (1999) Lack of immune stimulation by immobilized CpG-oligodeoxynucleotide. Antisense Nucleic Acid Drug Development 9:459-464.

Marshak-Rothstein, A. (2006) Toll-like receptors in systemic autoimmune disease. Nature Reviews Immunology 6:823-835.

Marshak-Rothstein, A, & Rifkin, IR. (2007) Immunologically active autoantigens: The role of Toll-like receptors in the development of chronic inflammatory disease. Annual Review of Immunology 25:419-441.

Nakano, S, Morimoto, S, Suzuki, S, Watanabe, T, Amano, H, & Takasaki, Y. (2010) Up-regulation of the endoplasmic reticulum transmembrane protein UNC93b in the B cells of patients with active Systemic Lupus Erythematosus. Rheumatology (Oxford) 49:876-881.

Napirei, M, Karsunky, H, Zevnik, B, Stephan, H, Mannherz, HG, & Moroy, T. (2000) Features of Systemic Lupus Erythematosus in DNase1-deficient mice. Nature Genetics 25:177-181.

Nishiya, T, & DeFranco, AL. (2004) Ligand-regulated chimeric receptor approach reveals distinctive subcellular localization and signaling properties of the Toll-like receptors. Journal of Biological Chemistry 279:19008-19017.

Park, B, Brinkmann, MM, Spooner, E, Lee, CC, Kim, YM, & Ploegh, HL. (2008) Proteolytic cleavage in an endolysosomal compartment is required for activation of Toll-like receptor 9. Nature Immunology 9:1407-1414.

Pisitkun, P, Deane, JA, Difilippantonio, MJ, Tarasenko, T, Satterthwaite, AB, & Bolland, S. (2006) Autoreactive B cell responses to RNA-related antigens due to TLR7 gene duplication. Science 312:1669-1672.

Randow, F, & Seed, B. (2001) Endoplasmic reticulum chaperone gp96 is required for innate immunity but not cell viability. Nature Cell Biology 3:891-896.

Ronnblom, L, & Alm, GV. (2001) A pivotal role for the natural interferon alpha-producing cells (plasmacytoid dendritic cells) in the pathogenesis of lupus. Journal of Experimental Medicine 194:F59-63.

Sano, H, & Morimoto, C. (1982) DNA isolated from DNA/anti-DNA antibody immune complexes in Systemic Lupus Erythematosus is rich in guanine-cytosine content. Journal of Immunology 128:1341-1345.

Sasai, M, Linehan, MM, & Iwasaki, A. (2010) Bifurcation of Toll-like receptor 9 signaling by adaptor protein 3. Science 329:1530-1534.

Sato, T, Yamamoto, M, Shimosato, T, & Klinman, DM. (2010) Accelerated wound healing mediated by activation of Toll-like receptor 9. Wound Repair Regeneration 18:586-593.

Sepulveda, FE, Maschalidi, S, Colisson, R, Heslop, L, Ghirelli, C, Sakka, E, Lennon-Dumenil, AM, Amigorena, S, Cabanie, L, & Manoury, B. (2009) Critical role for asparagine endopeptidase in endocytic Toll-like receptor signaling in dendritic cells. Immunity 31:737-748.

Tabeta, K, Hoebe, K, Janssen, EM, Du, X, Georgel, P, Crozat, K, Mudd, S, Mann, N, Sovath, S, Goode, J, Shamel, L, Herskovits, AA, Portnoy, DA, Cooke, M, Tarantino, LM, Wiltshire, T, Steinberg, BE, Grinstein, S, & Beutler, B. (2006) The UNC93B1 mutation 3d disrupts exogenous antigen presentation and signaling via Toll-like receptors 3, 7 and 9. Nature Immunology 7:156-164.

Takahashi, K, Shibata, T, Akashi-Takamura, S, Kiyokawa, T, Wakabayashi, Y, Tanimura, N, Kobayashi, T, Matsumoto, F, Fukui, R, Kouro, T, Nagai, Y, Takatsu, K, Saitoh, S, & Miyake, K. (2007) A protein associated with Toll-like receptor (TLR) 4 (PRAT4A) is required for TLR-dependent immune responses. Journal of Experimental Medicine 204:2963-2976.

Takeda, K, Kaisho, T, & Akira, S. (2003) Toll-like receptors. Annual Review of Immunology 21:335-376.

Tian, J, Avalos, AM, Mao, SY, Chen, B, Senthil, K, Wu, H, Parroche, P, Drabic, S, Golenbock, D, Sirois, C, Hua, J, An, LL, Audoly, L, La Rosa, G, Bierhaus, A, Naworth, P, Marshak-Rothstein, A, Crow, MK, Fitzgerald, KA, Latz, E, Kiener, PA, & Coyle, AJ. (2007) Toll-like receptor 9-dependent activation by DNA-containing immune complexes is mediated by HMGB1 and rage. Nature Immunology 8:487-496.

Verthelyi, D, Ishii, KJ, Gursel, M, Takeshita, F, & Klinman, DM. (2001) Human peripheral blood cells differentially recognize and respond to two distinct CpG motifs. Journal of Immunology 166:2372-2377.

Villanueva, E, Yalavarthi, S, Berthier, CC, Hodgin, JB, Khandpur, R, Lin, AM, Rubin, CJ, Zhao, W, Olsen, SH, Klinker, M, Shealy, D, Denny, MF, Plumas, J, Chaperot, L, Kretzler, M, Bruce, AT, & Kaplan, MJ. (2011) Netting neutrophils induce endothelial damage, infiltrate tissues, and expose immunostimulatory molecules in Systemic Lupus Erythematosus. Journal of Immunology 187:538-552.

Vollmer, J, Weeratna, R, Payette, P, Jurk, M, Schetter, C, Laucht, M, Wader, T, Tluk, S, Liu, M, Davis, HL, & Krieg, AM. (2004) Characterization of three CpG oligodeoxynucleotide classes with distinct immunostimulatory activities. Euopeanr Journal of Immunology 34:251-262.

Xu, Y, Tao, X, Shen, B, Horng, T, Medzhitov, R, Manley, JL, & Tong, L. (2000) Structural basis for signal transduction by the Toll/interleukin-1 receptor domains. Nature 408:111-115.

Yakubov, LA, Deeva, EA, Zarytova, VF, Ivanova, EM, Ryte, AS, Yurchenko, LV, & Vlassov, VV. (1989) Mechanism of oligonucleotide uptake by cells: Involvement of specific receptors? Proceedings of the National Academy of Science U S A 86:6454-6458.

Yamashita, T, Shimada, S, Guo, W, Sato, K, Kohmura, E, Hayakawa, T, Takagi, T, & Tohyama, M. (1997) Cloning and functional expression of a brain peptide/histidine transporter. Journal of Biological Chemistry 272:10205-10211.

Yang, Y, Liu, B, Dai, J, Srivastava, PK, Zammit, DJ, Lefrancois, L, & Li, Z. (2007) Heat shock protein gp96 is a master chaperone for Toll-like receptors and is important in the innate function of macrophages. Immunity 26:215-226.

Yasuda, K, Richez, C, Uccellini, MB, Richards, RJ, Bonegio, RG, Akira, S, Monestier, M, Corley, RB, Viglianti, GA, Marshak-Rothstein, A, & Rifkin, IR. (2009) Requirement for DNA CpG content in TLR9-dependent dendritic cell activation induced by DNA-containing immune complexes. Journal of Immunology 183:3109-3117.

Yasuda, K, Yu, P, Kirschning, CJ, Schlatter, B, Schmitz, F, Heit, A, Bauer, S, Hochrein, H, & Wagner, H. (2005) Endosomal translocation of vertebrate DNA activates dendritic cells via TLR9-dependent and -independent pathways. Journal of Immunology 174:6129-6136.

Yasutomo, K, Horiuchi, T, Kagami, S, Tsukamoto, H, Hashimura, C, Urushihara, M, & Kuroda, Y. (2001) Mutation of DNase1 in people with systemic lupus erythematosus. Nature Genetics 28:313-314.

6

Atherogenesis and Vascular Disease in SLE

Isabel Ferreira[1] and José Delgado Alves[1,2]
[1]*Systemic Immunomediated Diseases Unit*
Department of Medicine IV, Hospital Prof. Doutor Fernando Fonseca, Amadora
[2]*CEDOC-Centro de Estudos de Doenças Crónicas*
Faculdade de Ciências Médicas, Universidade Nova de Lisboa
Portugal

1. Introduction

SLE is the classical model of a chronic multi-systemic immune-mediated inflammatory disease. It affects mainly young women, a subgroup of the general population usually free of cardiovascular risk. Although survival rates have improved dramatically, mainly due to early diagnosis, improved treatment, and better management of complications, death rates for patients with SLE remain 3 to 5 times higher than in the general population (Haque & Bruce, 2009). Nevertheless, whilst the 5-year survival of SLE was below 50% in the 1950s, it is nowadays above 90% (Nikpour et al., 2005).

Atherosclerosis in SLE is a highly complex process with autoimmunity, local and systemic inflammation, and endothelial dysfunction playing critical roles in its initiation and propagation. In the particular case of SLE, the extremely intricate immune system deregulation involving all types of immune cells up to an increased autoantibody production seems to play a major role for the accelerated atheroma formation found in these patients.

Cardiovascular events are now the major cause of morbidity and mortality in SLE. The acceptance of the importance of vascular risk in this context came from the description of a bimodal mortality pattern (Urowitz et al., 1976), with the early peak (within 1 year of diagnosis) as a consequence of active lupus and its complications, and the later peak (more than 5 years after diagnosis) mainly attributable to atherosclerosis. SLE is now considered to be a coronary heart disease-risk equivalent, mainly due to accelerated atherosclerosis (Aranow & Ginzler, 2000; Bjornadal et al., 2004; Manzi et al., 1997; Esdaile et al., 2001; Fischer et al. 2004; Roman et al., 2003; Ward, 1999). This can be especially relevant in young women, where up to a 50-fold increase in cardiovascular risk over age and gender-matched controls has been reported (Manzi et al., 1997). In fact, the majority of those women were aged less than 55 years at the time of their first cardiac event.

Framingham risk factors do not explain entirely the atherosclerotic burden found in patients with SLE. Furthermore, traditional cardiovascular risk factors seem to be less important predictors of cardiovascular events than the activity of lupus (Esdaile et al., 2001). (see table 1).

The direct relation between conventional and SLE-related risk factors and the actual incidence of events has not been easy to establish for different reasons: most patients with

SLE are young or middle-age women, for whom the background rate of cardiovascular disease is low, SLE cohorts are small, the number of observed coronary heart disease events is also reduced, and may not provide statistical power for testing their associations with hypothetical SLE-specific risk factors (Karp et al., 2008). This is the main reason why recent studies are considering surrogate markers of cardiovascular risk, such as the presence of carotid plaques, coronary artery calcification and vascular stiffness.

TRADITIONAL RISK FACTORS	INFLAMMATION-RELATED RISK FACTORS	SLE-RELATED RISK FACTORS
Genetics Gender Post-menopausal status Hypertension Dyslipidemia Diabetes mellitus Smoking Obesity Homocysteine Sedentary life-style	Vascular endothelial growth factor Monocyte chemoattractant protein-1 TNF-α, IL-1, IL-6 VCAM-1, ICAM-1 Matrix -degrading proteases Acute phase reactants Vascular endothelial growth factor Monocyte chemoattractant protein-1 TNF-α, IL-1, IL-6 VCAM-1, ICAM-1 Matrix -degrading proteases	Duration of disease Disease activity Disease damage Corticosteroids Auto-antibodies Complement activation Lupus nephritis Increased oxidative stress

Table 1. Proposed cardiovascular risk factors in SLE

Both SLE-specific and non-specific mechanisms have been proposed to play a prominent role in the induction of premature vascular damage, but the exact etiology remains unclear. Chronic inflammation is a very appellative contributor for atherosclerosis, since the pathogenesis of the latter is, in part, mediated by inflammation (Ross, 1999).

A potential confounding factor is that clinically active lupus may also manifest itself with vascular inflammation and thrombosis in any vascular territory. However, when a significant large population is considered, premature vascular disease in SLE is not, as previously thought, just attributable to vasculitis. Actually, it presents mostly as premature atherosclerosis (Bacon et al., 2002; Ward, 1999), both clinically and histologically. Many authors believe that the rapid and progressive nature of vascular injury in patients with SLE makes this population ideal for the identification of mechanisms involved in general atherosclerosis and vascular damage.

This chapter aims at elucidating why patients with SLE are at high risk for cardiovascular events, what different types of vascular conditions may be more commonly found, and what treatments are more likely to help overcome such burden.

2. Burden of disease

Despite the fact that the overall survival of patients with SLE has reached over 90% in recent decades, the long term survival rate has not changed since the 1980s (Petri, 2002). SLE patients have mortality rates of 5-10% at 5 years and 15-30% at 10 years (Abu-Shakra et al., 1995; Jacobsen et al., 1998; Ståhl-Hallengren et al., 2000; Uramoto et al., 1999). This is particularly overwhelming in patients aged less than 55 years (Abu-Shakra et al., 1995). After the identification of the bimodal pattern of mortality in SLE, a more recent uptade from the Toronto group (Nikpour, 2005) showed that sudden death, congestive heart failure and vascular events are responsible for nearly 30% of late deaths in their SLE cohort. Currently, cardiovascular disease alone accounts for 20 to 30 % of deaths in patients with SLE (Rubin et al., 1985). Even with all-cause mortality declining during the last 20 years the risk of cardiovascular death remains unchanged. With the advent of more potent immunosuppressive and anti-inflammatory treatments, it is likely that the contribution of cardiovascular disease to morbidity and mortality in these patients will increase even further.

Using myocardial perfusion scintigraphy, subclinical coronary atherosclerosis can be present in 28-38% of patients with SLE (Manger et al., 2003; Sella et al., 2003) and the prevalence of symptomatic coronary heart disease (as defined by angina and myocardial infarction) ranges from 6,6% to 20% (Gladman & Urowitz, 1987; Jonsson et al., 1989; Manzi et al., 1997) . Women with SLE in the 35-44 year age group are over 50 times more likely to have a myocardial infarction than women of similar age in the Framingham Offspring Study (Manzi et al., 1997). The mean age at a first coronary event is 49 years in patients with SLE compared with 65-74 years in the general population, as the risk of development of coronary heart disease in the first decade after diagnosis is approximately 12% (Bruce et al., 1999).

There are significant racial disparities regarding age at the time of first hospital admission for a cardiovascular event and cardiovascular-related hospitalization resulting in death in patients with SLE (Scalzi et al., 2010). African-origin, in particular, is associated in an independent fashion with a worsened probability of survival.

The outcomes of hospitalization for acute myocardial infarction were thought to be identical between patients with and without SLE, despite women with SLE being less likely to undergo coronary artery bypass grafting (Ward, 2004). Whether this is due to a decreased need for the procedure or whether reflects a decreased referral or reduced access to the surgery, is not established. More recently it has been recognized that, like diabetes mellitus, SLE increases the risk of poor outcomes after acute myocardial infarction, and these patients should be considered for aggressive treatment. In fact, the risk for prolonged hospitalization is even higher for patients with SLE (OR 1.48, 95% CI 1.32-1.79) compared to those with diabetes mellitus (OR 1.30, 95% CI 1.28-1.32) (Shah et al., 2009).

Cerebrovascular disease has been identified in 2-15% of patients with SLE (Hermosillo-Romo & Brey, 2002; Manzi et al., 1999; Mok et al., 2001; Sanna et al., 2003), with a reported 2-10 times higher risk for stroke SLE (Jonsson et al., 1989; Manzi et al., 1997; Ward, 1999). A recent prospective study showed that the cumulative incidence of arterial thromboembolism in new-onset Caucasian SLE patients is 5,1%, with ischemic stroke and transient ischemic attack comprising 65% of them (Mok et al., 2005) . Cardiovascular risk is even higher in lupus patients who also have secondary antiphospholipid syndrome (APS), due to the additive effects of SLE- and APS-related risk factors. In fact, as APS is also related to accelerated atherosclerosis, it may be difficult to differentiate between SLE- and APS-associated risk factors in these patients.

3. Vascular disease in systemic lupus erythematosus

3.1 Atherosclerosis

3.1.1 Epidemiology

In cross-sectional studies, approximately one-third of patients with SLE has evidence of subclinical atheroma plaques in the carotid or coronary arteries (Asunuma et al., 2003) and autopsy findings have showed an even higher prevalence of subclinical atherosclerosis (Bulkley & Roberts, 1975). More than 20% of SLE patients who had been on steroids for more than one year before death had a 50% occlusion of at least one major coronary artery. In a cohort of women with SLE, in whom 15% had already a cardiovascular event, 40% had at least one focal carotid artery plaque, a higher frequency than would be expected among healthy women (Manzi et al., 1999). Not surprinsingly, the common carotid intima-media thickness (IMT) of patients with a history of cardiovascular disease is greater than that of SLE patients who had no such history and of healthy volunteers controls (Svenungsson et al., 2001). Using photon emission computed tomography (SPECT) and dual isotope myocardial perfusion imaging (DIMPI), 40% of all women with SLE and 35% of women with SLE and no history of coronary artery disease had abnormalities in myocardial perfusion, reinforcing the idea of a high prevalence of early coronary artery disease (Bruce et al., 2000). Also, coronary-artery calcification, as detected by electron-beam computed tomography (Roman et al., 2003), occurs more frequently and at a younger age in patients with SLE than in healthy controls. Aortic stiffness overall and at any level of the aortic artery was higher in patients with SLE than in controls, even after adjusting for age (Roldan et al., 2010). Furthermore, increased aortic stiffness seems to be an early manifestation of lupus vasculopathy that seems to precede the development of hypertension and atherosclerosis. Whether we consider the SLE context or not, better biomarkers for measuring disease burden are needed. They should be non-invasive, have a good sensitivity and specificity, predict disease in asymptomatic individuals and be available for widespread application.

In clinical practice, diagnosis of atherosclerosis is usually made after the presence of symptoms. Pre-symptomatic screening could identify subclinical disease, allowing for a more aggressive treatment of the different atherothrombotic risk factors.

3.1.2 Atheroma formation

Atherosclerosis is not an age-related process with passive accumulation of lipids in the vessel wall. It must be understood as a dynamic and complex biochemical and anatomical process. It is characterized by changes in lipoprotein metabolism, activation of the immune system and consequent proliferation of smooth-muscle cells, atheroma formation and arterial narrowing. In atheroma formation, inflammation and autoimmunity are at the forefront of the initiation, progression, and rupture of the plaque (Libby et al., 2010; van Leuven et al., 2008). Patients suffering from chronic inflammatory diseases have accelerated atherosclerosis, and the high level of inflammation to which patients with auto-immune diseases are exposed may induce and accelerate endothelial cell injury. Furthermore, biomechanic shear forces enhanced by classic cardiovascular risk factors, such as hypertension, hypercholesterolemia, diabetes and smoking are known to contribute to endothelium dysfunction (Ando & Yamamoto, 2011). In fact, the earliest manifestation of atherothrombosis can be the result of a single disturbance on the physiologic pattern of blood flow at an arterial bending on bifurcation site.

Endothelium regulates anti-inflammatory, mitogenic and contractility activities of the vessel wall; also, it has a role in the the hemostatic process within the vessel lumen. A dysfunctional endothelium is characterized by an increase in oxidative stress. It facilitates oxidation, the uptake of circulating lipoproteins by monocytes, and the migration of these cells to the vessel wall, resulting in the proliferation of smooth muscle cells. The expression of adhesion molecules (such as ICAM and VCAM) induces the binding of monocytes to the endothelial wall (Lusis, 2000). This, when submitted to shear stress forces is also susceptible to permeation and subendothelial accumulation of apolipoprotein-B-containing lipoproteins, such as low density lipoproteins (LDL) and remnant lipoproteins, that become targets for oxidative and enzymatic attack. After monocyte-endothelial binding takes place, the blood cells are internalized and differentiated into macrophages. Retained pro-atherogenic LDL leads to an enhanced selective leukocyte recruitment and attachment to the endothelial layer, further contributing to their transmigration across the endothelium into the intima. Lipoprotein uptake promotes the accumulation of lipid droplets in the cytoplasm of the macrophages, transforming them into foam cells. The consequent inflammatory response leads to the recruitment of more monocytes, T cells, mast cells and neutrophiles. A fibrous cap is produced by collagen secreting myofibroblasts that populate the intima, and the developing lesion is contained, most of the times, by a fibrous cap. At the beginning, the atherosclerotic lesions are asymptomatic and not at risk for rupture and induction of thrombosis. Atheroma lesions submitted to a chronic inflammatory state will become unstable and may result in an acute vascular event (Virmani et al., 2002). Within those plaques, apoptotic macrophages will suffer necrosis and perpetuate inflammation, with the formation of necrotic cores. These vulnerable or unstable plaques may rupture, exposing pro-coagulant and pro-thrombogenic molecules into the intima and initiating platelet activation and aggregation. This, in turn, will lead to thrombosis and to the clinical manifestation of atherothrombotic disease.

Inflammation plays a major role during all stages of atherosclerosis: endothelial dysfunction, endothelial and cytokine activation, recruitment of inflammatory cells, macrophage uptake of oxidized low-density lipoprotein (oxLDL), development of fatty streaks and fibrous plaque, and finally plaque rupture. Being so, it becomes obvious why SLE and atherosclerosis are so closely related.

3.1.3 Lipids and humoral response towards lipoproteins

Lipid abnormalities are one of the major contributors for atherosclerosis in SLE and different patterns of dyslipoproteinemia have been reported in this disease (Ilowite et al., 1988; Svenungsson et al., 2003). Dyslipoproteinemia in active lupus is characterized by depressed high density lipoprotein cholesterol and apolipoprotein A1 (ApoA1) with elevated very low density lipoprotein cholesterol (VLDL) and triglyceride; on the other hand, the dyslipoproteinemia associated with corticosteroid treatment is characterized by increased total cholesterol, VLDL, and triglycerides. The pattern of dyslipoproteinemia typical of SLE is closely related to disease activity. An enhanced activity in the TNFalpha/soluble TNF-receptor system seems to be an important underlying factor (Svenungsson et al., 2003).

Oxidative stress is also a key factor in atherogenesis, and it is increased in patients with SLE. Interactions between anticardiolipin (aCL) antibodies and anti-oxidant endothelial cells antibodies with the production of pro-oxidant substances suggestes that the interactive mechanisms linking plasma lipoproteins, the immune system, and the endothelium are one of the missing links that can unveil atheroma plaque formation in SLE. Oxidation profile in SLE is reflection of a pro-oxidant status and the presence of aCL antibodies is just one of the potential contributors. A direct effect of aCL antibodies with endothelial cells (inducing inducible nitric oxide synthase expression) leads to an enhanced peroxynitrite synthesis, a pro-oxidant substance, associated with vascular dysfunction and atherogenesis (Delgado Alves et al., 2005).

The primary lipid components involved in atherosclerosis are lipoproteins. Among these, low-density lipoprotein (LDL) and high-density lipoprotein (HDL) assume a central role. HDL are thought to have an anti-atherothrombogenic effect by stimulating endothelial nitric oxide and inhibiting oxidative stress and inflammation (Yuhanna et al., 2001), thus preventing LDL oxidation. LDL is the most pro-atherogenic lipoprotein, due to its ability to capture free radicals becoming itself a powerful pro-oxidant. HDL-associated ApoA1 has known anti-inflammatory properties (Ashby et al., 1998; Hyka et al., 2001) by promoting reverse cholesterol transport from macrophages *in vivo* as well as by blocking contact mediated activation of monocytes by T lymphocytes. Its anti-atherosclerotic actions is also associated with the stabilization of paraoxonase (James & Deakin, 2000). Paraoxonase is an anti-oxidant enzyme that prevents the formation of lipid peroxidation products, such as oxLDL. Higher paraoxonase activity is associated with a lower incidence of cardiovascular events (Soran et al., 2009).

HDL has several other antiatherogenic properties, including the transport of cholesterol from peripheral tissues to the liver. The concept that macrophage-cholesterol efflux has a significant role in cardiovascular disease prevention was recently suggested by the finding of a strong inverse association between HDL-mediated cholesterol efflux from macrophages, carotid intima media thickness (IMT) and the likelihood of coronary heart disease (Khera et al., 2011). These effects were shown to be independent of HDL-cholesterol level. Nevertheless, low levels of HDL increase the cholesterol burden and macrophage-driven inflammation, being strongly associated with the risk of coronary artery disease. Another condition that increases that risk involves the conversion of HDL to a dysfunctional form that is no longer cardioprotective (Barter et al., 2004), but instead acquire a pro-inflammatory and pro-oxidant phenotype promoting atherosclerosis (Delgado Alves et al., 2002, 2009). Regardless of all these data, the underlying mechanisms are still unclear, and no widely accepted methods for determining HDL function have been recognized. Other possible mechanisms for HDL dysfunction may be the increased glycation with the consequent ApoA1 multimerization and decreased phospholipid content (Parker & Cho, 2011). This proinflammatory form of HDL (piHDL) has been described in SLE (Navab et al., 2001) High levels of piHDL increases the risk of developing subclinical atherosclerosis in SLE (MacMahon et al., 2009).

A new concept has merged recently that might account for the higher risk of atherosclerosis in SLE: the humoral response towards HDL. It has been confirmed the presence of IgG antibodies towards HDL and its main protein component ApoA1 in patients with SLE. By interfering with the anti-atherogenic properties of HDL, anti-HDL and ApoA1 antibodies enhance oxidative stress and the consequent SLE-related atherosclerotic lesions. Anti-HDL antibodies are associated with decreased paraoxonase activity, increased biomarkers of endothelial dysfunction (nitric oxide, adhesion molecules VCAM-1 and ICAM-1), reduced total antioxidant capacity, and also increased disease-related damage and activity (Batuca et al., 2009). Both anti-HDL and anti-apolipoprotein A1 antibodies cross react with aCL. Theoretically, anti-HDL and anti-ApoA1 antibodies that cross react with aCL antibodies may contribute to endothelial dysfunction by favouring the oxidation of LDL.

Anti-ApoA1 antibodies have also been described in acute coronary syndromes (Vuilleumier et al., 2008), and they be potential markers of plaque instability (Montecucco et al., 2011).

LDL is the major cholesterol carrying lipoprotein in plasma and may exist in different forms. OxLDL injures cells in artery walls, and promotes atheroma formation (Colles et al., 2001; Hessler et al., 1979). Small dense LDL, when compared with its larger, normal-size counterpart, is more easily oxidized, has a higher affinity for extracellular matrix, and is subject to a higher degree of retention in the arterial wall (Berneis & Krauss, 2002; Hurt-Camejo et al., 2001; Packard & Sheperd, 1997). Also, smaller LDL has reduced binding to LDL receptors (Chapman et al., 1998) and a longer "half-life". These facts may lead to a greater degree of structural modification, which further increases its atherogenic profile.

In SLE, antibodies to oxidized LDL (anti-oxLDL) have been demonstrated in up to one half of patients with SLE (Romero et al., 1998). Also, anti-oxLDL antibody levels correlate with complement activation, disease activity scores, anti-double-stranded DNA antibody titres (Gómez-Zumaquero et al., 2004) and were found to facilitate the formation of foam cells(Matsuura et al., 2006)

3.1.4 Inflammation and acute response

It is already established that inflammation plays a pivotal role in the pathogenesis of atherosclerosis. It mediates several of the stages of atheroma development from initial leukocyte recruitment to eventual rupture of the unstable atherosclerotic plaque. SLE is characterized by a low-grade persistent pro-inflammatory state, present not only during flares but also during stable disease. The chronic burden of activated inflammatory mediators may have a considerable impact on endothelial cell function and blood coagulation. Several inflammatory circulating intermediates in SLE have been identified as highly atherogenic, such as IL-1, IL-6, IL-18, monocyte chemotatic protein 1, interferon γ and TNFα, among others (Asanuma et al., 2006; Blake &Ridker, 2001; Aringer & Smolen, 2004).

C-Reactive protein (CRP) is an acute phase protein that plays a major role in the regulation of the inflammatory response. It has been implicated in the promotion of both leukocyte adhesion and migration and also in vascular endothelial dysfunction by inducing adhesion molecules, chemokines and cytokines(Pasceri et al., 2000, 2001). Levels of C-reactive protein (CRP) have been shown to be predictive of cardiovascular disease in the general population (Ridker et al., 2002). High-sensitivity CRP and ICAM-1 have been associated with increased coronary artery calcification in SLE patients (Kao et al., 2008). The interaction of anti-monomeric CRP with monomeric CRP in blood vessel walls may also contribute to development of cardiovascular disease in SLE (O'Neill et al., 2007).

As compared with other auto-immune diseases, such as rheumatoid arthritis, the magnitude of CRP elevation is less important. It has been proposed that the relatively low CRP levels in SLE patients can be explained by increased clearance or decreased production of this protein. Autoantibodies to CRP in SLE patients support its increased clearance (Bell et al, 1998; Sjowall et al, 2004); however, the plasma clearance rate of CRP is the same in patients with active lupus and normal individuals, which makes this hypothesis less likely (Vigushin et al, 1993).

3.1.5 Insulin resistance and the metabolic syndrome

The metabolic syndrome is a new defined cluster of risk factors associated with increased insulin resistance, higher risk of developing type II diabetes mellitus and cardio and cerebrovascular events. It is an independent predictor of cardiovascular morbidity and mortality. These risk factors include abdominal obesity, pro-atherogenic dyslipidemia and elevated blood pressure. Even though individually these abnormalities may contribute little, as a risk-factor cluster it is very important and aggressive treatment should be considered in these patients. It is estimated that this syndrome may affect 20-25% of the overall population in the United States and the prevalence increases with age (Ford et al., 2002).

Insulin resistance is characterized by an impaired response to insulin in several insulin-sensitive tissue, such as muscle, liver, fat and endothelium (Simonson et al., 2005). Insulin has anti-inflammatory properties, mainly due to its ability to suppress several proinflammatory transcription factors, such as nuclear factor kappa-light-chain-enhancer of activated B cells (NF-κB) , early growth response protein 1 (Egr-1) and activator protein 1 (AP-1) (Aliada et al., 2002). Insulin resistance is a main contributor to the increased cardiovascular risk attributed to the metabolic syndrome (Hanley et al., 2002). There is a link between high levels of proinflammatory cytokines and cardiovascular disease through metabolic pathways. The exact mechanisms linking insulin resistance and inflammation are not fully established. A possible candidate is TNF- α. It is over-expressed in the adipose tissues of animal models of obesity (Hotamisligi et al., 1993). Adipose tissue act as an endocrine secretory gland, producing several inflammatory mediators, responsible for a pro-inflammatory state and thus to an increased cardiovascular risk (Després & Lemieux, 2006).

Tumor necrosis factor-α (TNF-α), IL-1β, IL-4, IL-6, IL-11, Interferon-γ (INF-γ), acting on sensitive adipocytes, can lead to the activation of inflammatory signaling cascades (Rajala & Sherer, 2003). As a response to fat activation, there is enhanced expression and secretion of several acute phase reactants and also mediators of inflammation, such as TNF-α, IL-1β, IL-6, IL-8, IL- 10, prostaglandin E2 (PGE2). Leptin, adiponectin, and resistin (Fain et al., 2004) can perpetuate in the highly pro-inflammatory state.

SLE is associated with an increased prevalence of the metabolic syndrome (El-Magdami et al., 2006). The frequency of metabolic syndrome amongst patients with SLE varies from 16,7% in Mexico(Zonana-Nacah e tal., 2008), 28,6 % in Argentina to 29,4 % in USA (Chung et al., 2007) and 32,1 % in Brazil (Telles et al., 2010), with other cohorts showing similar results. Other metabolic-associated changes such as insulin resistance, premature menopause, renal impairment and high triglyceridemia also occur more frequently in SLE. Controversy still remains regarding the exact role of metabolic syndrome in predicting long-term risk for coronary heart disease in SLE. The major benefit in recognising this syndrome in the context of SLE is related to the identification of patients more in need for lifestyle interventions and specific therapeutic approach.

There is no clear association between treatment with steroids and the development of metabolic syndrome (Telles et al., 2007. However, prednisone in dosages higher than 10 mg/ day and high dosages of intravenous methylprednisone has been previously associated with this condition (Négron et al., 2008). These findings are still not definitive as they can be a reflection of lupus activity and severity. In fact, low-dose steroids may still be of value, due to its anti-inflammatory effects.

3.1.6 Traditional risk factors for cardiovascular disease in SLE

A patient with SLE and cardiovascular disease has on average one less traditional risk factor than people in the general population with a similar cardiovascular condition (Bruce, 2005; Urowitz et al., 2007) and the baseline 10-year coronary heart disease and stroke risk (after adjusting for Framingham score) for all patients with SLE is 7.5–17-fold higher (Esdaile et al., 2001). This is one of the reasons why the relative importance of the individual traditional risk factors differs between patients with SLE and the general population.

Hypertension

Hypertension is a predictor of mortality and vascular events in SLE (Petri et al., 1992; Rahman et al., 2000). It is more common than in the general population with a relative risk of 2.59 (95% CI 1.79–3.75) (Bruce et al., 2003), independently of whatever treatment for SLE is being administred.

Smoking

Smoking, a well known risk factor for atherosclerosis, is not more frequent in patients with SLE than in the general population (RR 0.86, 95% CI 0.59–1.24) (Boyer et al., 2011), but in the Systemic Lupus International Collaborating Clinics registry (SLICC) (Urowitz et al., 2008) the prevalence of smokers increased from 13.7% at baseline to 18.7%.

Dyslipidemia

Hpercholesterolemia in lupus patients is associated with an 18-fold increased risk of myocardial infarction as compared with the general population (Fischer et al., 2004).

Body composition and low physical exercise

Patients with lupus are more likely to have a sedentary lifestyle, with consequent obesity and hypercholesterolemia (Petri et al., 1992). Low physical activity is associated with increased subclinical atherosclerosis and proinflammatory HDL levels in patients with SLE. Despite the common presence of fatigue as a symptom of the disease, there is reason to believe that exercise should be included in the rehabilitation of patients with mild to moderate SLE (Yuen et al., 2011). Exercise, if well tolerated, may reduce the risk of atherosclerosis in SLE (Volkmann et al., 2010).

3.1.7 Other risk factors

Treatment of SLE and its most common co-morbidities has become more and more complex with drug interactions and side effects becoming a very important issue. Apart from the classical complications of steroid and immunosuppressive treatment, new associations between drugs and clinical adverse effects have been identified. Azathioprine, as an example, was associated with arterial events (hazard ratio of 1.45 (95% CI 1.21–10.4) (Toloza et al., 2004) and with the presence of carotid plaques (Ahmad et al., 2004). Although we should keep these results in mind, the fact is that azathioprine is used in more active disease and it may be just a surrogate for more severe inflammation.

Hyperhomocysteinemia is a well known risk factor for cardiovascular disease and it is a possible marker of atherosclerosis progression and more-active lupus (Bultink et al., 2005; Kianai et al., 2007; Roman et al., 2007). It decreases the availability of endothelial cell-derived nitric oxide, impairs endothelial-dependent vasodilatation, induces oxidative stress, and increases the risk of thrombosis (Maron & Loscalzo, 2009). Homocystein actions on endothelial cells are partly mediated by asymmetric dimethylarginine (ADMA), an intrinsic inhibitor of nitric oxide synthase (Stuhlinger et al., 2003). High levels of ADMA have been described in patients with renal and heart failure, diabetes mellitus, hypertension, and acute coronary events and may predict stroke, coronary artery disease, and also cardiovascular-related death (Laier et al. 2008; Wilson et al., 2008). Among patients with SLE, higher ADMA levels are linked to a higher prevalence of cardiovascular disease.

Hyperuricemia correlates with arterial stiffness and inflammation markers in patients with SLE without symptomatic atherosclerotic disease. It has been showed that women with SLE and hyperuricemia have a high risk cardiovascular profile with metabolic syndrome and renal failure.

3.2 Vasculitis

In the absence of clinically significant coronary atherosclerosis, two other major mechanisms of vascular damage may occur: vasculitis and thrombosis.

The prevalence of vasculitis in SLE patients ranges from 11% to 20% (Cardinali et al., 2000; Wisnieki, 2000). Small vessels (both arteries and venules) of the skin are the most commoly involved (Gonzalez-Gay et al., 2005); medium-sized vessel involvement is less frequent (D'Cruz et al., 1993), and large vessel involvement is rare (Goldberger et al., 1992). Although vasculitis presents mainly as cutaneous lesions, the clinical spectrum is wide, and lifethreatening ischemic injury may result from vasculitis of medium-sized vessels in the gastrointestinal, cardiac, pulmonary, or cerebrovascular regions (D'Cruz, 1998).

Coronary vascular damage may be related to coronary arteritis, affecting preferentially small-size coronary arteries (Bulkley & Roberts, 1975) or, rarely, the medium-size coronary arteries (Bonfiglio et al., 1992); and/ or coronary artery thrombosis. Acute myocardial infarction due to coronary arteritis is reported in SLE, although the incidence is very low.

Immune complex deposition and complement activation play important roles in the pathogenesis of vasculitis in general and coronary arteritis in particular. In patients with both SLE and antiphospholipid syndrome, microvascular thrombi of the coronary circulation, with discrete atherosclerosis and vasculitis, have been observed (Brown et al., 1988).

The distinction between atherosclerosis and arteritis is a difficult task, because coronary vasculitis often occurs in the absence of a clinical SLE flare and also with minimal serologic evidence of disease activity (Wilson et al., 1992).

Central nervous system (CNS) vasculitis in the context of SLE is rare, although it has been found in autopsies in SLE in 7-12% of cases (Johnson & Richardson, 1968; Ellis & Verity, 1979).

Stroke (both ischaemic and haemorrhagic) and SLE cerebral vasculopathy are far more frequent. While ischaemic stroke in SLE is strongly associated to antiphospholipid syndrome, atherosclerosis (Bruce, 2005) and Libman-Sacks endocarditis (Moyassaki et al., 2007), factors that contribute to hemorrhagic stroke are less clear.

The predominant pathology finding in CNS vessels in SLE patients is a noninflammatory small vessel vasculopathy involving small arterioles and capillaries. At autopsy, 50% of the patients have cerebral vasculopathy, characterized by hyaline thickening and eosinophilia of the vessel wall, fibrinoid degeneration without vasculitis, and endothelial proliferation, sometimes accompanied by microhemorrhages (Devinsky et al., 1988; Ellison et al. 1993; Hanly et al., 1992).

3.3 Thrombosis

Thrombotic events are reported in 7-12% of patients with SLE (Somers et al., 1999). During the first year of disease, the incidence of both arterial and venous thrombotic events increases. Several reasons have been pointed out, and include aPL antibodies, circulating immune complexes, high levels of disease activity, and chronic inflammation (Manger et al., 2002). When associated with SLE, antiphospholipid syndrome is a relevant predictor of organ damage and death in patients (Ruiz-Irastorza et al., 2004). Anti-cardiolipin (aCL) antibodies, lupus anticoagulant (LAC) and anti-beta2-glycoprotein 1 antibodies (anti-B2GPI) are detected in approximately one-third of patients with SLE (Love & Santoro, 1990), especially in the context of the antiphospholipid syndrome. The best predictors for thrombotic events in SLE are persistent aPL antibodies, the presence of LAC (Somers et al., 2002), and high titers of aCL antibodies (Ginsburg et al., 1992).

Not all thrombotic phenomena are associated with the presence of aPL antibodies and some patients may develop venous and arterial thrombosis without aCL positivity. The relevance of traditional and SLE-related thrombotic risk factors in aPL positive patients is still under investigation. Most of the patients with SLE and aPL antibodies who developed thrombosis had other thrombotic risk factors (Erkan et al., 2007). Interestingly, after adjusting for other risk factors, SLE itself remains independently associated with thrombotic events (Bruce, 2005). Thrombosis is frequent in early SLE and is associated with a significant mortality; therefore, the identification of possible modifiable risk factors and the establishment of efficacious strategies of prevention and treatment are vital.

4. Treatment

The impact of cardiovascular disease has been under-recognized in the context of SLE, with limited attention on aggressive management of possible modifiable risk factors. Despite a general awareness of coronary vascular disease in SLE patients, physicians do not address risk factors in a comprehensive fashion. Also, the management of conventional cardiovascular risk factors such as diabetes mellitus, smoking, hypercholesterolemia and hypertension is not at the same level of non-SLE patients. This is reinforced by the fact that recruiting and retaining patients with SLE for clinical trials regarding preventive measures has been proven to be extremely difficult.

It is therefore of great importance to identify in each patient the modifiable risk factors and introduce in clinical practice guidelines to help clinicians reducing long-term cardiovascular morbidity and mortality. In this chapter, we analyze the potential impact of some of the most commonly used drugs in SLE and their effects in the cardiovascular system.

The general approach suggested in the overall population for primary and secondary prophylaxis of vascular disease should be proposed to every patient and should include (table 2):

4.1 Corticosteroids: Are they good or bad for lupus?

Corticosteroids still remain a first line treatment for lupus, despite having numerous detrimental side effects on blood pressure, blood glucose and lipid profile (Manzi et al., 2000). Corticosteroids have a particular deleterious effect on the heart (Bulkley et al., 1975). Prednisone dosage superior to 7,5 mg/d increases insulin levels, a risk factor for cardiovascular disease (Karp et al., 2008) and total cholesterol, triglycerides and apolipoprotein B levels increase significantly with a daily prednisone dose higher than 10 mg (Petri et al., 1992). The estimated 2-year coronary risk for a patient treated with anved an average dosage of 30 mg/day of prednisone for 1 year, is approximately 60% higher than it would be for a patient with the same levels of SLE activity and similar risk factors who received no corticosteroids (Karp et al., 2008).

When compared to a baseline chronic inflammatory status, low dose corticosteroids may exert an anti-inflammatory action which might be beneficial. In fact, such exposure may improve the lipid profile and increase insulin levels, whithout having a negative effect on blood pressure and atherosclerosis. A weak association between low-dose corticosteroids and cardiovascular risk factors has been established, and identified a dose-related trend for increasing major cardiovascular events (Ruyssen-Witrand et al., 2010). Furthermore, subclinical atherosclerosis is correlated with lower mean dose of corticosteroids and lesser immunossupressants (Roman et al., 2003).

Cholesterol	1. Screening: fasting lipid profile every year; 2. For LDL cholesterol <2.6 mmol/l: no treatment; 3. For LDL cholesterol 2.6–3.4 mmol/l: therapeutic lifestyle changes. 4. Consider statins when LDL is >3.4 mmol/l with or without other risk factors; or when LDL is persistently >2.6 mmol/l despite therapeutic lifestyle changes.
Hypertension	1. Blood pressure assessments at every visit to the outpatients clinic; 2. Ideal target is defined as blood pressure at <130mmHg systolic and <80mmHg diastolic. 3. If elevated blood pressure (>140 mmHg systolic or >90mmHg diastolic): lifestyle modification.; 4. If, despite previous measures, the blood pressure is persistently found to be elevated: start antihypertensive medication.
Diabetes mellitus	1. Regular testing for diabetes (1-2 /year); 2. In patients with a fasting glucose ≥6.1 mmol/l: glucose tolerance test and lifestyle changes; 3. Referral to a specialist in diabetes.
Weight control	1. Screening for obesity; 2. Lifestyle changes, exercise programmes and behavioral support; 3. If, despite efforts, obesity remains, refer to drug/ bariatric surgery by a multidisciplinary team.

Table 2. Summary of some therapeutic interventions.

There are some important limitations in addressing the role of steroids in cardiovascular risk. Corticosteroid use is more common in patients with moderate to severe disease (Bruce, 2006) and the duration of exposure to this drug may function as a surrogate for disease duration. Further work is needed to assess if there are doses or regimes of corticosteroid therapy that can optimise their anti-inflammatory effects whilst minimizing their multiple adverse effects.

4.2 Statins

Pleotropic actions of hydroxyl-3-methylglutaryl coenzyme A (HMG-CoA) inhibitors (statins) have been thourougly reported and is now accepted that their benefits go beyond cholesterol lowering and include immunomodulatory and immunossupressive properties. Statins inhibit HMG-CoA reductase, an enzyme that converts HMG-CoA to mevalonate, a fundamental step in cholesterol synthesis. The mevalonate pathway is involved in posttranslational modification of cell-signaling proteins during cell division and maturation, with inhibition of proinflammatory effects. It then promotes anti-inflammatory activities through the direct inhibition/activation of chemokyne, cytokine-, and acute-phase reactant-driven intracellular pathways in several cell types involved in inflammation. Statins modulate the activity of cells involved in both innate and adaptative immune responses, affecting the production of cytokines and cellular adhesion molecules (e.g. ICAM-a, IL-6, TNF-α, IL-1 and selectin levels (Mira & Mañes, 2009) and have an antithrombotic effect by

inhibiting platelet activation (Ferroni et al., 2006). In the general population, statins have shown efficacy in primary and secondary prevention of acute myocardial infarction and stroke (Amarenco et al., 2006; Ridker et al., 2008).
Following the identification of their mechanisms of action, statins became a potential drug for treating SLE patients despite cardiovascular involvement. Low dose rosuvastatin induced a significant reduction in LDL and CRP after 12 months treatment (Mok et al., 2011). In patients with low disease activity, rosuvastatin decreased plasma levels of endothelial activation markers such as P-selectin and VCAM-1. Unexpectedly, in 2011, the results from the Lupus Atherosclerosis Prevention Study (Petri et al., 2011) offered no evidence that atorvastatin could reduce markers of subclinical atherosclerosis or disease activity over 2 years and the anti-inflammatory effects of statins observed in the general population were not replicated in this SLE clinical trial. However, comments were raised regarding the homogeneity of both treatment arms which may limit the final interpretation. Importantly, there was no information about the treatments received by patients during the 2 years follow-up, regarding the use of prednisone, immunosupresive agents and hydroxychloroquine, all of them having a direct effect on inflammation and disease activity and potentially on subclinical atherosclerosis. Hence, the negative results in this clinical trial could be caused by an imbalance in the use of these drugs in both arms, rather than by the lack of efficacy of atorvastatin.

4.3 Low dose salicylic acid

Most of SLE patients with aPL, but without a history of thrombosis, do not receive any preventive therapeutic, while some receive low dose salicylic acid (ASA) (Kamashta, 2000). Prophylactic treatment with ASA in SLE patients may prevent both arterial and venous thrombotic manifestations, especially in patients with positive aPL (Wahl et al., 2000). In fact, ASA decreases the probability of thrombosis in asymptomatic individuals with aPL (Erkan et al., 2002). The use of low-dose ASA has been recommended by the expert committee in the recent European League Against Rheumatism guidelines for the management of SLE (Bertsias et al., 2008).

4.4 Hydroxychloroquine

Hydroxychloroquine is an anti-malarial drug also used to treat SLE, Sjögren's syndrome and other immune mediate diseases. Several mechanisms have been proposed to explain its beneficial effect, which is not fully established. Hydroxychloroquine can inhibit the binding of antiphospholipid antibody-β2-glycoprotein I complexes to phospholipid bilayers (Rand et al., 2008), reverse platelet activation induced by human IgG aPL antibodies (Espinola et al., 2002), and reduce of aPL antibody-induced thrombosis (Edwards et al., 1996). There is no consistent data regarding whether this antithrombotic effect is present both for arterial and venous events.
A beneficial effect on serum lipid levels, including patients taking corticosteroid therapy (Borba et al., 2001; Hodis et al., 1993; Sachet et al., 2007; Tam et al., 2000), was shown by a few observational studies. However, the strenght of evidence supporting a clinically meaningful beneficial effect was rated as low. Also, there is no data supporting any protective effect of this drug on the development of metabolic syndrome (Ruiz-Irastorza et al., 2010).

Regarding the effect of hydroxychloroquine on atherosclerosis, most studies are limited by the low consistency and lack of specific design (Ahmad et al., 2007; Maksimowicz-McKinnon et al, 2006). The effect was not quantified in most cases and the exposure to hydroxychloroquine has been heterogeneously defined, without taking into account the time of exposure or a possible dose effect.

Because of its beneficial effects on reducing SLE activity and mortality, most of the authors recommend hydroxychloroquine for most patients with SLE, starting as soon as the diagnosis is made. Its application for the specific prevention of thrombosis and treatment of atherosclerosis requires validation in future clinical trials.

4.5 B-cell depletion therapy

Rituximab, a drug that had no previously documented lipid-lowering effect, was recently investigated in patients with SLE who had failed standard immunosuppressive therapy (Pego-Reigosa et al., 2010). An increase in HDL cholesterol and a fall in the total cholesterol/HDL ratio and triglyceride levels was documented in a significant proportion of the 12 patients studied. Furthermore, this improvement in lipid profile mirrored a decrease in disease activity; this suggests a positive effect of rituximab related to a reduction in the overall high inflammatory status. Still, larger prospective studies should aim to evaluate if this observed favorable effect contributes to a lower incidence of cardiovascular events.

5. Conclusion

Patients with SLE are at increased risk for cardiovascular complications. Atherosclerosis occurs prematurely in patients with systemic lupus erythematosus and is independent of the traditional risk factors for cardiovascular disease. Premature atherosclerosis has emerged as a leading cause of morbidity and mortality in SLE. Traditional risk factors, such as hypertension, smoking, diabetes, obesity and dyslipidemia are common in SLE but they fail to explain entirely the atherosclerotic burden found in these patients. Increased understanding of the mechanisms underlying vascular damage, plaque formation and stability, and thrombosis, will greatly facilitate the long-term care of patients with lupus. The clinical profile of patients with lupus and atherosclerosis suggests a role for disease-related factors in atherogenesis and underscores the need better trials targeting atherosclerosis in a specific fashion.

An early identification of subclinical atherosclerosis in SLE is warranted to help to identify patients with higher risk to undergo major vascular complications, who might benefit from more aggressive treatment and lifestyle modifications.

6. References

Abu-Shakra, M, Urowitz, MB, Gladman, DD, et al. (1995). Mortality studies in systemic lupus erythematosus. Results from a single center. II. Predictor variables for mortality. *J Rheumatol*, Vol.22, No.7, (July 1995), pp. 1265-70, ISSN 1499-2752.

Aranow, C, Ginzler, EM. (2000). Epidemiology of cardiovascular disease in systemic lupus erythematosus. *Lupus*. Vol.9, No.3, (April 2000). pp.166–169, ISSN 1477-0962.

Asanuma, Y, Oeser, A, Shintani, AK, et al. (2003). Premature coronary-artery atherosclerosis in systemic lupus erythematosus. *N Engl J Med.* Vol.349, No.25, (December 2003), pp. 2407-2415, ISSN 1533-4406.

Ahmad, Y, Shelmerdine, J, Bodill, H, et al. (2007). Subclinical atherosclerosis in systemic lupus erythematosus (SLE): the relative contribution of classic risk factors and the lupus phenotype. *Rheumatology* (Oxford), Vol. 46, No.6, (June 2007), pp. 983–988, ISSN 1499-2752.

Amarenco, P, Bogousslavsky, J, Callahan, A 3rd, et al. (2006). Stroke Prevention by Aggressive Reduction in Cholesterol Levels (SPARCL) Investigators High-dose atorvastatin after stroke or transient ischemic attack. *N Engl J Med,* (August 2006), Vol.355, No.6, pp. 549-559, ISSN 1533-4406.

Ahmad ,Y, Bodill ,H, Shelmerdine ,J, et al. (2004). Antiphospholipid antibodies (APLA) contribute to atherogenesis in SLE. *Arthritis Rheum,* (2004), Vol. 50, Suppl. 1, pp. S191, ISSN 1529-013.

Aljada, A, Ghanim, H, Mohanty, P, et al. (2002). Insulin inhibits the pro-inflammatory transcription factor early growth response gene-1 (Egr-1) expression in mononuclear cells and reduces plasma tissue factor (TF) and plasminogen activator inhibitor-1 (PAI-1) concentrations. *J Clin Endocrinol Metab,* (March 2002), Vol.87, No.3, pp. 1419–1422, ISSN 1945-7197.

Asanuma,Y, Chung, CP, Oeser, A, et al. (2006). Increased concentration of proatherogenic inflammatory cytokines in systemic lupus erythematosus: relationship to cardiovascular risk factors. *J Rheumatol.* (March 2006), Vol.33, No.3, pp. 539-545, ISSN 1499-2752.

Aringer, M, Smolen, JS. (2004). Tumour necrosis factor and other proinflammatory cytokines in systemic lupus erythematosus: a rationale for therapeutic intervention. *Lupus,* (2004), Vol.13, Vol.5, pp. 344-347, ISSN 1477-0962.

Ashby, DT, Rye, KA, Clay, MA, et al. (1998). Factors influencing the ability of HDL to inhibit expression of vascular cell adhesion molecule-1 in endothelial cells. *Arterioscler Thromb Vasc Biol,* Vol.18, No.9, (September 1998), pp. 1450–1455, ISSN 0276-5047.

Ando, J, Yamamoto, K (2001). Effects of shear stress and stretch on endothelial function. *Antioxid Redox Signal,* (February 2011), ISSN 1523-0864.

Bacon, PA, Stevens, RJ, Carruthers, DM, et al. (2002). Accelerated atherogenesis in autoimmune rheumatic diseases. *Autoimmun Rev,* Vol.1, No.6, (December 2002), pp.338–347, ISSN 1568-9972.

Barter, PJ, Nicholls, S, Rye, KA, et al. (2004). Antiinflammatory properties of HDL. *Circ Res,* Vol.95, No.8, (October 2004), pp.764-772, ISSN 0009-7300.

Batuca, JR, Ames, PR, Amaral, M, et al. (2009). Anti-atherogenic and anti-inflammatory properties of high-density lipoprotein are affected by specific antibodies in systemic lupus erythematosus. *Rheumatology* (Oxford), (January 2009), Vol.48, No.1, pp. 26-31, ISSN 1499-2752.

Bell, SA, Faust, H, Schmid, A, et al. (1998). Autoantibodies to C-reactive protein (CRP) and other acute-phase proteins in systemic autoimmune diseases. *Clin Exp Immunol,* (September 1998), Vol.113, No.3, pp. 327–332, ISSN 1365-2249.

Berneis, KK, Krauss, RM. (2001). Metabolic origins and clinical significance of LDL heterogeneity. *J Lipid Res,* (September 2001), Vol.43, No.9, pp.1363–1379, ISSN 1539-7262.

Bertsias, G, Ioannidis, JP, Boletis, J, et al. (2008). Task Force of the EULAR Standing Committee for International Clinical Studies Including Therapeutics. EULAR recommendations for the management of systemic lupus erythematosus. Report of a Task Force of the EULAR Standing Committee for International Clinical Studies Including Therapeutics. *Ann Rheum Dis*, / February 2008), Vol. 67, No.2, pp. 195-205, ISSN 1468-2060.

Bjornadal, L, Yin, L, Granath, F, et al. (2004). Cardiovascular disease a hazard despite improved prognosis in patients with systemic lupus erythematosus: results from a Swedish population based study 1964–1995. *J Rheumatol*. Vol.31, No.4, (April 2004), pp. 713–719, ISSN 0263-7103

Blake, GJ, Ridker, PM. (2001). Novel clinical markers of vascular wall inflammation. *Circ Res*, (October 2001), Vol.89, No.9, pp. 763-771, ISSN 0009-7300.

Bonfiglio, TA, Botti, RE, Hagstrom, JWC. (1992). Coronary arteritis, occlusion and myocardial infarction due to lupus erythematosus. *Am Heart J*, (February 1992), Vol.183, No.2, pp.153-158, ISSN 0002-8703.

Boyer, JF., Gourraud, PA., Cantagrel, A, et al. (2011). Traditional cardiovascular risk factors in rheumatoid arthritis: A meta-analysis. *Joint Bone Spine*, (March 2011), Vol. 78, No.12, pp.179–183 (2011), ISSN 1297-319X.

Brown, JH, Doherty ,CC, Allen ,DC, et al. (1988). Fatal cardiac failure due to myocardial microthrombi in systemic lupus erythematosus. *Br Med J (Clin Res)*, (May 1988), Vol.296, No.6635, pp.1505-1510, ISSN 0267-0623.

Bruce, IN, Urowitz, MB, Gladman, DD, et al. (1999). Natural history of hypercholesterolemia in systemic lupus erythematosus. *J Rheumatol*, Vol.26, No.10, (October 1999), pp. 2137-2143, ISSN 1499-2752.

Bruce, IN, Burns, RJ, Gladman, DD, et al. (2000). Single photon emission computed tomography dual isotope myocardial perfusion imaging in women with systemic lupus erythematosus. I. Prevalence and distribution of abnormalities. *J Rheumatol*, Vol. 27, No.10, (October 2010), pp. 2372-2377. ISSN 1499-2752.

Bruce, IN, Urowitz, MB, Gladman, DD, et al. (2003). Risk factors for coronary heart disease in women with systemic lupus erythematosus: the Toronto Risk Factor Study. *Arthritis Rheum*, (November 2003), Vol.48, No.11, pp. 3159–3167, ISSN 1529-013.

Bruce IN. (2005). Atherogenesis and autoimmune disease: the model of lupus. *Lupus*, (2005), Vol.14, No.9, pp. 687–690, ISSN 1477-0962

Bruce IN. (2006). The influence of other drugs on coronary heart disease (CHD) risk in systemic lupus erythematosus. *Lupus*, (November 2006), Vol. 15, No.11, pp. suppl. 23-26, ISSN 1477-0962.

Bulkley, BH, Roberts, WC. (1975). The heart in systemic lupus erythematosus and the changes induced in it by corticosteroid therapy. A study of 36 necropsy patients. *Am J Med*, (February 1975), Vol.58, No.2, pp. 243-264, ISSN 0002-9343.

Bultink, EM, Teerlink, T, Heijst, JA, et al. (2005). Raised plasma levels of asymmetric dimethylarginine are associated with cardiovascular events, disease activity, and organ damage in patients with systemic lupus erythematosus. *Ann Rheum Dis*, (September 2005), Vol.64, No.9, pp. 1362–1365, ISSN 1468-2060.

Bultink, IE, Turkstra, F, Diamant, M, et al. (2008). Prevalence of and risk factors for the metabolic syndrome in women with systemic lupus erythematosus. *Clin Exp Rheumatol*, (January-February, 2008); Vol.26, No.1, pp. 32-38, ISSN 1593-098

Cardinali C, Caproni M, Bernacchi E, et al. (2000). The spectrum of cutaneous manifestations in lupus erythematosus—the Italian experience. *Lupus*, (2000), Vol.9, No.6, pp. 417–423, ISSN 1477-0962.

D'Cruz D. (1998). Vasculitis in systemic lupus erythematosus. *Lupus*, (1998), Vol.7, No.4, pp. 270–274, ISSN 1477-0962.

Chapman, MJ, Guerin, M, Bruckert, E. et al. (1998). Atherogenic, dense low-density lipoproteins: pathophysiology and new therapeutic approaches. *Eur Heart J*, (February 1998), Vol.19, Suppl.A, pp. A24–A30, ISSN 1522-9645.

Chung, CP, Avalos, I, Oeser, A, et al. (2007). High prevalence of the metabolic syndrome in patients with systemic lupus erythematosus: association with disease characteristics and cardiovascular risk factors. Ann Rheum Dis, (February 2007), Vol.66, No.2, pp. 208-214, ISSN 1468-2060.

Colles, SM, Maxson, JM, Carlson, SG,et al. (2001). Oxidized LDL-induced injury and apoptosis in atherosclerosis. Potential roles for oxysterols. *Trends Cardiovasc Med.* (April-May 2001), Vol.11, No.3-4, pp. 131-138, ISSN 1050-1738.

Costenbader, KH, Karlson, EW, Gall, V, et al. (2005). Barriers to a trial of atherosclerosis prevention in systemic lupus erythematosus. *Arthritis Rheum*, (October 2005), Vol.53, No.5, pp. 718-723, ISSN 1529-013.

D'Cruz, D, Cervera, R, Olcay Aydintug, A, et al. (1993). Systemic lupus erythematosus evolving into systemic vasculitis: a report of five cases. *Br J Rheumatol*, (February 1993), Vol.32, No.2, pp. 154–157, ISSN 1460-2172.

Delgado Alves, J, Ames, PR, Donohue, S, et al. (2002). Antibodies to high-density lipoprotein and beta2-glycoprotein I are inversely correlated with paraoxonase activity in systemic lupus erythematosus and primary antiphospholipid syndrome. *Arthritis Rheum*, Vol.46, No.10, (October 2002), pp. 2686-2694, ISSN 1529-013.

Delgado Alves, J, Kumar, S, Isenberg, DA. (2003). Cross-reactivity between anti-cardiolipin, anti-high-density lipoprotein and anti-apolipoprotein A-I IgG antibodies in patients with systemic lupus erythematosus and primary antiphospholipid syndrome. *Rheumatology* (Oxford), (July 2003), Vol. 42, No.7, pp. 893-899, ISSN 1499-2752.

Delgado Alves, J, Mason, LJ, Ames, PR, et al. (2005). Antiphospholipid antibodies are associated with enhanced oxidative stress, decreased plasma nitric oxide and paraoxonase activity in an experimental mouse model. *Rheumatology* (Oxford), Vol.44, No.10, (October 2005), pp.1238-44; ISSN 1462-0332.

Després, JP, Lemieux, I. (2006). Abdominal obesity and metabolic syndrome. *Nature*, (December 2006), Vol.14, No.444(7121), pp. 881-887, ISSN 0028-0836.

Devinsky, O, Petito, CK, Alonso, DR. (1088). Clinical and neuropathological findings in systemic lupus erythematosus: the role of vasculitis, heart emboli, and thrombotic thrombocytopenic purpura. *Ann Neurol*, (April 1988),Vol.23, No.4, pp.380–384, ISSN 0364-5134.

Edwards, MH, Pierangeli, S, Liu, X, et al. (1996), Hydroxychloroquine reverses thrombogenic properties of antiphospholipid antibodies in mice. *Circulation*, (December 1996), Vol.96, No.12, pp. 4380–4384, ISSN 0009-7322.

Ellis, SG, Verity, MA (1979) Central nervous system involvement in systemic lupus erythematosus: a review of neuropathologic findings is 57 cases, 1955-1977. *Semin Arthritis Rheum*, (February 1979), Vol.8, No.3, pp. 212-221, ISSN 0049-0172.

Ellison, D, Gatter, K, Heryet, A, et al. (1993). Intramural platelet deposition in cerebral vasculopathy of systemic lupus erythematosus. *J Clin . Pathol*, (January 1993), Vol.46, No.1, pp. 37–40, ISSN 0021-9738.

El Magadmi, M, Ahmad, Y, Turkie, W, et al. (2006). Hyperinsulinemia, insulin resistance, and circulating oxidized low density lipoprotein in women with systemic lupus erythematosus. *J Rheumatol*, (January 2006), Vol.33, No.1, pp.50-56, ISSN 1499-2752.

Erkan, D, Yazici, MG, Peterson, L, et al. (2002). A cross-sectional study of clinical thrombotic risk factors and preventive treatments in antiphospholipid syndrome. *Rheumatology* , (August 2002), Vol.41, No.8, pp. 924–929, ISSN 1462-0332.

Esdaile, JM, Abrahamowicz M, Grodzicky T, et al. (2001). Traditional Framingham risk factors fail to fully account for accelerated atherosclerosis in systemic lupus erythematosus. *Arthritis Rheum*, Vol.44, No.10, (October 2001), pp. 2331–2337, ISSN 1529-013.

Espinola, RG, Pierangeli, SS, Ghara, AE, et al. (2002). Hydroxychloroquine reverses platelet activation induced by human IgG antiphospholipid antibodies. *Thromb Haemost*, Vol.83, No. 3, pp. 518–522, ISSN 0340-6245.

Fain, JN, Madan, AK, Hiler, ML, et al. (2004). Comparison of the release of adipokynes by adipose tissue, adipose tissue matrix, and adipocytes form visceral and subcutaneous abdominal adipose tissue of obese humans. *Endocrinology*, (May 2004), Vol.145, No.5, 2273–2782, ISSN 1945-7170.

Ferroni, P, Basili, S, Santilli, F, et al. (2006). Low-density lipoprotein-lowering medication and platelet function. *Pathophysiol Haemost Thromb*, (2006), Vol. 35, No.3-4, pp. 346-354, ISSN 1424-8840.

Fischer, L. M., Schlienger, R. G., Matter, C.,et al. (2004). Effect of rheumatoid arthritis or systemic lupus erythematosus on the risk of first-time acute myocardial infarction. Am J Cardiol (January 2004), Vol.93, No.2, pp. 198–200, ISSN 0735-1097.

Ford, ES, Giles, WH, Dietz, WH. (2002). Prevalence of metabolic syndrome among US adults: findings from the third National Health and Nutrition Examination Survey. *JAMA*, (January 2002), Vol.287, No.3, pp. 356–359, ISSN 1538-3598.

Ginsburg, KS, Liang, MH, Newcomer, L, et al. (1992). Anticardiolipin antibodies and the risk for ischemic stroke and venous thrombosis. *Ann Intern Med*, (December 1992), Vol.117, No.12, pp. 997-1002, ISSN 1539-3704.

Gladman, DD, Urowitz, MB. (1987). Morbidity in systemic lupus erythematosus. *J Rheumatol Suppl*, Vol.14, (June 1987), pp. 223-226, ISSN 0380-0903.

Goldberger, E, Elder, RC, Schwartz, RA, (1992). Vasculitis in the antiphospholipid syndrome. A cause of ischemia responding to corticosteroids. *Arthritis Rheum*, (May 1992), Vol.35, No.5, pp. 569–572, ISSN 1529-013.

Gómez-Zumaquero, JM, Tinahones, FJ, De Ramón, E. (2004). Association of biological markers of activity of systemic lupus erythematosus with levels of anti-oxidized low-density lipoprotein antibodies. *Rheumatology* (Oxford), (April 2004), Vol.43, No.4, pp. 510-513, ISSN 1499-2752.

Gonzalez-Gay, MA, Garcia-Porrua, C, Pujol, RM. (2005). Clinical approach to cutaneous vasculitis. *Curr Opin Rheumatol*, (January 2005), Vol.17, No.1, pp. 56–61, ISSN 1531-6963.

Hanley, AJ, Williams, K, Stern, MP, et al. (2002). Homeostasis model assessment of insulin resistance in relation to the incidence of cardiovascular disease: the San Antonio Heart Study. *Diabetes Care*, (July 2002), Vol.25, No.7, pp.1177-1184, ISSN 1935-5548.

Hanly, JG, Walsh, NM, Sangalang, V. (1992). Brain pathology in systemic lupus erythematosus. *J Rheumatol*, (May 1992), Vol.19, No. 5, pp. 732–741, ISSN 1499-2752.

Harrison, MJ, Levy, R, Peterson, M, et al. (2007). Aspirin for primary thrombosis prevention in the antiphospholipid syndrome: a randomized, double-blind, placebo-controlled trial in asymptomatic antiphospholipid antibody-positive individuals. *Arthritis Rheum*, (July 2007), Vol.56, No.7, pp. 2382-2391, ISSN 1529-013.

Haque, S, Bruce, IN. (2009). Cardiovascular outcomes in systemic lupus erythematosus: big studies for big questions. *J. Rheumatol.* Vol.36, No.3, (March 2009), pp. 467–469, ISSN 1499-2752.

Harrison, MJ, Levy, R, Peterson, M, et al. (2007). Aspirin for primary thrombosis prevention in the antiphospholipid syndrome: a randomized, double-blind, placebo-controlled trial in asymptomatic antiphospholipid antibody-positive individuals. *Arthritis Rheum*, (July 2007), Vol.56, No.7, pp. 2382-2391, ISSN 1529-013.

Hermosillo-Romo, D, Brey, RL. (2002). Neuropsychiatric involvement in systemic lupus erythematosus. *Curr Rheumatol Rep*, Vol.4, No.4. (August 2002), pp. 337-344, ISSN 1534-6307.

Hessler, JR, Robertson, AL Jr, Chisolm, GM 3rd. (1979). LDL induced cytotoxicity and its inhibition by HDL in human vascular smooth muscle and endothelial cells in culture. *Atherosclerosis.* (March 1979), Vol.32, No.3, pp. 213- 229, ISSN 0021-9150.

Hotamisligil, GS, Shargill, NS, Spiegelman BM. et al. (1993). Adipose expression of tumor necrosis factor alpha: a direct role in obesity-linked insulin resistance. *Science*, (January 1993), Vol.259, No.5091, pp. 87–91, ISSN 1095-9203.

Hyka, N, Dayer, JM, Modoux, C et al. (2001). Apolipoprotein A-I inhibits the production of interleukin-1β and tumor necrosis factor-α by blocking contact-mediated activation of monocytes by T lymphocytes. *Blood.* Vol.97, No.8, (April, 2001), pp. 2381–2389, ISSN 1528-0020.

Hurt-Camejo, E, Camejo, G, Sartipy, P. (2001). Phospholipase: A2 and small, dense low-density lipoprotein. *Curr Opin Lipidol.* (October 2001), Vol.11, No.5, pp.465–471, ISSN 1473-6535.

Ilowite NT, Samuel P, Ginzler E, et a. (1988). Dyslipoproteinemia in pediatric systemic lupus erythematosus. *Arthritis Rheum.* Vol.31, No.7, (July 1988), pp. 859-863, ISSN 1529-013.

Jacobsen S, Petersen J, Ullman S, et al. (1998). A multicentre study of 513 Danish patients with systemic lupus erythematosus. II. Disease mortality and clinical factors of prognostic value. *Clin Rheumatol*, Vol.17, No.6, (June 1998), pp. 478-484, ISSN 1434-9949.

James, RW, Deakin, SP. (2004). The importance of high-density lipoproteins for paraoxonase-1 secretion, stability, and activity. *Free Radical Biol. Med*, Vol. 37, No. 12, (December 2004), pp.1986–1994, ISSN 0891-5849.

Johnson, RT, Richardson, EP. (1968). Theneurological manifestations of systemic lupus erythematosus: a clinical-pathological study of 24 cases and review of the literature. *Medicine* (Baltimore), Vol.47, No.4, pp. 337-369, ISSN 1536-5964.

Jonsson, H, Nived, O, Sturfelt, G. (1989). Outcome in systemic lupus erythematosus: a prospective study of patients from a defined population. *Medicine* (Baltimore), Vol.68, No.3, (May 1989), pp. 141-150, ISSN 1536-5964.

Khamashta, MA. (2000). Primary prevention of thrombosis in subjects with positive antiphospholipid antibodies. *J Autoimmun*, (September 2000), Vol.15, No.2, pp. 249-253, ISSN 1095-9157.

Karp, I, Abrahamowicz, M, Fortin, PR, et al. (2008). Recent corticosteroid use and recent disease activity: independent determinants of coronary heart disease risk factors in systemic lupus erythematosus? *Arthritis Rheum*, (February 2008), Vol.59, No.2, pp. 169-175, ISSN 1529-013.

Kao, AH, Wasko MC, Krishnaswami, S, et al. (2008). C-reactive protein and coronary artery calcium in asymptomatic women with systemic lupus erythematosus or rheumatoid arthritis. *Am J Cardiol*, (September 2008), Vol.102, No.6, pp. 755–760, ISSN 0002-9149.

Khera, A, Cuchel M, de la Llera-Moya M et al. (2011). Cholesterol efflux capacity, high-density lipoprotein function, and atherosclerosis. *N Engl J Med*, Vol.364, No.2, (January 2011), pp.127-135, ISSN 1533-4406.

Kianai, AN, Mahoney, JA, Petri, M. (2007). Asymmetric dimethylarginine isa marker of poor prognosis and coronary calcium in systemic lúpus erythematosus. *J Rheumatol*, (July 2007), Vol.34, No.7, pp. 1502–1505, ISSN 1499-2752

Lajer, M, Tarnow, L, Jorsal, A, et al. (2008). Plasma concentration of asymmetric dimethylarginine (ADMA) predicts cardiovascular morbidity and mortality in type 1 diabetic patients with diabetic nephropathy. *Diabetes Care*, (April 2008), Vol.31, No.4, pp. 747–752, ISSN 1935-5548.

Libby, P, Okamoto, Y, Rocha, VZ, et al. (2010). Inflammation in atherosclerosis: transition from theory to practice. *Circ J. Vol*, Vol.74, No.2, (February 2010), pp. 213-220, ISSN 1346-9843.

Love, PE, Santoro, SA. (1990). Antiphospholipid antibodies: anticardiolipin and the lupus anticoagulant in systemic lupus erythematosus (SLE) and in non-SLE disorders. Prevalence and clinical significance. *Ann Intern Med*, (May 1990), Vol.112, No.9, pp. 682-698, ISSN 1539-3704.

Lusis, AJ. (2000). Atherosclerosis. *Nature*. Vol. 407, No. 6801, (September 2000), pp. 233-241, ISSN 0028-0836.

Mackness, MI, Durrington, PN, Mackness, B. (2000). How high-density lipoprotein protects against the effects of lipid peroxidation. *Curr Opin Lipidol*. Vol.11, No. 4, (August 2000), pp. 383–388, ISSN 1473-6535.

Maksimowicz-McKinnon, K, Magder, L, Petri, M. (2006). Predictors of carotid atherosclerosis in systemic lupus erythematosus. *J Rheumatol*, Vol.33, No.12, (December, 2006), pp. 2458–2463, ISSN 1499-2752.

Manger, K, Kusus, M, Forster, C, et al. (2003). Factors associated with coronary artery calcification in young female patients with SLE. *Ann Rheum Dis*, Vol.62, No.9, (September 2003), pp. 846-850, ISSN 1468-2060.

Manger, K, Manger, B, Repp, R, et al. (2002). Definition of risk factors for death, end stage renal disease, and thromboembolic events in a monocentric cohort of 338 patients with systemic lupus erythematosus. *Ann Rheum Dis*, (December), Vol. 61, No.12, pp. 1065-70, ISSN 1468-2060.

Manzi, S, Meilahn, EN, Rairie, JE, et al. (1997). Age-specific incidence rates of myocardial infarction and angina in women with systemic lupus erythematosus: comparison with the Framingham Study. *Am J Epidemiol*, Vol.145, No.5, (March 1997), pp. 408-415, ISSN 1476-6256.

Manzi, S, Selzer F, Sutton-Tyrrell, K, et al. (1999). Prevalence and risk factors of carotid plaque in women with systemic lupus erythematosus. *Arthritis Rheum*, Vol. 42, No.1, (January 1999), pp. 51-60, ISSN 1529-013.

Manzi, S, Kuller, LH, Edmundowicz, D, et al. (2000). Vascular imaging: changing the face of cardiovascular research. Lupus, (2000), Vol.9, No.3, pp. 176-178, ISSN 1477-0962.

Maron, BA, Loscalzo, J. (2009). The treatment of hyperhomocysteinemia. *Annu Rev Med*. (July 2009), Vol.60, pp.39–54, ISSN 0785-3890.

Matsuura, E, Kobayashi, K, Tabuchi, M. (2006). Oxidative modification of low-density lipoprotein and immune regulation of atherosclerosis. *Prog Lipid Res*, (November 2006), Vol.45, No.6, pp. 466-486, ISSN 1873-2194.

McMahon, M, Grossman, J, Skaggs, B, et al. (2009). Dysfunctional proinflammatory high-density lipoproteins confer increased risk of atherosclerosis in women with systemic lupus erythematosus. *Arthritis Rheum*, (August 2009), Vol.60, No. 8, pp. 2428-2437, ISSN 1529-013.

Mira, E, Mañes, S. (2009). Immunomodulatory and anti-inflammatory activities of statins. *Endocr Metab Immune Disord Drug Targets*, (September 2009), Vol.9, No.3, pp. 237-247, ISSN 1871-5303.

Mok, CC, Lau, CS, Wong, RW. (2001). Neuropsychiatric manifestations and their clinical associations in southern Chinese patients with systemic lupus erythematosus. *J Rheumatol*, Vol.28, No.4, (April 2001), pp.766-771, ISSN 1499-2752.

Mok, CC, Tang, SS, To, CH, et al. (2005). Incidence and risk factors of thromboembolism in systemic lupus erythematosus: a comparison of three ethnic groups. *Arthritis Rheum*, Vol.52, No.9, (September 2005), pp. 2774-2782, ISSN 1529-013.

Mok, CC, Wong, CK, To, CH, et al. (2011). Effects of rosuvastatin on vascular biomarkers and carotid atherosclerosis in lupus: A randomized, double-blind, placebo-controlled trial. *Arthritis Care Res*, (June 2022), Vol.63, No.6, pp. 875-883, ISSN 0893-7524.

Montecucco, F, Vuilleumier, N, Pagano, S, et al. (2011). Anti-Apolipoprotein A-1 auto-antibodies are active mediators of atherosclerotic plaque vulnerability. *Eur Heart J*, (February 2011), Vol. 32, No.4, pp. 412-421, ISSN 1522-9645.

Moyssakis, I, Tektonidou, MG, Vasilliou, VA, et al.(2007). Libman-Sacks endocarditis in systemic lupus erythematosus: prevalence, associations, and evolution. *Am J Med*, (July 2007), Vol.120, No.7, pp. 636–642, ISSN 0002-9343.

Navab, M, Hama, SY, Hough, GP, (2001). A cell-free assay for detecting HDL that is dysfunctional in preventing the formation of or inactivating oxidized phospholipids. J *Lipid Res*, (August 2001), Vol.42, No. 8, pp. 1308-1317, ISSN 1539-7262.

Negrón, AM, Molina, MJ, Mayor, AM, (2008). Factors associated with metabolic syndrome in patients with systemic lupus erythematosus from Puerto Rico. *Lupus*, (April 2008), Vol.17, No.4, pp. 348-54, ISSN 1477-0962.

Nikpour, M, Urowitz, MB, Gladman, DD. (2005). Premature atherosclerosis in systemic lupus erythematosus. *Rheum Dis Clin North Am*, Vol.31, No.2, (May 2005), pp.329-354, ISSN 1558-3163.

O'Neill, SG, Isenberg, DA, Rahman, A. (2007). Could antibodies to Creactive protein link inflammation and cardiovascular disease in patients with systemic lupus erythematosus? Ann Rheum Dis, (August 2007), Vol.66, No.8, pp. 989–991, ISSN 1468-2060.

Packard, CJ, Shepherd, J. (1997). Lipoprotein heterogeneity and apolipoprotein B metabolism. *Arterioscler Thromb Vasc Biol,* (December 1997), Vol.17, No.12, pp. 3542–3556, ISSN 0276-5047

Pasceri, V, Willerson, JT, Yeh ET. (2000). Direct proinflammatory effect of C-reactive protein on human endothelial cells. *Circulation,* (October 2000), Vol.102, No.18, pp. 2165–2168, ISSN 0009-7322.

Pasceri, V, Cheng, JS, Willerson, JT, (2001). Modulation of C-reactive protein-mediated monocyte chemoattractant protein-1 induction in human endothelial cells by anti-atherosclerosis drugs. *Circulation,* (May 2001), Vol.103, No.21, pp. 2531–2534, ISSN 0009-7322.

Park, KH, Cho, KH. (2011). High-density lipoprotein (HDL) from elderly and reconstituted HDL containing glycated apolipoproteins A-I share proatherosclerotic and prosenescent properties with increased cholesterol influx. *J Gerontol A Biol Sci Med Sci.* (May 2011), Vol. 66, No.5, pp. 511-520, ISSN 1079-5006.

Petri ,M, Spence ,D, Bone, LR, et al. (1992). Coronary artery disease risk factors in the Johns Hopkins Lupus Cohort: prevalence, recognition by patients, and preventive practices. *Medicine* (Baltimore), (September 1992), Vol.71, No.5, pp. 291-302. ISSN 1536-5964.

Petri, M. (2002). Epidemiology of systemic lupus erythematosus. *Best Pract Res Clin Rheumatol,* Vol.16, No.5, (December 2002), pp.847-858, ISSN 1521-6942.

Petri, MA, Kiani, AN, Post, W, et al (2011). Lupus Atherosclerosis Prevention Study (LAPS). *Ann Rheum Dis,* (May 2011), Vol.70, No.5, pp. 760-765, ISSN ISSN 1468-2060.

Pego-Reigosa, JM, Lu, TY, Fontanillo, MF, et al. (2010). Long-term improvement of lipid profile in patients with refractory systemic lupus erythematosus treated with B-cell depletion therapy: a retrospective observational study. *Rheumatology* (Oxford), Vol. 49, No.4, (October 2010), pp. 691-696; SSN 1499-2752.

Rahman, P., Aguero, S., Gladman, D. D., et al. (2000). Vascular events in hypertensive patients with systemic lupus erythematosus. *Lupus,* (2000), Vol.9, No.9, pp. 672–675, ISSN 1477-0962.

Rajala, MW, Sherer, PE. (2003). Minireview: the adipocyte at the crossroads of energy homeostasis, inflammation, and atherosclerosis. *Endocrinology,* (September 2003), Vol.144, No.9, 3765–3773, ISSN 1945-7170.

Rand, JH, Wu, XX, Quinn, AS, et al. Hydroxychloroquine directly reduces the binding of antiphospholipid antibody–β2-glycoprotein I complexes to phospholipid bilayers. *Blood,* Vol.112, No.5, pp. 1687–1695, ISSN 1528-0020.

Ridker, PM, Rifai, N, Rose L, et al. (2002). Comparison of C-reactive protein and low-density lipoprotein cholesterol levels in the prediction of first cardiovascular events. *N Engl J Med,* (November 2002), Vol.347, No.20, pp.1557–1565, ISSN 1533-4406.

Ridker, PM, Danielson, E, Fonseca FA, et al. (2008). JUPITER Study Group Rosuvastatin to prevent vascular events in men and women with elevated C-reactive protein. *N Engl J Med,* (November 2008), Vol.329, No.20, pp. 2195-2207, ISSN 1533-4406.

Roldan, CA, Joson, J, Qualls, CR, et al. (2010). Premature aortic stiffness in systemic lupus erythematosus by transesophageal echocardiography. *Lupus.* Vol.19, No.14, (December 2010), pp.1599-1605, ISSN 1477-0962.

Roman, MJ, Shanker, BA, Davis, A, et al. (2003). Prevalence and correlates of accelerated atherosclerosis in systemic lupus erythematosus. *N Engl J Med,* (December 2003), Vol.349, No.25, pp. 2399-2406, ISSN ISSN 1533-4406.

Roman, MJ, Crow, MK, Lockshin, MD, et al. (2007). Rate and determinants of progression of atherosclerosis in systemic lupus erythematosus. *Arthritis Rheum,* (October 2007), Vol.56, No.10, pp.3412–3419, ISSN 1529-013.

Romero, FI, Amengual, O, Atsumi, T. et al. (1998). Arterial disease in lupus and secondary antiphospholipid syndrome: association with anti-beta2-glycoprotein I antibodies but not with antibodies against oxidized low-density lipoprotein. *Br J Rheumatol,* (August 1998), Vol.37, No.8, pp. 883-888, ISSN 1460-2172.

Ross R. (1999). Atherosclerosis--an inflammatory disease. *N Engl J Med,* Vol.340, No.2, (January 1999), pp. 115-26, ISSN 1533-4406.

Rubin, LA, Urowitz, MB, Gladman DD. (1985). Mortality in systemic lupus erythematosus: the bimodal pattern revisited. *Q J Med,* Vol.55, (April 1985), pp. 87-98, ISSN 1460-2393.

Ruiz-Irastorza, G, Egurbide, MV, Ugalde, J, et al. (2004). (High impact of antiphospholipid syndrome on irreversible organ damage and survival of patients with systemic lupus erythematosus. *Arch Intern Med,* (January 2004), Vol.164, No.1, pp. 77-82, ISSN 1538-3679.

Ruiz-Irastorza G, Ramos-Casals, M, Brito-Zeron, P, et al. (2010). Clinical efficacy and side effects of antimalarials in systemic lupus erythematosus: a systematic review. *Ann Rheum Dis,* Vol.69, No.1, (January 2010), pp. 20-28, ISSN 1468-2060.

Ruyssen-Witrand, A, Fautrel, B, Sarauxc, A, et al. (2010).Cardiovascular risk induced by low-dose corticosteroids in rheumatoid arthritis: a systematic literature review. *Joint Bone Spine,* (January 2010), pp. 23-30, ISSN 1297-319X.

Sabio, JM, Vargas-Hitos, JA, Mediavilla, JD, et al. (2010). Correlation of asymptomatic hyperuricaemia and serum uric acid levels with arterial stiffness in women with systemic lupus erythematosus without clinically evident atherosclerotic cardiovascular disease. *Lupus,* (April 2010), Vol.19, No.5, pp. 591-598, ISSN 1477-0962.

Sachet, J, Borba, E, Bonfa, E, et al. Chloroquine increases low-density lipoprotein removal from plasma in systemic lupus patients. *Lupus,* Vol.16, No.4, (2007), pp. 273–278, ISSN 1477-0962.

Sanna, G, Bertolaccini, ML, Cuadrado, MJ, et al. (2003). Neuropsychiatric manifestations in systemic lupus erythematosus: prevalence and association with antiphospholipid antibodies. *J Rheumatol,* Vol.30, No.5, (May 2003), pp. 985-992, ISSN 1499-2752.

Scalzi, LV, Hollenbeak, CS, Wang, L. (2010). Racial disparities in age at time of cardiovascular events and cardiovascular-related death in patients with systemic lupus erythematosus. *Arthritis Rheum,* Vol.62, No.9, (September 2010), pp. 2767-2775, ISSN 1529-013.

Sella, EM, Sato, EI, Leite, WA, et al. (2003). Myocardial perfusion scintigraphy and coronary disease risk factors in systemic lupus erythematosus. *Ann Rheum Dis,* Vol.62, No.11, (November 2003), pp.1066-1070, ISSN 1468-2060.

Shah, MA, Shah, AM, Krishnan, E. (2009). Poor outcomes after acute myocardial infarction in systemic lupus erythematosus. *J Rheumatol,* Vol.36, No.3, (March 2009), pp. 570-575, ISSN 1499-2752.

Simonson, GD, Kendall, DM. (2005). Diagnosis of insulin resistance and associated syndromes: the spectrum from the metabolic syndrome to type 2 diabetes mellitus. *Coron Artery Dis*, (December 2005), Vol.16, No.8, pp. 465–472, ISSN 1473-5830.

Sjowall, C, Bengtsson, AA, Sturfelt, G, et al. (2004). Serum levels of autoantibodies against monomeric C-reactive protein are correlated with disease activity in systemic lupus erythematosus. *Arthritis Res Ther*, (December 2004), Vol. 6, No.2, pp. R87–R94, ISSN 1478-6362

Ståhl-Hallengren, C, Jönsen, A, Nived, O, et al. (2000). Incidence studies of systemic lupus erythematosus in Southern Sweden: increasing age, decreasing frequency of renal manifestations and good prognosis. *J Rheumatol*. Vol.27, No.3, (March 2000), pp. 685-691, ISSN 1499-2752.

Somers, E, Magder, LS, Petri, M, et al. (1999). Morbidity and mortality in systemic lupus erythematosus during a 5-year period. A multicenter prospective study of 1,000 patients. European Working Party on Systemic Lupus Erythematosus. *Medicine* (Baltimore), (May 1999), Vol.78, No.3, pp.167-175, ISSN 1536-5964.

Somers, E, Magder, LS, Petri, M. (2002). Antiphospholipid antibodies and incidence of venous thrombosis in a cohort of patients with systemic lupus erythematosus. *J Rheumatol*, (December 2002), Vol.29, No.12, pp. 2531-2536, ISSN 1499-2752

Soran, H, Younis, NN, Charlton-Menys, V, et al. (2009). Variation in paraoxonase-1 activity and atherosclerosis. *Curr Opin Lipidol*, Vol. 20, No.4, (August 2009), pp.265–274, ISSN 1473-6535.

Stuhlinger, MC, Oka, RK, Graf, EE, et al. (2003). Endothelial dysfunction induced by hyperhomocysteinemia: role of asymmetric dimethylarginine. *Circulation*, (August 2003), Vol.108, No.8, pp. 933–938, ISSN 0009-7322.

Svenungsson, E, Jensen-Urstad, K, Heimburger, M, et al. (2001). Risk factors for cardiovascular disease in systemic lupus erythematosus. *Circulation*, Vol. 104, No.16, (October 2001), pp. 1887-1893, ISSN 0009-7322.

Svenungsson, E, Gunnarsson, I, Fei, GZ, et al. (2003). Elevated triglycerides and low levels of high-density lipoprotein as markers of disease activity in association with up-regulation of the tumor necrosis factor alpha/tumor necrosis factor receptor system in systemic lupus erythematosus. *Arthritis Rheum*, Vol. 48, No. 9, (September 2003), pp. 2533-2540, ISSN 1529-013.

Telles, R, Lanna C, Ferreira, G, et al. (2010). Metabolic syndrome in patients with systemic lupus erythematosus: association with traditional risk factors for coronary heart disease and lupus characteristics. Lupus, (June 2010), Vol.19, No.7, pp.803-809, ISSN 1477-0962.

Toloza, SM, Uribe, AG, McGWin, G Jr, et al. (2004). Systemic lupus erythematosus in a multiethnic US cohort (LUMINA). XXIII. Baseline predictors of vascular events. *Arthritis Rheum*, (October 2004), Vol.50, No.10, pp. 3947–3957, ISSN 1529-013.

Tuhrim S. (2004). Antiphospholipid antibodies and stroke. *Curr Cardiol Rep*, (March 2004), Vol.6, No.2, pp.130–134, ISSN 1534-3170.

Uramoto KM, Michet CJ Jr, Thumboo J, et al. (1999). Trends in the incidence and mortality of systemic lupus erythematosus, 1950-1992. *Arthritis Rheum*, Vol.42, No.1, (January 1999), pp. 46-5, ISSN 1529-013.

Urowitz, MB, Bookman, AA, Koehler, BE, et al. (1976). The bimodal mortality pattern of systemic lupus erythematosus. *Am J Med*, Vol.60, No.2, (February 1976), pp.221-225, ISSN 0002-9343.

Urowitz, MB., Ibanez, D, Gladman, DD. (2007). Atherosclerotic vascular events in a single large lupus cohort: prevalence and risk factors. *J. Rheumatol*, (January 2007), Vol.34, No.1, pp. 70–75, ISSN 1499-2752.

Urowitz, MB, Gladman, D, Ibañez, D, et al. (2008). Systemic Lupus International Collaborating Clinics. Accumulation of coronary artery disease risk factors over three years: data from an international inception cohort. *Arthritis Rheum*, (February 2008), Vol.59, No.2, pp. 176–180, ISSN 1529-013.

van Leuven, SI, Franssen, R, Kastelein, JJ, et al. (2008). Systemic inflammation as a risk factor for atherothrombosis. *Rheumatology* (Oxford), Vol.47, No.1, (January 2008), pp. 3-7, ISSN 1499-2752.

Virmani, R, Burke, AP, Kolodgie, FD, et al. (2002). Vulnerable plaque: the pathology of unstable coronary lesions. *J Interv Cardiol*. Vol.15, No.6, (December 2002), pp. 439–446, ISSN 1540-8183.

Vlachoyiannopoulos, PG, Karassa, FB, Karakostas, KX, et al. (1993). Systemic lupus erythematosus in Greece. Clinical features, evolution and outcome: a descriptive analysis of 292 patients. *Lupus*, (1993), Vol.2, No.5 , pp. 303–312, ISSN 1477-0962.

Volkmann, ER, Grossman JM, Sahakian, LJ, et al. (2010). Low physical activity is associated with proinflammatory high-density lipoprotein and increased subclinical atherosclerosis in women with systemic lupus erythematosus. *Arthritis Care Res*, (February 2010), Vol.62, No.2, pp. 258-265, ISSN 2151-4658.

Vuilleumier N, Charbonney, E, Fontao, L, et al (2008). Anti-(apoA-1) IgG are associated with high levels of oxidized low-density lipoprotein in acute coronary syndrome. *Clin Sci*. (July 2008), Vol.115 ,No.1 ,pp. 25-33, ISSN 1470-8736.

Vigushin, DM, Pepys, MB, Hawkins, PN. (1993). Metabolic and scintigraphic studies of radioiodinated human C-reactive protein in health and disease. *J Clin Invest*, (April 1993), Vol.91, No.4, pp. 1351–1357, ISSN 1558-8238.

Wahl, DG, Bounameaux, H, de Moerloose, P, et al. (2000). Prophylactic antithrombotic therapy for patients with systemic lupus erythematosus with or without antiphospholipid antibodies: do the benefits outweigh the risks? A decision analysis. *Arch Intern Med*, (July 2000), Vol.160, No. 3, pp. 2042–2048, ISSN 1538-3679.

Ward, MM. (1999). Premature morbidity from cardiovascular and cerebrovascular diseases in women with systemic lupus erythematosus. *Arthritis Rheum*, Vol.42, No.2, (February 1999), pp. 338–346, ISSN 1529-013.

Ward, MM. (2004). Outcomes of hospitalizations for myocardial infarctions and cerebrovascular accidents in patients with systemic lupus erythematosus. *Arthritis Rheum*, Vol.50, No.10, (October 2004), pp. 3170-3176, ISSN 1529-013.

Wilson ,VE, Eck ,SL, Bates ,ER. (1992). Evaluation and treatment of acute myocardial infarction complicating systemic lupus erythematosus. *Chest*, (February 1992), Vol.101, No.2, pp. 420–424, ISSN 1931-3543.

Wilson Tang ,WH, Tong ,W, Shrestha ,K, et al. (2008). Differential effects of arginine methylation on diastolic dysfunction and disease progression in patients with chronic systolic heart failure. *Eur Heart J*, (October 2008), Vol.29, No.20, pp. 2506–2513, ISSN 1554-2815

Wisnieski ,JJ. (2000). Urticarial vasculitis. *Curr Opin Rheumatol*, (January 2000), Vol.12, No.1, pp.24–31, ISSN 1531-6963

Yuen, H, Holthaus, K, Kamen ,DL, (2011). Using Wii Fit to reduce fatigue among African American women with systemic lupus erythematosus: A pilot study. *Lupus*, (June 2011), ISSN 1477-0962.

Yuhanna ,IS, Zhu, Y, Cox ,BE, et al. (2001). High density lipoprotein binding to scavenger receptor-BI activates endothelial nitric oxide synthase. *Nat Med*, Vol.7, No.7, (July 2001), pp. 853-857, ISSN 1078-895.

Zonana-Nacach, A, Santana-Sahagún, E, Jiménez-Balderas, FJ, et al. (2008). Prevalence and factors associated with metabolic syndrome in patients with rheumatoid arthritis and systemic lupus erythematosus. *J Clin Rheumatol*, (April 2008), Vol.14, No.2, 74-77, ISSN 1536-7355

7

Tyrosine-Based Monitoring of Glucocorticoid Therapy of Systemic Lupus Erythematosus

I. T. Rass
Center of Theoretical Pharmacology, Russian Academy of Sciences, Moscow Russia

1. Introduction

The present chapter considers only one aspect of glucocorticoid therapy of patients with systemic lupus erythematosus (SLE): a possibility of using blood level of tyrosine for monitoring glucocorticoid therapy. Thus, problems of SLE etiology and pathogenesis, as well as numerous schemes of SLE therapy are beyond the limits of this chapter. In the chapter normal catabolism of tyrosine and some congenital disturbances in catabolism of this amino acid are considered. But in the great majority of cases, specific features of tyrosine catabolism allow us to admit that tyrosine content in blood should be determined by the liver functional competence, in particular, its ability to synthesize an adaptive enzyme tyrosine aminotransferase and by entrance into the liver of glucocorticoids, natural hormones or glucocorticoid preparations. This chapter also presents experimental data obtained on adrenalectomized rats and observations on children with adrenogenital syndrome which clearly demonstrate blood tyrosine dependence on glucocorticoids and support the idea of using blood tyrosine content as a promising laboratory parameter for monitoring glucocorticoid therapy, similar to blood glucose for insulin. Some observations on glucocorticoid therapy in patients with SLE compared with changes in their blood tyrosine level which were earlier published only in Russian are presented, as well as the imaginary tyrosine-based monitoring of these cases.

2. Approaches to treatment of systemic lupus erythematosus

Systemic lupus erythematosus (SLE) seems to be the most striking example of using corticosteroid, or glucocorticoid, preparations in non-endocrine diseases as the most powerful anti-inflammatory, immunosuppressive, anti-allergic, antitoxic, etc. agents. Sixty years ago glucocorticoids allowed clinicians to radically change the fate of patients with SLE – this collagen disease stopped to be virtually lethal (Dubois, 1974; Schroeder & Euler, 1997; Ioannou & Isenberg, 2002; Goldblatt & Isenberg, 2005; Nived et al., 2008). In modern schemes of SLE treatment glucocorticoids are usually combined with various other preparations: cyclophosphamide, mycophenolate mofettil, rituximab, cyclosporine, azathioprine, etc. (Ntali et al., 2009; Ponticelli et al., 2010). In addition to their specific effects, all these preparations are given, in particular, in order to lower the dose of steroids, however, up to now glucocorticoids remain the cornerstone in the schemes of SLE treatment. Therefore, in SLE all problems associated with using glucocorticoid preparations in non-endocrine diseases are clearly pronounced and still urgent: the unpredictability of efficiency of glucocorticoids and nearly inevitable serious side effects, difficulties and sometimes even the impossibility to abolish glucocorticoids, and glucocorticoid resistance of some patients - such was the situation at the beginning of the "steroid era" and it is nearly the same nowadays, and the same problems are still urgent.

Since 1966, life-threatening exacerbations of SLE are sometimes treated by pulse-therapy - intravenous injection of very high doses of glucocorticoid preparations - up to 1 mg methylprednisolone daily for three days. However, the rapid immunosuppressive effect is often accompanied by various infections. But this regimen of pulse-therapy has been formed historically, although it is not excluded that lower doses of glucocorticoids would be similarly effective (Badscha & Edwards, 2003; Franchin & Diamond, 2006).

It is obvious that the existent schemes of using glucocorticoids in SLE are far from optimal, and to specify and refine therapeutical approaches there are some attempts to compare the glucocorticoid efficiency in SLE with different individual characteristics of the patients, such as the number and type of glucocorticoid receptors (Li et al., 2010; Deng & Tsao, 2010; Oakley & Cidlowski, 2011), titers of antibodies to double-stranded DNA (Rahman & Isenberg, 2008), specific features of T- and B-cells, etc. It seems clear that responsiveness to glucocorticoids should be associated with some individual specific features of the patients. Moreover, glucocorticoid sensitivity is not steady in the same patient, but can vary from time to time and can be much more changeable than it has been believed earlier (De Rijk & Sternberg, 1997).

It is rather strange but a very essential aspect of action of glucocorticoid preparations has been neglected during the whole period of using glucocorticoids in clinical medicine. It is extremely important that glucocorticoid preparations, as discriminated from all other pharmaceuticals used in the treatment of SLE, are synthetic copies of *natural products* of the organism - of glucocorticoid hormones synthesized in the adrenal cortex. Glucocorticoid preparations possessing the unique combination of therapeutic properties also inevitably retain the features of their natural prototypes, i.e. they are directly or indirectly involved in regulation of many if not all physiological processes and metabolic reactions and their using interferes the negative feedback regulation in the hypothalamus-pituitary-adrenocortical system. Therefore, it should be noted and emphasized that the inevitable complications of glucocorticoid therapy really are not "side effects", on the contrary, they are natural manifestations of just hormonal properties of glucocorticoid preparations, either of their excess or of induced disorders in the feedback regulation of the hypothalamus-pituitary-adrenocortical system. Possibly, this neglecting was reasoned by a surprising and somewhat discouraging discovery in the beginning of "the glucocorticoid era" that the therapeutical effect of glucocorticoid preparations did not depend on the level of a patient's own hormones?

However, not the level of glucocorticoid hormones should be important, but the tissue provision with these hormones, especially on taking into account that glucocorticoids are hormones of virtually total action. Nevertheless, for glucocorticoids there is no parameter to characterize the tissue provision with these hormones (or with glucocorticoid preparations) and to determine the real need in them of a subject under various circumstances, in particular, under stress situations or in disease. This is especially important because glucocorticoids play a determinative role in stress situations. For glucocorticoids an indirect parameter is required *which would be similar to blood glucose for insulin.*

Naturally, this parameter must be easily determinable in blood, have rather narrow normal limits in healthy persons, and clearly depend on glucocorticoids, natural hormones or preparations. In particular, the glucocorticoid-dependent hepatic enzyme tyrosine aminotransferase and the resulting tyrosine level in blood which is directly determined by the activity of this enzyme deserve a special attention.

3. Blood tyrosine levels in some non-endocrine diseases

In the late 1950s Japanese researchers of the Nishimura group found increased levels of tyrosine in blood and urine of patients with collagen diseases (Nishimura et al., 1958; Nishimura et al., 1961) and supposed that disorders in tyrosine catabolism could be a biochemical basis of these diseases. These reports stimulated intensive studies on tyrosine catabolism in collagenoses and some other diseases, especially in Russia. As it was reasonably to expect, tyrosine catabolism was disturbed in patients with liver disorders, such as infectious hepatitis, chronic hepatitis, and liver cirrhosis, and blood tyrosine level was two-threefold increased in them (Levine & Kohn, 1967; Powell & Axelsen, 1972; Nordlinger et al., 1979).

The hypothesis about the role of tyrosine catabolism disorders in pathogenesis of collagen diseases was not confirmed, but very interesting observations were described, in particular, by A.S. Kainova (Kainova, 1974): tyrosine levels in blood of patients with rheumatism decreased to normal values on successful hormonal and/or medicamentous therapy, and abolishment of glucocorticoid preparations in some cases was accompanied by an increase in the blood tyrosine level.

4. Observations on blood tyrosine levels and glucocorticoid treatment in patients with SLE

Systemic Lupus Erythematosus (SLE) was a problem for the Clinics of Therapy and Occupational Diseases, I Moscow Medical Institute, where I entered as a biochemist in 1968 and had been working until 1978. Naturally, the disorders in tyrosine metabolism observed by Nishimura et al. in patients with collagen diseases and observations by Kainova on blood tyrosine changes in patients with rheumatism seemed to me a possible biochemical approach to start my study on SLE.

Sixteen healthy donors (14 women and 2 men in the age from 20 to 40 years old) were used for determination the normal level of blood tyrosine, and it was found to be 16.2 ± 0.9 μg/ml. Note, that the repeated measurements of blood tyrosine levels in the same donors gave virtually the same values, i.e. it occurred to be rather a stable parameter.

Altogether 80 patients with SLE, 70 women and 10 men in the age range from 16 to 53 years old, were observed at 134 hospitalizations over the period of 1973–1976. Some patients were under observation repeatedly. The patients were not selected previously basing on their case history and severity and character of the disease. Tyrosine was determined in the serum from blood samples taken from patients with SLE at 8.00–8.30 a.m. on the empty stomach, usually once during 7-14 days over the period of hospitalization. The work was not a part of a previously approved plan of investigations, therefore, no blood samples were taken specially to determine the tyrosine content. Initially, levels of tyrosine and of its transamination product *p*-oxyphenylpyruvic acid were determined in parallel samples of blood and 24-h urine. The determination of tyrosine was performed spectrophotometrically by the method of Udenfriend & Cooper (1952), *p*-oxyphenylpyruvic acid was determined as described in the work (Knox & Pitt , 1957). It was shown that the increase in blood tyrosine level was caused by disturbance in transamination (Rass, 1976), whereas the further stages of tyrosine oxidation in the patients under study were virtually unaffected.

Changes in blood tyrosine in every patient were compared with the clinical and laboratory data recorded in their case histories after the patients' discharge from the hospital, with a special attention to using glucocorticoid preparations, i.e. a kind of the retrospective experiment was performed. The results were published in Russian in the work (Rass et al., 1977). Thirty-six patients were observed in the state of clinical remission; blood tyrosine was in normal limits in 23 of them and was steadily elevated in three patients (two of them had the affected liver); 28 patients obtained a supporting dose of glucocorticoids (not more than 15 mg prednisolone per day).

In 44 patients with SLE short-term "splashes" in blood tyrosine level were observed, and the retrospective analysis revealed that these "splashes" occurred simultaneously with some extraordinary events, such as a concurrent infection, aggravation of symptoms, or on the other day of a severe diagnostic procedure (e.g. the kidney biopsy), during the reaction to a new preparation, etc. Thus, these "splashes" were associated with a "stress-situation" when the need in glucocorticoid hormones was increased and in healthy subjects the synthesis of glucocorticoid hormones should increase. Thus, in a patient with chronic SLE who obtained 5 mg/day prednisolone as a supporting dose over the period of 50 days of hospitalization blood tyrosine values were 25, 20, 22 μg/ml, and a "splash" to **53** μg/ml was recorded on the day after the diagnostic intravenous urography. At the other hospitalization two years later this patient obtained the daily dose of 10 mg prednisolone and had blood tyrosine level of 8 μg/ml (possibly, the supporting dose of 10 mg prednisolone/day was too high - the previous supporting dose of 5 mg/day seemed sufficient to maintain the level of blood tyrosine in normal limits of 20-25 μg/ml). Similar "splashes" in blood tyrosine level were also observed in patients with glomerulonephritis under similar situations.

A very demonstrative was an attempt to even slightly lower the dose of glucocorticoid preparations in a clinically steroid-dependent patient with subacute SLE (Fig. 1). This "splash" in blood tyrosine was observed concurrently with the aggravation of her condition. In this patient the high background content of tyrosine was thought to be associated with the liver affection.

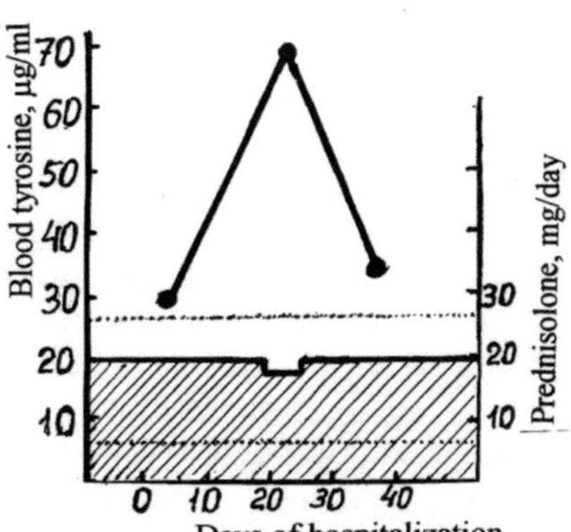

Fig. 1. Changes in the blood tyrosine content in a clinically steroid-dependent 40-year-old patient with subacute SLE. The attempt to decrease the dose of prednisolone was associated with an aggravation of the patient's condition. Dotted lines here and in the further Figures show normal limits of blood tyrosine contents.

"Splashes" in blood tyrosine were also observed in some patients with SLE at the alternate-day scheme of hormonal treatment on the next morning after glucocorticoid-free day.

But comparing results of glucocorticoid therapy with the initial level and behavior of blood tyrosine in patients with SLE seems to be the most interesting and informative. Changes in blood tyrosine upon prescribing or increasing the dose of glucocorticoids (40-60 mg/day calculated per prednisolone) because of SLE exacerbation were followed in 32 patients. Glucocorticoid preparations were prescribed according to the conventional schemes. The post-discharge analysis of the case histories revealed that to 20 patients glucocorticoids were prescribed at the significantly increased level of blood tyrosine (49.1 ± 0.8 μg/ml as compared to 16.2 ± 0.9 μg/ml in 16 healthy donors) and an essential improvement of clinical and laboratory parameters was recorded in 17 of them. In 13 patients this improvement was accompanied by a decrease in blood tyrosine, and this decrease was recorded before appearance of signs of Cushing's syndrome; in four patients with markedly affected liver functions the level of blood tyrosine remained elevated although their general condition became somewhat better. It should be noted that the "improvement" in all cases concerned only parameters of SLE activity, and side effects were considered as inevitable.

Twelve patients were given glucocorticoids on the background of normal blood tyrosine (≤ 26.5 μg/ml); glucocorticoids were inefficient in nine of them, and in four patients signs of Cushing's syndrome appeared very rapidly. Some improvement was recorded in three patients but this improvement could be due to other preparations given to them concurrently with glucocorticoids: azathioprine, heparin, cyclophosphamide, etc.

Let us consider some real cases.

Patient M., 27 years old, suffering from SLE for nine years was hospitalized because of aggravation of chronic SLE. Blood tyrosine at the first determination was 47.5 μg/ml. She was given prednisolone (30 mg/day) and antibiotics because of catarrhal state, however, 20 days later the immunologic activity was still present, as well as arthralgia and myalgia, blood tyrosine remains increased - 40 μg/ml; because of a continued aggravation of her condition 15 days later the prednisolone dose was increased to 40 mg/day, and *in a week a pronounced clinical improvement was recorded, together with a decrease in the blood tyrosine level to normal (25 μg/ml)*. She received 40 mg/day prednisolone for 20 days, and then the lowering prednisolone dose was started - and blood tyrosine slightly increased. The patient was discharged with the improved clinical and laboratory data (Fig. 2).

The following case (Fig. 3) presents a 21-year-old patient Zh., suffering of SLE during five years. She received long-term courses of prednisolone earlier in the maximal dose of 30 mg/day. A progressing osteonecrosis was observed. This time she was hospitalized because of an acute flare. At the first determination blood tyrosine level was somewhat increased (34.0 μg/ml), on the next day she was prescribed with prednisolone - 45 mg/day, and this dose was maintained *during 20 days. Five days* after the beginning of glucocorticoid therapy blood tyrosine decreased to 20.0 μg/ml, and *two days later a moon-like face appeared and elevations of arterial pressure up to 170/100 mm Hg* were recorded. GG therapy for 1.5 months was considered to be unfavorable; moreover, pains in femoral joints increased. Clinical improvement in this patient was obtained on prescribing heparin.

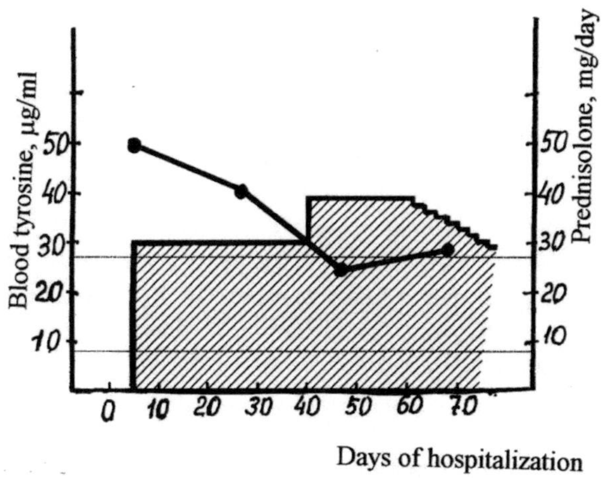

Fig. 2. Changes in the blood tyrosine content and regimen of glucocorticoid therapy (hatched) in a 27-year-old patient with chronic SLE.

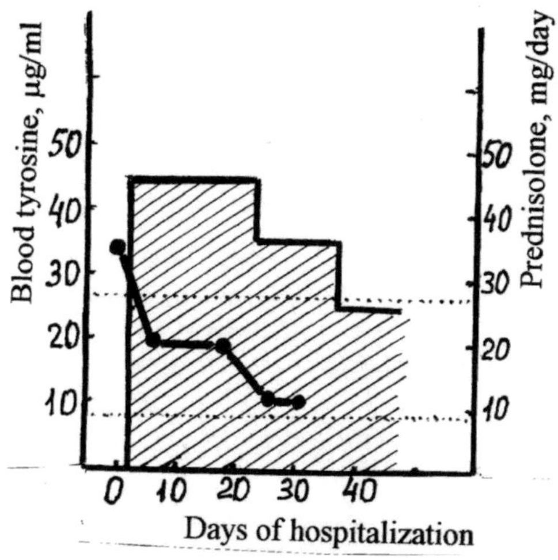

Fig. 3. Changes in the blood tyrosine content and regimen of glucocorticoid therapy (hatched) in a 21-year-old patient with chronic SLE.

Figure 4 shows changes in blood tyrosine level observed at withdrawal syndrome in a 22-year-old patient P. with subacute SLE (Fig. 4). The patient was in the state of a relative clinical and laboratory remission at the supporting dose of prednisolone (15 mg/day) for rather a long time. Such a rapid abolishment of prednisolone at the hospitalization in 1974 was forced by development of a pronounced aseptic osteonecrosis of femoral heads, and this abolishment was associated with a sharp aggravation of SLE symptoms associated with a sharp increase in blood tyrosine level.

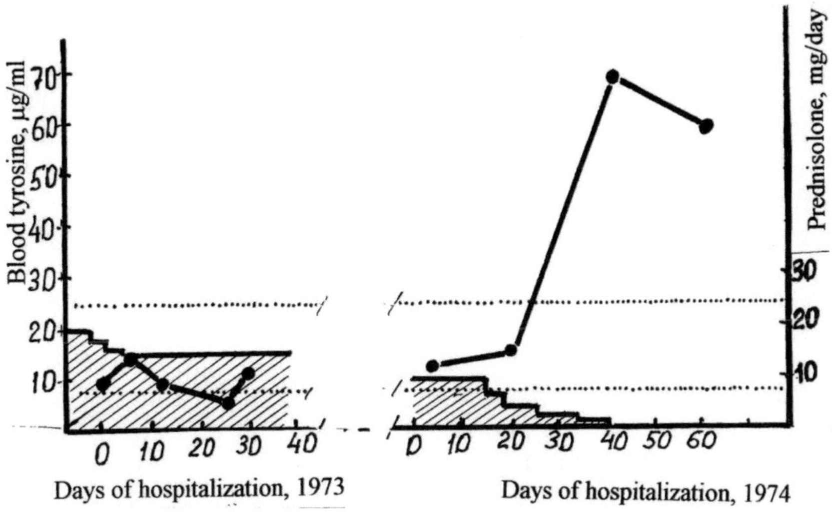

Fig. 4. Blood tyrosine levels and regimen of glucocorticoid therapy in a patient with subacute SLE during two hospitalizations, at the state of relative remission in 1973, and at withdrawal syndrome in 1974.

Thus, a certain association obviously occurred between the therapeutic effect of glucocorticoid preparations and their regulatory effect manifested by changes in the blood level of tyrosine. Moreover, such association cannot be occasional, exclusive, or SLE-specific, because the dependence of tyrosine catabolism on glucocorticoids is fundamentally the same in humans and in other mammals. Such an association must be significantly most common. In particular, blood tyrosine level was also increased in patients with bronchial asthma (not receiving glucocorticoids) during the period of attacks and was normal during the state of remission (Rass et al., 1978).
If so, may be blood tyrosine content can be used as a representative index of action of glucocorticoid hormones on metabolism, as an index of tissue provision with these hormones, and of real need of a subject in these hormones? May be blood tyrosine level can be used as a parameter (index) of glucocorticoid action, similarly to blood glucose which is a parameter of insulin action?

5. Tyrosine catabolism and blood tyrosine level as an index of glucocorticoid hormone action

This idea induced by observations on changes in blood tyrosine levels and regimens of glucocorticoid therapy in patients with SLE was for the first time published in the above-mentioned work (Rass et al., 1977) and was theoretically considered in the paper (Rass, 1978); then this idea was confirmed by experimental studies on adrenalectomized rats (Rass, 1980; Rass, 1983) and by observations on children with adrenogenital syndrome receiving long-life substitutive glucocorticoid therapy (Rass et al., 1979). In 1991 the hazard of glucocorticoid hormone application in non-endocrine diseases was considered to be mainly due to the absence of a test for sufficiency and real need in these hormones, and introduction of blood tyrosine as such a test was proposed as a safety basis for the individualized strategy of glucocorticoid therapy (Piruzian & Rass, 1991). However, all these works were published only in Russian, and this apparently promising idea remained virtually not called for until the review (Rass, 2010) was published in English.

Let us consider some specific features of tyrosine catabolism, especially those which allow us to consider the blood level of this amino acid as a promising laboratory parameter for monitoring glucocorticoid therapy.

Tyrosine is produced in the organism as a result of hydrolysis of food protein immediately or after hydrolysis of phenylalanine. About 30% of produced tyrosine is used for synthesis of catecholamines, melanin, and thyroid hormones, a portion is used for renewal of tissue proteins, and more than 60% is oxidized in the liver (Knox, 1955). And the first reaction in the major oxidation pathway of tyrosine is its transamination with alpha-ketoglutaric acid under the influence of tyrosine aminotransferase with production of *p*-oxyphenylpyruvic acid. Then *p*-oxyphenylpyruvic acid is oxidized under the influence of the appropriate oxidase in the presence of ascorbic acid with production of 2,5-dioxyphenylpyruvic, or homogentisic acid. The terminal products of the major pathway of tyrosine oxidation are acetoacetic and fumaric acids (Fig. 5).

Most frequently, tyrosine content in blood is determined using its reaction with alpha-nitroso-beta-naphthol with a subsequent recording by spectrophotometry (Udenfriend & Cooper, 1952) or by fluorimetry (Grenier & Laberge, 1974; Gavrilov et al., 1998). In some works HPLC (Kand'ar & Zakova, 2009), ion-exchange chromatography (Allard et al., 2004), and gas chromatography - mass-spectrometry (Deng et al., 2002) are also used. In some of the above-listed works tyrosine was determined in blood samples dried on filter paper discs.

The interest for determination of tyrosine level in blood is caused by necessity of early diagnosis of congenital disturbances of phenylalanine–tyrosine catabolism which result in severe disorders in the mental and physical development of the affected children. Phenylketonuria is caused by deficiency of the enzyme phenylalanine hydroxylase and is characterized by an extremely low level of blood tyrosine (< 0.05 μg/ml), tyrosinosis which is caused by an insufficient elimination of *p*-oxyphenylpyruvate acid due to deficiency of the appropriate oxidase (Scriver, 1967; Cerone at al., 1997) is manifested by a stable hypertyrosinemia up to 100 μg/ml, and in Richner–Hanhart syndrome caused by an inborn insufficiency of tyrosine aminotransferase blood tyrosine level can reach 600 μg/ml (Goldsmith, 1978; Natt et al., 1992). Incidence of phenylketonuria throughout the world is, on average, 1 : 15'000, and of the two other disorders in tyrosine catabolism are, respectively, 1 : 100'000 and 1 : 250'000, but in Canada they are recorded more frequently.

Tyrosine aminotransferase is an adaptive enzyme synthesized by the liver cells in response to entrance of the substrate - tyrosine, but for the substrate induction of this enzyme the entrance of glucocorticoids in the liver is necessary (Rosen and Nichol, 1963; Gelehrter, 1973; Thompson, 1979). Synthesis of hepatic tyrosine aminotransferase is a well-known example of the so-called gene-mediated action of glucocorticoids, and this enzyme is the most demonstrative and beloved object for studies of such effects of glucocorticoids (Sun at al., 1998; Grange et al., 2001; Hazra et al., 2007). Tyrosine aminotransferase is also used for testing on cell cultures and on intact and adrenalectomized animals of newly synthesized preparations which are expected to have less adverse effects than "classic" glucocorticoid preparations (Schacke et al., 2004; Zimmermann et al., 2009). The synthesis of tyrosine aminotransferase quantitatively depends on glucocorticoids, but being a hepatic enzyme, it cannot be determined in blood. However, tyrosine aminotransferase is a key enzyme in the major pathway of tyrosine catabolism and its activity determines the level of free tyrosine in blood. As a result, blood tyrosine level also depends on glucocorticoids (and, naturally, also on the functional competence of the liver cells).

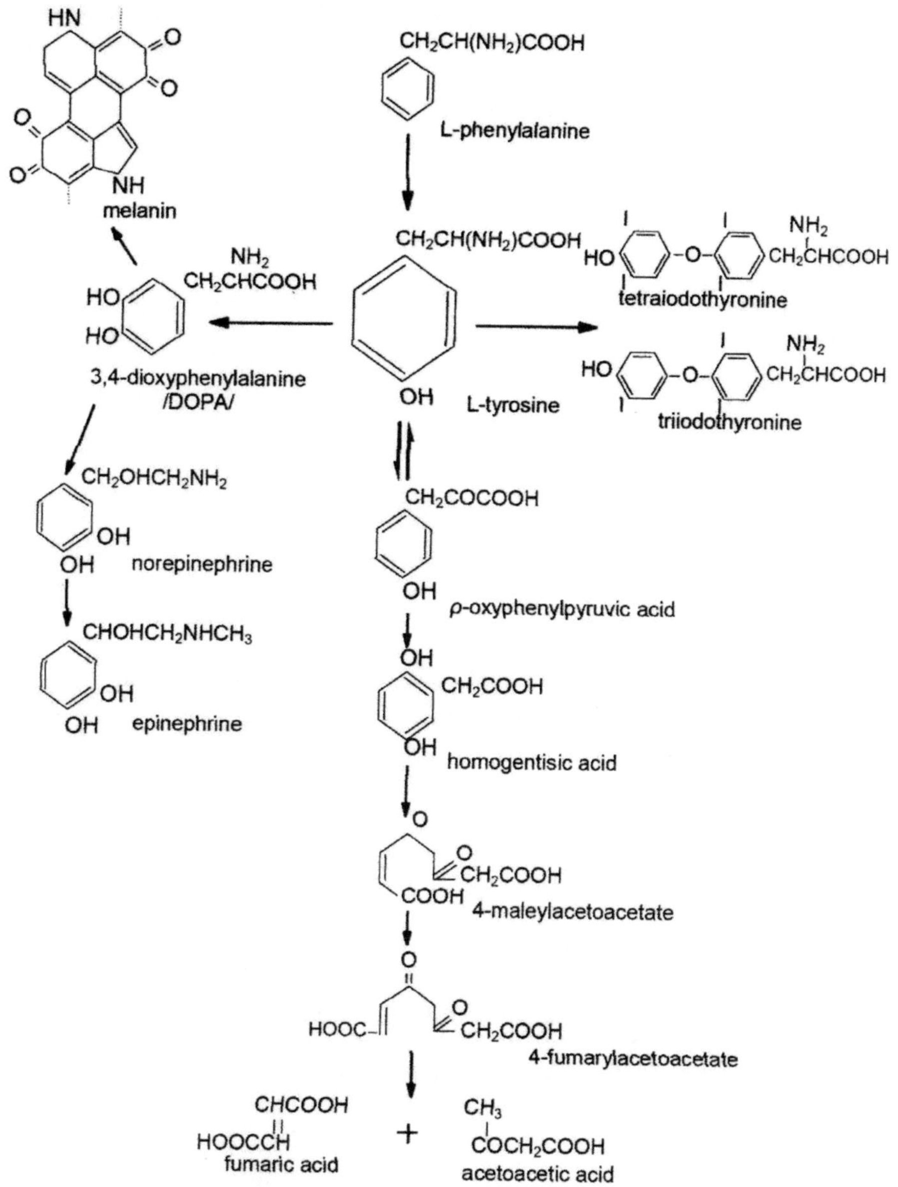

Fig. 5. Tyrosine catabolism (Scheme).

Due to substrate induction of tyrosine aminotransferase, even on tenfold increase in protein amount in the diet the blood content of tyrosine increases no more than by 50% above the basal level (Scriver et al., 1971), whereas circadian variations in blood tyrosine level mainly depending on circadian variations in production of natural glucocorticoids are in the limit of ± 25% (Wurtman et al., 1968).

But in the majority of cases and under real conditions an increase in blood tyrosine can be mainly determined by two factors: 1) a functional inferiority of the liver leading to a disturbed reception of glucocorticoids and inability of the liver cells to synthesize some enzymes including tyrosine aminotransferase, and 2) an insufficient entrance of glucocorticoids in the liver. As a result, under conditions of physiological rest, in the absence of extreme fluctuations in the diet, and on determination on the empty stomach in the morning the levels of free tyrosine in blood are similar in healthy animals and humans and do not depend on age and sex (Table 1).

Subjects under study	The number of subjects	μg/ml
Men	91	**13.0** ± 2.7
Women	103	**12.3** ± 2.4
Boys 6-18 yr	75	**12.3** ± 1.8
Girls 6-18 yr	65	**11.4** ± 2.0

Table 1. Blood tyrosine levels in humans, after (Armstrong & Stave, 1973a)

Moreover, it should be noted that blood samples taken from the same subjects (35 boys and 26 girls) four times over the period of 3–3½ years displayed characteristic individual patterns for the most of plasma amino acids, in particular, the content of blood tyrosine was virtually constant in the same subject (Armstrong & Stave, 1973b). We have also observed virtually the same values of blood tyrosine level in the samples taken repeatedly from the same healthy donors, as well as in blood samples from patients with SLE on supporting dose of glucocorticoids in the state of remission.

Injection of glucocorticoid preparations induced a 20–40% dose-dependent decrease in blood tyrosine in both animals and humans (Rivlin & Melmon, 1965; Betheil et al., 1965), and this decrease was the most pronounced 4-5 h after the injection, i.e. at the maximum of the glucocorticoid-induced synthesis of tyrosine aminotransferase. A decrease in the content of blood tyrosine was also recorded under stress conditions (Nemeth, 1978), obviously, due to a well-known increase in the glucocorticoid production by the adrenal cortex. Effects of hydrocortisone injection to healthy volunteers recorded by changes in the blood tyrosine levels and in the peripheral lymphocyte counts were considered as manifestations of genomic and nongenomic effects of glucocorticoids, respectively (Derks et al., 1999).

It is interesting to note that injections of hepatotoxins caused in rats an increase in the level of blood tyrosine, and the more pronounced was the liver necrosis the higher was this increase (Clayton et al., 2007).

6. Blood tyrosine content is an index of tissue provision with glucocorticoids: Confirmation on the experimental and clinical models

The dependence of blood tyrosine content on glucocorticoids was demonstrated experimentally on adrenalectomized rats (Rass, 1980; Rass, 2010). In intact rats blood tyrosine level was 15.0 ± 1.4 μg/ml. After bilateral adrenalectomy the blood level of tyrosine began to increase and reached, on average, 37.9 ± 6.4 μg/ml on the 5th day concurrently with the worst condition of the animals; then blood tyrosine level began to decrease most likely

due to synthesis of corticosterone in the brown fat tissue in response to the increased synthesis of ACTH after adrenalectomy; on the 10th day blood tyrosine level was the same as initially (under conditions of physiological rest!). Thus, the tyrosine level in blood manifested a pronounced dependence on production of natural glucocorticoids.
Starting from the 7th day after the operation, adrenalectomized rats were injected daily intraperitoneously with hydrocortisone in the dose of 2 mg per kg body weight (this dose approximately corresponded to the supporting dose 15 mg/day of prednisolone). Daily injections of hydrocortisone during 20 days resulted in a decrease in the tyrosine level in blood to undeterminable level, the abolishment of the injections and their absence during 5 days caused an increase in blood tyrosine, and the recommencement of hydrocortisone injections (5 mg per kg body weight) was accompanied by a decrease in blood tyrosine (Fig. 6).

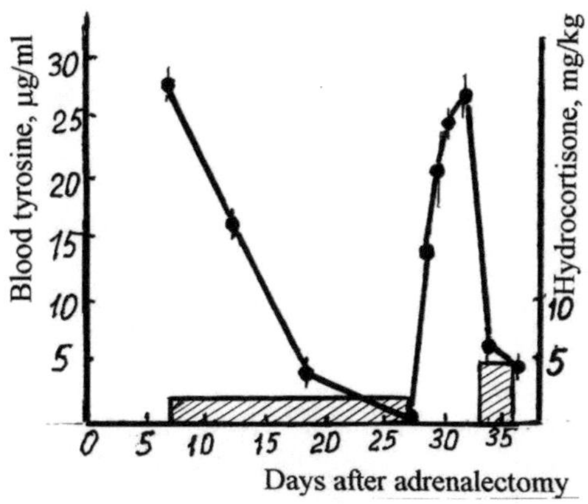

Fig. 6. Changes in tyrosine content in blood of adrenalectomized rats subjected to daily injections of hydrocortisone (hatched), upon abolishment of the injections, and on their recommencement.

And it seems that the only clinical situation exists (the model was recommended by Prof. M.A. Zhukovsky) which allows a physician (endocrinologist) to control the entrance of glucocorticoids in the organism and to some degree assess the adequacy of tissue provision with glucocorticoids to real needs of just this patient. This unique situation is presented by adrenogenital syndrome (synonyms: congenital adrenal hyperplasia, congenital virilizing adrenal cortex dysfunction) in children. The disease is caused by a genetically determined deficiency of glucocorticoid biosynthesis enzymes in the adrenal cortex, most frequently of 21-beta-hydroxylase, and a resulting shift to synthesis of androgens, mainly of dehydroepiandrosterone. The decreased production of glucocorticoids induces an increased synthesis of ACTH in the adenohypophysis that permanently stimulates the adrenal cortex with a resulting surplus synthesis of androgens (Brooks, 1979). The excess of androgens is displayed by a characteristic clinical picture: an abnormal structure of external sex organs, an accelerated body growth with an overdevelopment of masculine type muscles during the first years of life, the early arresting of growth because of premature ossification of tubular bones, etc. In the affected girls a picture of pseudohermaphroditism is developed.

The lifelong substitutive glucocorticoid therapy is the only pathogenetically reasonable treatment of this disease (Lo et al., 1999; Stikkelbroeck et al., 2003; Hughes, 2007). Glucocorticoid preparations break the vicious circle: recompensing the shortage of endogenous glucocorticoids they inhibit synthesis of ACTH responsible for overproduction of androgens. Glucocorticoid therapy started as early as possible after the birth and the appropriate dose can provide the normal physical and sexual maturation of the affected children according to their genetic sex, with a possibility of normal pregnancy and labor in females. The dose of glucocorticoids must be strictly individualized, and it can vary from 2.5 to 15 mg prednisolone per day.

On the other hand, changes in the clinical picture observed in children with adrenogenital syndrome - the rate of growth, ossification, and sexual maturation - allow a physician to relatively objectively and faultlessly estimate the correctness of the dose. In adult patients with this syndrome and in other conditions which obviously require the substitutive glucocorticoid therapy, after bilateral adrenalectomy or in chronic hypocorticism of various etiology, the dose of glucocorticoids can be prescribed only "according to the patient's self-feeling". According to B. Lukert (Lukert, 2006), "The problem for the clinician is the lack of objective criteria for determining adequate, but not excessive doses of glucocorticoids… In current practice, the clinician must rely on surrogate markers of glucocorticoid excess (early changes of Cushing's syndrome) rather than definitive end points".

Our study was performed with participation of 38 children with virilizing adrenogenital syndrome (33 girls and five boys of 3–18 years old hospitalized in the Pediatric Department of the Institute of Experimental Endocrinology and Chemistry of Hormones, the USSR Academy of Medical Sciences). Tyrosine levels were determined in blood samples taken in the morning on empty stomach and compared with clinical picture which characterized the degree of compensation of the genetic defect. The results were published in Russian (Rass et al., 1979) and republished in English in the review (Rass, 2010). The main results are presented in Fig. 7.

Figure 7 shows that in 17 children with adrenogenital syndrome at the complete clinical compensation blood contents of tyrosine were the same as in healthy donors (16 adults and seven children of 7–13 years old). In a girl with signs of Cushing's syndrome blood tyrosine was below the normal level. In untreated patients and in non-compensated patients because of irregular treatment blood tyrosine was significantly increased. In three non-compensated patients a pronounced melanodermia was observed along with the normal level of blood tyrosine, i.e. a part of excessive tyrosine was not oxidized through the major pathway but was converted into melanin (compare with the Scheme in Fig. 5!). Prescribing glucocorticoids resulted in "whitening" of such patients. Normalization of skin color in patients with hypocorticism upon taking glucocorticoids was also described in the literature (Snell, 1967).

In two compensated patients who initially displayed normal levels of blood tyrosine, transient increases to 29.0 and 45.0 μg/ml were recorded in association with a concurrent acute respiratory disease. Obviously, these increases are very alike "splashes" observed in patients with SLE, and can be explained by increased requirements for glucocorticoid hormones under conditions of stress or concurrent disease. Such observations justify the empirical recommendation to increase the dose of glucocorticoid preparations in the case of stress situations.

Two previously untreated girls were prescribed with glucocorticoids, and the determinations of blood tyrosine levels were helpful for choosing the optimal dose. Note that in patients with hypocorticism an acute withdrawal of the substitutive hydrocortisone injections resulted on the next day in a 25-30% increase in the level of blood tyrosine, whereas the levels of other amino acids remained virtually unchanged (Christiansen et al., 2007). The data presented in this section show that the normal level of blood tyrosine seems to indicate a sufficient provision of tissues and glucocorticoid-dependent reactions and processes with these hormones, whereas an increased level of blood tyrosine seems to be due to insufficient level of glucocorticoids. This seems rather clear for endocrine diseases.

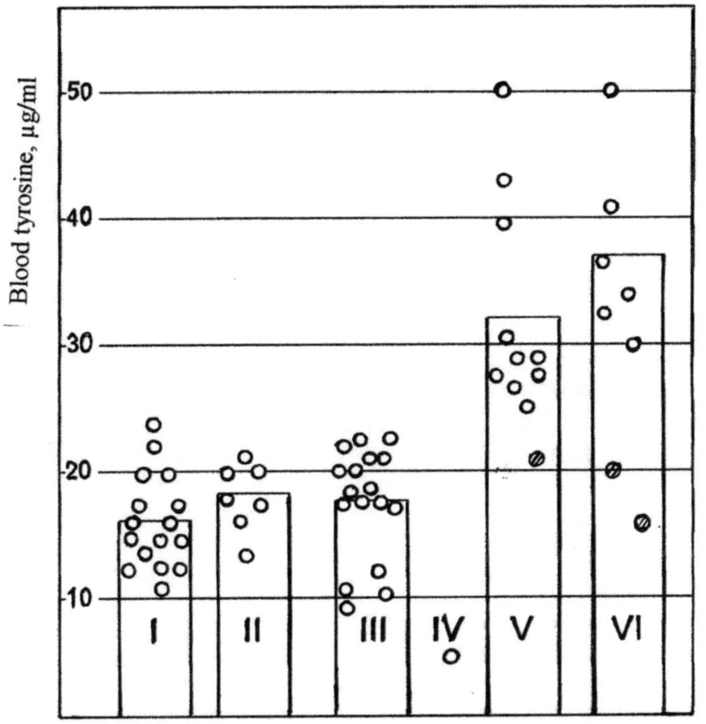

Fig. 7. Tyrosine contents in blood of healthy donors and children with adrenogenital syndrome. The columns present arithmetic means for the corresponding groups; the circles show individual values: I) healthy adults; II) healthy children; III) patients with the complete clinical compensation; IV) a girl patient with overdosed glucocorticoids; V) irregularly treated non-compensated patients; VI) untreated patients. Hatched circles in the columns V and VI show patients with a pronounced melanodermia.

However, it is also reasonable to expect that blood content of tyrosine could be a promising candidate for the role of an indirect marker for prescribing the correct dose in non-endocrine diseases. Unfortunately, for non-endocrine diseases there are no similar data, nevertheless, let us admit that blood tyrosine level could be used as an index of tissue provision and real need in glucocorticoid hormones (or glucocorticoid preparations) – in our patients with SLE described in the Section 4.

7. The imaginary tyrosine-based monitoring of glucocorticoid therapy in the above-presented cases of SLE (reconsideration of cases presented in Figs. 2–4)

Thus, keeping in mind the blood tyrosine as an index of the real need in glucocorticoids, let us look again at Figs. 2–4 and *imagine* the tyrosine-based monitoring of glucocorticoid treatment in these patients with SLE.

Fig. 2 – the imaginary monitoring. The patient M. was prescribed with 30 mg prednisolone daily on the background of a rather high initial level of blood tyrosine (47.5 µg/ml); she received this dose during 35 days without a pronounced clinical effect and on retention of the increased blood tyrosine (40.0 µg/ml). The improvement was achieved as soon as a week after increasing the prednisolone dose to 40 mg/day and this improvement was accompanied by normalization of blood tyrosine. The patient continued to receive 40 mg prednisolone for the following 15 days. Thus, in total, the patient M. received *30-40 mg prednisolone daily within two months.* But, taking into account the initial high level of blood tyrosine, as well as its retention at the second determination 20 days later, *it would have been reasonable to give her 40 mg prednisolone earlier and to start lowering the dose on normalization of blood tyrosine, i.e. the course of hormonal therapy could be much shorter.*

Fig. 3 – the imaginary monitoring. The increased level of blood tyrosine (34 µg/ml) at the first determination on the next day after the hospitalization could be a kind of "splash" - the reaction to hospitalization-associated procedure. The patient was prescribed 45 mg prednisolone per day and obtained this dose for 20 days. Blood tyrosine became normal very rapidly - on the 5th day after the hospitalization (even *earlier than the recorded in the case history appearance of the moon-like face and elevations in blood pressure*!) and continued to decrease to very low level during the treatment with glucocorticoids. After 1.5 months, glucocorticoid therapy was qualified as unfavorable. Was it a case of steroid-resistance or simply a manifestation of a sufficient provision with own hormones? In any case, *this patient did not need such a prolonged and rather intensive glucocorticoid therapy.*

Fig. 4 – the imaginary monitoring. Withdrawal syndrome in a 22-year-old patient with subacute SLE. The normal blood tyrosine level during the hospitalization the year before at the supporting dose of prednisolone 15 mg/day made it possible to think about at least *of decreasing the supporting dose of glucocorticoids, or even of trying to abolish hormonal preparations the year earlier!*

8. And the real successful course of glucocorticoid therapy *without side effects*

The next case (Fig. 8) exemplifies a successful course of glucocorticoid therapy performed by Dr. I.A. Borisov (described in detail in the work (Rass et al., 1977)) in a 48-year-old patient E. who had been suffering of SLE for 12 years. This hospitalization was because of a serious flare of SLE after an acute respiratory disease. *All previous courses of glucocorticoids in this patient resulted in a rapid development of Cushing's syndrome.* On the entrance blood tyrosine was 45-79 µg/ml. She was given prednisolone (40 mg/day) within a week and then transferred to alternate-day scheme of the dose lowering (the increase in blood tyrosine to 100 µg/ml was recorded in the morning two days after the abolishment of daily prednisolone). The alternate-day scheme was started from daily dose of 75 mg with a stepwise decreasing to 25 mg/day (combined with methindol on prednisolone-free days). Blood tyrosine decreased to the normal level (16 μg/ml) alongside with a general improvement of all clinical and laboratory data. The increase in the blood tyrosine level to 35 μg/ml concurrently with the SLE activation was recorded when prednisolone was replaced by decortilene; then a respiratory disease was associated with blood tyrosine increases to 30–45 μg/ml; and prednisolone was prescribed again in the daily dose of 30 mg during a week followed by the alternate-day lowering the prednisolone dose starting from 55 mg. The patient was discharged with an essential improvement *without any side effect of glucocorticoid therapy.*

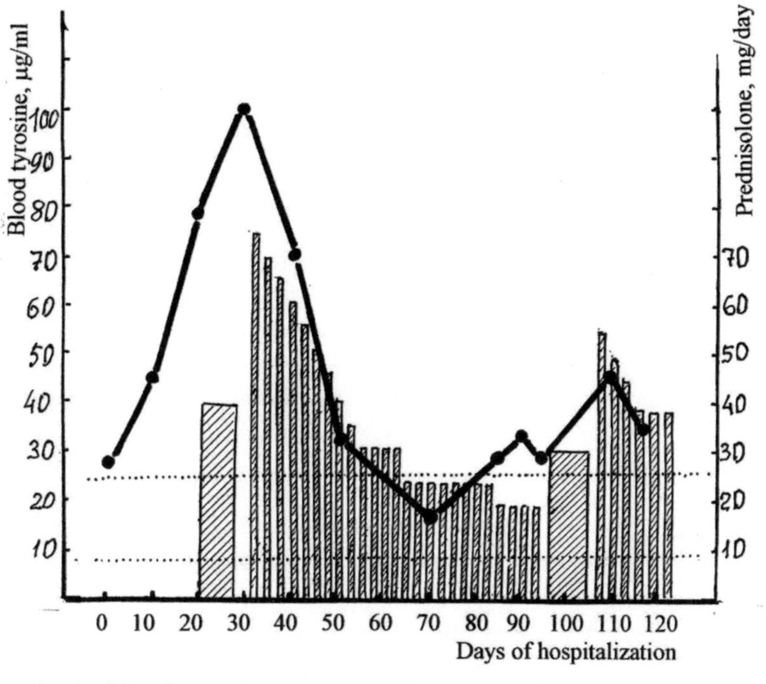

Fig. 8. Changes in the blood tyrosine content and regimen of glucocorticoid therapy (hatched) in a 48-year-old patient with SLE.

It should be underlined that in this case two specific hormonal features of the glucocorticoid preparations were taken into account: the organism's provision with glucocorticoids characterized by blood tyrosine level and using the alternate-day scheme for lowering the dose of hormonal preparation dose to promote the recovery of the negative feedback regulation in the hypothalamus-pituitary-adrenocortical system.

9. Conclusion

Preparations of glucocorticoid hormones for more than 60 years remain one of cornerstones of modern medicine as the most effective anti-inflammatory drugs also possessing anti-allergic, immunosuppressive, antitoxic, and anti-shock properties. Glucocorticoid preparations are widely used in all fields of clinical medicine and are virtually indispensable, although very serious complications are associated with their application. The number of works concerning glucocorticoid treatment of various diseases is innumerable. However, despite the extreme importance and indispensability of glucocorticoid preparations, up to now there is no objective laboratory parameter, similar to blood glucose for insulin, which would allow a clinician to foresee the effect of hormonal therapy in a given patient and realize a reasonable monitoring of the dose of glucocorticoid preparations.

The problem of safety of glucocorticoid therapy arose concurrently with the first usage of glucocorticoids by Dr. P. Hench and colleagues in 1948 (Hench et al, 1949) and difficulties which should be inevitable on using glucocorticoids were predicted and described in their large publication (Hench et al., 1950). Unfortunately, multiple refined studies on glucocorticoids by biochemists, geneticists, endocrinologists, physiologists, although very informative, are not frequently intersected with real need of clinical medicine.

Just the permanent critical state of glucocorticoid therapy made me reconsider my old works published in Russian in 1976–1983 which remained unnoticed and unknown. And only the publication in English (Rass, 2010) has attracted the attention to the still urgent problem of absence of a laboratory parameter extremely required for glucocorticoid therapy of both endocrine and non-endocrine diseases.

I hope that rather an easy determination of blood tyrosine level will be at last used as a suitable laboratory parameter for many situations in clinical medicine, endocrinology, and physiology of the hypothalamus–pituitary–adrenal cortex system. In physiology blood tyrosine determination can supplement measurements of levels of the hormonal participants of this system by data on adequacy of this system functioning to the organism's needs under different situations.

And finally some speculations.

The comparison of therapeutic effect of glucocorticoid preparations in SLE with their regulatory influence on the blood tyrosine level suggests that the therapeutic action of these preparations cannot be conditioned by an exclusive combination of pharmacological properties; on the contrary, the unique combination of therapeutic properties of these preparations is caused by retention of specific hormonal properties.

Glucocorticoid hormones are essentially responsible for supporting homeostasis - they directly or indirectly participate in regulation of the majority (if not all) biochemical reactions and physiological processes. They are hormones of total action and of vital importance. But in addition to supporting homeostasis under conditions of health and physiological rest, glucocorticoid hormones play a very important and sometimes a decisive role under conditions of stress or disease when, as a rule, their secretion increases. Under stress situations or in disease glucocorticoid hormones can realize their effects acting via the evolutionary selected best pathways, and, no doubt, a certain optimum of the adrenal cortex activity must exist for every subject (a human or animal) under extraordinary conditions. However, it seems that the optimum of this individual adrenocortical response can be revealed not by determination of functions of the hypothalamus-pituitary-adrenocortical system links, but only using a result of this system activity - an indirect glucocorticoid-dependent parameter, which can indicate whether this response is sufficient or not just for the concrete subject in a specific situation.

Glucocorticoid preparations retain the fundamental features of their natural prototypes, including their physiological and regulatory functions and can act via the same pathways. Therefore, it seems very likely that glucocorticoid therapy in non-endocrine diseases must imitate the optimal hormonal response of a given patient under conditions of disease - as if his adrenals could realize such a response. Glucocorticoid therapy must compensate an insufficient response of the patient's own adrenals, it can be life-saving within these limits and dangerous beyond them. The determination of blood tyrosine level which is a manifestation of the regulatory effect of glucocorticoid can allow a clinician to assess the correspondence of the hormonal provision to real needs of the patient.

10. References

Allard, P.; Cowell, L., Zytkovicz, T., Korson, M. & Ampola, M. (2004). Determination of Phenylalanine and Tyrosine in Dried Blood Specimens by Ion-Exchange Chromatography Using the Hitachi L-8800 Analyzer. *Clinical Biochemistry*, Vol.37, No.10, (October 2004), pp. 857-862, ISSN 0009-9120

Armstrong, M. & Stave, U. (1973). A Study of Plasma Free Amino Acid Levels. II. Normal Values for Children and Adults. *Metabolism*. Vol.22, No.4, (April 1973), pp. 561-569, ISSN 0026-0495

Armstrong, M. & Stave, U. (1973). A Study of Plasma Free Amino Acid Levels. IV. Characteristic Individual Levels of the Amino Acids. *Metabolism*. Vol. 22, No.6, (June 1973), pp. 821-825, ISSN 0026-0495

Badsha, H. & Edwards, C. (2003). Intravenous Pulses of Methylprednisolone for Systemic Lupus Erythematosus. *Seminars in Arthritis and Rheumatism*. Vol.32, No.6, (June 1973), pp. 1370-377, ISSN 0049-0172

Betheil, J.; Feigelson, M. & Feigelson, P. (1965). The Differential Effect of Glucocorticoids on Tissue and Plasma Amino Acid Levels. *Biochemica et Biophysica Acta*. Vol.104, No. 1, (January 1965), pp. 92-97, ISSN 0006-3002

Brooks, R. (1979). Biosynthesis and Metabolism of Adrenocortical Steroids. In: *The Human Adrenal Gland*, V.H.T. James, (Ed.), 67-92, ISBN 0861963628, Academic Press, London

Cerone, R; Holme, E., Schiaffino, M., Caruso, U., Maritano, L. & Romano, C. (1997). Tyrosinemia Type III: diagnosis and ten-year follow-up. *Acta Paediatrica*. Vol.86, No.9, (September 1997), pp. 1013-1015, ISSN 0340-6717

Christiansen, J.J.; Djurhuus, C., Gravholt, C., Iversen, P., Christiansen, J.S., Schmitz, O., Weeke, J., Lunde, J., Jergensen, J. & Meller, N. (2007). Effects of Cortisol on Carbohydrate, Lipid, and Protein Metabolism: Studies of Acute Cortisol Withdrawal in Adrenocortical Failure. *Journal of Clinical Endocrinology and Metabolism*. Vol.92, No.9, (September 2009), pp. 3553-3559, ISSN 0021-972X

Clayton, T.; Lindon, J., Everett, J., Charuel, C., Hanton, G., Le Net, L., Provost, J. & Nicholson, J. (2007). Hepatotoxin-Induced Hypertyrosinemia and Its Toxicological Significance. *Archive of Toxicolology*. Vol.81, No.3, (March 2007), pp. 201-210, ISSN 0340-5760 (doi)

Deng, Y. & Tsao, B. (2010). Genetic Susceptibility to Systemic Lupus Erythematosus in the Genomic Era. *National Reviews of Rheumatology.* Vol. 6, No.12, (December 2010), pp. 683-692, ISSN 1759-4790

De Rijk, R. & Sternberg, E. Corticosteroid Resistance and Disease. (1997) *Annals of Medicine.* Vol.29, No.1, (January 1997), pp. 79-82, ISSN 0785-3890

Derks, M; Dubois, E.F., Koomans, P. & Boxtel, C. (1999). Effect of Hydrocortisone on Plasma Tyrosine Concentration and Lymphocyte Counts in Healthy Volunteers. *Clinical Drug Investigations.* Vol.18, No.5, (November 1999), pp. 391-401. ISSN 1058-4838

Dubois, E.L. (1974). *Lupus Erythematosus.* 2nd Edition, ISBN 0781793947, University of Southern California Press, Los Angeles, USA

Franchin, G. & Diamond, B. (2006). Pulse Steroids: How Much is Enough? *Autoimmunity Reviews.* Vol. 5, no. 2, (February 2006), pp. 111-113, ISSN 0022-1767

Gavrilov, V.; Lychkovskii, E., Shostak, E. & Konev, S. (1998). Fluorescence Assay of Tyrosine in Blood Plasma. *Journal of Applied Spectroscopy.* Vol. 65, No. 3, (March 1998), pp. 379-384, ISSN 0021-9037

Gelehrter, T. (1973). Mechanisms of Hormonal Induction of Enzymes. *Metabolism.* Vol.22, No.1, (January 1973), pp. 85-100, ISSN 0026-0495

Godblatt, F. & Isenberg, D. (2005). New Therapies for Systemic Lupus Erythematosus. *Clinical and Experimental Immunology.* Vol.140, No.2 (May 140), pp. 205-212, ISSN 0268-3369

Goldsmith, L. (1978). Molecular Biology and Molecular Pathology of a Newly Described Molecular Disease - Tyrosinemia II (the Richner-Hanhart Syndrome). *Experimental Cell Biology.* Vol.46, No.1-2, (January-February 1978), pp. 96-113, ISSN 0304-3568

Grenier, A. & Laberge, C. (1974). A Modified Automated Fluorimetric Method for Tyrosine Determination in Blood Spotted on Paper: A Mass Screening Procedure for Tyrosinemia. *Clinica et Chimica Acta.* Vol.57, No.1, (January 1974), pp. 71-75, ISSN 0022-2275

Hazra, A.; Pyszeznsli, N., DuBois, D., Almon, R. & Jusko, W. (2007). Modeling Receptor/Gene-Mediated Effect of Corticosteroids on Hepatic Tyrosine Aminotransferase Dynamics in Rats: Dual Regulation by Endogenous and Exogenous Corticosteroids. *Journal of Pharmacokinetetics and Pharmacodynamics.* Vol.34, No.5, (May 2007), pp. 643-647, ISSN 0344-5704

Hench, P.; Kendall, E., Slocumb, C. & Polley, H. (1949). The Effect of a Hormone of the Adrenal Cortex (17-Hydroxy-11-dehydrocorticosterone, Compound E) and of Pituitary Adrenocorticotrophic Hormone on Rheumatoid Arthritis. Preliminary Report. *Proceedings of the Staff Meetings of Mayo Clinic.* Vol.24, No.1, (January 1949), pp. 181-197, ISSN 1462-0324

Hench, P.; Kendall, E., Slocumb, C. & Polley, H. (1950). Effect of Cortisone Acetate and Pituitary ACTH on Rheumatoid Arthritis, Rheumatic fever, and Certain Other conditions; Studies in Clinical Physiology. *Archives of Internal Medicine.* Vol.85, No.4, (April 1950), pp. 545-666, ISSN 1462-0324

Hughes, I. (2007). Congenital Adrenal Hyperplasia: a Lifelong Disorder. *Hormone Research.* Vol. 68, Supplement 5, pp. 84-89, DOI 000110585

Ioannou, Y, & Isenberg, D. (2002). Current Concepts for the Management of Systemic Lupus Erythematosus in Adults: a Therapeutic Challenge. *Postgraduated Medicne Journal.* Vol.78, No.924, (July 2002), pp. 599-606, ISSN 0032 - 5473

Kainova, A. (1974) Amino Acid Metabolism in Patients with Collagen Diseases. *Voprosy Revmatizma.* 1974; Vol.14, No.1, pp. 68-73, ISSN 0040-3660

Kand'ar, R. & Zakova, P. (2009). Determination of Phenylalanine and Tyrosine in Plasma and Dried Blood Samples Using HPLC with Fluorescence Detection. *Journal of Chromatography. B. Analytic Technology for Biomedical Life Sciences.* Vol.877, No.30, (November 2009), pp. 3926-3929, ISSN 1873-376X

Knox, W. (1955). Metabolism of Phenylalanine and Tyrosine. In: *Symposium on Amino Acid Metabolism.* pp. 836-866, ISSN 0022-3166, Baltimora, USA, April 1955.

Knox, W. & Pitt, B. (1957). Enzymic Catalysis of the Keto-enol-Tautomerization of Phenylpyruvic Acid. *Journal of Biological Chemistry.* Vol.225, No.2, (April 1957), pp. 675-688, ISSN 0021-9258

Levine, R. & Kohn, H. (1967). Tyrosine Metabolism in Patients with Liver Diseases. *Journal of Clinical Investigations.* Vol.46, No.12, (December 1967), pp. 2012-2030, ISSN 0021-9738

Li, X; Zhang, F., Zhang, J. & Wang, J. (2010). Negative Relationship between Expression of Glucocorticoid Receptor alpha and Disease Activity: Glucocorticoid Treatment of Patients with Systemic Lupus Erythematosus. *Journal of Rheumatolology.* Vol.37, No.2, (March 2010), pp. 316-321, ISSN 0315-162X

Lo, J.; Schwitzgebel, V., Tyrrell, V., Fitzgerald, P., Kaplan, S., Conte, F. & Grumbach, M. (1999). Normal Female Infants Born of Mothers with Classic Congenital Adrenal Hyperplasia due to 21-Hydroxylase Deficiency. *Journal of Clinical Endocrinology and Metabolism.* Vol.84, No.3, (March 1999), pp. 930-936, ISSN 0021-972X

Lukert, B. (2006) Glucocorticoid Replacement – How Much is Enough? *Journal of Clinical Endocrinology and Metabolism.* Vol.91, No.3, pp. 793-794, ISSN 0021-972X

Natt, E.; Kida, K., Odievre, M., Di Rocco, M. & Scherer G. (1992). Point Mutations in the Tyrosine Aminotransferase Gene in Tyrosinemia Type II. *Proceedings of the National Academy of Sciences of USA.* Vol.89, No.19, (October 1992), pp. 9297-9301, ISSN 0027-8424

Nemeth, S. (1978). The Effect of Stress or Glucose Feeding on Hepatic Tyrosine Aminotransferase Activity and Liver and Plasma Tyrosine Level of Intact and Adrenalectomized Rats. *Hormone and Metabolism Research.* Vol.10, No.2, (March 1978), pp. 144-147, ISSN 0018-5043

Nishimura, N.; Yasui, M., Okamoto, H., Kanazawa, M., Kotaka, Y. & Shibata, Y. (1958). Intermediary Metabolism of Phenylalanine and Tyrosine in Diffuse Collagen Diseases. *Archives of Dermatology.* 1958; Vol.77, No.2, (February 1958), pp. 255-262, ISSN 0003-4819

Nishimura, N.; Maeda, K., Yasui, M., Okamoto, H., Matsukawa, M. & Toshina, H. (1961). Phenylalanine and Tyrosine in Collagen Diseases. *Archives of Dermatology.* Vol.83, No.4, (April 1961), pp. 644-652, ISSN 0003-4819

Nived, O.; Sturfelt, G. & Bengtsson, A. Improved Lupus Outcome. We Are Doing a Good Job, But Could We Do Better? (2008). *Journal of Rheumatology.* Vol.59, No.2, (February 2008), pp. 176-180, ISSN 0315-162X

Nordlinger, B.; Fulenwider, J., Ivey, J., Faraj, B., Ali, F., Kutner, M., Henderson, J. & Rudman, D. (1979). Tyrosine Metabolism in Cirrhosis. *Journal of Laboratory and Clinical Medicine.* Vol.94, No.6, (December 1979), pp. 832-840, ISSN 0022-2143

Ntali, S.; Tzanakakis, M., Bertsias, G. & Boumpas, D. (2009). What's New in Clinical Trials in Lupus? *International Journal of Clinical Rheumatology.* Vol.4, No.4, (April 2009), pp. 473-485, ISSN 1462-0324

Oakley, R. & Cidlowski, J. (2011). Cellular Processing of the Glucocorticoid Receptor Gene and Protein: New Mechanisms for Generating Tissue Specific Action of Glucocorticoids. *Journal of Biological Chemistry.* Vol.286, No.5, (February 2011), pp. 3177-3184, ISSN 0270-7306.

Piruzian, L. & Rass, I. (1991). The Safety Problem and a Physiological Strategy for Using Glucocorticoid Hormones. *Izvestiya Akademii Nauk SSSR, Seriya Biologicheskaya.* No.5, (October 1991), pp. 735-743, ISSN 0002-3329

Ponticelli, C.; Glassock, R. & Moroni, G. (2010). Induction and Maintenance Therapy in Proliferative Lupus Nephritis. *Journal of Nephrology.* Vol.23, No.1, (January 2010), pp. 9-16, ISSN 0250-8095.

Powell, L. & Axelsen, E. (1972). Corticosteroids in Liver Diseases: Studies on the Biological Conversion of Prednisone to Prednisolone and Plasma Protein Binding. *Gut.* Vol.13, No.9, (September 1972), pp. 690-696, ISSN 0003-4819

Rahman, A. & Isenberg, D. (2008) Severe Lupus Erythematosus. *New England Journal of Medicine.* Vol.358, No. 9, (September 2009), pp. 929-939, ISSN 0961-2033.

Rass, I. (1976). Character of Tyrosine Metabolism Disorder in Systemic Lupus Erythematosus. *Voprosy Revmatizma.* Vol.16, No.4, (April 1976), pp. 21-23, ISSN 0040-3660

Rass, I. (1978). The Usage of Corticosteroid Hormones and Tyrosine Metabolism. *Patologicheskaya Fiziologiya.* No.2, pp. 87-91, ISSN 0040-3660

Rass, I. (1980). Changes in Blood Tyrosine Content in Rats upon Adrenalectomy and on Substitution Injection of Hydrocortisone. *Doklady Akademii Nauk SSSR.* Vol.250, No.6, (June 1983), pp. 1497-1499, ISSN 0869-5652

Rass, I. (1983). Changes in Blood Tyrosine Levels in Response to Stress in Intact and Adrenalectomized Rats. *Byulleten Eksperimental'noi Biologii i Meditsiny.* Vol.95, No.3, (March 1983), pp. 29-31, ISSN 0365-9615

Rass, I. (2010). Blood Content of Tyrosine is an Index of Glucocorticoid Action on Metabolism, *Biochemistry (Moscow).* Vol.75, No.3, (March 2010), pp. 353-366, ISSN 0006-2979

Rass, I.; Borisov, I., Nikishova, T. & Sura, V. (1977). Blood Tyrosine Dynamics and Treatment with Corticosteroids in Systemic Lupus Erythematosus. *Terapevticheskii Arkhiv.* Vol.59, No.8, (August 1977), pp. 110-115, ISSN 0040-3660

Rass, I.; Bunyatyan, A., Kornev, B. & Turusina, T. (1978). Tyrosine, 11-Oxycorticosteroids, and Cortisol in Blood of Patients with Bronchial Asthma. *Terapevticheskii Arkhiv.* Vol.60, No.11, (November 1978), pp. 98-101, ISSN 0040-3660

Rass, I.; Kuznetsova, E. & Zhukovskii, M. (1979). Blood Tyrosine as an Index of Adequacy of the Glucocorticoid Substitution Therapy in Congenital Adrenal Cortex Dysfunction in Children. *Pediatriya.* Vol.58, No.9, (September 1979), pp. 26-29, ISSN 0031-403X

Rivlin, R. & Melmon, K. (1965). Cortisone-Provoked Depression of Plasma Tyrosine Concentration: Relation to Enzyme Induction in Man. *Journal of Clinical Investions.* Vol.44, No.3, (March 1965), pp. 1690-1698, ISSN 0021-9738

Rosen, F. & Nichol, C. (1963). Corticosteroids and Enzyme Activity. *Vitamins and Hormones.* Vol.21, No.1, (January 1963), pp. 135-214, ISSN 0042-7543

Schacke, H.; Schottelius, A., Docke, W., Strehlke, P., Jaroch, S., Schmees, N., Rehwinkel, H., Hennekes, H. & Khusru, A. (2004). Dissociation of Transactivation from Transrepression by a Selective Glucocorticoid Agonist Leads to Separation of Therapeutic Effects from Side Effects. *Proceedings of National Academy of Sciences of USA.* Vol.101, No.1, (January 2004), pp. 227-232, ISSN 0027-8424

Schroeder, J. & Euler, H. (1997). Recognition and Management of Systemic Lupus Erythematosus. *Drugs.* Vol.54, No.3, (March 1997), pp. 422-434, ISSN 1525-6359

Scriver, C. (1967). The Phenotypic Manifestions of Hereditary Tyrosinemia and Tyrosyluria. A Hypothesis. *Canadian Medical Association Journal.* Vol.97, No.18, (October 1967), pp. 1045-1101, ISSN 0003-4819

Scriver, C.; Clow, C. & Lamm, P. (1971). Plasma Amino Acids. Screening, Quantitation, and Interpretation. *American Journal of Clinical Nutrition.* Vol.24, No.7, (July 1971), pp. 826-890, ISSN 0002-9165

Snell, R. (1967). Hormonal Control of Pigmentation in Man and Other Mammals. *Advances in Biology of Skin.* Vol. 8, No. 4, (April 1967), pp. 447-466, ISSN 0906-6705

Stikkelbroeck, N.; van't Hof Grootenboer, B., Hermus, A., Otten, B., & van't Hof, M. (2003). Growth Inhibition by Glucocorticoid Treatment in Salt Wasting 21-Hydroxylase Deficiency: in Early Infancy and (Pre)puberty. *Journal of Clinical Endocrinology and Metabolism.* Vol.88, No.7, (July 2003), pp. 3525-3530, ISSN 0021-972X

Sun, Y.; DuBois, D., Almon, R., Pyszeznsli, N. & Jusko, W. (1998). Dose-Dependence and Repeated-Dose Studies for Receptor/Gene-mediated Pharmacodynamics of Methylprednisolone on Glucocorticoid Receptor Down-regulation and Tyrosine Aminotransferase Induction in Rat Liver. *Journal of Pharmacokinetics and Biopharmacology.* Vol. 26, No.6, (June 1998), pp. 619-648, ISSN 0090-466X

Thompson, E. (1979). Glucocorticoid Induction of Tyrosine Aminotransferase in Cultured Cells. In: *Glucocorticoid Hormone Action,* J. D. Baxter & G. G. Rousseau, (Eds.), 203-213, Springer Verlag, ISBN 038708973X Berlin/Heidelberg/New York

Udenfriend, S. & Cooper J. (1952). The Chemical Estimation of Tyrosine and Tyramine. *Journal of Biological Chemistry.* Vol.196, No.1, (January 1952), pp. 227-233, ISSN 0022-1767

Wurtman, R.; Rose, C., Chou, C. & Larin, F. (1968). Daily Rhythms in the Concentration of Various Amino Acids in Human Plasma. *New England Journal of Medicine.* Vol.279, No.1, (January 1968), pp. 171-175, ISSN 1759-4790

Zimmermann, C.; Avery, W., Finelli, A., Farwell, M., Fraser, C. & Borisy, A. (2009). Selective Amplification of Glucocorticoid Anti-inflammatory Activity through Synergistic Multi-target Action of a Combination Drug. *Arthritis Research and Therapy.* Vol.11, No.1, (January 2009), pp. 12-26, ISSN 1759-4790

8

Embryonic and Placental Damage Induced by Maternal Autoimmune Diseases - What Can We Learn from Experimental Models

Zivanit Ergaz[1] and Asher Ornoy[2]
[1]*Laboratory of Teratology, Israel Canada Institute of Medical Research Hebrew University Hadassah Medical School, Jerusalem Department of Neonatology, Hadassah-Hebrew University Hospital Mount Scopus, Jerusalem*
[2]*Laboratory of Teratology, Israel Canada Institute of Medical Research, Hebrew University Hadassah Medical School, Jerusalem, Israel and Israeli Ministry of Health Israel*

1. Introduction

Autoimmune diseases may have an adverse effect on reproduction and pregnancy outcome. Systemic Lupus Erythematosus (SLE) is associated with a wide variety of antibodies to different cell body components, mostly antiphospholipid antibodies. These are a heterogeneous group of antibodies that bind to negatively charged phospholipids and/or serum phospholipid binding proteins. Antiphospholipid syndrome (APLs) may occur as primary APLs or in association with autoimmune diseases. During normal pregnancy maternal immunity and hormones allow fetal survival, but when these mechanisms are impaired it may have a detrimental effect on the fetus. Pregnancies in women with APLs can be complicated by a high rate of pregnancy loss, pre-eclampsia, fetal growth restriction, prematurity and fetal distress. Disease flare during pregnancy predicts adverse fetal outcome (Kwok et al., 2011). The mechanisms underlying the recurrent abortions and fetal loss among women suffering from SLE are not completely elucidated. Thrombotic placental events may explain only some of the miscarriages. In vitro cell culture of placental trophoblast cell lines with IgG from patients suffering from APLs showed that APLs/ anti-β2-glycoprotein I antibodies / anti-β 2 globulin antibodies might disrupt the annexin coverage of thrombogenic anionic surfaces on the trophoblast and endothelial cell monolayers and lead to Factor X and prothrombin activation (Rand et al., 1997). However histopathological findings suggestive of thrombosis cannot be detected in the majority of the placentas from women suffering from APLs (Levy et al., 1998, Meroni et al., 2008). It has been suggested that antiphosholipids may be responsible for a local acute inflammatory response mediated by complement activation and neutrophil infiltration that eventually leads to fetal loss. Circulating antiphospholipid antibodies occurring at about 40% of SLE patients are associated with fetal loss. Some investigators regard APLs as a marker for recurrent abortions and not necessarily as their primary cause. Lupus anticoagulants, anticardiolipin and anti-β2-glycoprotein I antibodies are typically found among the patients. Complement activation was shown to play a role in antiphospholipid antibody - mediated fetal loss associated with inflammatory process, when C4d, a degradation product of C4 was demonstrated in human placenta of SLE patients (Cohen et al., 2011), as well as diminished number of T regulatory cells, associated with pregnancy loss and pre-eclampsia (Tower et al., 2011). Circulating microparticles that expose phospholipids in the outer membrane and induce coagulation via tissue factor have been associated with lupus anticoagulants and poor obstetric outcome (Alijotas-Reig et al., 2009). Other reports indicate that enhanced oxidative stress could be linked to autoimmune diseases; however, there is lack of data about anti oxidant status of the placenta and embryos during pregnancy in women suffering from autoimmune diseases.

2. The role of experimental animal studies in evaluation of pregnancy complications among women suffering from autoimmune diseases

As more than one mechanism of pathogenesis exists for fetal damage in autoimmune diseases, experimental animal models can be used to isolate the different causative effects. Evaluation of the role of different antibodies and molecules can be obtained by direct injection or induction of antibodies production in the pregnant animals and evaluation of the resultant effect on the embryos and fetuses. In such case the effect is evaluated in normal animals rather than being secondary to an autoimmune disease.

Previous published studies revealed fetal damage induced by various antibodies. A smaller litter size was demonstrated after the injection to pregnant BALB/C mice with a human cytomegalovirus -peptide-induced monoclonal antiphospholipid (Gharavi et al., 2004). Fetal heart block and bradycardia were evidenced in a murine model as a result of maternal autoantibodies to Ro and La antigen induced by maternal immunization (Suzuki et al., 2005). In addition maternal immunization with DNA memitope in mice led to the induction of autoantibodies that bind DNA and the N-methyl-D-aspartate receptor in the maternal circulation leading to increased neocortical cell death in the fetal brain and subsequent delayed acquisition of neonatal reflexes and cognitive impairments in the adult offspring. In this model the antibodies that were detected in the fetal neocortex outside of blood vessels evidenced their transport through fetal circulation until binding to the fetal brain (Lee et al., 2009). We previously found that the immunization of BALB /C mice with mouse laminin-1 was followed by the development of anti-laminin-1 antibodies. A double fetal resorption rate and lower fetal and placental weight was found in the laminin-1 immunized group compared with controls. Resorption rate was highest in the subgroup of animals with very high levels of anti-laminin-1 (Matalon et al., 2003). Other molecules were also found to have direct embryotoxic effects. The injection of a low-molecular weight fraction of boiled human serum containing antiphospholipid antibodies that had been obtained from women with antiphospholipid syndrome to pregnant rats at day 5 - 6 of pregnancy resulted in increased embryonic apoptosis 2 to 4 hours after the injection (Halperin et al., 2008).

3. In vitro systems to evaluate sera toxicity in autoimmune diseases

To try to evaluate the different mechanisms that lead to poor obstetric outcome we practiced three in vitro systems that use sera obtained from patients suffering from autoimmune diseases and recurrent abortions as culture media.

3.1 In vitro development of pre-implantation mice embryos in culture

Mouse blastocysts obtained from the uterine horns before implantation at 3.5 days of gestation can be cultured for up to 10 days and reach the developmental stage equivalent of 9.5 to 10 days of gestation in utero, or one-half of the total gestational period. At that early somite stage, the blood circulation in the yolk sac is not yet established and the anterior neuropore is open. The limb buds and the primordia of the lung, liver, and pancreas are not yet present (Chen & Hsu, 1982).

The technology in brief: Female mice are treated with gonadotropins followed 48 h later by Human Chorionic Gonadotropin in order to cause super-ovulation. The mice are mated with males and insemination is verified the following morning by the finding of a copulation plug in the vagina (day 0). Late morula-early blastocyst stages are obtained by flushing the uterine horns with culture medium 3 days after mating. Embryos are removed from several mice, pooled in an embryological watchglass, washed and transferred to fresh medium. A group of 8-10 embryos are placed in drops with Eagle's medium supplemented with 50% or 80% human serum. L Glutamine is added to the medium in a concentration of 2 mM/cc. Embryos are cultured in a humidified atmosphere in unaerobic conditions under paraffin drops. They are checked before incubation, after 24 and 72 hours or other incubation times under an inverted microscope to determine the developmental stage. The parameters used as criteria for assessing the rate of development and differentiation of embryos are namely, hatching of blastocysts from the zona pellucida, their adhesion to the substratum, and outgrowth and spreading on the surface (Abir et al., 1990).

Using this method, one can examine direct effects of the sera from women with recurrent abortions on early pre-implantation embryos.

3.2 In vitro development of early somite stage rat embryos in culture

The early somite rat embryo culture allows the investigation of the embryotoxicity of various teratogens in face of the difficulty to perform studies on mammalian embryos while in utero (New et al., 1976). It is an in vitro method to evaluate teratogenicity of various chemicals (i.e. different drugs and chemicals) as the tested compounds are added to the culture medium and the embryos cultured during organogenesis (New et al., 1976). The various agents can be evaluated either individually or in combination. Adverse embryonic outcomes (malformations or embryolethality) were shown to be directly related to the serum concentration of the compound being tested and can be compared to the serum concentration in the human. Moreover, as embryos can also be cultured directly on human serum, it may serve as a tool to investigate the direct effects of sera from women with different diseases on embryonic development. Additionally, the early somite rat embryo culture model can allow the evaluation of success of various treatment modalities and thus may be an important tool to predict the outcome of the pregnancy. This can be achieved due to the yolk sac (the chorioallantoic placental equivalent at this stage in rat pregnancy) which provides a large surface area for nutritional and respiratory exchange between the embryo and the culture medium. Previous studies proved that rat conceptuses explanted at 9.5-12.5 days, when the embryo develops from the early neurula to the late tail bud stage, can be maintained in vitro for 48 hours with almost 100% survival and growth that is indistinguishable from that occurring in vivo.

The technology in brief: Pregnant female rats are euthanized on day 9.5 to 12.5 of pregnancy when sperm finding is considered to be day 0. The embryos are cultured for 28-48 hours at

37°C in rotating bottles, and supplemented with gas mixtures: day-1: 20% Oxygen, 75% N2, 5% CO2, and day-2: 40% oxygen, 55% N2, and 5% CO2. After 28-48 hours of culture the embryos are examined under a dissecting microscope and scored according to the method described by Brown et al (Brown & Fabro, 1981) and us (Abir & Ornoy, 1996, Abir et al., 1994). Only embryos with a beating heart are examined for yolk sac size and circulation, axial rotation, neural tube closure, presence of telencephalic vesicles, optic and otic vesicles, number of somites, body size, and presence of gross anomalies. The use of morphological scoring system provides an index for embryonic development proportional to the embryonic age and aids in the detection of anomalies induced by the different teratogens. The embryos and yolk sacs are kept for different morphological, biochemical and molecular studies.

The possible direct effects of the sera from women with autoimmune diseases can be examined on cultured rat embryos using sera or IgG obtained from women with SLE/APLs as the culture medium, and analyzing the effects these sera has on embryonic growth, rate of anomalies, and ultrastructural yolk sac damage compared to sera from control healthy women and control rats.

3.3 Human placental explants in culture

The use of first trimester chorionic villi explants cultures has the advantage over cell culture of being the in vivo source of extravillous trophoblast and the preservation of topological and functional villous-extravillous trophoblast inter-relationships. It was demonstrated that first trimester villous explants maintained on Matrigel or rat tail collagen support the villous explants differentiation, migration and hormone production in 98 per cent of cultures (Genbacev et al., 1992). The study of placental explants in culture, where no blood circulation exists, enabled the evaluation of the direct effects of different sera on the placenta, thus exposing the mechanisms of placental damage other than placental infarcts, thrombosis and vasculopathy.

The technique in brief: Placental tissue of 5.5–7.5 weeks of gestation are transferred on sterile gauze in an ice-cold phosphate-buffered saline and then removed to a Petri dish and rinsed in phosphate buffered saline. Placental tissue is dissected from deciduas and fetal membranes for inspection under a dissecting microscope. Explants of approximately 10 mg wet weight are transferred into Millicell-CM culture dish insert (Millipore, Bedford, MA), which has been previously layered with polymerized Matrigel® (Collaborative Research, Bedford, MA). The inserts are then placed in 24-well culture dishes. Explants are placed in incubator (5% CO2) for 60 min at 39°C to evaporate phosphate buffered saline droplets to assist in villi adherence to the thin layer of Matrigel®. Cultures are incubated overnight in an incubator with 5% CO2. Twelve hours from the initiation of culture 400 µl of different types of different sera enriched with 1 mg glucose/ml are added directly to the inserts. Both the media from the insert (top) and the well (bottom) are changed every 48 hr, collected, and stored at -20°C until assayed. Villous explants are inspected daily using an inverted phase-contrast microscope for general cellular integrity, cellular proliferation, and outgrowth. The explants remain in culture for 4 days. At the end of the experiment, villi with supporting Matrigel® are dissected out using surgical blades and kept for morphological, immunohistochemical biochemical and molecular studies, and the media is removed for the analysis of major hormones secreted by the placental tissue.

To evaluate the possibility that in SLE/APLs at least some of the antibodies may directly damage placental trophoblastic cells, consequently causing fetal damage that may lead to intrauterine growth restriction or fetal death and to evaluate therapeutic interventions we used human placental explants in culture.

4. In vitro studies of embryotoxicity of sera from women with recurrent abortions on pre-implantation mice in culture

4.1 The embryotoxicity of sera from women with recurrent abortions on pre-implantation mice in culture

Mouse blastocysts 3.5-day-old at late morula stage and inside the zona pellucida, were cultured for 72 h in 50% or 80% sera from women with recurrent abortions. In embryos cultured in sera from women with recurrent abortions, 53.2% did not reach blastocystic development, compared to 33.6% of the embryos grown on sera from women after only one miscarriage and 8.2% and 12% on control sera from women following delivery of a normal infant or on sera obtained from women in the second trimester of a normal pregnancy respectively. When sera from women with miscarriages were divided into "high risk'"(50% or more embryotoxicity) and "low risk"(less than 50% embryotoxicity) sera, the "high risk" sera from two or more miscarriages caused an average of 72.1% undevelopment (i.e. not reaching the blastocystic stage), while the "low risk" sera from the same group caused 33.6% undevelopment. The "high risk" sera from one miscarriage were embryotoxic to 55.8% of the blastocysts and the "low risk" sera from the same group caused only 8.7% undevelopment similar to the controls (Abir et al., 1990).

4.2 The limitations of the pre-implantation rat culture

The limitations of this method is that it is impossible to evaluate even early post-implantation periods that equivalents early organogenesis. It cannot be used for the study of growth restriction and for the effects of teratogens which affect the embryo in later stage. In addition, the small embryonic size limits the possibility to perform various biochemical and genetic studies and does not allow the investigation of the effect of the different chemicals on isolated organs.

In conclusion: More pre-implantation mouse blastocytes failed to reach blastocystic development when cultured in sera obtained from women with recurrent abortions compared to those cultured in control sera.

5. In vitro studies of the embryotoxicity of sera from patients suffering from systemic lupus erythematosus/antiphospholipid syndrome on early somite rat embryos in culture

5.1 The role of IgG antibodies in recurrent abortions

To test the hypothesis that IgG antibodies from women with recurrent abortions may be responsible for the miscarriage, sera from women one day after an abortion were used as culture media for 10.5 days old embryos and compared to human control sera obtained from women either during a second trimester of a normal pregnancy or a day after normal delivery. Anomalies rate increased from 22% among controls to 47% among embryos cultured in sera from women who had a history of one abortion and to 54% among embryos cultured in sera from women who had a history of two abortions or more. Anomalies included mainly microcephaly, open neural tube, lack of eyes and cardiac anomalies. The difference between the sera was more prominent when the sera were classified as low- less than 50% anomalies compared to high-more than 50%. The high rate of anomalies was particularly characteristic to the highly teratogenic sera while in the other sera anomalies rate was similar to controls. This difference may indicate a basic difference between the two sera groups: one that has a factor(s) that is teratogenic in this model and the other that induces abortions in a different mechanism that is not relevant to this model.

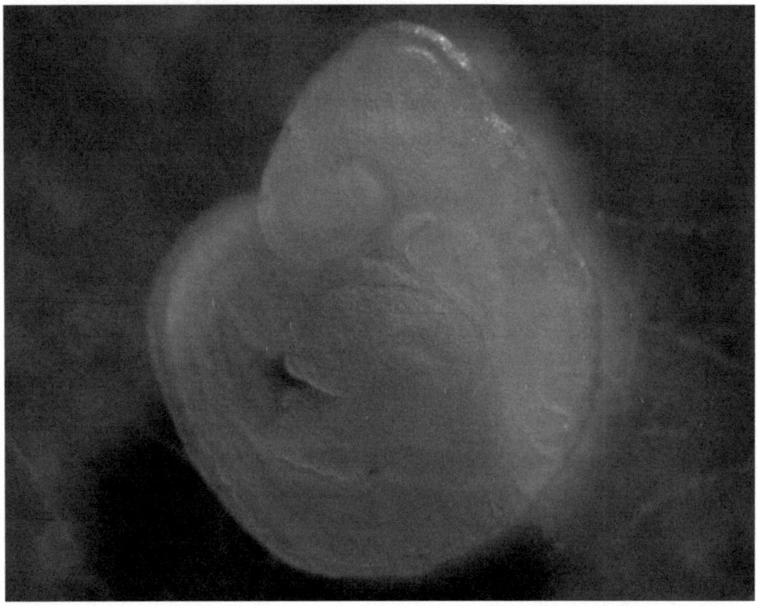

Fig. 1. Early somite 10.5 days rat embryo after 28 hours in culture: normal embryo

To further evaluate whether the embryotoxic factor in this model is IgG, we used high risk sera and control sera, separated the IgG fraction and exchanged it between the sera. We defined three groups: one in which IgG from controls corrected the anomalies induced by the toxic sera, and the IgG from toxic sera induced anomalies in the embryos cultured in the control sera, the second in which control sera did not reduce the rate of anomalies but the IgG induced anomalies in the controls, and the third in which no effect was demonstrated after IgG exchange. We assumed that in these embryos a different factor was responsible for the teratogenicity. When the yolk sacs were evaluated by transmission electron microscopy we found a morphological damage represented by fewer microvilli and more inclusions in the entodermal epithelial cell in the sacs from embryos cultured in high risk sera (Abir et al., 1993).

5.2 The role of IgG antibodies in intra-uterine growth restriction

Besides recurrent abortions and fetal death, a main morbidity among infants of mothers suffering from autoimmune diseases is intra-uterine growth restriction. To investigate the role of the IgG antibodies on embryonic and fetal growth we evaluated the effect of high levels of antiphospholipid and anti DNA antibodies on 11.5 days rat embryos in culture, a stage when most of the organs have already been formed. Reduced fetal growth and yolk

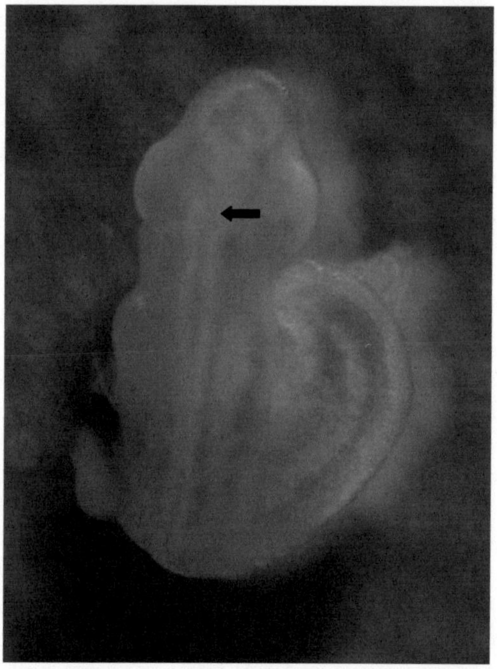

Fig. 2. Early somite 10.5 days rat embryo after 28 hours in culture: arrow-open neural tube

sac diameter were found in embryos cultured in media containing IgG from women suffering from SLE / recurrent abortions, compared to IgG from controls or medium without IgG. When we evaluated the role of the different IgG fractions (anticardiolipin-β2 glycoprotein, antiphosphatidylserine, anti-double stranded DNA, anti-laminin, anti-thyroglobulin and anti-pyruvate dehydrogenase) compared to controls, only embryos that were cultured in sera positive for anti-cardiolipin were significantly smaller than the embryos cultured in sera containing normal IgG fractions. The embryos cultured in medium containing anticardiolipin/ anti DNA/ antiphosphatidylserine had a smaller yolk sac. However, embryos cultured in sera from SLE patients with a history of recurrent abortions were also smaller even when they were negative for antiphosphatydilserine. In spite of the fact that in these experiments the embryos were cultured towards the end of organogenesis when many of the organs have already been formed, 15.6% of the embryos exposed to IgG purified from women suffering from SLE / recurrent abortions had anomalies, while only 8.7% of the embryos exposed to IgG purified from sera of healthy women were malformed. There was a significant difference in the development of the brain and branchial bars between embryos that were exposed to patients' IgG and those exposed to IgG that was purified from healthy women. There was also a significant reduced somite number among the experimental group embryos (Matalon et al., 2002).

5.3 The effect of IgG antibodies on the yolk sac

The embryos at the early somite stage are surrounded by their yolk sac and by their ectoplacental cone which is the trophoblastic part of the cellular complex at the embryonic pole of the blastocyst. The ectoplacental cone is responsible for the invasion into the decidua. To evaluate the mechanism by which IgG affects the yolk sac, 11.5 days old embryos were cultured in two human IgG2 monoclonal antiphosphatidylserine antibodies

(HL5B, RR7F). The antiphosphatidylserine antibodies were associated with implantation failure in previous studies with mainly trophoblastic injury by inhibition of syncytium formation, decreased human chorionic gonadatropin (hCG) production, and disturbed trophoblast invasion (McIntyre, 2003). The HL5B monoclonal antibody was generated from a primary antiphospholipid syndrome patient with multiple central ischemic events and the RR7F monoclonal antibody was generated from SLE patient with high titers of circulating antiphosphatidylserine and anticardiolipin antibodies, with no history of thrombosis or fetal loss. Both antibodies showed reactivity against phosphatidylserine and cross-reactivity with cardiolipin but lacked reactivity against β2-glycoprotein and did not have a lupus anticoagulant activity. Embryos cultured in both sera had reduced yolk sac diameter without significant difference in the rate of anomalies. Apoptotic processes were found in some of the giant cells and in most of the cells located in the area between the mature giant cells to the small cytotrophoblastic mononuclear cells. More apoptotic cells were counted within the ectoplacental giant cells exposed to anti phosphatidylserine in comparison with cells that were exposed to the control human IgG. More than 19% of the giant cells that were exposed to HL5B (from the patient with multiple ischemic events) underwent apoptosis, while only 12.7%of the cells exposed to RR7F (from the patient with high titers of circulating antiphosphatidylserine and anticardiolipin, with no thrombosis neither fetal loss) and 7.3 and 9.6% of the cells exposed to the control IgG or the experimental medium alone underwent apoptosis. Both antibodies stained the ectoplacental cone in the rat embryos most strongly with the moderately larger cell layer. Cytotrophoblastic mononuclear cells, which are located in the center of the ectoplacental cone, were not stained. The control antibodies did not stain the ectoplacental cone at all. Immunofluorescence staining proved that the anti phosphatidylserine monoclonal antibodies, reacted with 11.5-day ectoplacental cone cells (Matalon et al., 2004).

5.4 The embryotoxicity of oxidative stress

The role of oxidative damage in disease activity among patients suffering from autoimmune diseases has become more evident in the last decade (Wang et al., 2010). Reactive Oxygen Species (ROS) have been implicated in causing immunogenic modifications in the DNA and causing oxidative damage that may lead to various autoimmune and degenerative diseases. Excessive ROS production which disturbs redox status, may damage macromolecules and modulate the expression of a variety of immune and inflammatory molecules leading to inflammatory processes and affecting tissue damage (Nathan, 2002).

The role of oxidative stress in SLE was demonstrated in various studies including: an association of the oxidative stress parameters with the pro-inflammatory cytokines (Shah et al., 2011b); exposure of purified human dsDNA resulting in ROS production that led to changes in the primary structure of the dsDNA that rendered it highly immunogenic when injected into rabbits (Al Arfaj et al., 2007); a positive correlation between apoptotic cell numbers and ROS production and increased numbers of apoptotic cells positively correlating with lipid peroxidation in SLE patients (Shah et al., 2011a). The Conflicting results on antioxidant enzyme activities may be due to continued oxidative stress and measurement of different components of the antioxidant system at different disease stages (Ames et al., 1999, Whitaker & Knight, 2008, Zaken et al., 2000). However the role of oxidative stress in recurrent fetal death and growth restriction is unclear.

Despite medical treatment, women with autoimmune diseases suffer from increased rate of pregnancy complication. We tried to determine if during remission there is a relation between the clinical history of the SLE patients (i.e. recurrent abortions and/or thromboembolic event) and the morphologic and functional damage which their sera induce on the 10.5 days rat embryos and yolk sac in culture. We used as culture media sera from SLE /APLs patients during remission (The APLs patients were at least one year free of clotting events and the SLE patients had SLEDAI (Systemic lupus erythematosus disease activity index-a commulative clinical and laboratory index with higher scores representing increased disease activity) 2000 less than 4 and compared it to control human sera. The survival of the embryos cultured in sera of SLE /APLs women decreased significantly from 87.5% to 70.9% in comparison to embryos cultured in control sera. There was a positive correlation between survival rate, the neurological developmental stage (calculated by summing the score given for the caudal neural tube, hind, mid and forebrain) and number of somites. Additionally a significant positive correlation between the growth parameters was demonstrated among the embryos cultured in sera from patients and controls: the larger embryos had larger yolk sacs; had higher general and neurologic developmental score and more somites, implying more mature embryos. (Ergaz et al., 2010). A high rate of anomalies in embryos cultured in sera from women with recurrent spontaneous abortions (Abir et al., 1994) or following the addition to the culture medium of purified IgG from SLE and APLs patients (Abir & Ornoy, 1996), differed from the study using sera obtained from non-pregnant patients in remission, where there was no increase in the rate of anomalies compared to controls. It can be speculated therefore, that the teratogenicity of the sera reflected the patient's high-activity disease state (Clowse et al., 2005). Delayed neurological system development when the brain structures development were behind the other embryonic systems was the predominant finding in correlation with clinical studies published in the medical literature that reported learning and memory impairment among offspring of mothers with SLE (Urowitz et al., 2008, Ross et al., 2003) and the finding that the main anomalies in our previous studies were neural tube defects (Abir et al., 1994). We speculate that the low activity of the disease allowed high survival and low anomalies rate in most of the sera but some sera remained teratogenic due to factors that were still active despite remission. We defined two sera groups: "toxic" sera with over-all survival rate under ⅔ and those cultured in "non-toxic" sera with over-all survival above ⅔. In order to define the characteristics of the "toxic" sera we analyzed the correlations between the survival rate, the growth parameters, maternal laboratory findings regarding APLs and the clinical history of the patients. We did not find a correlation between sera toxicity and: the diagnosis of APLs; The levels of the specific antibodies (anti-double stranded DNA, anti-single stranded DNA and the antiphospholipid antibodies: anti cardiolipin, anti-β2 glycoprotein, antiphosphatidylserine, antiphosphatidylcholine and antiphosphatidylethanolamine) which were high compared to human controls. There was no significant correlation between the survival rate and any specific antibody measured in those sera, the history of recurrent abortions and toxemia and the history of thrombo-embolic attacks. The yolk sac function was evaluated by measuring the 14C sucrose endocytic index which did not differ between the controls and SLE/APLs non toxic sera, this is explained by the fact that we studied the index only in "non toxic" sera.

To evaluate the antioxidant defense mechanisms which include a variety of intracellular enzymes we evaluated superoxide dismutase, catalase like activity, and low molecular weight antioxidants. The low molecular weight antioxidants includes lypophilic and hydrophilic molecules like glutathione, carnosine, ascorbate (vitamin C), tocopherol (vitamin E), carotenoids (vitamin A), bilirubin, uric acid and flavonoids, which act directly with various reactive oxygen species, DNA repair enzymes and methionine sulphoxide reductase that repair or remove reactive oxygen species-damaged biomolecules (Ornoy et al., 1999). Our previous studies on the reducing power of the low molecular weight antioxidants in control rat embryos and yolk sacs revealed only one peak 1 at 560-620 mvolts on 9.5-11.5 days of gestation and an additional peak (peak 2) at 950-970 mvolts first appearing on day 11.5 of gestation (Zaken et al., 2000), which is the day we ended our culture. The major components of peak 1 as measured by HPLC are ascorbic and uric acids, Tryptophan, carnosine, melatonine (Beit-Yannai et al., 1997) and thioacetic acid (Chevion et al., 2000) were found to be the major components of peak 2 in the rat brain . The low molecular weight antioxidants were evaluated by cyclic voltametry (Zaken et al., 2000). Most of the embryos cultured in the "toxic" SLE / APLs sera did not have the peak 2 of the low molecular weight antioxidants. The lack of the peak 2 in the present study may be the reflection of the delayed embryonic maturation as the embryos were smaller and less developed. This is similar to our finding of decreased low molecular weight antioxidants demonstrated by the absence of peak 2, in 10.5 days embryos cultured for 28 hours under diabetic conditions (Zaken et al., 2000). There was also a positive correlation between a lower peak 1 of low molecular weight antioxidants and recurrent abortions in the embryos cultured in the SLE / APLs sera that was not related to sera toxicity. Catalase and superoxide dismutase activity did not vary between the groups. It is unknown whether the oxidative insult has a similar effect on the different developing organs. We evaluated the oxidative stress in the total embryo, while the different organs and systems in the rat embryo may have different expressions under similar circumstances (Dubnov et al., 2000). The normal levels of the anti oxidant enzymes evaluated may indicate that sera toxicity is not related to oxidative stress. We did not find any past clinical history or laboratory finding that was in correlation with the sera embryotoxicity. The possible causes for the high embryotoxicity of about half of the sera in remission are currently unknown.

5.5 The effect of maternal medical treatment on sera teratogenicity

The role of some treatment modalities was evaluated by rat embryo cultures in sera from women with and without medications. We examined 10.5 days old embryos cultured in sera from women suffering from SLE complicated by recurrent abortions, either untreated women, or treated with steroids and aspirin and compared the results to embryos cultured in sera from control women and to a pool of control rat sera. Untreated sera resulted in 45.1% death rate compared to 29.8% in treated sera, 3.9% in control human and 5.1% in control rat serum. Malformation rate decreased from 73.3% in untreated sera to 37.5% in treated sera, 10.2% in human controls and 5.4% in rat controls. Malformations were mostly in the heart, brain, limbs and tail (Ornoy et al., 1998). Thus, treatment that improves pregnancy outcome also reduces the embryotoxic effects of the sera.

5.6 The effect of maternal medical treatment on the extent of yolk sac damage

Transmission electron microscopy of the yolk sacs revealed an increase in intracellular inclusions and decrease in microvilli number in both experimental groups, embryos cultured in sera from treated or untreated patients compared to controls. Scanning electron microscope revealed abnormally large entodermal cells, a decreased number of microvilli with sometimes crater formation (Ornoy et al., 1998). The anticoagulant treatment reduced fetal anomalies rate but did not improve yolk sac damage implying that yolk sac damage is only a component in the different factors leading to fetal damage.

5.7 The limitations of the early somite rat embryo culture system

By using the early somite rat embryo culture system we evaluated the direct effect of sera from patients suffering from autoimmune diseases and analyzed the levels of the different sera variables during flare and remission. The impact of the different sera was not universal, and only some of the sera caused embryonic damage. Since the antiphospholipid antibodies were proven as the cause of embryotoxic effect only in some of the sera, we believe that other mechanisms are involved in the teratogenic effect and growth restriction as well. A disadvantage of this in vitro testing are also the limited culture time and limited period of embryogenesis that is undertaken in the commonly used culture system which restricts the range of embryotoxicity that can be induced. It may, therefore, render the testing system unsuitable for teratogens that are likely to exert their major toxicological effect very early or late in gestation (Webster et al., 1997). Additionally we evaluated embryonic growth, structural anomalies and yolk sac function. Infants of mothers who suffer from SLE experience mainly intra-uterine growth retardation, which may be more prominent at the final pregnancy stages not in correlation with the pregnancy stage of early somite rat embryos. The lack of change in oxidative stress parameters may reflect the evaluation of the embryo as a whole. It is unknown whether the oxidative insult has a similar effect on the different developing organs. The different organs and systems in the rat embryo may have different expressions under similar circumstances as shown in another murine model (Dubnov et al., 2000).

In conclusion: Early somite rat embryos cultured in sera from women who suffered from autoimmune diseases had lower survival rate, increase anomalies rate and delayed maturation as reflected by their lower morphological score and less developed anti-oxidant system. The damage was related to IgG antibodies only in some of the embryos. Morphologic yolk sac damage was constant and did not improve with maternal medical treatment.

6. Placental explants studies

6.1 The effect of SLE/APLs sera on placental explants

At the early somite stage the yolk sac is the equivalent of the human chorioallantoic placenta. The inhibition of yolk sac growth even without inhibition of embryonic growth, as well as ultrastructural damage to the yolk sac endothelial cells may indicate that the primary insult or at least a major insult in SLE /APLs and recurrent abortions may be damage to the placenta.

We therefore examined the effects of sera from the patients on early human placental explants obtained from interruptions of normal 5.5 to 7.5 week-old pregnancies (because of psychosocial reasons), and compared to the effects of sera from healthy women and of a chemically defined medium. Placental explants cultured on sera from untreated non-pregnant women with SLE/APLs demonstrated a significant decrease in the trophoblastic cell proliferation rate compared with non-pregnant control women (Ornoy et al., 2003). Placental extracts cultured in SLE/APLs had a higher rate of apoptosis, and reduced βhCG secretion in correlation with antiphospholipid antibodies levels. The sera were analyzed for the presence and quantification of anti-double stranded DNA, anti-single stranded DNA and antiphospholipid antibodies (anti cardiolipin, anti-β2glycoprotein, antiphosphatidylserine, antiphosphatidylcholine and antiphosphatidylethanolamine) and Anti-Ro and anti-La. High levels of all the different antiphospholipid atibodies and both anti-dsDNA and anti-ssDNA

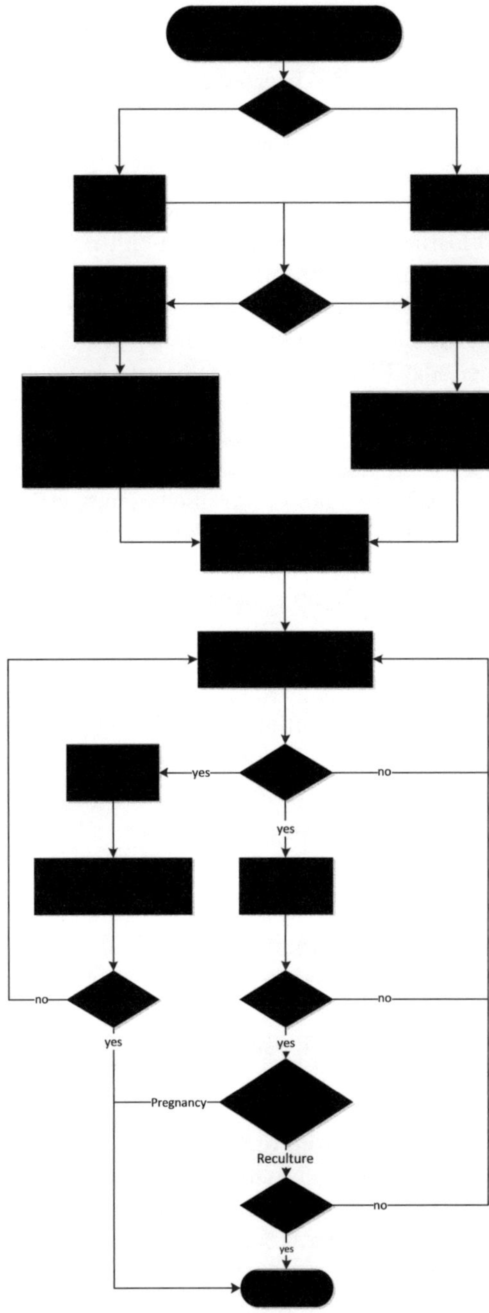

(1) More specific, embryotoxic in 2/3 of the sera.
(2) Less specific but allows to investigate the multi factorial mechanisms of embryotoxicity.
(3) Evaluate blastocystic development.
(4) Evaluate: Embryonic survival, score, anomalies rate and yolk sac apoptosis.
(5) Evaluate trophoblastic cell proliferation, apoptosis and βhCG secretion.

Fig. 3. In vitro cultures as an aid in clinical decisions making for recurrent abortions

showed a trend towards reduction in βhCG secretion by the placental extracts in culture. Titers of anti-Ro and anti-La did not correlate with a reduction in the βhCG levels, probably because anti-Ro and anti-La antibodies exert their effect on pregnancy by a passively transferred autoimmune disease in fetuses or newborns, causing neonatal lupus and not through placental damage. There was no specific single antibody that could be identified to cause the placental damage, but rather a combination of different antibodies was responsible for the cumulative damage, in accordance with the inconsistent findings of the effects of the different antiphospholipid antibodies (Schwartz et al., 2007).

6.2 The effect of maternal medical treatment on the degree of damage induced in placental explants

When we evaluated the impact of maternal treatment with steroids and/or aspirin on placental explants, treatment significantly increased proliferation rate compared with the untreated group but remained significantly lower than that found in the control non-pregnant women. Additionally, a significant increase in the rate of the trophoblastic cell apoptosis was demonstrated compared to explants cultured in sera from treated or control women. The apoptotic rate, however, was still significantly higher in the treated group than that found in the control human group (Yacobi et al., 2002).

6.3 The limitations of the placental explants culture system

The placental explants system allows the investigation of the direct effect of sera on trophoblastic proliferation. This system where only young human placental explants are cultured does not seem to enable the investigation of late pregnancy damage induced by the various mechanisms. Additionally it does not allow the investigation of growth parameters which tend to impact the fetus at later pregnancy stages.

In conclusion: Placental explants culture in SLE/APLs sera had decreased trophoblastic cells proliferation, a higher rate of apoptosis, and reduced βhCG secretion in correlation with antiphospholipid antibodies levels, and increased yolk sac trophoblastic cell apoptosis.

7. Conclusions

The pathophysiology of fetal loss and growth restriction among patients suffering from SLE/APLs is still an open question that needs to be studied. The pre-implantation murine and early somite rat embryo culture offers a model for evaluation of the direct effect of the different antibodies and molecules on survival and growth at different time points during pregnancy. The concomitant evaluation of the yolk sac function allows the investigation of those molecules on the rodent's placental equivalent. The addition of the human early placental extracts culture improves the understanding of the disturbance to early placental differentiation, migration and hormone production induced by similar teratogens.

8. Future research possibilities

New molecules associated with fetal death, embryotoxicity and growth failure were discovered in the last years. The direct effect of those molecules can be evaluated in vitro on placental explants, murine pre-implantation embryos and on early somite rat embryos in culture in order to isolate the impact that each molecule has, solely or in combination with other molecules on pregnancy outcome. The evaluation of the pathological, immunological and biochemical parameters of the cultured embryos may add more clues to the multi-factorial mechanism of fetal damage among women suffering from autoimmune diseases. The understanding of those mechanisms may help to develop new treatment modalities which can also be evaluated in this model.

9. References

Abir R, Zusman I, Ben Hur H, Yaffe P, & Ornoy A. The effects of serum from women with miscarriages on the in vitro development of mouse preimplantation embryos. Acta Obstet Gynecol Scand. 1990;69(1):27-33.

Abir R, Ornoy A, Ben Hur H, Jaffe P, & Pinus H. IgG exchange as a means of partial correction of anomalies in rat embryos in vitro, induced by sera from women with recurrent abortion. Toxicol In Vitro. 1993 Nov;7(6):817-26.

Abir R, Ornoy A, Ben Hur H, Jaffe P, & Pinus H. The effects of sera from women with spontaneous abortions on the in vitro development of early somite stage rat embryos. Am J Reprod Immunol. 1994 Sep;32(2):73-81.

Abir R, & Ornoy A. Teratogenic IgG from sera of women with spontaneous abortions seem to induce anomalies and yolk sac damage in rat embryos. A possible method to detect abortions of immunologic origin. Am J Reprod Immunol. 1996 Feb;35(2):93-101.

Al Arfaj AS, Chowdhary AR, Khalil N, & Ali R. Immunogenicity of singlet oxygen modified human DNA: implications for anti-DNA antibodies in systemic lupus erythematosus. Clin Immunol. 2007 Jul;124(1):83-9.

Alijotas-Reig J, Palacio-Garcia C, & Vilardell-Tarres M. Circulating microparticles, lupus anticoagulant and recurrent miscarriages. Eur J Obstet Gynecol Reprod Biol. 2009 Jul;145(1):22-6.

Ames PR, Alves J, Murat I, Isenberg DA, & Nourooz-Zadeh J. Oxidative stress in systemic lupus erythematosus and allied conditions with vascular involvement. Rheumatology (Oxford). 1999 Jun;38(6):529-34.

Beit-Yannai E, Kohen R, Horowitz M, Trembovler V, & Shohami E. Changes of biological reducing activity in rat brain following closed head injury: a cyclic voltammetry study in normal and heat-acclimated rats. J Cereb Blood Flow Metab. 1997 Mar;17(3):273-9.

Brown NA, & Fabro S. Quantitation of rat embryonic development in vitro: a morphological scoring system. Teratology. 1981 Aug;24(1):65-78.

Chen LT, & Hsu YC. Development of mouse embryos in vitro: preimplantation to the limb bud stage. Science. 1982 Oct 1;218(4567):66-8.

Chevion S, Roberts MA, & Chevion M. The use of cyclic voltammetry for the evaluation of antioxidant capacity. Free Radic Biol Med. 2000 Mar 15;28(6):860-70.

Clowse ME, Magder LS, Witter F, & Petri M. The impact of increased lupus activity on obstetric outcomes. Arthritis Rheum. 2005 Feb;52(2):514-21.

Cohen D, Buurma A, Goemaere NN, Girardi G, le Cessie S, Scherjon S, et al. Classical complement activation as a footprint for murine and human antiphospholipid antibody-induced fetal loss. J Pathol. 2011 Mar 10.

Dubnov G, Kohen R, & Berry EM. Diet restriction in mice causes differential tissue responses in total reducing power and antioxidant compounds. Eur J Nutr. 2000 Feb;39(1):18-30.

Ergaz Z, Mevorach D, Goldzweig G, Cohen A, Patlas N, Yaffe P, et al. The embryotoxicity of sera from patients with autoimmune diseases on post-implantation rat embryos in culture persists during remission and is not related to oxidative stress. Lupus. 2010 Dec;19(14):1623-31.

Genbacev O, Schubach SA, & Miller RK. Villous culture of first trimester human placenta--model to study extravillous trophoblast (EVT) differentiation. Placenta. 1992 Sep-Oct;13(5):439-61.

Gharavi AE, Vega-Ostertag M, Espinola RG, Liu X, Cole L, Cox NT, et al. Intrauterine fetal death in mice caused by cytomegalovirus-derived peptide induced aPL antibodies. Lupus. 2004;13(1):17-23.

Halperin R, Elhayany A, Ben-Hur H, Gurevich P, Kaganovsky E, Zusman I, et al. Pathomorphologic and immunohistochemical study on the devastation of rat embryos by antiphospholipid antibody positive serum. Am J Reprod Immunol. 2008 Dec;60(6):523-8.

Kwok LW, Tam LS, Zhu T, Leung YY, & Li E. Predictors of maternal and fetal outcomes in pregnancies of patients with systemic lupus erythematosus. Lupus. 2011 May 4.

Lee JY, Huerta PT, Zhang J, Kowal C, Bertini E, Volpe BT, et al. Neurotoxic autoantibodies mediate congenital cortical impairment of offspring in maternal lupus. Nat Med. 2009 Jan;15(1):91-6.

Levy RA, Avvad E, Oliveira J, & Porto LC. Placental pathology in antiphospholipid syndrome. Lupus. 1998;7 Suppl 2:S81-5.

Matalon ST, Shoenfeld Y, Blank M, Yacobi S, Blumenfeld Z, & Ornoy A. The effects of IgG purified from women with SLE and associated pregnancy loss on rat embryos in culture. Am J Reprod Immunol. 2002 Nov;48(5):296-304.

Matalon ST, Blank M, Matsuura E, Inagaki J, Nomizu M, Levi Y, et al. Immunization of naive mice with mouse laminin-1 affected pregnancy outcome in a mouse model. Am J Reprod Immunol. 2003 Aug;50(2):159-65.

Matalon ST, Shoenfeld Y, Blank M, Yacobi S, von Landenberg P, & Ornoy A. Antiphosphatidylserine antibodies affect rat yolk sacs in culture: a mechanism for fetal loss in antiphospholipid syndrome. Am J Reprod Immunol. 2004 Feb;51(2):144-51.

McIntyre JA. Antiphospholipid antibodies in implantation failures. Am J Reprod Immunol. 2003 Apr;49(4):221-9.

Meroni PL, Gerosa M, Raschi E, Scurati S, Grossi C, & Borghi MO. Updating on the pathogenic mechanisms 5 of the antiphospholipid antibodies-associated pregnancy loss. Clin Rev Allergy Immunol. 2008 Jun;34(3):332-7.

Nathan C. Points of control in inflammation. Nature. 2002 Dec 19-26;420(6917):846-52.

New DA, Coppola PT, & Cockroft DL. Comparison of growth in vitro and in vivo of post-implantation rat embryos. J Embryol Exp Morphol. 1976 Aug;36(1):133-44.

Ornoy A, Yacobi S, Avraham S, & Blumenfeld Z. The effect of sera from women with systemic lupus erythematosus and/or antiphospholipid syndrome on rat embryos in culture. Reprod Toxicol. 1998 Mar-Apr;12(2):185-91.

Ornoy A, Zaken V, & Kohen R. Role of reactive oxygen species (ROS) in the diabetes-induced anomalies in rat embryos in vitro: reduction in antioxidant enzymes and low-molecular-weight antioxidants (LMWA) may be the causative factor for increased anomalies. Teratology. 1999 Dec;60(6):376-86.

Ornoy A, Yacobi S, Matalon ST, Blank M, Blumenfeld Z, Miller RK, et al. The effects of antiphospholipid antibodies obtained from women with SLE/APS and associated pregnancy loss on rat embryos and placental explants in culture. Lupus. 2003;12(7):573-8.

Rand JH, Wu XX, Andree HA, Lockwood CJ, Guller S, Scher J, et al. Pregnancy loss in the antiphospholipid-antibody syndrome--a possible thrombogenic mechanism. N Engl J Med. 1997 Jul 17;337(3):154-60.

Ross G, Sammaritano L, Nass R, & Lockshin M. Effects of mothers' autoimmune disease during pregnancy on learning disabilities and hand preference in their children. Arch Pediatr Adolesc Med. 2003 Apr;157(4):397-402.

Schwartz N, Shoenfeld Y, Barzilai O, Cervera R, Font J, Blank M, et al. Reduced placental growth and hCG secretion in vitro induced by antiphospholipid antibodies but not by anti-Ro or anti-La: studies on sera from women with SLE/PAPS. Lupus. 2007;16(2):110-20.

Shah D, Aggarwal A, Bhatnagar A, Kiran R, & Wanchu A. Association between T lymphocyte sub-sets apoptosis and peripheral blood mononuclear cells oxidative stress in systemic lupus erythematosus. Free Radic Res. 2011a May;45(5):559-67.

Shah D, Wanchu A, & Bhatnagar A. Interaction between oxidative stress and chemokines: Possible pathogenic role in systemic lupus erythematosus and rheumatoid arthritis. Immunobiology. 2011b Apr 13.

Suzuki H, Silverman ED, Wu X, Borges C, Zhao S, Isacovics B, et al. Effect of maternal autoantibodies on fetal cardiac conduction: an experimental murine model. Pediatr Res. 2005 Apr;57(4):557-62.

Tower C, Crocker I, Chirico D, Baker P, & Bruce I. SLE and pregnancy: the potential role for regulatory T cells. Nat Rev Rheumatol. 2011 Feb;7(2):124-8.

Urowitz MB, Gladman DD, MacKinnon A, Ibanez D, Bruto V, Rovet J, et al. Neurocognitive abnormalities in offspring of mothers with systemic lupus erythematosus. Lupus. 2008;17(6):555-60.

Wang G, Pierangeli SS, Papalardo E, Ansari GA, & Khan MF. Markers of oxidative and nitrosative stress in systemic lupus erythematosus: correlation with disease activity. Arthritis Rheum. 2010 Jul;62(7):2064-72.

Webster WS, Brown-Woodman PD, & Ritchie HE. A review of the contribution of whole embryo culture to the determination of hazard and risk in teratogenicity testing. Int J Dev Biol. 1997 Apr;41(2):329-35.

Whitaker BD, & Knight JW. Mechanisms of oxidative stress in porcine oocytes and the role of anti-oxidants. Reprod Fertil Dev. 2008;20(6):694-702.

Yacobi S, Ornoy A, Blumenfeld Z, & Miller RK. Effect of sera from women with systemic lupus erythematosus or antiphospholipid syndrome and recurrent abortions on human placental explants in culture. Teratology. 2002 Dec;66(6):300-8.

Zaken V, Kohen R, & Ornoy A. The development of antioxidant defense mechanism in young rat embryos in vivo and in vitro. Early Pregnancy. 2000 Apr;4(2):110-23.

9

A Rabbit Model of Systemic Lupus Erythematosus, Useful for Studies of Neuropsychiatric SLE

Rose G. Mage[1] and Geeta Rai[2]
[1]*Laboratory of Immunology, NIAID, National Institutes of Health*
[2]*Department of Molecular and Human Genetics, Faculty of Science*
Banaras Hindu University, Varanasi
[1]*US*
[2]*India*

1. Introduction

The aim of this review is to present in one place a summary of the development of a rabbit model of SLE conducted using pedigreed rabbits bred and selected at the National Institute of Allergy and Infectious Diseases (NIAID), NIH. We provide an overview of the knowledge gained by using rabbits *(Oryctolagus cuniculus)* as models for SLE, and eliciting autoantibodies typical of those produced by patients with SLE. We present here summaries of work by ourselves and coauthors that can contribute to improved understanding of neuropsychiatric SLE (NPSLE) (Sanches-Guerro et al., 2008). Our gene expression studies (Rai, et al., 2010) and extensive evaluations of autoantibody responses coupled with observed clinical symptoms of animals immunized against peptides from the Smith antigen (Sm) or the NMDA glutamate receptor have shown promise to improve understanding NPSLE.

An overview of immune system development, genetic diversity of immunoglobulin genes and somatic diversification during B-cell development in rabbits can be found in a review by Mage et al., (2006) and reference therein. Investigations of autoantibodies found in patients with NPSLE and the problems of diagnosis and specific treatments are addressed in other chapters in this volume.

2. Our model

2.1 Earlier studies of SLE models by other laboratories using rabbit

We set out to develop a model of SLE in pedigreed rabbits because an earlier report showed that immunization of non-pedigreed rabbits with peptides such as PPPGMRPP, derived from the Sm B/B′ subunit of the spliceosomal Smith autoantigen led to epitope spreading, SLE-like autoantibody production and clinically observed seizures. This peptide sequence is one of the major regions of reactivity in SLE patients and may mimic the peptide PPPGRRP from the EBNA-1 component of Epstein-Barr virus (EBV) (James et al., 1995). Another study attempted to reproduce this report but only found some evidence for epitope spreading with no suggestion of induced autoimmunity (Mason et al., 1999). We hypothesized that the different results may have been obtained because small numbers of rabbits were studied, and there may have been different genetic susceptibilities among outbred rabbits studied by the two groups. Since our work already depended on breeding and maintenance of immunoglobulin allotype-defined pedigreed rabbits, we were in a position to pursue this idea further. In addition to using the MAP-8-PPPGMRPP immunogen used in these previous studies (termed SM-MAP-8 in the following sections), we chose a new immunogen termed GR-MAP-8 based on a report by DeGiorgio et al (2001) that some anti-DNA antibodies cross-react with the NMDA glutamate receptor.

2.2 The model in pedigreed rabbits

We established a rabbit model of Systemic Lupus Erythematosus (SLE) in which peptide immunization led to lupus-like autoantibody production including anti-Sm, -RNP, -SS-A, -SS-B and -dsDNA. Some neurological symptoms in form of seizures and nystagmus were observed (Rai et al., 2006). The animals were selectively bred within the colony of pedigreed, immunoglobulin allotype-defined but non-inbred rabbits at the NIAID. We continued breeding responders from the first three groups studied (Rai et al., 2006, 2010, Puliyath et al., 2008, Yang et al., 2009a,b). Details about genetics, gene expression and cellular studies are in the sections below. The genetic heterogeneity of the pedigreed animals studied may correspond to that found among patients of a given ethnicity.

2.2.1 Methods

Rabbits: All rabbit experimentation and immunization protocols were reviewed and approved by the Animal Care and Use committees of the NIAID, NIH and of Spring Valley Laboratories where the animals were bred, housed and monitored. The animals' designations, sexes, and allotypes at the V_H a immunoglobulin heavy chain and Cκ b light chain loci are summarized in Tables 1A and B. Rabbits of groups 1, 3, 4, 5 and 6 received peptides (SM or GR) synthesized on MAP-8 branched lysine backbones and rabbits of group 2 received the peptides on MAP-4. BB indicates control rabbits that received backbone alone. SM animals received MAP-peptide derived from the sequence of the Smith antigen spliceosomal B/B' complex. GR animals received MAP-peptide derived from the NMDA glutamate receptor sequence.

Antigens: The peptide immunogens "GR" and "SM" used for the initial rabbit immunizations (Rai et al., 2006), were synthesized on branched lysine MAP-8 and MAP-4 backbones (BB) (AnaSpec) The SM peptide sequence PPPGMRPP corresponds to major antigenic regions at 191-198, 216-223 and 231-238 of the nuclear protein Sm B/B′ (James et al, 1995). The GR peptide sequence DEWDYGLP corresponds to a known rabbit sequence of an extracellular epitope of the NR2b subunit of neuronal postsynaptic NMDA receptor. The MAP-BB without peptide was used as a control antigen. For subsequent studies, (Puliyath et al., 2008, Yang et al., 2009b, Rai et al. 2010), MAP-8 was the BB of choice because it appeared to elicit more diverse autoantibody responses.

Immunization: Rabbits each received subcutaneous (s.c.) injections of one of the MAP-peptides or control BB (0.5 mg/0.5 ml, in borate buffered saline, pH 8.0) emulsified with 0.5 ml of complete Freund's adjuvant (CFA). Boosts were given s.c. at 3-week intervals with the same antigen concentration emulsified with incomplete Freund's adjuvant (IFA). Controls that received only CFA followed by IFA were included in one study (Yang et al., 2009b). Sera collected immediately before immunization (pre-immune) and 1 week after each boost (post-boost) were stored at -20°C in multiple aliquots for assays.

Rabbit ID	Rabbit no.	Allotype	Sex
Group 1			
SM1	XX129-3	a1/1, b4/5	M
SM2	2XX127-4	a1/1, b5/5	F
SM3	2XX288-2	a1/1, b9/9	M
SM4	1XX288-4	a1/1, b5/9	F
SM5	2XX127-2	a1/1, b9/9	M
SM6	2XX92-06	a1/1, b9/9	F
GR7	XX129-5	a1/1, b4/5	M
GR8	2XX127-5	a1/1, b9/9	F
GR9	1XX288-3	a1/1, b5/5	M
GR10	2XX288-6	a1/1, b5/9	F
BB11	2XX127-1	a1/1, b5/5	M
BB12	1XX78-8	a1/1, b9/9	F
Group 2			
SM13	LL191-1	a1/1, b4/5	M
SM14	LL191-2	a1/1, b5/5	F
SM15	2LL179-1	a1/1, b9/9	M
SM16	1LL163-3	a1/1, b9/9	F
SM17	LL164-4	a1/1, b9/9	F
GR18	1LL178-2	a1/1, b9/9	M
GR19	1LL178-3	a1/1, b4/4	F
GR20	1LL178-4	a1/1, b9/9	F
GR21	1LL178-5	a1/1, b4/9	M
GR22	1LL178-6	a1/1, b4/9	F
GR23	1LL178-8	a1/1, b4/4	F
BB24	LL164-1	a1/1, b9/9	M
BB25	LL164-3	a1/1, b9/9	F
BB26	2LL179-3	a1/1, b5/9	M
BB27	1LL163-4	a1/1, b5/9	F
Group 3			
GR28	LL108-1	a1/1, b5/9	M
GR29	LL108-3	a1/1, b5/5	F
GR30	LL108-4	a1/1, b9/9	F
BB31	2LL179-2	a1/1, b9/9	M
Group 4			
SM32	1QQ299-2	a1/1, b5/5	M
SM33	1QQ299-3	a1/1, b4/5	F
SM34	6QQ299-1	a1/1, b4/9	M
SM35	6QQ299-2	a1/1, b4/5	F
GR36	3QQ299-1	a1/1, b4/5	M
GR37	3QQ299-2	a1/1, b5/9	M
GR38	3QQ299-4	a1/1, b5/9	M
GR39	4QQ299-1	a1/1, b5/9	M
GR40	5QQ299-2	a1/1, b5/9	F
GR41	5QQ299-3	a1/1, b5/5	F
BB42	1QQ299-1	a1/1, b5/5	M
BB43	5QQ299-4	a1/1, b5/5	F
BB44	6QQ299-3	a1/1, b4/9	F
PB45	1QQ173-1	a1/1, b5/9	M
PB46	1QQ173-2	a1/1, b5/5	M
PB47	1QQ173-3	a1/1, b5/5	M

Table 1. A. Designations of sexes and allotypes of Groups 1-4.
PB45, 46, and 47 received injections with phosphate buffered saline only.

Group 5			
GR 48	UA345-1	a2/2, b9k/9k	M
GR49	1UA344-1	a1/2, b9k/9k	M
GR50	1UA344-5	a1/2, b9k/9k	F
GR51	1YY119-6	a1/1, b9/9	F
GR52	1YY119-8	a1/1, b9/9	F
GR53	2YY119-6	a1/1, b9/9	M
GR54	2YY299-5	a1/1, b4/9	F
GR55	2YY299-3	a1/1, b4/9	F
GR56	UA345-2	a1/2, b4/9k	M
GR57	1UA344-2	a1/2, b5/9k	M
GR58	1UA344-6	a2/2, b5/9k	F
GR59	1YY119-7	a1/1, b9/9	F
GR60	1YY327-2	a1/1, b5/9	M
GR61	2YY327-9	a1/1, b4/5	F
GR62	2YY299-4	a1/1, b4/9	F
GR63	2YY119-8	a1/1, b9/9	F
BB64	UA345-4	a2/2, b9k/9k	F
BB65	2UA344-1	a1/2, b9k/9k	F
BB66	1UA344-3	a2/2, b5/9k	M
BB67	2YY327-8	a1/1, b4/5	M
BB68	UA345-6	a1/2, b4/9k	F
BB69	1YY327-4	a1/1, b5/9	F
BB70	1YY119-5	a1/1, b9/9	M
BB71	2YY119-7	a1/1, b9/9	M
Group 6			
GR72	UA345-5	a2R3/2R3, 4/9k	F
GR73	UA269-3	a1/1, b4/9k	F
BB74	6YY328-4	a1/1, b5/9	M
BB75	2YY125-6	a1/2, b9k/9k	M
CF1	6YY328-3	a1/1, b5/9	M
CF2	1UA161-1	a1/1, b9/9	M
GR76	2YY119-9	a1/1, b9/9	F
GR77	UA269-1	a1/1, b4/5	M
BB78	YY118-6	a1/1, b9/9	M
BB79	1UA161-2	a1/1, b9/9	M
CF3	1YY125-4	a2/2, b4/9k	M
CF4	2YY125-4	a2/2, b5/9k	M
GR80	XA345-1	a1/2, b9/9k	F
GR81	2UA14-2	a1/1, b5/9	F
BB82	XA346-2	a1/1, b9/9	M
BB83	2UA14-3	a1/1, b5/9k	F
CF5	XA345-2	a1/2, b9/9k	F
GR84	XA234-2	a1/2, b5/9	F
GR85	XA346=1	a1/1, b9/9	M
BB86	XA234-2	a1/2, b5/9	M
B87	3XA203-2	a1/ali	M
CF6	2XA344-2	a1/1, b9/9	F
CF7	1XA344-1	a1/1, b9/9	M

Table 1. B. Designations of sexes and allotypes of Groups 5 and 6.

Clinical Assessments: Rabbits were housed in a separate room equipped with video surveillance so that abnormal behavior such as seizure activity and other neurological dysfunctions could be detected. They were observed daily and also received periodic complete health evaluations. Hematology using a Bayer Advida, model 120 hematology analyzer and blood chemistry assessments of each rabbit were carried out in a Veterinary diagnostic laboratory (Antech Diagnostics, Lake Success NY).

ELISA for anti-peptide antibodies, anti-dsDNA and autoantibodies to nuclear antigens: Serum antibody responses to the MAP-peptides and control immunogens were measured by solid phase ELISA as previously described (Rai et al 2006). "Polystyrene 96-well plates (Corning Inc, Corning, NY, Cat # 3590) were coated with 50 μl/well of either SM-, GR- or BB- (MAP-8 or MAP-4) at 10 μg/ml in bicarbonate buffer, (pH 9.6) and incubated overnight at 4^{0}C. Plates were washed three times with PBS (pH 7.2) containing 0.1% Tween 20 and blocked with 100 μl blocking solution for 1 hr at 37^{0}C (Quality Biological Inc, Gaithersburg, MD). Wells were then incubated 1 hr, at 37^{0}C with 50 μl/well of sera titrated by four-fold dilutions in blocking solution, washed 5 times, incubated for 1 hr at 37^{0}C with 50 μl of a 1:2000 dilution (0.4 ng/μl) of affinity-purified horseradish peroxidase conjugated (HRP) goat anti-rabbit IgG (H+L) secondary antibody (Jackson Immunoresearch Laboratories Inc., West Grove, PA), developed with 3, 3', 5, 5'- tetramethylbenzidine (TMB) (Inova Diagnostics, Inc., San Diego, CA) and the resulting OD read at 450 nm."

Commercially available human diagnostic kits (INOVA Diagnostics) were adapted and used to assay serum autoantibodies to total extractable nuclear Ags (ENA) and to component Ags Sm, Rnp, SS-A, SS-B. Assays for autoantibodies to calf thymus dsDNA were adapted similarly using two different commercially available kits (Vidia, Vestec (Kit A); Zeus scientific, NJ (Kit B). Briefly, 100 μl rabbit sera diluted 1:100 in the proprietary sample diluents were added to antigen-coated wells and incubated for 60 min. at 37°C (Kit A) or 30 min. at RT (Kit B). Wells were then washed, incubated for 60 min. at 37°C (Kit A) or 30 min at RT (Kit B) with secondary antibody HRP-goat anti-rabbit IgG Fc (Jackson Immunoresearch Laboratories, Inc.) and developed with TMB for reading OD at 450 nm. For groups 5 and 6, anti-dsDNA, -ANA, -RNP and -Sm were assayed with the Quantalite kits (Inova Diagnostics) substituting affinity purified HRP-goat anti-rabbit IgG Fc for the anti-human secondary reagent (Puliyath et al., 2008, Yang et al., 2009b).

Detection of anti-nuclear antibodies (ANA) by indirect immunofluorescence: Commercially available slides coated with fixed Hep-2 cells (Antibodies Inc., Davis, CA) were incubated with rabbit antisera diluted 1:20 in 5% goat serum (Jackson Immunoresearch Laboratories Inc.) for 30 min. at RT. ANA binding was detected by fluorescence microscopy following 30 min incubation at RT with 12.5 ng/μl of FITC-goat anti-rabbit IgG Fc (Southern Biotech Inc., Birmingham, AL). Fluorescent binding patterns were compared with reference pictures provided by Antibodies, Inc.

Flow cytometry: Anti-human antibodies that cross reacted with rabbit B-cell activation factor (BAFF) (biotin conjugated goat anti-human BAFF polyclonal antibody), transmembrane activator and CAML interactor (TACI) (biotin conjugated goat anti-human TACI polyclonal antibody)(Antigenix, America, Inc.), BAFF receptor (BR3) (purified goat anti-human BR3 antibody) (R&D systems) were used for staining. Briefly, purified PBMCs were incubated on ice for 40 min with primary antibody before washing twice with cold PBS containing 1% FCS, then subsequent incubation with various secondary reagents or secondary antibodies. For BR3 detection, a biotinylated donkey anti-goat IgG was used as secondary antibody. Biotinylated antibodies were visualized by PE-conjugated streptavidin (Jackson ImmunoResearch laboratories, Inc.). After washing, cells were analyzed using a FACS-Calibur flow cytometer (BD Pharmingen) and FlowJo analytical software (Tree Star). Cells were gated on the side scatter x forward scatter (SSCxFSC) profiles to include both small and large lymphocytes, as well as monocytes but exclude red blood cells and granulocytes; dead cells were excluded by propidium iodide staining. Rabbit IgM$^+$ B cells were detected by FITC-conjugated goat anti-rabbit IgM (Southern Biotechnology Associates).

Gene Expression studies: *RNA extraction and synthesis of cDNA and cRNA*

Peripheral white blood cells (PWBCs) were lysed with TRIzol (Invitrogen, CA) and total RNA was extracted using RNAeasy Mini columns following the manufacturer's instructions (Qiagen, CA). The cRNA probes were prepared from mRNA using the Affymetrix gene chip eukaryotic small sample target labeling protocol assay version II (Affymetrix, Santa Clara, CA) using 2 cycles of cDNA synthesis and *in vitro* transcription (IVT) reactions. The cRNA thus obtained was used in the final IVT cycle for obtaining biotinylated cRNA using CTP and UTP (EnzoBioarray, Enzo Life Sciences, Farmingdale, NY) (Rai et al 2010).

Microarray analysis Affymetrix U95A human microarray chips were used and hybridization of the labeled cRNA was carried out according to the manufacturer's recommended protocol. Non-normalized MAS5 signals were used to compare raw probeset intensity values between human and rabbit samples. Final rabbit study analyses were conducted with expression values summarized using dChip, log2 transformed and Loess normalized using an R package (http://www.elwood9.net/spike). Analyses of the gene sets were done using Database for Annotation, Visualization and Integrated Discovery (DAVID) (http://david.abcc.ncifcrf.gov/knowledgebase/) and Ingenuity Pathways Analysis (IPA) (Ingenuity Systems, Mountain View, CA; www.ingenuity.com).

Quantitative real time PCR: Quantitative real time PCR analysis of mRNAs was performed on a 7900HT Sequence Detection System (Applied Biosystems). The cDNA synthesized from isolated PWBCs was directly used as template for real-time PCR by using TaqMan 2x PCR Master Mix Reagents Kit (Applied Biosystems). Each sample from three independent experiments was run in duplicate. The unit number showing relative mRNA levels in each sample was determined as a value of mRNA normalized against Peptidylprolyl isomerase A (PPIA). RT-PCR data were analyzed by using the $2^{-\Delta\Delta C_T}$ method. Based on its uniform expression among rabbit groups in the microarray analysis, rabbit peptidylprolyl isomerase A (*PPIA*; cyclophilin A) was selected as the housekeeping gene control and used for the calculation of ΔC_T. Where rabbit sequences were unavailable, primers were designed after searching for rabbit sequences with corresponding human gene sequences in the database containing the trace archives of the whole genome shotgun sequence of the rabbit (*Oryctolagus cuniculus*) generated by the Broad Institute of MIT and Harvard University (NCBI trace archive: cross- species Megablast at http://www.ncbi.nlm.nih.gov/blast/ tracemb.shtml) and in assemblies of rabbit scaffolds at Ensembl and UCSC (see NCBI Rabbit Genome Resources site) at: http://www.ncbi.nlm.nih.gov/projects/genome/guide/rabbit/

2.2.2 Genetics and autoantibody responses

Figure 1 shows the pedigree and an overview of antibody responses of the rabbits immunized and selectively bred during the project to develop a rabbit model of SLE. There were 31 1- to 2-year-old rabbits in the initial studies (Rai et al., 2006). Rabbits of groups 2 or

3 were descendants of rabbits of groups 1 or 2 and/or their siblings. Rabbits that did not respond with autoantibody production after immunization during this initial study by Rai et al., (2006) are not shown. The fourth group was described in Rai et al., (2010) and their mRNA included along with mRNA from the first three groups for gene expression profiling of a total of 46 pedigreed control- or immunized-rabbits as detailed below (section 2.2.3). Controls that received only phosphate buffered saline are designated PB. Because the GR peptide generally elicited better autoantibody responses than the SM peptide, the two subsequent groups [5 (Puliyath et al., 2008) and 6 (Yang et al., 2009b)] were immunized with GR-MAP-8 or control BB-MAP-8. The final 6th group also included controls that received complete followed by incomplete Freund's adjuvant but no MAP-BB or MAP-peptide, to investigate whether adjuvants alone led to any autoantibody production (designated CF).

An overview of autoantibody responses, and the relationships of males (squares) and females (circles) in six immunization groups is shown in Figure 1. The four quadrants indicate post-immunization elevations of levels of anti-dsDNA (upper left), anti-Sm and/or anti-RNP (lower left), ANA by IFA (upper right) and ANA by ELISA (lower right). For the 5th (Puliyath et al. 2008) and 6th groups (Yang et al., 2009b), darker shades indicate high autoantibody responses. The large circles and squares represent the 6th group developed from selective breeding using responders from earlier groups. Figure originally published by Yang et al., (2009b) Investigations of a rabbit (*Oryctolagus cuniculus*) model of systemic lupus erythematosus (SLE), BAFF and its receptors. *PLoS ONE* Vol. 4, 2009.

The selective breeding led to subsequent progeny (groups 5 and 6) exhibiting more consistent autoantibody production. In the pedigree, we can trace the ancestry of some responder rabbits back to the first high responders (SM1 and GR9) that also exhibited seizures. For example, GR54 and GR55 from litter 2YY299 had high-responder grandsires SM1 and SM15 (Puliyath et al. 2008). The model developed using selectively bred pedigreed rabbits remains a promising one for further genetic investigations.

As is found in human sera (Li et al., 2011), some rabbits had detectable pre-immune anti-nuclear antibodies (ANA) by ELISA. ANA of sixteen of twenty-four rabbits in group 5, including four immunized with only MAP-8 backbone had an increased ELISA value (delta OD) above pre-immune of 1.0 or more optical density units after the third boost. Anti-dsDNA increased in 12/24 rabbits after the fifth or seventh boost (Puliyath et al., 2008). Figure 2 shows examples of indirect immunofluorescence (ANA-IFA) studies of some sera from group 6 (Yang et al. 2009b). As in human SLE sera, the ANA-IFA patterns reflect responses to one or more autoantigens in different individuals. Littermates that received GR peptide such as UA269-3 and -1 (GR73 and GR77) developed similar patterns after the 3rd boost. ANA staining with sera of littermates XA346-1 and -2 (GR85 and BB82) resulted in different patterns. GR85 serum exhibited some cytoplasmic and peripheral nuclear staining not seen with the serum of BB82. Puliyath et al., (2008) also noticed that GR-immunized littermates had similar ANA-IFA staining patterns but that BB immunized animals' patterns generally differed.

2.2.3 Gene expression studies

We extended the information about the rabbit model of SLE by microarray-based expression profiling of mRNA from peripheral blood leukocytes following peptide immunization (Rai et al., 2010). Data obtained in studies of gene expression in the first four groups of immunized rabbits were deposited in the Gene Expression Omnibus and became

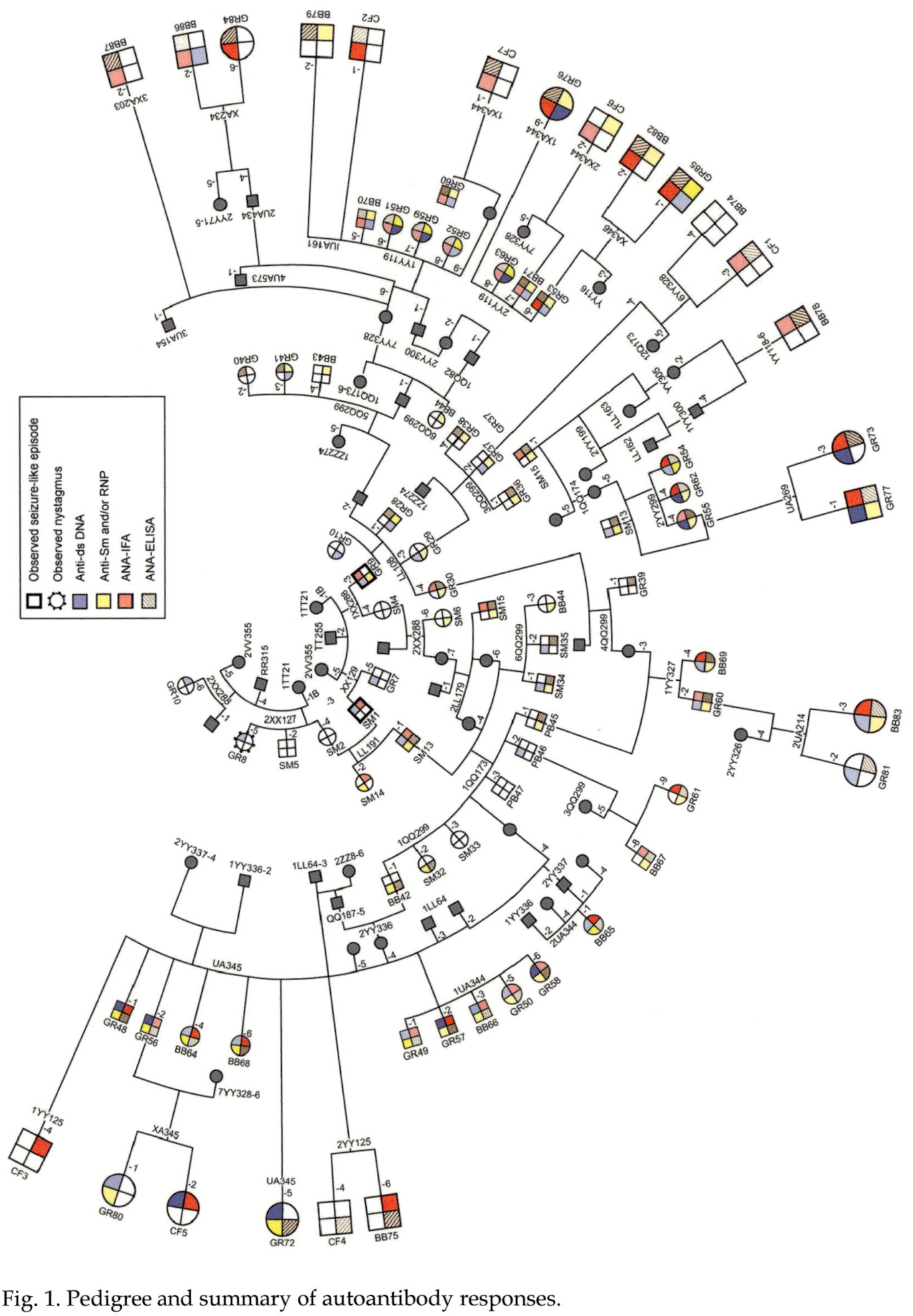

Fig. 1. Pedigree and summary of autoantibody responses.

public on Jul 23, 2010 at the NCBI website: http://www.ncbi.nlm.nih.gov/geo/query/acc.cgi?acc=GSE23076
Experiment type: Expression profiling by array. GEO accession: Series GSE23076 Query DataSets for GSE23076

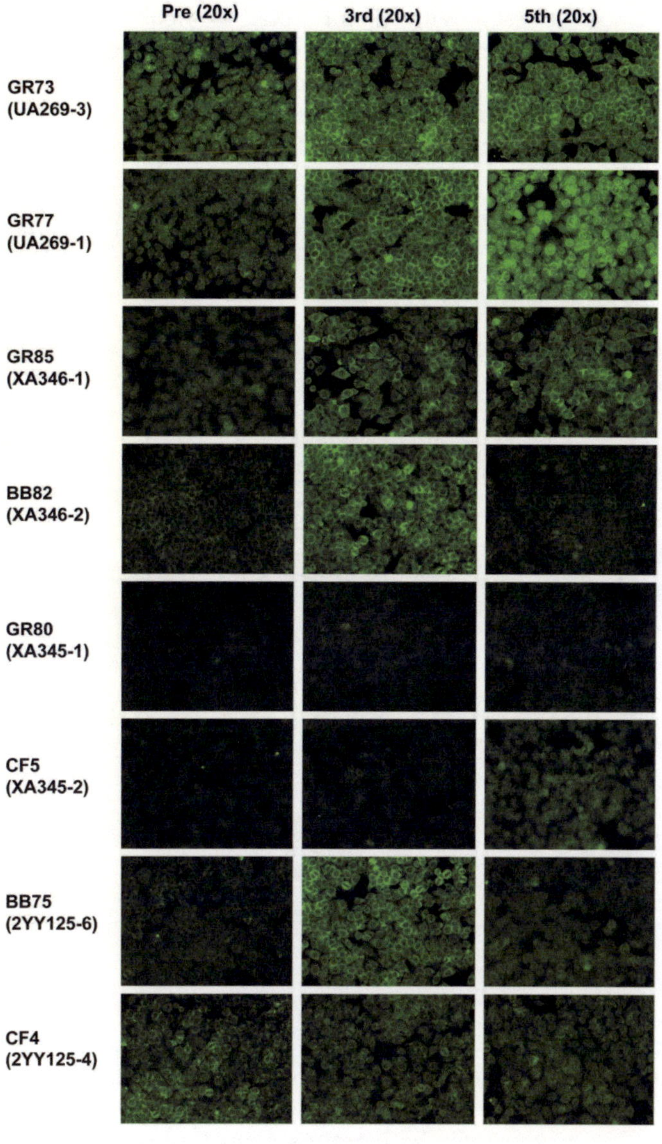

Fig. 2. Examples of indirect ANA-IFA assays of pre- and post-immune sera. Figure originally published by Yang et al., (2009b) Investigations of a rabbit (*Oryctolagus cuniculus*) model of systemic lupus erythematosus (SLE), BAFF and its receptors. *PLoS ONE* Vol.4, 2009.

At the time of the gene expression studies, microarrays specific for study of gene expression profiles were not available for rabbits. We therefore first conducted comparisons of identically prepared rabbit and human cRNA binding to the Affymetrix U95 microarray available for human gene expression analyses. We showed that the human microarray could be used with rabbit cRNA to yield information on genetic pathways activated and/or suppressed in autoantibody-producing immunized rabbits. After demonstrating that human expression arrays could be used with rabbit RNA to yield information on molecular pathways, we designed a study evaluating gene expression profiles in a total of 46 rabbits from 4 groups of the pedigreed control and immunized rabbits. We discovered unique gene expression changes associated with lupus-like serological patterns in immunized rabbits. Our results also demonstrated that caution must be applied when choosing the structure of the carrier Multiple Antigen Peptide (MAP-peptide) for immunization. We discovered that using MAP-4 rather than MAP-8 significantly altered patterns of immune response and gene expression.

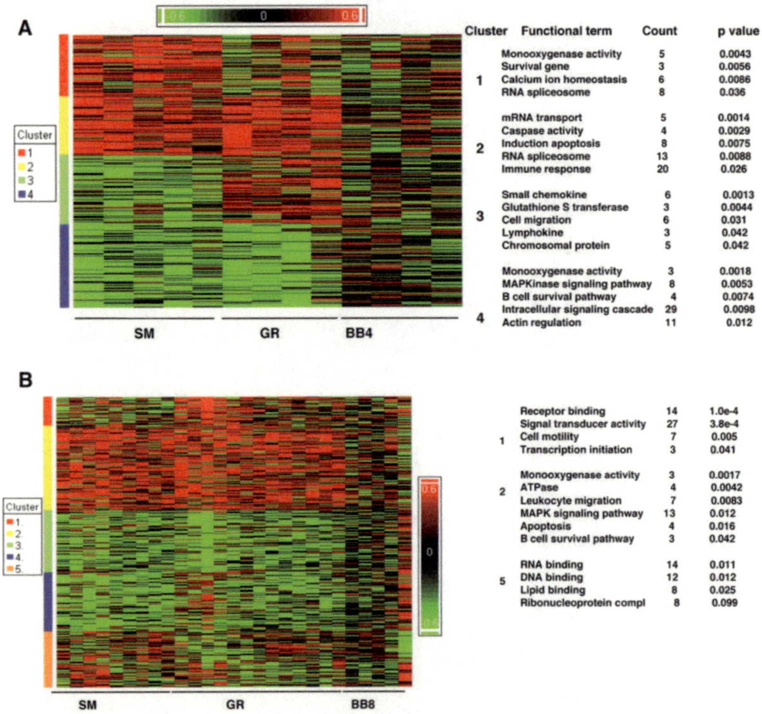

Fig. 3. Gene expression patterns differ when the backbone of immunogen is MAP-4 (A) or MAP-8 (B). In panel A, Cluster 1 genes were overrepresented in the SM group, Cluster 2 were common to both, Cluster 3 genes were overexpressed in the GR group and Cluster 4 genes were decreased in expression in both groups. Count indicates the number of different genes associated with each functional term. Figure modified from one originally published in The Journal of Immunology. Rai, G., Ray S., Milton, J., Yang, J., Ren, P., Lempicki, R., and Mage, R.G. 2010. Gene expression profiles in a rabbit model of systemic lupus erythematosus autoantibody production. J. Immunol. 185:4446-4456. Copyright © [2010] The American Association of Immunologists, Inc.

Figure 3 shows that distinct patterns and clusters of functionally related genes were found to be upregulated when peptides SM or GR on MAP-4 backbone (A) were used as immunogens compared to when MAP-8 backbone was used (B) (Rai et al., 2010). Validation of gene expression data by quantitative real-time PCR was conducted for two genes for which primer sequences were available beta2-microglobulin (B2M) and p-21-protein (Cdc42/Rac)-activated kinase 1 (PAK1) (Figure 6 in Rai et al., 2010). These genes appear in the interactive pathway shown in Figure 4 below. Among the genes significantly upregulated in SLE rabbits were those associated with NK cytotoxicity, antigen presentation, leukocyte migration, cytokine activity, protein kinases, RNA spliceosomal ribonucleoproteins, intracellular signaling cascades, and glutamate receptor activity (Rai et al., 2010).

Functional Annotation	p-Value	Number of molecules
Inflammatory Disorder	1.6E-11	25
Immunological Disorder	3.1E-11	23
Rheumatic Disease	5.4E-11	19
Autoimmune Disease	2.7 E-08	18
Rheumatoid Arthritis	1.7E-06	13
Glomerulonephritis	2.6E-06	5
Inflammation	2.5E-05	7
Lupus Nephritis of Mice	3.2E-04	3

Table 2. The top functional annotations found using Ingenuity Pathways Analysis (IPA) in comparisons of upregulated genes of rabbits making anti-dsDNA to those only making other anti-nuclear antibodies.

Figure 4 and Table 2 summarize the patterns of upregulated gene expression found in the rabbits from the three groups immunized with MAP-8-peptides that made anti-dsDNA compared to those that only made other anti-nuclear antibodies. Twenty-five genes associated with inflammatory disorders were significantly upregulated in expression. Subsets of these were associated with various immunological disorders in the IPA databases including Autoimmune, Rheumatic, and inflammatory diseases. The results linked increased immune activation with up-regulation of components associated with neurological and anti-RNP responses, demonstrating the utility of the rabbit SLE model to uncover biological pathways related to SLE-induced clinical symptoms, including NPSLE. We suggested that our finding of distinct gene expression patterns in rabbits that made anti-dsDNA should be further investigated in subsets of SLE patients with different autoantibody profiles (Rai et al., 2010). In Figure 4, the connecting lines indicate direct interactions among the products of these genes. The shapes classify the proteins found as transmembrane receptors e.g. CD 40, cytokines/growth factors, e.g. CCL2, kinases, e.g. TYK2, peptidases, e.g. MMP9, other enzymes, e.g. ARF1 and transcriptional regulators, e.g. STAT5B. Genes shown were common to the pathways listed in Table 2 that were upregulated in the anti-dsDNA positive rabbits. Figure 4 was modified from one originally published in the Journal of Immunology. Rai, G., Ray S., Milton, J., Yang, J., Ren, P., Lempicki, R., and Mage, R.G. 2010. Gene expression profiles in a rabbit model of systemic lupus erythematosus autoantibody production. J. Immunol. 185:4446-4456. Copyright © [2010] The American Association of Immunologists, Inc.

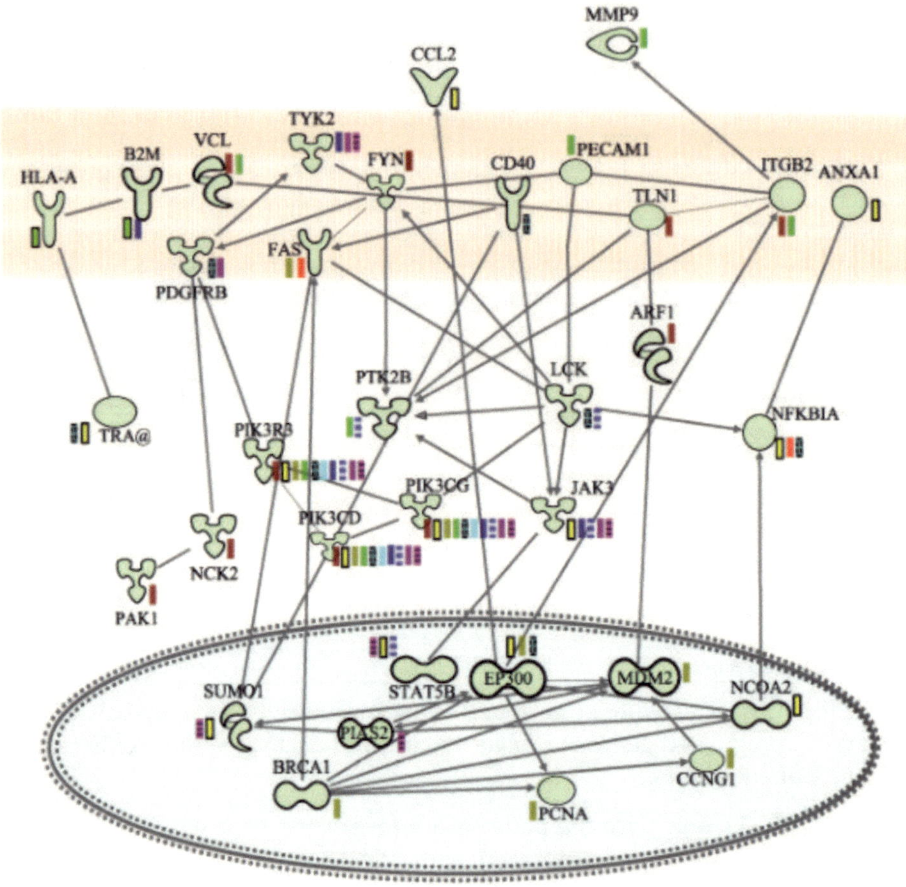

Fig. 4. Interactive pathway network of upregulated genes in anti-dsDNA positive rabbits.

2.2.4 Rabbit BAFF

Our laboratory described the expression and localization of rabbit B-cell activating factor (BAFF also termed BLys, TNFSF13b TALL1, zTNF4) and its receptor BR3 in cells and tissues of the rabbit (Yang et al., 2009a). In addition to its important role in B-cell development and survival, disease activity in human lupus patients has been reported to correlate with serum BAFF levels (reviewed in Groom et al., 2007) and with elevated expression of mRNA for BAFF and two BAFF receptors, BR3 and transmembrane activator and CAML interactor (TACI) in PBMC of lupus patients (Petri et al, 2008). We therefore also investigated BAFF and its receptors in our rabbit model of SLE (Yang et al., 2009b). We previously concluded that BAFF detected on B cells by flow cytometry represented BAFF bound to its receptors on the cells (Yang et al, 2009a). An independent study (Yeramilli, & Knight, 2010) also reported that BAFF-binding receptors on rabbit B-cells are occupied by endogenous soluble BAFF. These authors' studies also suggested that B cells in rabbit could produce BAFF. With the small number of total animals available in group 6 (Table 1B), and no reagents available to detect levels of serum BAFF, we could only measure BAFF on cell surfaces by flow cytometry. These studies found decreased surface expression of BAFF, BR3 and TACI after immunization and boosting

in most animals. However, two rabbits that produced high anti-dsDNA responses (GR76 and GR77) developed higher percentages of BAFF/CD14 and BR3/CD14 positive cells. We did observe consistently lower mean fluorescence intensities of staining of TACI on PBMC and lower percentages of TACI positive cells. We suggested that since TACI is a negative regulator of B cells in mouse and man, perhaps the decrease in TACI in the rabbits producing autoantibodies had allowed autoreactive B cells to escape regulation.
At the time these studies were conducted, clinical trials targeting BAFF/BLys and its receptors were in progress. With the FDA approval of Benlysta® (belimumab) in March, 2011, this monoclonal antibody, that inhibits binding of BLys/BAFF to receptors on B cells, became the first United States FDA approved treatment for SLE in over fifty years. Unfortunately, the clinical trials did not include SLE patients with severe active central nervous system lupus or nephritis. Post-approval trials will be required before this treatment can be recommended for these cohorts of patients.

2.3 Future prospects

2.3.1 Detection of autoantibodies to other antigens including neuroantigens in the rabbit model

In our rabbits, the development of severe symptoms may not yet have occurred because many were euthanized to make room for immunization and testing of their progeny and for tissue collection. For example, although nephritis was not observed, our gene expression studies identified upregulation of genes associated with Glomerulonephritis and also found in mice with Lupus Nephritis (Table 2 and Figure 4). Protein arrays containing microbial and autoantigens have been used to extend information on patients' serum profiles beyond the standard tests used in diagnosis (see for example, Robinson et al., 2002; Quintana et al., 2004; Li et al., 2005; Fattal et al. 2010). Recently, Li et al, (2011) used protein microarrays to determine risk factors for ANA positivity in healthy persons and concluded that serum profiles of autoantibodies can potentially identify healthy individuals with potential to develop lupus and other autoimmune diseases. Their observations extended the widely quoted earlier observations by Arbuckle et al, (2003) that autoantibodies develop as much as ten years before the clinical onset of SLE. In a NOD mouse model of cyclophosphamide-accelerated diabetes, Quintana et al (2004) used a protein microarray to predict from autoantibody repertoires, resistance or susceptibility to the development of diabetes before the induction with cyclophosphamide. Recently Fattal et al, (2010) applied the same technology to studies of SLE patients and controls. They reported highly specific SLE profiles that typically show increases in IgG binding to dsDNA, single-stranded DNA, Epstein–Barr virus, and hyaluronic acid. Interestingly, a healthy control subject who had the SLE antibody profile was later found to develop clinical SLE. Decreases in some specific IgM reactivities to autoantigens observed in this and earlier studies (Li et al., 2005) suggest that some natural IgM autoantibodies may play a protective role. A project to determine the antibody profiles of the rabbits' serum IgG and IgM, purified anti-dsDNA, and anti-peptide on protein microarrays carrying microbial and self antigens including those from the central and peripheral nervous system is in progress.

2.3.2 NPSLE and anti-NMDA glutamate receptors

The suggestion from extensive studies in the laboratory of Betty Diamond that some anti-dsDNA antibodies may react with the NMDA receptor and contribute to neurological manifestations in some lupus patients (DeGiorgio et al. 2001; Kowal et al, 2004), has led to numerous follow-up studies by the Diamond group, (Diamond & Volpe, 2004) and others. A recent editorial (Appenzeller, 2011) provides an updated overview of controversies in the field and discusses the accompanying paper by Gono et al., (2011) who report new analyses of 107 patients' sera for cross-reactivities of anti-dsDNA with a peptide derived from the sequence of the human NMDA receptor 2A (NR2A) compared with the similar peptide from human NR2B. They suggest that the sensitivity for detection of autoantibodies is greater with the NR2A peptide although their ELISA results directly comparing serum reactivities with each peptide were correlated with high significance ($r = 0.94$; $P<0.0001$). They conclude that assays of sera for anti-NR2A antibodies may be a better predictor of NPSLE than assays for NR2B and suggest that mixed results from other similar studies may be explained by small numbers of patients (Husebye et al., 2005) or less sensitive assays. We chose the GR peptide used in our immunization protocol based on the human sequence of NR2B because the rabbit sequence was not yet known. However, we knew that this sequence was highly conserved in several species including mouse, rat, dog, cow and chicken.

2.3.3 Rabbit genomics

Future studies of rabbit autoimmune and infectious diseases will benefit from the availability of a high quality draft rabbit genome sequence and assembly at ~7 x coverage recently completed at the Broad Institute, Boston (OryCun2.0). The donor was from a partially inbred strain. NCBI maintains a Rabbit Genome Resources website: http://www.ncbi.nlm.nih.gov/projects/genome/guide/rabbit/

Rabbit genomic sequences and assemblies from the ENCODE Project, with ~ 1% of rabbit genomic sequence from a different, outbred NZW animal are also available in GenBank. The selection of peptides for future immunization studies in rabbits can benefit from searching these resources.

3. Conclusion

The work described in this review documents that rabbits have a strong genetic component that leads to predisposition to production of autoantibodies similar to those found in SLE patients including those with NPSLE. Breeding and selection for consistent autoantibody production in the rabbit model can be accomplished over a few generations. When one of us (RGM) retired to Emeritus status at NIAID, the pedigreed colony was no longer maintained. Some animals related to those studied were distributed to others. In addition, although the pedigreed colony was dispersed, there is sperm available from two male breeders rabbits LL191-1 (SM13) and 1UA344-1 (GR49). In particular male SM13 and his progeny in the breeding scheme shown in Figure 2 generated numerous responders that made autoantibodies similar to those found in human Lupus patients. Cryovials of sperm from these animals are currently stored at the Twinbrook 3 facility of the Comparative Medicine Branch (CMB) of NIAID in liquid nitrogen storage tanks, and monitored weekly by their personnel. Further contact information can be obtained at the website of the CMB, of the NIAID, NIH at: http://www.niaid.nih.gov/LabsAndResources/labs/aboutlabs/cmb/Pages/default.aspx.

4. Acknowledgment

This research was supported by the Intramural Research Program of the NIH, NIAID. All coauthors of the papers from the laboratory made valuable contributions to the current understanding of the rabbit model of SLE. We appreciate the major contributions of Cornelius Alexander, Laboratory of Immunology, NIAID as well as the veterinary staff at Spring Valley Laboratories who provided invaluable technical assistance. We thank Jeff Skinner for statistical analyses, Mariam Quiñones for help with IPA analyses and figures, and Folake Soetan and Rami Zahr for assistance with preparation of some figures. We dedicate this chapter to the memory of Dr. Barbara A. Newman who was a major contributor to this research.

5. References

Appenzeller, S.; (2011) NR2 antibodies in neuropsychiatric systemic lupus erythematosus. *Rheumatology (Oxford).* Vol. 50 (February 2011) Epub ahead of print doi:10.1093/rheumatology/ker015

Arbuckle, M.R.; McClain. M.T., Rubertone, M. V., Scofield, R. H., Dennis, M.D., James, J.A., & Harley, J.B. (2003) Development of autoantibodies before the clinical onset of systemic lupus erythematosus. *N. Engl. J. Med.,* Vol. 349, No. 16 pp. 1526-1533.

DeGiorgio, L. A.; Konstantinov, K. N, Lee, S. C., Hardin, J. A., Volpe, B. T. & Diamond, B. (2001) A subset of lupus anti-DNA antibodies cross-reacts with the NR2 glutamate receptor in systemic lupus erythematosus. *Nat. Med.* Vol.7, No.11 (November 2001), pp. 1189–1193.

Diamond, B.; & Volpe, B. T. (2004). Cognition and immunity: antibody impairs memory. *Immunity* Vol.21 No.2, (August 2004). pp. 179–188.

Fattal, I.; Shental, N,, Mevorach, D., Anaya, J.M., Livneh, A., Langevitz, P., Zandman-Goddard, G., Pauzner, R., Lerner, M., Blank, M., Hincapie, M.E., Gafter, U., Naparstek, Y., Shoenfeld, Y., Domany, E., & Cohen IR. (2010) An antibody profile of systemic lupus erythematosus detected by antigen microarray. Immunology. 2010 Vol.130, No.3, (July 2010) pp. 337-343.

Groom, J.R.; Fletcher, C.A., Walters, S.N., Grey, S.T., Watt, S.V., Sweet, M.J., Smyth, M.J., Mackay, C.R., & Mackay, F. (2007) BAFF and MyD88 signals promote a lupuslike disease independent of T cells. *J. Exp. Med.* Vol. 204, No. 8, (August 2007) pp.1959-1971.

Gono, T.; Kawaguchi, Y., Kaneko, H., Nishimura, K., Hanaoka, M., Kataoka, S., Okamoto, Y., Katsumata, Y., & Yamanaka, H. (2011) Anti-NR2A antibody as a predictor for neuropsychiatric systemic lupus Erythematosus. *Rheumatology* Vol.50 (January 2011) Epub ahead of print. doi:10.1093/rheumatology/keq408 ISSN 1462-0332.

Husebye, E. S.; Z. M. Sthoeger, M. Dayan, H. Zinger, D. Elbirt, M. Levite, & E. Mozes. (2005). Autoantibodies to a NR2A peptide of the glutamate/NMDAreceptor in sera of patients with systemic lupus erythematosus. *Ann. Rheum. Dis.* 64, No.8 (August 2005) pp. 1210–1213.

James, J. A.; Gross, T., Scofield, R. H. & Harley, J. B. (1995). Immunoglobulin epitope spreading and autoimmune disease after peptide immunization: Sm B/B -derived PPPGMRPP and PPPGIRGP induce spliceosome autoimmunity. *J. Exp .Med.* Vol.181, No.2 (February 2005), pp. 453–461.

Kowal, C.; DeGiorgio, L. A., Nakaoka, T., Hetherington, H., Huerta, P. T., Diamond, B. & Volpe, B. T. (2004). Cognition and immunity: antibody impairs memory. *Immunity* Vol.21 No.2, (August 2004). pp. 179–188.

Li Q.Z.; Xie C., Wu, T., Mackay, M., Aranow, C., Putterman, C., & Mohan, C. (2005) Identification of autoantibody clusters that best predict lupus disease activity using glomerular proteome arrays. *J Clin Invest.* Vol.115, No. 12, (December 2005) pp.3428–3439.

Li, Q.Z.; Karp, D.R., Quan, J., Branch, V.K., Zhou. J., Lian, Y., Chong, B.F., Wakeland, E.K., & Olsen, N.J. (2011). Risk factors for ANA positivity in healthy persons. *Arthritis Research & Therapy* 2011 13 No.2 (March 2011):R38.

Mage, R.G.; Lanning,D., & Knight, K.L. (2006). B cell and antibody repertoire development in rabbits: the requirement of gut-associated lymphoid tissues. *Develop. Comp. Immunol.* Vol.30, No.1-2, (January February 2006) pp.137-153.

Mason, L.J.; Timothy, L.M., Isenberg, D.A., & Kalsi, J.K. (1999) Immunization with a peptide of Sm B/B' results in limited epitope spreading but not autoimmune disease. *J. Immunol.* Vol.162, No.9, (May, 1999) pp. 5099-5105.

Petri, M.; Stohl, W., Chatham, W., McCune, W.J., Chevrier, M., Ryel, J., Recta, V., Zhong, J., & Freimuth, W. (2008) Association of plasma B lymphocyte stimulator levels and disease activity in systemic lupus erythematosus. *Arthritis Rheum.* Vol.58, No. 8 (August, 2008) pp.2453-2459.

Puliyath, N.; Ray, S., Milton, J., & Mage R. G. (2008) Genetic contributions to the autoantibody profile in a rabbit model of systemic lupus erythematosus (SLE). *Vet. Immunol. Immunopathol.* Vol.125, No.3-4, (October 2008), pp. 251-267.

Quintana, F.J.; Hagedorn, P.H., Elizur. G., Merbl. Y., Domany, E., & , Cohen I.R. (2004) Functional immunomics: microarray analysis of IgG autoantibody repertoires predicts the future response of mice to induced diabetes. *Proc Natl Acad Sci USA* Vol.101, Suppl 2 (October 2004) pp. 14615-14621.

Rai, G.; Ray, S., Shaw, R. E., DeGrange, P. F., Mage, R. G., & Newman, B. A. (2006). Models of systemic lupus erythematosus: Development of autoimmunity following peptide immunizations of noninbred pedigreed rabbits. *J. Immunol.* Vol.176, No.1 (January 2006), pp. 660-667.

Rai, G.; Ray S., Milton, J., Yang, J., Ren, P., Lempicki, R., & Mage, R.G. (2010). Gene expression profiles in a rabbit model of systemic lupus erythematosus autoantibody production. *J. Immunol.* Vol.185, No.7 (October 2010), pp. 4446-4456.

Robinson, W.H.; DiGennaro, C., Hueber, W., Haab, B.B., Kamachi, M., Dean, E.J., Fournel, S., Fong, D., Genovese, M.C., de Vegvar, H.E., Skriner, K., Hirschberg, D.L., Morris, R.I., Muller, S., Pruijn, G.J., van Venrooij, W.J., Smolen, J.S., Brown, P.O., Steinman, L., & Utz, P.J. (2002) Autoantigen microarrays for multiplex characterization of autoantibody responses. Nature Medicine Vol. 8, No. (March 2002), pp. 295-301.

Sanchez-Guerrero, J.; Aranow, C., Mackay, M., Volpe, B. & Diamond, B.(2008) Neuropsychiatric systemic lupus erythematosus reconsidered. *Nature Clinical Practice Rheumatology* Vol 4. No. 3 (March 2008) pp. 112-113.

Yang, J.; Pospisil, R. & Mage, R.G. (2009a). Expression and localization of rabbit B-cell activating factor (BAFF) and its specific receptor BR3 in cells and tissues of the rabbit immune system. *Develop. Comp. Immunol.* Vol.33, No.5 (May 2009), pp. 697-708.

Yang, J.; Pospisil, R., Ray, S., Milton, J., & Mage, R. G. (2009b) Investigations of a rabbit (*Oryctolagus cuniculus*) model of systemic lupus erythematosus (SLE), BAFF and its receptors. *PLoS ONE* Vol.4, No.12, (December 2009) e8494, Open Access online.

Yeramilli, V.A. & Knight, K.L (2010) Requirement for BAFF and APRIL during B Cell Development in GALT. *J. Immunol.* Vol. 184, No. 10 (May 2010) pp. 5527-5536.

Part 2

Clinical Aspects of SLE

10

How to Avoid Delay in SLE Diagnosis and Management

Hani Almoallim[1,2], Esraa Bukhari[2], Waleed Amasaib[2] and Rania Zaini[1]
[1]*Umm Alqura University, Makkah*
[2]*King Faisal Specialist Hospital, Jeddah*
Saudi Arabia

1. Introduction

Systemic lupus erythematosus (SLE) is a wide spectrum disease with many clinical manifestations. Lack of awareness of the disease itself, with its common and rare presentations results in significant delay in diagnosis and consequently serious compromise of patients' care.

Physical examination will always retain its importance as the most common diagnostic test used by doctors and as an essential tool for modern practice(Joshua, Celermajer et al. 2005). Findings from proper musculoskeletal (MSK) examination is extremely useful in diagnosing rheumatologic disorders especially where gold standard diagnostic tests are lacking. From this perspective there should be much emphasis on basic bedside skills among clinicians searching for arthritis. Asking about morning stiffness and joint swelling are simple enough to pick up early arthritis (Paget 2007). Performing an active range of motion testing of joints as a screening method would pick up limitations in joints mobility from active arthritis. In real practice, the picture is not simple as such. Despite the impact of MSK disorders on health care, rheumatological diseases are often overlooked or inadequately assessed by doctors (Jones, Maddison et al. 1992). This chapter will explore some of the issues around this complex clinical and educational problem.

SLE (the disease of thousand faces) is not only affecting the joints. Major organ involvement can be the first presenting symptom(s) and/or sign(s). Knowledge of some of the common presenting features of SLE apart from arthritis would help greatly in early recognition of this multisystem disease. Renal, central nervous system (CNS), and cardiovascular system (CVS) are commonly affected in SLE patients. Knowing the risk factors, early detection and close folllow up will have positive impact on patient's outcome. This chapter will discuss some of the clinical issues arising while managing SLE patients that are commonly overlooked by clinicans. Late onset SLE and other rare associations like Kikuchi Fujimoto disease will be disscussed in this chapter as well.

2. Deficiencies in musculoskeletal examination skills

MSK symptoms are the most common health complications that require medical attention, accounting to 20% of both primary care and emergency-room visits (Rasker 1995). In a health survey, MSK disorders were ranked first in prevalence as the cause of chronic health problems, long term disabilities, and consultations with a health professional (Badley, Rasooly et al. 1994). In Saudi Arabia, MSK disorders is the second major cause of outpatients visit in primary care centers and private clinics (MOH 2009). A number of different medical specialties are involved in treating patients with musculoskeletal complaints, including general practitioners, family physicians, internists, orthopedic and surgeons, working in teams with other health professionals, but often without a multispecialty focus. In order to truly improve the outcome of treatment for musculoskeletal conditions, it is important that experts in the various specialties work more closely together and look for commonality of approach, as they often treat the same patients but from different angles.

Despite the high prevalence of musculoskeletal disorders in all fields of clinical practice, studies show a lower level of competence and confidence in MSK cognitive and clinical skills (including physical examinations) across clinicians (Akesson, Dreinhofer et al. 2003; Almoallim, Khojah et al. 2007; Beattie, Bobba et al. 2008). Also, a continuous neglect of musculoskeletal examination skills in clinical practice is observed. We reported a case of SLE with active arthritis where the diagnosis was delayed for seven days after hospital admission due to the lack of basic skills in MSK examination (Almoallim, Khojah et al. 2007). The patient in the report presented to the emergency room with fever and pancytopenia and apparently the focus of the treating medical team was mainly on these presenting findings. This might had restricted the clerking done on admission to "hematology and infectious diseases" while what should had been done was a complete history and thorough physical examination regardless of initial impression. Musculoskeletal assessment should be a part of routine clerking (Lillicrap, Byrne et al. 2003). Assuring such attitude among clinicians will prevent unnecessary delay in diagnosis. If a simple musculoskeletal screening examination focused mainly on range of motion testing to assess function was done, this patient's active arthritis would have been picked up on admission. This would have initiated early search for a rheumatological disease and start treatment without a delay.

Despite this impact of MSK disorders on health care, rheumatological diseases are often overlooked or inadequately assessed by doctors (Jones, Maddison et al. 1992). Thus, patients with complaints about bones and joints are often ignored and their problems underestimated by doctors. In a study among 200 general medical inpatients in a teaching hospital, it was found out that the signs and symptoms of MSK disorder which were recorded in the hospital notes was only 5.5% and 14% respectively. This compared poorly with recorded examinations of other systems and regions for example, cardiovascular symptoms were recorded in 100% of the cases; respiratory and abdominal symptoms were recorded in 99%, the nervous system , skin and female breasts symptoms were recorded in 77% and 13% respectively (Doherty, Abawi et al. 1990). In another report, only 40%of patients admitted to general medicine ward had the history of their MSK symptoms recorded and only 14.5% of these patients received comprehensive MSK examination (Ahern, Soden et al. 1991). Furthermore, 80% of symptomatic patients received either no treatment for their rheumatic disorders, or treatment that was regarded as suboptimal or inappropriate (Ahern, Soden et al. 1991). Another report showed even a higher percentage of patients – 63% of all patient admitted to general medicine ward- had MSK symptoms or its signs, but relevant MSK history was missed in 49% of the patients records, while signs were missed in 78%; 42% of those with MSK conditions would have benefitted from additional treatment (Lillicrap, Byrne et al. 2003). A more recent report reviewed 150 patient notes in three different hospitals from the acute admission wards for medicine and surgery and the medical assessment unit. Factors considered included whether GALS screenings had taken place, documentation of MSK examinations and assessment of confidence of junior doctors in assessing MSK conditions. GALS screenings were performed in 4% of patients on the medical assessment unit, 7% in acute medical and 0% in acute surgical patients on admission. Examination of the MSK system yielded better results with 16%, 22% and 10% on each of the respective wards. Interviews with junior doctors found 10% routinely screening for MSK conditions, despite 87% feeling confident in taking MSK histories (Sirisena, Begum et al.).

Matzkin et al. (2005) indicated that the majority (79%) of the study respondents including medical students, residents, and staff physicians failed the basic MSK cognitive examination. This suggests that training in MSK medicine is inadequate in both medical school and in most residency training programs. Worldwide, undergraduate and postgraduate medical teaching of MSK disorders is currently brief and not directly relevant to the knowledge and skills commonly required for the management of these conditions in an outpatient setting.

In undergraduate education, inadequate MSK education has been reported. Medical students spend very few hours on the MSK system, both in basic science and in clinical training. It is quite common for students to leave medical schools without being able to make a general assessment of the musculoskeletal system. On the other hand, it would be considered a total neglect if a medical graduate is incompetent at adequately assessing the heart or lungs. Harvard medical students have reported general dissatisfaction of their confidences in examining MSK system as compared to their skills in examining pulmonary system (Day, YEh et al. 2007). They suggested more time to be devoted to MSK medicine and more integration between pre-medical and clinical courses.

The American Association of Medical Colleges claims that most medical schools do not effectively educate future physicians on MSK medicine in spite of the increasing prevalence of MSK conduction across medical practice ((AAMC) 2005). The obvious discrepancy between the magnitude of MSK conditions and physicians competences, which mostly stemmed from the educational deficiencies at the medical schools, is maintained across years ((AAMC) 2005; Day, YEh et al. 2007; Clark, Hutchison et al. 2010). Akesson and colleagues (2003) argued that teaching at the undergraduate and graduate programmes is not adequate and the resulting competence does not reflect the impact of these conditions on individuals and society. A comprehensive study reviewing the curricula of all Canadian medical schools indicated that directors of undergraduate MSK programmes felt dissatisfied with the curricular time devoted to MSK education (Pinney and Regan 2001). In a comprehensive study based on a national survey in Saudi Arabia using the Delphi technique, internal medicine knowledge and skills competencies including rheumatology were determined and prioritized (Almoallim 2010). Table 1 represents only rheumatological skills competencies that were identified. Note that the score of 3: indicates must know the topic, 2: should know the topic, 1: interesting to know the topic. It was decided in this research that any competency with a score ≥ 2.2 should be considered a core competency. Table 2 represents overall disease ratings with the number of competencies identified for each disease. Such findings would help greatly in designing educational programmes and assessment methods based on priorities and it will help in determining what skills for rheumatological diseases should be taught. It is a common recommendation among experts to give proper attention to training in MSK conditions for both undergraduate and postgraduate training programmes.

In the postgraduate programme the same limitation was highlighted since the 1980s: Goldenberg et al (1985) reported that the majority of directors of residency programs thought that many basic skills and techniques were not taught adequately and that the training of their rheumatology residents was not equal to that of residents in cardiology or gastroenterology. General dissatisfactions of MSK training was reported among the internal medicine residents and family practice. United States residents expressed their dissatisfaction of their competence in performing MSK examinations at various parts of the body and revealed that to the inadequate or poor training (Clawson, Jackson et al. 2001).

2.1 Possible obstacles toward an appropriate MSK medical practice

Previous studies suggested many reasons related to MSK poor clinical skills and physical examinations in particular (Clawson, Jackson et al. 2001; Akesson, Dreinhofer et al. 2003; (AAMC) 2005; Matzkin, Smith et al. 2005; Day, YEh et al. 2007; Dequeker, Esselens et al. 2007; Thompson 2008; MOH 2009; Clark, Hutchison et al. 2010):

- Vague training of MSK in undergraduate programmes;
- Underestimate the prevalence of MSK conditions and its impact on individuals and society
- MSK is not considered as main competence among medical graduates because it is not a life threatening condition.
- Number of different specialties involved in treating patients with MSK conditions do not share common approach regardless of specialties interventions,
- Lack of a proper teaching in MSK is essential in the low competence in MSK generally and physical examinations
- Lack of summative evaluation of MSK physical examination contributes to medical graduate low level of competencies
- The lack of holistic approach and the focus of specialties
- The lack of standardize approach to the clinical assessment of MSK problems whether presenting to primary care, rheumatology or orthopedics that give a benchmark for this competency.
- The disparity in the approach to examination between rheumatologists and orthopaedic surgeons mostly leads to poor performances in MSK physical examinations
- The lack of appropriate teaching and evaluation of MSK because the physical examination teachers are not skilled in MSK examinations and thus bone and joint diseases are not screened.

2.2 Global initiative toward MSK medicine

The global initiative to disseminate awareness to MSK wellbeing had made the World Health Organization (WHO) designate the years 2000 to 2010 as Bone and Joint Decade (Lidren 2003). In the light of the worldwide commitment, the focus increases on the responsibility of medical education and training programmes in providing adequate musculoskeletal education. Therefore, global consensus among international experts from different specialties and organizations developed a recommendation for MSK teaching in undergraduate medical education (Woolf, WAlsh et al. 2004).

A standardized approach to the clinical assessment of a musculoskeletal problem is suggested by Wolf and Akesson (2008): such a standardized approach will be conducted whether the patient is presenting to primary care, rheumatology or orthopedics. It also will provide a benchmark for this competency and can also be used as a teaching aid (Woolf and Åkesson 2008). The issue is whether this kind of standardization would be widely accepted by different displines or not.

SN	RHEUMATOLOGICAL DISEASES (SKILLS COMPITENCIES)	EXPERT RATING
1	To demonstrate competency skills in obtaining comprehensive history from patient with rheumatological disorders	**2.60**
2	To demonstrate competency skills in applying general principle of joint examination (screening exam, inspection, palpation, range of motion, & special tests) in musculoskeletal examination	**2.50**
3	To demonstrate competency skills in performing comprehensive musculoskeletal examination including (the hands & wrists, elbows, shoulders, TMJ, the neck, spine & sacroiliac joints, knees, hips, ankles & feet).	**2.20**
4	To interpret the ANAs results	**1.80**
5	To interpret synovial fluid analysis results including polarized light microscopy	**1.70**
6	To demonstrate competency skills in obtaining comprehensive history from patient with back pain.	**2.30**
7	To identify on plain x-ray of joints findings consistent with RA.	**1.90**
8	To demonstrate competency skills in examining patient with RA.	**2.30**
9	To identify on plain x-ray findings consistent with spondyloarthropathies.	**1.70**
10	To identify on plain x-ray findings consistent with crystal related joint disease.	**1.70**
11	To identify on plain x-ray findings consistent with JRA.	**1.30**
12	To demonstrate competency skills in examining patient with crystal-related joint disease.	**1.60**
13	To demonstrate competency skills in examining patient with SLE.	**2.30**
14	To demonstrate competency skills in examining patient with scleroderma.	**1.80**
15	To demonstrate competency skills in examining patient with rheumatic fever.	**2.30**
16	To demonstrate competency skills in examining patient with soft tissue rheumatism.	**1.50**
17	To demonstrate competency skills in obtaining comprehensive history from patients suspected to have vasculitis.	**2.00**
18	To demonstrate competency skills in examining patient with nerve entrapment syndrome.	**1.70**
19	To demonstrate competency skills in eliciting physical signs consistent with spondyloarthropathies.	**1.60**
20	To demonstrate competency skills in performing joint aspiration.	**1.00**

Table 1. Rheumatological diseases (skills compitencies)

GALS (Gait, Arms, Legs and Spine) a locomotor screening was developed and validated as a rapid screening protocol / system for MSK with the aim for a quick identification of significant abnormalities (Doherty, Dacer et al. 1992). Various spectrums of health specialties could utilize this screening routine before specific examination and teach it to trainees and medical students. Tabe 3 represents a quick screening tool for MSK disorders adopted from (Woolf and Akesson 2008).

KNOWLEDGE COMPETENCIES BREAKDOWN	MEAN WEIGHTED RESPONSE	NO.OF IDENTIFIED COMPETENCIES
Approach To The Patient With Joint Pain	1.91	13
Approach To The Patient With Low Back Pain	2.00	6
Rheumatoid Arthritis	2.12	14
Spondyloarthropathies(SpA)	1.89	17
Crystal Related Joint Disease	1.95	16
Osteoarthritis	2.36	7
Bacterial Septic Arthritis	2.32	6
Systemic Lupus Erythematosus	2.13	9
Scleroderma	1.65	6
Inflammatory Myopathies(Polymyositis &Dermatomyositis)	1.69	7
Sjogren's Syndrome	1.65	4
Vasculitis	1.78	8
Juvenile Rheumatoid Arthritis (Juvenile Idiopathic arthritis)	1.74	5
Miscellaneous Syndromes	0.90	1
TOTAL		119

Table 2. Disease Specific Ratings For Rheumatological Diseases

3. Late onset SLE

It is true that most SLE patients are in the child bearing age but SLE can occur in elderly. SLE has always been considered a disease of the young. Little attention has been given to late onset disease. In contrast with childhood disease, studies on elderly SLE patients are scarce (Boddaert, Huong et al. 2004). Late onset disease is the type of SLE whose manifestations begin after the age of 50 in majority of the studies (Boddaert, Huong et al. 2004; Karoubi Nordon, Hayem et al. 2007; Rovensky and Tuchynova 2008) or after the age of 65 (Pu, Luo et al. 2000). SLE should be considered in the differential diagnosis while dealing with certain clinical settings in elderly population. Clincians recognizing this clinical entity will help greatly to assure early diagnosis of SLE and avoid unnecessary delay in diagnosis and management.

Screening questions		
1	"Do you suffer from any pain or stiffness in your arms, legs, neck or back?"	
2	"Do you have any swelling of your joints?"	
3	"Do you have any difficulty with washing and dressing?"	
4	"Do you have any difficulty with going up or down stairs or steps?"	
Screening examination		
Gait		Observe the patient walking forwards for a few meters, turning and walking back again. Recognize abnormalities of the different phases—heel strike, stance phase, toe-off and swing phases. Look for abnormalities of the movement of arms, pelvis, hips, knees, ankles and feet.
Inspection of standing patient		View the patient from the front, side and back, looking for any abnormalities, particularly of posture and symmetry. Apply pressure in the midpoint of each supraspinatus and roll an overlying skin fold to examine for tenderness.
Spine		Ask the patient to flex the neck laterally to each side. Place several fingers on the lumbar spinous processes and ask the patient to bend forward and attempt to touch their toes whilst standing with legs fully extended, observing for normal movement and feeling for expansion of space between spinous processes.
Arms		ask the patient to place both hands behind their head and then move elbows right back, then straighten the arms down the side of the body and bend elbows to 90° with palms down and fingers straight. Turn hands palms up and make a tight fist with each hand, then place, in turn, the tip of each finger onto the tip of the thumb. Squeeze the metacarpals from second to fifth cautiously for tenderness.
Legs		get the patient to recline on a couch, then flex, in turn, each hip and knee while holding and feeling the knee. Passively rotate the hip internally. With the leg extended and resting on the couch, press down on the patella while cupping it proximally to examine for tenderness or swelling of the knee. Squeeze all metatarsals and then inspect the soles of the feet for callosities.

Table 3. Quick screening tool for msk disorder

Overall, the incidence of late-onset SLE is low, but there are variable numbers reported in the literature, ranging from as low as 3.7% (Costallat and Coimbra 1994) and to as high as 20.1% (Jacobsen, Petersen et al. 1998). This may be related to the different ethnic backgrounds included in the studies and the variable definitions of late-onset SLE. Most of the literature indicated that the sex ratio declines with age in SLE. In a pooled analysis of 714 cases of late-onset SLE reported in the literature and 4700 young SLE patients, the female to male ratio observed with age in SLE was 4.4:1 vs. 10.6:1 respectively (Boddaert, Huong et al. 2004). This probably reflects the relationship between SLE and estrogen status which decline in the elderly.

Late onset SLE is not a well studied disease and it has distinct clinical features. Although the disease activity and major organ involvement is less than in the early onset disease, it can cause more morbidity and mortality. In one study, there were significant number of patients with late onset SLE who died during the research period which may be related to the comorbidities and the use of medication which are age related rather than the disease itself (Bertoli, Alarcon et al. 2006). Skin manifestations, photosensitivity, Raynaud phenomenon, arthritis, nephritis and neuropsychiatric manifestations were less frequent in comparison with young SLE patients. In late-onset SLE, a higher occurrence of pulmonary involvement, serositis, and Sjögren's syndrome were observed (Boddaert, Huong et al. 2004; Rovensky and Tuchynova 2008).

There are variable findings in the literature about the occurrence of anti ds DNA antibodies in late-onset SLE (Padovan, Govoni et al. 2007; Rovensky and Tuchynova 2008). These antibodies did not correlate with organ complications of late-onset disease in one study (Padovan, Govoni et al. 2007). A higher prevalence of rheumatoid factor, anti-Ro and anti-La antibodies were observed in late-onset SLE. However, lower prevalence of anti-RNP antibodies and hypocomplementemia were observed as well (Maddison 1987; Belostocki and Paget 2002; Boddaert, Huong et al. 2004; Padovan, Govoni et al. 2007).

In general, late onset SLE is characterized by a lower disease activity (Costallat and Coimbra 1994; Boddaert, Huong et al. 2004). This fact does not exclude significant morbidity associated with it. The seriuosness of some clinical presentations may preclude clinicians from considering autoimmune diseases as an etiology in their work up. This may result in unncessary delay in diagnosing late onset SLE. We reported a case of late onset SLE in a 65 year old female patient, previously healthy, who presented with progressive paraplegia and sensory level at T4 (Almoallim, Bukhari et al. 2009). MRI showed extensive transverse myelitis (TM) involving the thoracic spine. Antinuclear antibodies (ANA), anti-double stranded DNA antibodies (Anti ds DNA) and lupus anticoagulant were all positive. The diagnosis was delayed for a month after hospital admission due to lack of awareness of basic work up to diagnose SLE. Obviously, SLE was not considered in the basic differential diagnosis of this patient. What had been required was simply considering SLE as a possible etiology then ordering ANA as a screening tool for SLE.

4. Neuropsychiatric manifestations of SLE (NPSLE)

NPSLE may still present a very difficult diagnostic challenge for clinicians (Joseph, Lammie et al. 2007). Neurologic features at the onset of SLE is regarded rare, occurring only in approximately 3% in some studies and up to 24% in others (Joseph, Lammie et al. 2007). NPSLE affects more than half of SLE patients. It ranges in severity from mild symptoms like headache to severe neurological dysfunction. Clinicians particularly general internists and neurologists who are dealing primarily with patients presenting with complex neurological presentations should consider autoimmune diseases and particularly SLE in their diffrential diagnosis. Awarness of the 19 neuropsychiatric syndromes defined by ACR as an associated feature with NPSLE is essential. (See corresponding chapters for further details).

The most prevalent symptoms are headache, seizures, mood disorders and cerebrovascular disease. Regarding headaches, data showed that there was no significant difference in the prevalence of tension type headache and migraine between the SLE patient and the general population (Mitsikostas, Sfikakis & Goadsby, 2004).

Simple or complex attention, memory, reasoning, executive skills, language, visual-spatial processing and psychomotor speed are normal cognitive functions, and any significant deficit in one or all of these functions is defined as cognitive dysfunction by ACR. These dysfunctions are usually underestimated and require careful testing to avoid unnecessary delay in diagnosis.

Guillain-Barre syndrome (GBS), myasthenia gravis (MG), plexus injury, TM, aseptic meningitis and autonomic dysfunctions are less frequent and rare neurological manifestation associated with SLE. GBS is an acute, rapidly progressive, autoimmune demylinating polyneuropathy resulting in symmetric, ascending paralysis that can be severe involving the respiratory muscles and require mechanical ventilation. This disease is relatively rare among SLE patients as it is only associated in 7 out of 1100 GBS cases in an early study (Leneman 1966). MG is another autoimmune disorder affecting the proximal, bulbar and extraocular muscles due to antibodies directed against the post synaptic acetylcholine receptors resulting in weakness of the muscles. Among 78 patients with this disease, 6 patients (7.7%) had SLE (Sthoeger, Neiman et al. 2006). It was concluded in this study that MG patients should be evaluated for the coexistence of SLE, and assessment for MG is suggested in lupus patients with unexplained muscular weakness. Various case reports showed the association between them (Vaiopoulos, Sfikakis et al. 1994; Bhinder, Majithia et al. 2006). The prevalence of TM in SLE patients is 1-2% (Kovacs, Lafferty et al. 2000). It can occur as the initial manifestation of SLE in up to 39% or within the first five years of a diagnosis of SLE in 42% of the total patient population analyzed in one study (Kovacs, Lafferty et al. 2000). The predominant presentation of TM in SLE is a sensory level commonly in the thoracic region, spastic paraparesis and sphincter disturbance (Kovacs, Lafferty et al. 2000; D'Cruz, Mellor-Pita et al. 2004). TM as a presenting feature of late onset SLE is rare. Few cases were reported; one patient out of 15 in a report of TM as a presenting feature for SLE (D'Cruz, Mellor-Pita et al. 2004), two patients out of 14 in an older series about TM in SLE (Kovacs, Lafferty et al. 2000) and two case reports (Chen, Lai et al. 2004; Almoallim, Bukhari et al. 2009).

5. How to avoid delay in diagnosis and management of renal involvment in SLE?

Lupus nephritis (LN) is one of the most worrisome and potentially serious complication of SLE and a delay in rcognition and treatment of LN lead to significant morbidity and mortality. LN occurs in 40 to 70% of SLE patients (Cameron,1999a; Seligman et al, 2002) especially in the first year after diagnosis during the first three months (Eilertsen et al,2011).

Early searching for renal involvment in SLE is crucial to prevent it from progression. The goal of clinicians taking care of lupus patients is to identify individuals with signs of early renal disease who are at risk for renal damage. Appropriate treatment can be initiated early to prevent inflammatory lesions from progression to sclerotic ones (end stage LN).

There are simple parameters that should be followed in each clinical visit to pick up early disease. Clinicians should monitor blood pressure, urine analysis and possibly renal function test and anti ds DNA antibodies in each clinical visit. The following are abnormal parameters that suggest renal involvement and mandate biopsy: elevated anti ds DNA antibodies and decreased C4 were more commonly seen in proliferative lupus nephritis compared with non proliferative lupus nephritis (Wen, 2011), hematuria (>5 red blood cells per high power field on urine microscopy), nephrotic (>3.5 g protein/24hrs) or subnephrotic range proteinuria (>0.5g protein/24hrs),or protein/creatinine ratio (>1.0), casts (>5 haemogranular or red blood cast), elevated urea and creatinine and elevated blood pressure (BP>140/90 mmHg).

There is a clear need to consider kidney biopsy early on in the course of the disease to help guide therapy and suggest long term prognosis. Kidney biopsy can determine the degree and severity of renal involvment through established histopathological guidelines. Determining the stage of kidney disease have a signigicant impact on determining response to therapy. Most nephrologists agree that kidney biopsy is worthwhile in SLE patients with abnormal urine analysis and/or reduced renal function. They suggest that kidney biopsy should be performed as soon as clinical signs of renal involvment are evident in order to accelerate treatment decisions and minimize risk of inflamation induced irreversible renal damage (Contreras et al, 2002). Delaying kidney biopsy is unfortunately a practice that is still observed among some rheumatologists and nephrologists. Lack of adequately trained nephrologists/radiologists who can perform kidney biopsy safely might be a factor that explains this delay. Less frequent follow up visits for lupus patients due to overwhelmed rheumatology practices in some parts of the world is another possible factor. Poor monitoring, inadequate control of lupus disease activity, and lack of awareness of the need to consider kidney biopsy are all other possible factors.

It was demonstrated early on in the literature in a cohort of 87 patients with LN that delay between the detection of the onset of renal disease and renal biopsy was a significant predictor at the time of a first renal biopsy for subsequent renal insufficiency (relative risk 4.9; 95% confidence interval 1.7 to 14.5; $p < 0.001$) and death due to lupus renal involvement (relative risk 6.7; 95% confidence interval 2.1 to 21.2; $p < 0.001$) (Esdaile, Joseph et al. 1994). Delaying therapy, because of presumably mild disease, is often associated with increased glomerular injury and fibrosis and therefore a lesser response to immunosuppressive drugs (Esdaile, Joseph et al. 1994). Several other recent studies reported that a delay in renal biopsy(and therapy) is a strong independent predictor of poor outcome in LN (Faurscho et al,2006; Fiehn et al, 2003). Sometimes significant renal disease (stage 3, 4 and 5) can be found in renal biopsy even in the absence of impired renal function or even in the presence of low level of protienuria (urine:protien/creatinine ratio < 1.0)(Christopher-Stine et al, 2006). A full discussion on issues related to kidney biopsy in SLE is presented in another chapter in this book.

5.1 Control of risk factors in lupus nephritis

An important goal for proper medical care for lupus patient, particularly from a renal perspective is the control of risk factors such as protienuria, hypertension, dyslipidemia and diet control.

5.1.1 Proteinuria and hypertension

Heavy proteinuria is a common feature of patients with proliferative LN and progressive renal impairment (Dubois et al, 1987). Serial studies by the Stanford group demonstrated that heavy proteinuria is a predictor of progressive renal impairment (Buckheit et al, 1997). Therefore, reduction of proteinuria independent of reduction in blood pressure is associated with subsequent beneficial effect on the progression of renal disease (Lewis et al, 1993; Maschio et al, 1996; Petersen et al, 1995; The Gisen Group 1997). Early intervention on proteinuria has a major impact in preventing the progression of kidney disease in SLE.

Aggressive reduction of proteinuria should be a goal for any clinician taking care of LN patients.

A number of reports indicated that aggressive treatment of hypertension inhibits progressive renal injury (Petersen et al, 1995; Brazy et al, 1990; Rosansky et al, 1990). Few mmHg reduction in blood pressure value does matter on the long term. The hypertension detection and follow-up programs showed that patients whose BP was 129/86 mmHg versus 130/90 mmHg had greater preservation of renal function (Shulman et al, 1989). It should be recognized that hypertension is also a strong risk factor for developing atherosclerosis which lead to increased risk of heart attacks and strokes. This is to add to the extreme importance of controlling hypertension in lupus patients.

5.1.2 Dyslipidemia

Dyslipidemia is a common feature of lupus patients treated with steroids and also with progressive renal injury and nephrotic syndrome. There is a strong relation in LN patients between cholesterol concentration and proteinuria. There are several reports in non-diabetic renal disease with proteinuria that relate increase cholesterol and triglyceride to an increase in loss of renal function (Apperloo, de Zeeukw & de Jong,1994; Maschio et al, 1989; Samuelsson et al, 1993). Hydroxyl-3-methylglutaryl coenzyme A (HMG-CoA) inhibitors (statins) are beneficial in lowering low density lipoprotien (LDL) cholesterol. Fish oils and fibric acid analogs are helpful in lowering triglyceride and raising high density lipoprotien (HDL) cholesterol and should be considered in patients with dyslipidemia. Again, it is hoped that this issue should not be neglected by clinicians taking care of lupus patients.

5.2 The role of angiotensin converting enzyme inhibitors in patients with lupus nephritis

Angiotensen converting enzyme inhibitors (ACEI) represent a class of drugs used to treat many common diseases like hypertension, heart failure, post myocardial infarction, and microalbuminuria in diabetic patients and nowadays is also used in SLE for many purposes. They work by inhibiting the angiotensin converting enzyme that is responsible for converting angiotensin 1 to angiotensin 2. ACEI have an anti-inflamatory property as angiotensin 2 has pro-inflamatory effect on the cells of different organ system. ACE has been found to be high in synovial fluid (Veal et al, 1992) and rheumatoid nodule in rheumatoid arthritis patients (Goto et al, 1992) which suggest its role in the inflammation. In SLE patients, ACEI have an end organ protection effect by its multiple effects on hypertension and protienuria. ACEI delay the occurence of renal involvment and are associated with decreased risk of disease activity in patients with SLE (Duran-Barragan et al, 2008). This is an impressive and important finding that should alert all clinicans taking care of lups patients to be aware of this valuable effect on patients outcome. Every effort should be spent to assure that LN patients are maintained on these drugs. Lupus patients are chronic steroid users which make them liable for hypertension, diabetes mellitus (DM) ,and coronary artery disease (CAD). Numerous studies have shown beneficial effects of using ACEI in the management and prevention of these conditions. Unfortunately, many clinicians including rheumatologists tend not to use ACEI/ARBs (angiotensin receptors blockers) commonly in SLE patients or they delay introducing them early in the course of the disease. One possible reason for this delay is that physicians tend to focus more on acute and dramatic presentations of SLE rather than monitoring risk factors that would show benefical effects on the long term. Therefore, a comprehensive approach to care for lupus patients should be followed.

6. Cardiovascular involvement in SLE

SLE is associated with a variety of cardiovascular manifestations; some are life threatening (including myocardial infarction) and others are much less serious. Threre are several risk factors for heart related conditions, many of which can be avoided. Cardiovascular disease is a major cause of morbidity and mortality in SLE.

Pericarditis remains the most common cardiovascular disease in SLE and occur in 12- 48% (Moder, Miller & Tazelaar, 1999). It should be included in the differential diagnosis of SLE patients presenting with shortness of breath, low grade fever,pleuritic chest pain and/or dry cough. ANA test should be ordered for any young lady in childbearing age with pleuritic chest pain. This is to avoid delaying the diagnosis of SLE as pericarditis can be a presenting feature. Other less frequent cardiac manifestations of SLE are myocrditis (which is usually silent), endocarditis with one characteristic but rare presentation as Libman-Sack endocarditis known as verrucous non bacterial thrombotic endocarditis, valvular disease, arrhythmias, pulmonary hypertension, and systemic hypertension.

6.1 SLE and accelarated atherosclerosis

Today with SLE patients living longer due to more effective drug therapies, CAD has become a leading cause of late mortality in SLE. Women with aged 35-44 were found to have 50 times more risk of myocardial infarctions than aged matched controls (Mazni et al, 1997). Several case-control studies, both autopsy studies and myocardial perfusion studies have consistently shown a 30-40% prevelance of sub-clinical CAD in SLE patient (Korkmaz, Cansu & Kasifoqlu, 2007). Despite an increasing appreciation of the importance of cardiovascular disease in SLE, recognition of traditional risk factors have been noted to be suboptimal. As an example, in one academic rheumatology practice, deficits in knowledge and management of cardiac risk factors were observed among both SLE patients and their physicians (Costenbader et al, 2004). This is again to emphasize the point of increase awareness of this serious issue in lupus patients. Lack of comprehensive approach to care for SLE patients may lead to significant delay in diagnosing a reversible cardiac risk factor. Obviously, this will result in delay in management and increase in cardiac morbidity and mortality.

Many cases with SLE have evidence of subclinical accelerated atherosclerosis (figure 1). It is related to both traditional and non traditional risk factors for CAD. The traditional risk factors are demographics, family history, smoking, hypertension, DM, and dyslipidemia, while the non traditional risk factors include chronic inflammation, presence of autoantibodies, prolonged vascular inflamation, corticosrteroid use (10 mg change in prednisolone lead to change in mean arterial pressure of 1.1 mmHg after adjustment for age, weight and antihypertensive drug use, and 10 mg increase in prednisolone was associated with a mean weight change of 5.50 ±1.23 (Petri, 2000)), renal disease and antiphospholipd antibodies. One factor that has repeatedly been shown to affect the prevelance of CAD in SLE is active disease. Appropriate management of active SLE is one of the best preventitive measures. Due to the high prevelance of CAD in SLE patient, SLE itself should be viewed as a CAD risk factor in the same way as DM is (Bradley, 2009; Shah, Shah & Krishnan, 2009).

SLE patients should have an annual fasting blood glucose and a urinalysis at every clinic visit to assess for protienuria, glucosuria and hematuria. Patients with evidence of impaired glucose tolerance should undergo dietary changes to prevent frank diabetes from developing. Blood pressure(BP) should be followed at every clinical visit with a goal BP of less than 130/80 mmHg. For prehypertensive patients, the physician first should try therapeutic lifestyle changes (exercise and diet modification) and assess renal function. If blood pressure is consistently above 140/90 mmHg, despite therapeutic lifestyle changes, then antihypertensive medications should be started with prefarable drugs such as ACEI. The cholesterol recommandation for lupus patients are more stringent than those for the average patients. Lupus patients should have an annual fasting lipid profile with a goal LDL <100 mg/dl (<2.6 mmol/L) (Wajed et al, 2004). Statin therapy is indicated for LDL>130 mg/dl (> 3.4 mmol/L) even in those without traditional CAD risk factors. Statins have been shown to directly improve endothelial function even in patient with normal lipid profile (Vaughan et al, 2000; Laufs et al, 1998). Also, these patients should be counseled on smoking cessation and weight reduction if their BMI >25. Low dose aspirin should be considered for those patients with traditional risk factors and those that are antiphospholipid antibody positive (Erkan et al, 2002; Bertsias et al, 2008; Wahl et al, 2000). Screening patients at higher risk by non invasive techniques like carotid Duplex or Single Photon Emission Computed Tomography-Dual Isotope Myocardial Perfusion Imaging (SPECT-DIMPI) can help in early detection of subclinical atherosclerosis (Sella et al, 2003). To prevent long-term cardiovascular consequences, these patients should be treated aggressively, both to control their primary lupus disease activity and to minimize modifiable CAD risk factors. Life style modification, weight reduction, statins for hyperlipidemia, controlling blood pressure, controlling DM and minimizing the glucocorticoids use all these can minimize the CAD in SLE patients.

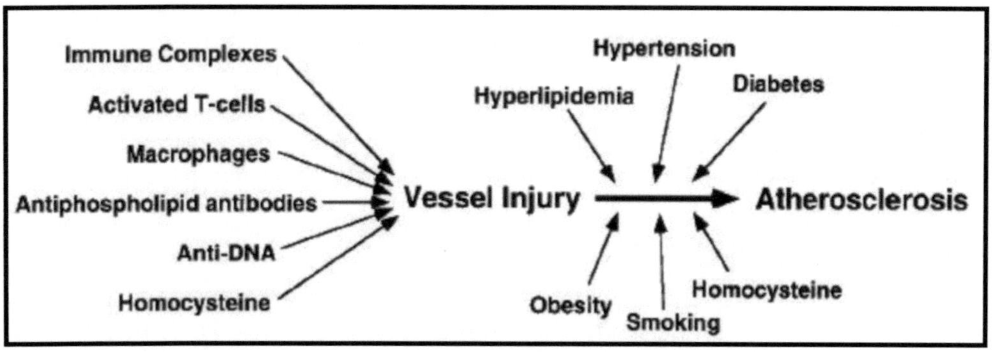

Fig. 1. Two-stage model of accelerated atherosclerosis in SLE (Petri, 2000)

7. The role of antimalarial drugs in SLE

Currently, there is over-emphasis from many international authorities in SLE on the need to maintain all lupus patients on antimalarial drugs (AMD). This is based on the abundance of data that confirm their huge beneficial effects in SLE. They are one of the most widely tolerated medications used in the treatment of SLE since 1955 (Scherbel, Schuchter & Harrison, 1957; Tye et al, 1959). They are safe even during pregnancy. Like any other medication, they have their side effects. However, an antimalarial drug like hydroxychloroquine (HCQ) on a daily low dose has no or mild side effects and serious complications are rare. Ocular toxicity is the most important toxicity of HCQ, so regular ophthalmological check up is important. Chloroquine is found to have more side effects than hydroxychloroquine. Nowadays, AMD are not only used for patients with organ damage or patients with active disease but they are essential and key treatment for all patients with SLE. They should be started alone or with other medications once the diagnosis is made. A recent data showed the beneficial effects not only on the disease itself but on many other factors. For this reason, AMD should never be stopped in patients with SLE. Over the last decades many studies were done on AMD (especially HCQ) and it showed that HCQ has an effect in lowering fasting glucose and calculated insulin resistance (Penn et al, 2010) and reducing insulin degradation (Smith et al, 1987). There is significant reduction in total cholesterol, triglyceride (TG), LDL and very low density lipoprotein(VLDL) and significant increase in high density lipoprotein (HDL) level among patients using AMD and prednisolone than those with prednisolone alone (Borba & Bonfa, 2001; Rahman, 1999; Tam et al, 2000). As the HCQ showed its effect on glycemic control and lipid profile, it might decrease the risk for atherosclerosis. In addition, HCQ inhibits platelet aggregation and adhesion (Petri, 1996) so it is a mild anticoagulant and can decrease the risk of thrombosis (both arterial and venous) in patients with SLE (Kaiser, Cleveland & Criswell, 2009; Wallace, 1987) but this effect is still under trials. Data showed protective effect of HCQ on the BMD especially on the spine (Mok, Mak & Ma, 2005). Lupus activity was significantly reduced among patients who were using HCQ, and can reach up to 50% in some studies (Ruiz-Irastorza et al, 2010). It has positive impact on the survival and can protect against irreversible organ damage. As SLE and other rheumatological diseases affect female in child bearing age and they will have concerns regarding taking medications during pregnancy. HCQ does not appear to have effect on the fetus and it is not associated with any congenital anomalies. In addition data showed that its use during pregnancy decreases lupus activity. Other non-rheumatological specialities like nephrology and obstetrics and gynaecology may underestimate the clinical value of continuing AMD in all SLE patients. LN patients who are followed exclusively by nephrologists are not maintained on HCQ as observed in some centres unfortunately. This is probably because some believe that HCQ is not considered as one of the standard therapies for LN. However, AMD are standard therapies for SLE.

8. Rare manifestations of SLE

One of the approaches to avoid delay in SLE diagnosis and management is to recognize rare presentations of SLE. Fever of unknown origin is an example of this. Fever by itself is very common in SLE. It may affect up to 50% of SLE patients as a sign of active disease (Petri, 2002). Patients with SLE frequently develop abnormalities in one or more of the three blood cell lines. Awareness of different hematological abnormalities affecting SLE patients is essential. The association between idiopathic thrombocytopenic purpura (ITP), thrombotic thrombocytopenic purpura (TTP) and SLE should be noted. Rare entities like Kikuchi-Fujimoto's disease (KFD) or histiocytic necrotizing lymphadenitis (a benign, self-limited disease of unknown etiology which affects mainly young women, characterized by localized lymphadenopathy, predominantly in the cervical region, fever and leukopenia) has been reported in association with SLE. It can present before, at the same time, or after the clinical appearance of KFD (Boddaert, Huong et al. 2004).

8.1 Kikuchi-Fujimoto disease

Kikuchi-Fujimoto disease (KFD) or Necrotizing Lymphadenitis is a rare, benign, self-limited disease that was first reported in Japan in 1972. It affects the female predominantly with female to male ratio 4:1 (Al Salloum, 1998; Dorfman, 1987; Lopez et al, 2000). It usually resolves spontaneously between one and four months (Santana et al, 2005) and up to six months in another study (Kucukardali et al, 2007). Although it is benign, there are reported cases of disease progression and mortality rate can reach up to 2.1% (Kucukardali et al, 2007). KFD is found to be associated with many comorbid diseases; SLE was the most frequently associated with it. Among 224 cases with KFD, 32 of them had SLE. Of these, eighteen (56%) had both diseases together, six (19%) developed SLE later, four (12%) already had SLE previously and four (12%) had incomplete SLE as they did not meet the ACR criteria for SLE (Kucukardali, Solmazgul et al. 2007).

8.2 Thrombotic Thrombocytopenia Purpura (TTP)

TTP is a life threatening condition in which there is platelet aggregation that result in microangiopathic haemolytic anaemia (MAHA) and thrombocytopenia. It presents with the pentad of MAHA, thrombocytopenia, fever, acute renal failure and neurological manifestations. SLE is one of its secondary causes and it correlates with disease activity (Cheung, 2006*)* but rarely occurs as a first manifestation although there was a reported case in which a patient was diagnosed to have TTP and SLE simultaneously (Vasoo, Thumboo & Fong, 2002). Making the diagnosis of TTP in SLE patient is difficult as classical TTP symptoms may be due to SLE disease activity. The diagnosis of TTP can be established by the presence of thrombocytopenia, fragmented red blood cells (schistocytes) in blood film, increase billirubin and lactate dehydrogenase, high urea and creatinine, normal coagulation profile and negative Coomb's test. It is important to rule out other serious conditions like disseminated intravascular coagulation (DIC) and intracranial haemorrhage (thrombocytopenia and neurological manifestation) by ordering coagulation profile and CT head respectively. The hallmark of TTP is detection fragmented RBC's in blood film. It is mandatory to have a peripheral smear conducted in any SLE patient presenting with new onset of anemia and thrombocytopenia. It is obvious that early diagnosis and aggressive treatment can make a huge difference in outcome.

8.3 Immune Thrombocytopenic Purpura (ITP)

ITP is a disease characterized by the presence of antibodies against platelets. This results in early clearance of platelets particularly by the spleen, and decreases their life span from 7-10 days to few hours. It presents by symptoms related to decrease platelet count as petechial haemorrhage, easy bruising, gum bleeding or epistaxis and menorrhagia in women. Intracranial bleeding is rare. ITP is a diagnosis of exclusion as more serious conditions like haematological malignancies must be ruled out first especially in people more than 60 years of age. It is characterized by presence of low platelet and normal haemoglobin and white blood cells count (WBC) except if there is concomitant iron deficiency anaemia or anaemia of chronic disease, normal PT and PTT, decrease platelet or presence of giant platelet in peripheral blood film and increase the number of megakaryocyte in bone marrow. An association between ITP and SLE has been recognized for decades and it can be the first manifestation in some patients with SLE (Jun, et al, 2008; Mestanza-Peralta et al, 1997). It has been estimated that 3-15% of patients with apparently isolated ITP go on to develop SLE (Karpatkin, 1980).

8.4 Fever of Unknown Origin (FUO)

FUO is a documented fever of >38°C on several occasions, for> 3 weeks without reaching the diagnosis after the initial diagnostic workup (Abdelbaky et al., 2011). FUO remains an important health problem that requires demanding efforts in order to reach the diagnosis despite the presence of advanced technology. Infections, connective tissue diseases, neoplasms are major causes that should be first ruled out before thinking about other causes. It was shown that among 100 patients with FUO, 50% were found to have infections, 24% were found to have connective tissue diseases (33.3% of them diagnosed as SLE, 20.8% familial Mediterranian fever, 16.6% rheumatoid arthritis, 12.5% Still's disease & rheumatic fever and 4.3% Behcet's disease/ Chron's disease), no cause was identified in 11%, while the remaining 8% and 7% were found to have miscellaneous causes and neoplasia respectively (Abdelbaky et al, 2011).

How to avoid delay in SLE diagnosis and management?	Action plan
1. Consider SLE in the differential diagnosis of multisystemic presentations.	• Order screening ANA.
2. Assure screening for MSK abnormalities in all acutely ill patients.	• Ask about joint pain, swelling and morning stiffness. • Perform simple active range of motion test as a screening tool for MSK abnormalities.
3. Be aware of neurological manifestations of SLE (seizure, stroke, TM, MG, GBM, etc).	• Include in your work-up screening ANA. • Educate clinicians taking care of neurological diseases about this.
4. Be aware of CAD risk factors in SLE patients	• Life style modifications, weight reduction, check BP in every clinic visit, annual fasting blood glucose, statins for LDL>130mg/dl,
5. to decrese disease activity and possibly to decrease the risk of atherosclerosis.	• Maintain all patients on HCQ
6. Fever is common in SLE and it might be a presenting feature.	• Order screening ANA.
7. Be aware of different hematological abnormalities related to SLE (cytopenias, ITP, KFD, TTP).	• Order screening ANA. • Order peripheral smear for any SLE patient with new onset anemia and thrombocytopenia.
8. SLE can still affect elderly population.	• Order screening ANA as appropriate to the clinical presentation. • Educate clinicians taking care of elderly patients about this.

Table 4. Some recommended steps to avoid delay in SLE diagnosis and management

9. Conclusion

We discussed in this chapter several issues that can face clinicians in their daily work with SLE patients. Our aim was to focus on how to prevent delay in SLE diagnosis and management. Table 4 represents some recommended steps that might help in this regard. Enhancing MSK examination skills among clinicans in general is an international concern. This clearly will result in early detection of patients with clinical evidence of arthritis including SLE. There are several clinical settings and presentations where SLE should be considered. Late-onset SLE can affect elderly patients with few differences than classical SLE patients. NPSLE represents a diagnositic challenge to clinicians. There are 19 neuropsychiatric syndromes defined by ACR as an associated feature with NPSLE. Delay in considering kidney biopsy in SLE patients once indicated results in poor renal outcomes. Adjusting risk factors for renal disease like proteinuria, hypertension and dyslipidemia is vaguely considered by some clinicans. The leading cause of mortality in SLE is cardiac. Clinicans taking care of SLE patients should put prevention of cardiac morbidities and mortalities an important goal in their management agenda. With new modalities of treatment and the wide use of AMD since 1955 there is significant improvement in survival and quality of life in patients with SLE. Therefore, all lupus patients should be maintained on AMD like HCQ. SLE can present initially with a variety of hematological maifestations like ITP , TTP and KFD. SLE should be in the differenrtial diagnosis of FUO.

10. Acknowledgments

The work to produce this chapter was supported by Alzaidi's Chair of research in rheumatic diseases- Umm Alqura University.

11. References

Association of American Medical Colleges (2005) *Contemporary issues in medicine.* Washington, DC: Musculoskeletal Medicine Education.

Abdelbaky, M.S. et al (2011) Prevalence of connective tissue diseases in Egyptian patients presenting with Fever of unknown origin. *Clinical Medicine Insights. Arthritis & Musculoskseletal Disorders,* 4, pp.33-41.

Ahern, M.J. et al (1991) The musculo-skeletal examination: a neglected clinical skill. *Australian New Zealand Journal of Medicine,* 21(3), pp.303-306.

Akesson, K., Dreinhofer, K.E., & Woolf, A.D. (2003) Improved education in musculoskeletal conditions is necessary for all doctors, *Bulletin of the World Hlealth Organization,* 81(9), pp.677-683.

Almoallim, H. (2010) Knowledge and Skills Competencies for the Undergraduate Internal Medicine Curriculum in Saudi Arabia. [Internet] Available from : http://services.aamc.org/30/mededportal/servlet/s/segment/mededportal/?subid=8177 .

Almoallin, H. et al (2009) Transverse myelitis as a presenting feature of late onset systemic lupus erythematosus. *Annals of Saudi Medicine,* 29 (2), pp.156-167.

Almoallim, H. et al (2007) Delayed diagnosis of systemic lupus erythematosus due to lack of competency skills in musculoskeletal examination. *Clinical Rheumatology*, 26 (1), pp.131-133.

Al Salloum, A.A. (1998) Kikuchi's disease and systemic lupus erythematoisus in a Saudi child. *Annals of Saudi Medicine*, 18(1), pp.51-53.

Apperloo, A.J., de Zeeuw, D. & de Jong, P.E. (1994) Discordant effects of enalapril and lisnopril on systemic and renal hemodynamics. *Clinical Pharmacology and Therapeutics*, 56 (6 Pt.1), pp.647-658.

Badley, E.M., Rasooly, I. & Webster, G.K. (1994) Relative importance of musculoskeletal disorders as a cause of chronic health problems, disability, and health care utilization: findings from the 1990 Ontario Health Survey. *Journal of Rheumatology*, 21(3), pp.505-514.

Beattie, K.A. et al (2008) Validation of the GALS musculosketal screening exam for use in primary care: a pilot study. *BMC Musculoskeletal Disorders*, 9, pp.115.

Belostocki, K.B. & Paget, S.A. (2002) Inflammatory rheumatologic disorders in the elderly. Unusual presentations, altered outlooks. *Postgraduate Medicine*, 111 (4), pp.72-74.

Bertoli, A.M. et al (2006) Systemic lupus erythematosus in a multiethnic US cohort. XXXIII. Clinical [corrected] features, course, and outcome in patients with late-onset disease. *Arthritis and Rheumatism*, 54(5), pp.1580-1587.

Bertsias, G. et al (2008) EULAR recommendations for the management of systemic lupus erythematosus. Reprot of a Task Force of the EULAR Standing Committee for International Clinical Studies Including Therapeutics. *Annals of the Rheumatic Diseases*, 67(2), pp.195-205.

Bhinder, S., Majithia, V. & Harisdangkul, V. (2006) Myasthenia gravic and systemic lupus erythematosus: truly associated or coincidental - two case reports and review of the literature. *Clinical Rheumatology*, 25(4), pp.555-556.

Boddaert, J. et al. (2004) Late-onset systemic lupus erythematosus: a personal series of 47 patients and pooled analysis of 714 cases in the literature. *Medicine (Baltimore)*, 83(6), pp.348-359.

Borba, E.F. & Bonfa, E. (2001) Longterm beneficial effect of chloroquine diphosphate on lipoprotein profile in lupus patients with and without steroid therapy. *Journal of Rheumatology*, 28(4), pp.780-785.

Bradley, I. (2009) Systematic lupus erythematosus and premature coronary artery disease. [Online] Available from: http://www/clinicalcorrelations.org/?p=4593 [Accessed 9 August 2011]

Brazy, P.C. & Fitzwilliam, J.F. (1990) Progressive renal disease: role of race and antihypertensive medications. *Kidney International*, 37(4), pp.1113-1119.

Buckheit, J.B. et al (1997) Modeling of progressive glomerular injury in humans with lupus nephritis. *American Journal of Rheumatology*, 273 (1 Pt.2), pp.F158-F169.

Bulkley, B.H, & Roberts, W.C. (1975) The heart in systemic lupus erythematosus and the changes induced in it by corticosteroid therapy. A study of 36 necropsy patients. *American Journal of Medicine*, 58(2), pp.243-264.

Cameron, J.S. (1999a) Lupus nephritis. *Journal of the American Society of Nephrology*, 10(2), pp.413-424.

Cameron, J.S. (1999b) Lupus nephritis: an historical perspective 1968-1998. *Journal of Nephrology*, 12(Suppl 2), pp.S29-S41.

Chen, H.C. et al (2004) Longitudinal myelitis as an initial manifestation of systemic lupus erythematosus. *American Journal of the Medical Sciences*, 327(2), pp.105-108.

Cheung, W.Y. (2006) Thrombotic thrombocytopenic purpura and systemic lupus erythematosus-distinct entities or overlapping syndromes? *Transfusion & Apheresis Science*, 34(3), pp.263-266.

Christopher-Stine, L, et al (2007) Renal biopsy in lupus patients with low levels of proteinuria. *Journal of Rheumatology*, 34(2), pp.332-335.

Clark, M.L., Hutchison, C.R. & Lockyer, J.M. (2010) Musculoskeletal education: a curriculum evaluation at one univeristy. *BMC Medical Education*, 10, p.93.

Clawson, D.K., Jackson, D.W. & Ostergaard, D.J. (2001) It's past time to reform the musculoskeletal curriculum. *Academic Medicine*, 76(7), pp.709-710.

Colpan, A. et al (2007) Fever of unknown origin: analysis of 71 consecutive cases. *American Journal of the Medical Sciences*, 334(2), pp.92-96.

Contreras, G. et al. (2002) Lupus nephritis: a clinical review for practicingg nephrologists. *Clinical Nephrology*, 57(2), pp.95-107.

Costallat, L.T. & Coimbra, A.M. (1994) Systemic lupus erythematosus: clinical and laboratory aspects related to age at disease onset. *Clinical and Experimental Rheumatology*, 12(6), pp.603-607.

Costenbader, K.H. et al (2004) Cardiac risk factor awareness and management in patients with systemic lupus erythematosus. *Arthritis & Rheumatism*, 51(6), pp.983-988.

Day, C.S. et al (2007) Musculoskeletal medicine: an assessment of the attitudes and knowledge of medical students at Harvard Medical School. *Academic Medicine*, 82(5), pp.452-457

D'Cruz, D.P. et al (2004) Transverse myelitis as the first manifestation of systemic lupus erythematosus or lupus-like disease: good functional outcome and relevance of antiphospholipid antibodies. *Journal of Rheumatology*, 31(2), pp.280-2285.

Dequeker, J., Esselens, G. & Westhovens, R. (2007) Educational issues in rheumatology. The musculoskeletal examination: a neglected skill. *Clinical Rheumatology*, 26(1), pp.5-7.

Doherty, M., Abawi, J. & Pattrick, M. (1990) Audit of medical inpatient examination: a cry from the joint. *Journal of the Royal College of Physicians of London*, 24(2), pp.115-118.

Doherty, M. et al (1992) The "GALS" locomotor screen. *Annals of the Rheumatic Diseases*, 51(10), pp.1165-1169.

Dorfman, R.F. (1987) Histiocytic necrotizing lymphadenitis of Kikuchi and Fujimoto. *Archives of Pathology & Laboratory Medicine*, 111(11), pp.1026-1029.

Dubois, E.L & Wallace, D.J. Clinical and laboratory manifestations of systemic lupus erythematosus. *In* Wallace, D.J. & Dubois, E.L. eds. *Dubois lupus erythomatosus*. 3rd ed. Philadelphia: Lea & Febiger. pp. 317-449.

Duran-Barragan, S. et al (2008) Angiotensin-converting enzyme inhibitors delay the occurrence of renal involvement and are associated with a decreased risk of disease activity in patients with systemic lupus erythematosus—results from

LUMINA (LIX): a multiethnic US cohort. *Rheumatology (Oxford),* 47(7), pp.1093-1096.

Eilertsen, G.O. et al (2011) Decreaedd incidence of lupus nephritis in northern Norway is linked to increased use of antihypertensive and anticoagulant therapy. *Nephrology, Dialysis , Transplantation,* 26(2), pp.520-627.

Erkan, D. et al (2002) A cross-sectional study of clinical thrombotic risk factors and preventive treatments in antiphospholipid syndrome. *Rheumatology (Oxford),* 41(8), pp.924-929.

Esdaile, J.M. et al (1994) The benefit of eaerly treatment with immunosuppressive agents in lupus nephritis. *Journal of Rheumatology,* 21(11), pp.2046-2051.

Faurschou, M. et al (2006) Prognostic factors in lupus nephritis: diagnostic and therapeutic delay increases the risk of terminal renal failure. *Journal of Rheumatology,* 33(8), pp.1563-1569.

Fiehn, C. et al (2005) Lack of evidence for inhibition of angiogenesis as a central mechanism of the antiarthritic effect of methotrexate. *Rheumatology International,* 25(2), pp.108-113.

The GISEN Group (1997) Randomised placebo-controlled trial of effect of ramipril on decline in glomerular filtration rate and risk of terminal renal failure in proteinuric, non-diabetic nephropathy. *Lancet,* 349 (9069), pp.1857-1863.

Goldenberg, D.L. et al (1985) Rheumatology training at internal medicine and family practice residency programs. *Arthritis & Rheumatism,* 28(4), pp.471-476.

Goto, M. et al., (1992) Constitutive production of angiotensin convertiing enzyme from rheumatoid nodule cells under serum free conditions. *Annals of the Rheumatic Diseases,* 51(6), pp.741-742.

Haider, Y.S. & Roberts, W.C. (1981) Coronary arterial disease in systemic lupus erythematosus; quantification of degrees of narrowing in 22 necropsy patients (21 women) aged 16 to 37 years. *American Journal of Medicine,* 70(4), pp.775-781.

Hochberg, M.C. et al (1985) Systematic lupus erythematosus: a review of clinico-laboratory features and immunogenetic markers in 150 patients with emphasis on demographic subsets. *Medicine (Baltimore),* 64(5), pp.285-285.

Jacobsen, S. et al (1998) A multicentre study of 513 Danish patients with systemic lupus erythematosus.I. Disease manifestations and analyses of clinical subsets. *Clinical Rheumatology,* 17(6), pp.568-477.

Jones, A., Maddison, P. & Doherty, M. (1992) Teaching rheumatology to medical students: current practice and future aims. *Journal of the Royal College of Physicians of London,* 26(1), pp.41-43.

Joseph, F.G., Lammie, G.A. & Scolding, N.J. (2007) CNS lupus: a study of 41 patients. *Neurology,* 69 (7), pp.644-654.

Joshua, A.M., Celermajer, D.S. & Stockler, M.R. (2005) Beauty is in the eye of the examiner: reaching agreement about physical signs and their value. *Internal Medicine Journal,* 35(3), pp.178-187.

Jun, S.E., Park, S.S. & Lim, Y.T. (2008) Prevalence and clinical significance of the positive antinuclear antibody in chhildren with idiopathic thrombocytopenic purpura. *Korean Journal of Pediatrics,* 51(11), pp.1217-1221.

Kaiser, R., Cleveland, C.M. & Criswell, LA. (2009) Risk and protective factors for thrombosis in systemic lupus erythematosus: results from a large, multi-ethnic cohort. *Annals of the Rheumatic Diseases*, 68(2), pp.238-241.

Karoubi Nordon, E. et al (2007) Late onset systemic lupus erythematosus: a new approach. *Lupus*, 16(12), pp. 1011-1014.

Karpatkin, S. (1980) Autoimmune thrombocytopenic purpura. *Blood*, 56(3), pp.329-343.

Korkmaz, C., Cansu, D.U. & Kasifoqlu, T. (2007) Myocardial infarction in young patients (< or =35 years of age) with systemic lupus erythematosus: a case report and clinical analysis of the literature. *Lupus*, 16(4), pp.289-297.

Kovacs, B. et al (2000) Transverse myelopathy in systemic lupus erythematosus: an analysis of 14 cases and review of the literature. *Annals of the Rheumatic Diseases*, 59(2), pp.120-124.

Kucukardali, Y. et al (2007) Kikuchi-Fujimoto disease: analysis of 244 cases. *Clinical Rheumatology*, 26(1), pp. 50-54.

Laufs, U. et al (1998) Upregulation of endothelial nitric oxide synthase by HMG CoA reductase inhibitors. *Circulation*,, 97(12), pp.1129-1135.

Leneman, F. (1966) The Guillain-Barre syndro+me. Definition, etiology, and review of 1,100 cases. *Archives of Internal Medicine*, 118(2), pp.139-144.

Lewis, E.J. et al (1993) The effect of angiotensin-converting-enzyme inhibition on diabetic nephropathy. *New England Journal of Medicine*, 329(20), pp.1456-1462.

Lidgren, L. (2003) The bone and joint decade 2000-2010. *Bulletin of the World Health Organization*, 81(9), p.629.

Lillicrap, M.S., Bryne, E. & Speed, C.A. (2003) Musculoskeletal assessment of general medical in-patients—joints still crying out for attention. *Rheumatology (Oxford)*, 42(8), pp.951-954.

Lopez, C. et al (2000) Kikuchi-Fujimoto necrotizing lymphadenitis associated with cutaneous lupus erythematosus: a case report. *American Journal of Dermatopathology*, 22(4), pp.328-333.

Maddison, P.J. (1987) Systemic lupus erythematosus in the elderly. *Journal of Rheumatology Supplements*, 14 (Suppl 13), pp.182-187.

Manzi, S. et al (1997) Age-specific incidence rates of myocardial infarction and angina in women with systemic lupus erythematosus: comparison with the Framingham Study. *American Journal of Epidemiology*, 145(5), pp.408-415.

Maschio, G. et al (1996) Effect of the angiotensin-converting enzymee inhibitorr benazepril on the progression of chronic renal insufficiency. *New England Journal of Medicine*, 334(15), pp.939-945.

Maschio, G. et al (1989) Serum lipids in patients with chronic renal failure on long-term, protein-restricted diets. *American Journal of Medicine*, 87(5N), pp.51N-54N.

Matzkin, E. et al (2005) Adequacy of education in musculoskeletal medicine. *Journal of Bone & Joint Surgery (American)*, 87(2), pp.310-314.

Mestanza-Peralta, M. et al (1997) Thrombocytopenic purpura as initial manifestation of systemic lupus erythematosus. *Journal of Rheumatology*, 24(5), pp.867-870.

Ministry of Health (2009) *The Annual Health Report – 1430H*. Riyadh: Ministry of Health.

Mitsikostas, D.D., Sfikakis, P.P. & Goadsby, P.J. (2004) A meta-analysis for headache in systemic lupus erythematosus: the evidence and the myth. *Brain*, 127(Pt.5), pp.1200-1209.

Moder, K.G., Miller, T.D. & Tazelaar, H.D. (1999) Cardiac involvement in systemic lupus erythematosus. *Mayo Clinic Proceedings*, 74(3), pp.275-284.

Mok, C.C., Mak, A. & Ma, K.M. (2005) Bone mineral density in postmenopausal Chinese patients with systemic lupus erythematosus. *Lupus*, 14(2), pp.106-112.

Padovan, M. et al (2007) Late onset systemic lupus erythematosus: no substantial differences using different cut-off ages. *Rheumatology International*, 27(8), pp.735-741.

Paget, S. (2007) The European League Against Rheumatism guidelines for early arthritis. *Nature Clinical Practice Rheumatology*, 3(7), pp.374-375.

Penn, S.K. et al (2010) Hydroxychloroquine and glycemia in women with rheumatoid arthritis and systemic lupus erythematosus. *Journal of Rheumatology*, 37(6), pp.1136-1142.

Peterson, J.C. et al (1995) Blood pressure control, proteinuria, and the progression of renal disease. *Annals of Internal Medicine*, 123(10), pp.754-762.

Petri, M. (1996) Hydroxychloroquine use in the Baltimore Lupus Cohort: effects on lipids, glucose and thrombosis. *Lupus*, 5 (Suppl 1), pp.S16-S22.

Petri, M. (2000) Detection of coronary artery disease and the role of traditional risk factors in the Hopkins Lupus Cohort. *Lupus*, 9(3), pp.170-175.

Petri, M. (2002) Epidemiology of systemic lupus erythematosus. *Best Practice & Research Clinical Rheumatology*, 16(5), pp.847-858.

Pinney, S.J. & Regan, W.D. (2001) Educating medical students about musculoskeletal problems. Are community needs reflected in the curricula of Canadian medical schools? *Journal of Bone & Joint Surgery (American)*, 83-A(9), pp.1317-1320.

Pu, S.J. et al (2000) The clinical features and prognosis of lupus with disease onset at age 65 and older. *Lupus*, 9(2), pp.96-100.

Rahman, P. (1999) The cholesterol lowering effect of antimalarial drugs is enhanced in patients with lupus taking corticosteroid drugs. *Journal of Rheumatology*, 26(2), pp.325-330.

Rasker, J.J. (1995) Rheumatology in general practice. *British Journal of Rheumatology*, 34(6), pp.494-497.

Rosansky, S.J. et al (1990) The association of blood pressure levels and change in renal function in hypertensive and nonhypertensive subjects. *Archives of Internal Medicine*, 150(10), pp.2073-2076.

Rovensky, J.. & Tuchynova, A. (2008) Systemic lupus erythematosus in the elderly. *Autoimmunity Reviews*, 7(3), pp.235-239.

Ruiz-Irastorza, G. et al (2010) Clinical efficacy and side effects of antimalarials in systemic erythematosus: a systematic review. *Annals of the Rheumatic Diseases*, 69(1), pp.20-28.

Samuelsson, O. et al (1993). Apolipoprotein-B-containing lipoproteins and the progression of renal insufficiency. *Nephron*, 63(3), pp.279-285.

Santana, A. et al (2005). Kikuchi-Fujimoto's disesase associated with systemic lupus erythematosus: case report and review of the literature. *Clinical Rheumatology*, 24(1), pp.60-63.

Scherbel, A.L., Schuchter, S.L. & Harrison, J.W. Comparison of effects of two antimalarial agents, hydroxychloroquine sulfate and chloroquine phosphate, in patients with rheumatoid arthritis. *Cleveland Clinic Quaterly*, 24(2), pp.98-104.

Seligman, V.A. et al (2002) Demographic differences in the development of lupus nephritis: a retrospective analysis. *American Journal of Medicine*, 112(9), pp.726-729.

Sella, E.M. et al (2003) Myocardial perfusion scintigraphy and coronary disease risk factors in systemic lupus erythematosus. *Annals of the Rheumatic Diseases*, 62(11), pp.1066-1070.

Shah, M.A., Shah, A.M. & Krishnan, E. (2009) Poor outcomes after acute myocardial infarction in systemic lupus erythematosus. *Journal of Rheumatology*, 36(3), pp.570-575,

Shulman, N.B. et al (1989) Prognostic value of serum creatinine and effect of treatment of hypertension on renal function. *Hypertension*, 13 (Suppl 5), pp.I80-I90.

Sirisena, D. et al (2011) Musculoskeletal examination—an ignored aspect. Why are we still failing the patients? *Clinical Rheumatology*, 30(3), pp.403-407.

Smith, G.D. et al (1987) Effect of chloroquine on insulin and glucose homoeostasis in normal subjects and patients with non-insulin dependent diabetes mellitus. *British Medical Journal (Clinical Research Edition)*, 294(6570), pp.465-467.

Sthoeger, Z. et al (2006) High prevalence of systemic lupus erythematosus in 78 myasthenia gravis patients: a clinical and serologic study. *American Journal of Medical Sciences*, 33(1), pp.4-9.

Tam, L.S. et al (2000) Effect of antimalarial agents on the fasting lipid profile in systemic lupus erythematosus. *Journal of Rheumatology*, 27(9), pp.142-145.

Thompson, A.E. (2008) Improving undergraduate musculoskeletal education: a continuing challenge. *Journal of Rheumatology*, 35(12), pp.2298-2299.

Tye, M.J. et al (1959) Lupus erythematosus treated with a combination of quinacrine, hydroxychloroquine and chloroquine. *New England Journal of Medicine*, 260(2), pp.63-66.

Vaiopoulos, G. et al (1994) The association of systemic lupus erythematosus and myasthenia gravis. *Postgraduate Medicine Journal*, 70(828), pp.741-745.

Vasoo, S., Thumboo, J. & Fong, K.Y. (2002) Thrombotic thrombocytopenic purpura in systemic lupus erythematosus: disease activity and the use of cytotoxic drugs. *Lupus*, 11(7), pp. 443-450.

Vaughan, C.J., Gott, A.M. & Basson, C.T. (2000) The evolving role of statins in the management of atherosclerosis. *Journal of the American College of Cardiology*, 35(1), pp.1-10.

Veale, D. et al (1992) Production of angiotensin converting enzyme by rheumatoid synovial membrane. *Annals of the Rheumatic Diseases*, 51(4), pp.476-480.

Wahl, D.G. et al (2000) Prophylatic antithrombotic therapy for patients with systemic erythematosus with or without antiphospholipid antibodies: do the benefits outweigh the risks? A decision analysis. *Archives of Internal Medicine*, 160 (13), pp.2042-2048.

Wajed, J. et al (2004) Prevention of cardiovascular disease in systemic lupus erythematosus—proposed guidelines for risk factor management. *Rheumatology*, 43(1), pp.7-12.

Wallace, D.J. (1987) Does hydroxychloroquine sulfate prevent clot formation in systemic lupus erythematosus? *Arthritis & Rheumatism*, 30(12), pp.1435-1436.

Wen, Y.K. (2011) Renal biopsy findings in new-onset systemic lupus erythematosus with clinical renal disease. *International Urology & Nephrology* 00: 1-6 (accessed 8 August 2011)

Woolf, A.D., & Akesson, K. (2008) Primer: history and examination in the assessment of lusculoskeletal problems. *Nature Clinical Practice Rheumatology,* 5 (1), pp.26-33.

Woolf, A.D., Walsh N.E. & Akesson, K. (2004) Global core recommendations for a musculoskeletal undergraduate curriculum. *Annals of the Rheumatic Diseases*, 63(5), pp.517-524.

11

Kidney Manifestation of Systemic Lupus Erythematosus

Wael Habhab
Umm Alqura University, Makkah
Saudi Arabia

1. Introduction

Kidney disease secondary to SLE can affects up to 50% of patients with SLE and largely mediated by deposition of immune complex in the kidneys (1) (2).
The clinical diagnosis of lupus nephritis is usually made following a diagnostic kidney biopsy in the presence of proteinuria and/or hematouria,positive serology,and extrarenal manifestation of SLE. The presence of kidney disease is the most important predictor of morbidity and mortality in the patients with SLE.
Several demographic,serologic,and genetic risk factors are associated with an increased risk for developing kidney disease. Patient with lupus nephritis are more likely than SLE patients without kidney involvement to have a family history of SLE,anemia,high anti-dsDNA antibody titer,and hypocomplementemia. Children with SLE develop nephritis more frequently than adults and so do males.

2. Pathogenesis

Autoimmunity plays a major role in the pathogenesis of lupus nephritis. The immunologic mechanisms include production of autoantibodies directed against nuclear elements. These autoantibodies form pathogenic immune complexes. Deposition of these immune deposits in the kidneys initiates an inflammatory response by activating the complement cascade and recruiting inflammatory cells that can subsequently be observed on biopsy specimens.
Glomerular thrombosis is another mechanism that may play a role in pathogenesis of lupus nephritis, mainly in patients with antiphospholipid antibody syndrome, and is believed to be the result of antibodies directed against negatively charged phospholipid-protein complexes.

3. Symptoms and signs of lupus nephritis

Clinically lupus nephritis varies in its expression mild ,asymptomatic proteinuria to an overt nephrotic syndrome or acute nephritis associated with rapidly progressive azotemia. Glomerulonephritis is uncommonly the sentinel manifestation of SLE.
The key challenge for the clinician is to detect clinically significant lupus nephritis befor the appearance of the overt disease.

Patients can present with proteinuria during regular follow up. Hypertention is more common in patient with diffuse prolifrative lupus nephritis compared with focal prolifrative lupus nephritis or membranous lupus nephritis. Edema is an other presentation of lupus nephritis.

4. Prognostic factors

Different factors have been identified to predict the prognosis of lupus nephritis (3).
Histological factors:

- Histological class IV(diffuse proliferative LN)
- High activity and chronicity on Biopsy
- Crescents and interstitial fibrosis
- Segmental necrotizing lesion

Clinical Predictors:

- Hypertension
- Anemia
- high baseline creatinine
- high base line proteinuria
- Delay in therapy

Epidemiological Predictors

- Low socioeconomic status
- African American Race

5. Classification of Lupus Nephritis (LN)

Types of lupus nephritis

Renal biopsy is essential for the staging the type and the severity of lupus nephritis and planning the treatment.

Indication of renal biopsy

Renal biopsy is indicated in patients who have one or both of the following clinical manifestations:

- Protein excretion greater than 500 mg/day.
- An active urinary sediment with hematuria (five or more red blood cells per high power field, most of which are dysmorphic) and often pyuria and cellular casts. The urine may be contaminated with vaginal blood in menstruating women. Red cells from this source are not dysmorphic.

Lupus patients who have an inactive sediment and less than 500 mg/day of proteinuria are unlikely to have focal or diffuse proliferative or membranous lupus nephritis (LN). They may have minimal mesangial or mesangial proliferative disease, neither of which requires immunosuppressive treatment.

Such patients should be followed for evidence of progressive disease such as increasing proteinuria, emergence of an active sediment, and/or an increase in serum creatinine. These manifestations suggest transformation to a more severe lesion and warrant renal biopsy.

In patients with an inactive sediment and less than 500 mg/day of proteinuria, it is advisable to do a urinalysis every three to six months for three years; every three months is preferred in patients with anti-double-stranded DNA antibodies and/or hypocomplemententemia.

The initial classification is WHO that have been modified in 1982 and 1995(4).The most recent classification is ISN/RPS 2004(international society of nephrology and renal pathology society) (5).

DESIGNATION	DESCRIPTION
Class I: Minimal mesangial LGN	Near-normal glomeruli by LM; mesangial deposits are present by IF and/or EM
Class II: Mesangial proliferative LGN	Mesangial hypercellularity and matrix expansion, with mesangial deposits by IF and EM
Class III: Focal LGN	<50% of glomeruli display active or inactive segmental (<50% of the tuft) or global (>50% of the tuft) endocapillary proliferation or sclerosis; predominantly mesangial and subendothelial deposits are present on IF and EM
Class IV: Diffuse LGN	>50% of glomeruli have endocapillary or extracapillary glomerulonephritis;predominantly mesangial and subendothelial deposits are present on IF and EM; two subsets are defined
Class IV-S: Segmental diffuse LGN	>50% of affected glomeruli have segmental lesions
Class IV-G: Global diffuse LGN	>50% of affected glomeruli have global lesions
Class V: Membranous LGN	Capillary loop thickening in association with predominantly subepithelial deposits by IF and EM
Class VI: Advanced sclerosis	>90% of glomeruli are obsolescent, with substantial activity in remaining glomeruli

Table 1. International Society of Nephrology—Renal Pathology Society, 2004 Classification of Lupus Glomerulonephritis

Characteristic clinical features of patients with the various classes of pathology can be summarized as follows:

- Class I, Minimal mesangial lupus glomerulonephritis (LGN)—normal urine or microscopic hematuria
- Class II, Mesangial proliferative LGN—microscopic hematuria and/or low-grade proteinuria
- Class III, Focal proliferative LGN—nephritic urine sediment and subnephrotic proteinuria
- Class IV, Diffuse proliferative LGN—nephritic and nephrotic syndromes, hypertension, azotemia
- Class V, Membranous LGN—nephrotic syndrome
- Class VI, Sclerosing disease—hypertension and reduced kidney function

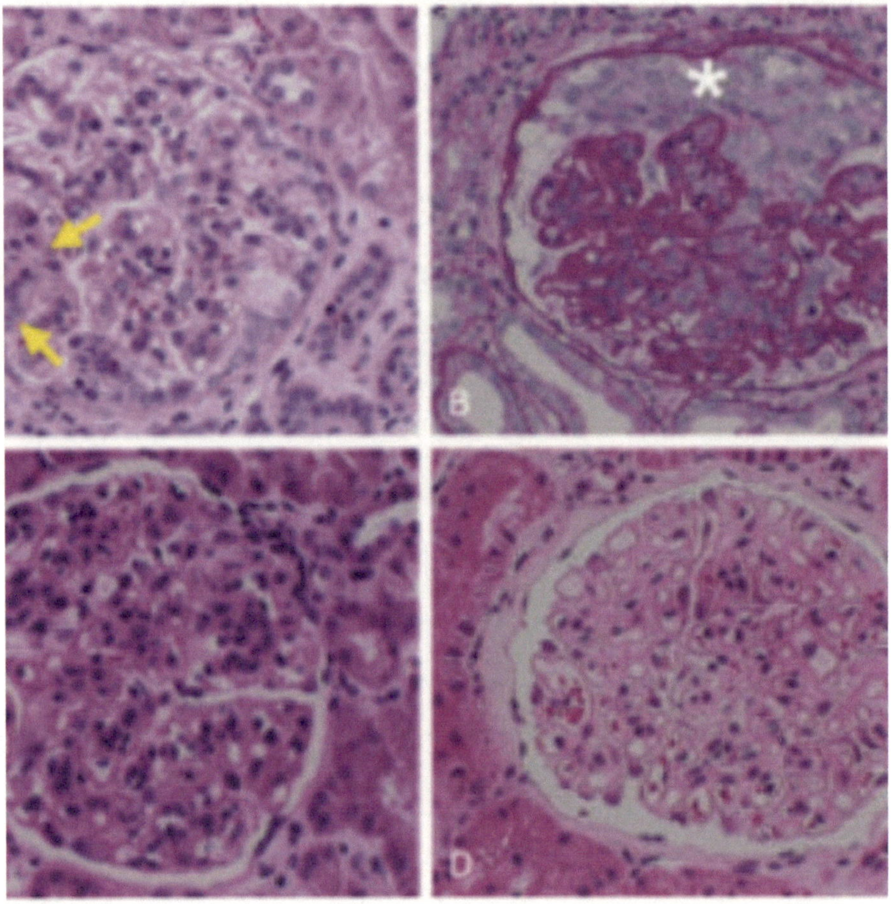

EM, electron microscopy; IF, immunofluorescence; LGN, lupus glomerulonephritis; LM, light microscopy

Fig. 1. Light microscopic changes in lupus glomerulonephritis (LGN). A, Segmental proliferative LGN. The glomerulus shows a discrete segmental lesion with karyorrhexis and necrosis *(gold arrows)*; the remaining capillary loops are patent with only mild mesangial expansion (hematoxylin and eosin stain). B, Global proliferative LGN with an extracapillary cellular crescent *(asterisk)*; the integrity of the glomerular tuft is compromised by proliferation and thickening of the capillary loops (hematoxylin and eosin stain). C, Pure global proliferative LGN (hematoxylin and eosin stain). D, Membranous LGN; capillary loops are uniformly thickened (hematoxylin and eosin stain).

6. Treatment of lupus nephritis

Treatment depends mainly on the clinical presentation and the pathological classification of LN. The treatment usually consists of two phases, the induction phase and the maintenance phase. The total duration of treatment around two years but it can varies based on the clinical response. But all patients need to be on non-immunosuppressive therapy.

Non-immunosuprressive therapy

Angiotensin inhibition - Administration of an angiotensin converting enzyme (ACE) inhibitor or an angiotensin II receptor blocker (ARB) is recommended in virtually all patients with proteinuric chronic kidney disease, since such therapy may significantly reduce the rate of disease progression, acting at least in part by lowering the intraglomerular pressure. The recommended goal for protein excretion is at least a 60 percent reduction from the baseline value and optimally less than 500 to 1000 mg/day. Patients with baseline protein excretion below 500 mg/day do not appear to benefit from angiotensin inhibition.(21).

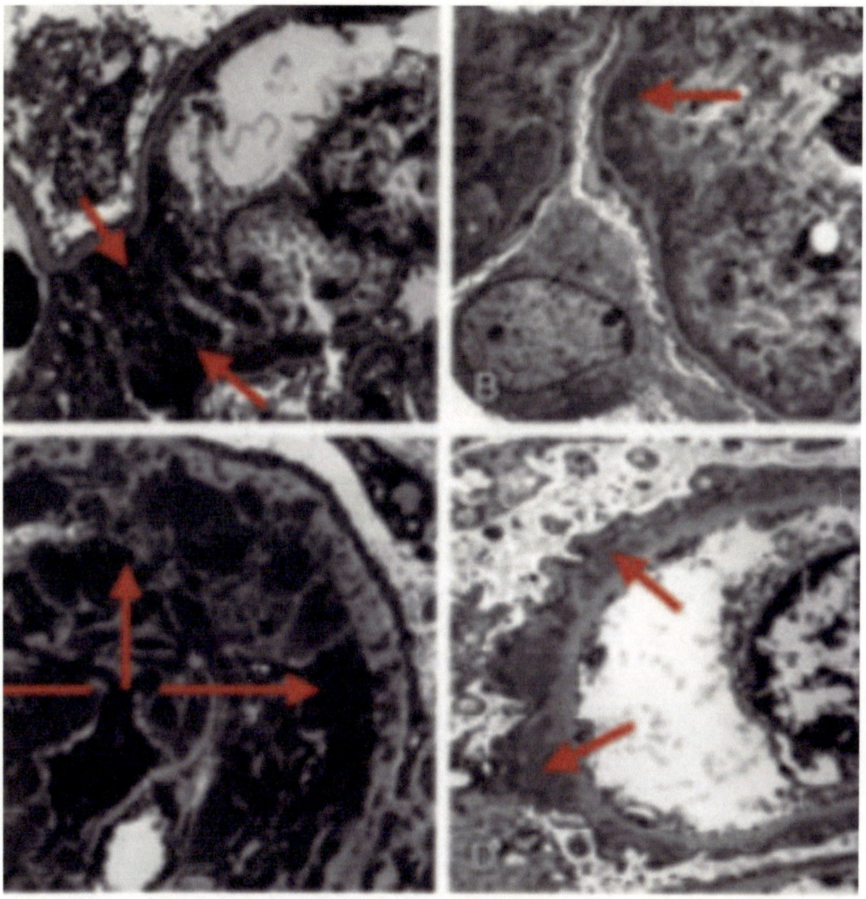

Fig. 2. Ultrastructural changes in lupus glomerulonephritis (LGN). A, Mesangial proliferative LGN; electron-dense deposits corresponding to immune complexes are concentrated in mesangial region *(red arrows)*. B and C, Continuum of subendothelial and intraluminal electron-dense deposits characteristic of proliferative forms of LGN *(red arrows)*. D, Subepithelial electron-dense deposits characteristic of membranous LGN *(red arrows)*.

Blood pressure control - The goal blood pressure in patients with any form of proteinuric chronic kidney disease is less than 130/80 mmHg, if the proteinuria is more than 3.5g/day the target is less than 125/70. Reaching this goal can slow the progression of proteinuric chronic kidney disease. It may also provide cardiovascular protection, since chronic kidney disease is associated with a marked increase in cardiovascular risk. BP control through rennin angiotensin aldosterone(RAAS) blockade is a cornerstone of conservative therapy in lupus nephritis. The RAAS, and its pharmacologic blockade, may play a role in the pathogenesis and prognosis of SLE independent of its effects on systemic BP and glomerular hemodynamics. A number of animal studies have highlighted the inflammatory components of the RAAS and the potential benefits of RAAS blockade in reducing or eliminating this inflammation in lupus nephritis (22).
Lipid lowering - Hyperlipidemia, with often dramatic elevations in the serum cholesterol concentration, is commonly present in patients with nephrotic syndrome. Although control of serum LDL cholesterol is the main indication for statin therapy, there is some evidence in patients with chronic kidney disease that it may also slow the progression of the underlying renal disease (22).

7. Immunosuppressive therapy

Different immunosuppressive medication can be used as induction and/or maintenance therapy as follows:

induction	maintaince
cyclophosphamide	**cyclophosphamide**
Mycophenolate mofetil	Mycophenolate mofetil
Rituximab	**Rituximab**
Steroids	**Steroids**
	Cyclosporine
	Azathioprine

1. Steroids

During the induction phase Methylprednisolone in doses of 7mg/kg/day as intravenous pulse therapy for three days followed by 1 mg/kg/day for 4-6 weeks to be tapered during the maintenance phase slowly according to the clinical response (6).it is usually used in combination with other drugs.

2. Cyclophosphamide

The most studied in lupus nephritis. The data for using Cyclophosphamide is coming mainly from two major randomized control trial. The first one is the National Institutes of Health (NIH) study(6), which used cyclophsphamide as intravenous monthly doses for 6 consecutive months, starting at a dose of 0.5g/m2 body surface not to exceed 1g/m^2. After the first 6 months .pulse cyclophosphamide is given every 3 months for a total of 24 months. The second trial is EURO Lupus trial (7) (8).intravenous cyclophosphamide is given every 2 weeks in a fixed dose of 500 mg for 6 doses, followed by Azathioprine (2mg/kg/day) to finish 30 months of treatment.

The downside of treatment with cyclophosphamide is the side effect profile associated with it including leucopenia, increase risk of infection, hemorrhagic cystitis ,hair loss and increase risk of malignancy.

Both regimen were equally effective in various renal and extra-renal outcomes. The low dose regimen(Euro-lupus) had less toxicity with significantly less sever and total infections as a complication of treatment(8).

During the treatment with cyclophsphamide physician need to monitor the patient with biweekly WBC count during the first six months them monthly and adjust the dose if the WBC count drop below 3000 mm2.

Mycophenolate mofetil l(MMF)

The active component of MMF, mycophenolic acid, is an inhibitor of inosine 5'-monophosphate dehydrogenase, the rate-controlling enzyme in *de novo* biosynthesis of guanosine triphosphate, used by antigen-activated B cells and T cells. Mycophenolic acid exhibits a selective antiproliferative effect on lymphocytes with anti-inflammatory effects and a profound effect on autoantibody production by B cells.

Because of its favorable safety profile, there has been great interest in the use of Mycophenolate mofet(MMF) as both induction and maintenance therapy(9)(10)(16). Since 2000 two controlled trials comparing induction therapy with MMF versus cyclophosphamide have indicated comparable rates of renal remission and short term renal survival but fewer side effects in patients treated with MMF. The best data are from international trial (ALMS) that compared MMF in a dose of 3g/day as induction therapy for six months with monthly intravenous Cyclophosphamide(IVC) for six doses (11). Overall response rates similar with MMF and IVC in all renal and non-renal parameters. In this trial MMF in a dose of 1g twice daily for 36 months was superior to Azathioprine in 2mg/kg/day as maintenance therapy.

MMF can be used in a dose of 3g/day in divided dose for 6 months as induction therapy followed by 1g twice daily for 36 months as maintenance therapy.

Cyclosporine (CSA)

The available data suggest that CSA may be a useful drug in patients with lupus nephritis showing persistent sever proteinuria after induction therapy or intolerance to other immunosuppressive drugs (12).

Azathioprine(AZA)

The role of AZA is much less established as induction therapy. The available data support the use of AZA as maintenance therapy for 24-30 months (7) (12).

preferred in women who are in complete remission and want to become pregnant. Cyclosporine is an alternative if azathioprine is not tolerated. MMF has a boxed warning because of an increased risk of congenital malformations and spontaneous abortion.

Rituximab

An anti-CD20 monoclonal antibody that depletes B cells, is useful in inducucing remissions in some patients. Currently rituximab is used for refractory or non-responder cases, alone or in combination with other immunosuppressive agents (13)(17)

Plasmapheresis

Randomized trials showed no add benefit value of plasmapheresis to immunosuppressive therapy in patient with lupus nephritis (14) (15). However, plasmapheresis may have a role in selected patients, such as those with severe crescentic LN who require dialysis (especially those with concomitant ANCA, extrapolating from the MEPEX trial of patients with Wegener's granulomatosis) or those with proliferative LN and thrombotic thrombocytopenic purpura with antiphospholipid antibodies.

The above mentioned lines of treatment usually indicated for class three and four.

Treatment of membranous lupus nephritis still controversial. Most of the clinical trial included patients with focal or diffuse proliferative lupus nephritis.

In general patients with membranous lupus nephritis who have normal renal function and subnephrotic proteinuria may not require intensive immunosuppressant while patient with high grade nephrotic syndrome or abnormal renal function or mixed membranous and proliferative lesions on biopsy which may be present at diagnosis or develop later need to be treated with immunosuppressant.

The only randomized trial limited to patients with pure lupus MN, the National Institutes of Health (NIH) trial, showed equivalent efficacy with cyclophosphamide plus glucocorticoids and cyclosporine plus glucocorticoids [18]. There were trends with cyclosporine toward higher rates of both remission (83 versus 60 percent at one year) and of relapse after the cessation of therapy (60 percent within 36 months versus 20 percent within 50 months.

A randomized trial (ALMS) compared MMF with cyclophosphamide in 370 patients with LN, including 60 with pure membranous LN [11]. The primary outcome was a prespecified reduction in the urine protein-to-creatinine ratio to less than 3 or by at least 50 percent. Secondary outcomes included stabilization or improvement of the serum creatinine, reduction of protein excretion to less than 0.5 g/day, and attainment of inactive urinary sediment. At 24 weeks, there was no difference in the two groups in the percentage of patients with pure membranous LN who achieved either the primary or secondary outcome.

8. In summary

1. lupus nephritis stage III and IV with active disease(high creatinine and/or proteinuria > 500 mg/day and/or active sediment: should be treated with cyclophosphamide intravenous as monthly dose for six months as induction therapy followed by cyclophosphamide intravenous every 3 months to finish 24 months.
2. The other approach to treat stage 3 and 4 lupus nephritis is to use cyclophosphamide intravenous in a fixed dose 500 mg every 2 weeks for six doses as induction therapy followed by MMF in a dose of 1 mg orally twice daily for 36 months which has been superior to Azathioprine as maintenance therapy. This approach is preferable to the former approach because the risk of side effect is much less.
3. If the patient can not take cyclophosphamide or prefer not to, MMF can be used in a dose of 3g/day in divided dose for six months as induction therapy followed by MMF in a dose of 1-2 g/day for 36 months as maintenance dose.
4. For stage 5 lupus nephritis with active disease(nephritic range proteinuria,active sediment and/or abnormal renal function, can be treated with oral cyclosporine in a

dose of 5mg/kg /day in divided doses but the dose need to be adjusted if the creatinine is rising. this treatment need to be continued for one year.

Intra venous Cyclophosphamide can be used (0.5-1.0g/m2) given every other month for one year.

If patient can not tolerate cyclosporine or cyclophosphamide,MMF can be used as it was beneficial in ALMS trial. It can be used in dose of 3g/day for 6 months then to be reduced to 1-2g/day.

9. Criteria for clinical reemission

Most of the clinical trials defined complete remission can be defined by the following criteria,

1. Inactive urinary sediment defined as ≤5 red blood cells per high power field, ≤5 white blood cells per high power field, a reading of 0 to 1+ on the urine dipstick for heme, and no red cell casts.
2. Normalization of the serum creatinine and protein excretion below 500 mg/day.

Partial remission can be defined by reduction of proteinuria by 50% or more.

10. Kidney transplantation in patient with lupus nephritis

If patient with lupus nephritis progress to ESRD and require dialysis, data suggest that renal transplant has better outcome than dialysis in such patients. (19)

Long-term patient and graft survivals were similar in SLE and non-SLE renal transplant recipients. The risk for thrombotic complications was greater among SLE patients (19).

Patients need to be clinically and serologically inactive at the time of transplant.

The rate of clinically recurrent disease in the renal transplant of 2.0 to 9.0 percent in patients with lupus nephritis, which is thought to reflect, diminished immunologic activity (20). The incidence of recurrent symptoms of systemic lupus was also low at 5.7 percent.

11. Experimental therapy

Several studies involving novel therapeutic agents for lupus nephritis are underway. The agents being evaluated in these studies are summarized in Table 24-3. The Web site www.clinicaltrials.gov is a potentially useful resource in searching for studies that may be recruiting patients, along with information about eligibility and exclusion criteria.

12. Prognosis

The prognosis of class III and IV proliferative lupus nephritis has improved, from a 5-year renal survival rate of less than 20% during the period 1960-1980 to a rate of more than 80% during 1980-2000. This improvement in prognosis has been ascribed mostly to increasing use of cyclophosphamide. Although preliminary data based on achievement of renal remission suggest that mycophenolate mofetil may have comparable benefits, it remains to be established whether mycophenolate mofetil will achieve comparable long-term renal survival.

Monoclonal Antibodies (Targets)
Rituximab (CD20, B cells)[* † ‡]
Epratuzumab (CD22, B cells)[*]
MEDI-545 (interferon-α)[‡]
Belimumab (BLyS cytokine)[‡]
Tocilizumab (interleukin-6 receptor)[‡]
Infliximab (tumor necrosis factor)[* ‡]
Costimulation Inhibitors
CTLA4-Ig, abatacept, belatacept (CD80/86)[‡]
Tolerogens
Abetimus, LJP-394 (anti-DNA)[‡]
Hematopoietic stem cell transplants

* Case reports.
† Case series.
‡ Ongoing clinical trials.

Table 2. Experimental Therapies for Systemic Lupus Erythematosus and Lupus Nephritis

13. Acknowledgments

The work to produce this chapter was supported by Alzaidi's Chair of research in rheumatic diseases- Umm Alqura University.

14. References

[1] Clinical features of SLE. In: Textbook of Rheumatology, Kelley, WN, et al (Eds), WB Saunders, Philadelphia 2000.

[2] Baranowska-Daca E, Choi YJ, Barrios R, Nassar G, Suki WN, Truong LD, Nonlupus nephritides in patients with systemic lupus erythematosus: a comprehensive clinicopathologic study and review of the literature, Hum Pathol. 2001;32(10):1125-35.

[3] Appel G, Cameron JS in Comprehensive clinical Nephrology 2007.

[4] Tan EM,Cohen AS,Fries JF:The 1982 revised criteria for the classification of systemic lupus erythematosus.Artheritis Rheum25:1271,1982.

[5] Weening JJ, D'Agati VD, Schwartz MM, Seshan SV, Alpers CE, Appel GB, Balow JE, Bruijn JA, Cook T, Ferrario F, Fogo AB, Ginzler EM, Hebert L, Hill G, Hill P, Jennette JC, Kong NC, Lesavre P, Lockshin M, Looi LM, Makino H, Moura LA, Nagata M, International Society of Nephrology Working Group on the Classification of Lupus Nephritis, Renal Pathology Society Working Group on the Classification of Lupus Nephritis, The classification of

glomerulonephritis in systemic lupus erythematosus revisited, Kidney Int. 2004;65(2):521-30.

[6] Gourley MF, Austin HA 3rd, Scott D, Yarboro CH, Vaughan EM, Muir J, Boumpas DT, Klippel JH, Balow JE, Steinberg AD, Methylprednisolone and cyclophosphamide, alone or in combination, in patients with lupus nephritis. A randomized, controlled trial, Ann Intern Med. 1996;125(7):549-57.

[7] Houssiau FA, Vasconcelos C, D'Cruz D, Sebastiani GD, Garrido Ed Ede R, Danieli MG, Abramovicz D, Blockmans D, Mathieu A, Direskeneli H, Galeazzi M, G?l A, Levy Y, Petera P, Popovic R, Petrovic R, Sinico RA, Cattaneo R, Font J, Depresseux G, Cosyns JP, Cervera R, Immunosuppressive therapy in lupus nephritis: the Euro-Lupus Nephritis Trial, a randomized trial of low-dose versus high-dose intravenous cyclophosphamide, Arthritis Rheum. 2002;46(8):2121-31.

[8] Houssiau FA, Ann Rheum Dis 2009.

[9] Contreras G, Pardo V, Leclercq B, Lenz O, Tozman E, O'Nan P, Roth D, Sequential therapies for proliferative lupus nephritis, N Engl J Med. 2004;350(10):971-80.

[10] Zhu B, Chen N, Lin Y, Ren H, Zhang W, Wang W, Pan X, Yu H, Mycophenolate mofetil in induction and maintenance therapy of severe lupus nephritis: a meta-analysis of randomized controlled trials, Nephrol Dial Transplant. 2007;22(7):1933-42.

[11] Appel GB, Contreras G, Dooley MA, Ginzler EM, Isenberg D, Jayne D, Li LS, Mysler E, S?nchez-Guerrero J, Solomons N, Wofsy D, Aspreva Lupus Management Study Group, Mycophenolate mofetil versus cyclophosphamide for induction treatment of lupus nephritis, J Am Soc Nephrol. 2009;20(5):1103-12.

[12] Moroni G, Doria A, Mosca M, Alberighi OD, Ferraccioli G, Todesco S, Manno C, Altieri P, Ferrara R, Greco S, Ponticelli C, A randomized pilot trial comparing cyclosporine and azathioprine for maintenance therapy in diffuse lupus nephritis over four years, Clin J Am Soc Nephrol. 2006;1(5):925-32.

[13] R.Furie, R. J. Looney[2], B. Rovin[3], Kevin M. Latinis[4], G. Appel[5], J. Sanchez-Guerrero[6], F.C. Fervenza[7], R. Maciuca[8], P. Brunetta[9], D. Zhang[8] and J. Garg[8], [1]North Shore-LIJ Health System, Lake Success, NY, [2]University of Rochester, Rochester, NY, [3]Ohio State, Columbus, OH, [4]KS Univ Med Ctr, Kansas City, KS, [5]Columbia, New York, NY, [6]Inst Nacional, Mexico City DF, Mexico, [7]Mayo Clinic, Rochester, MN, [8]Genentech, South San Francisco, CA, [9]Genentech, Inc., South San Francisco, CA,ACR,2009

[14] Berden JH, Lupus nephritis, Kidney Int. 1997;52(2):538-58.

[15] Lewis EJ, Hunsicker LG, Lan SP, Rohde RD, Lachin JM, A controlled trial of plasmapheresis therapy in severe lupus nephritis. The Lupus Nephritis Collaborative Study Group, N Engl J Med. 1992;326(21):1373-9.

[16] Ginzler E, Appel G,N Eng J Med,Nov.2005.

[17] Melander C, Sall?e M, Trolliet P, Candon S, Belenfant X, Daugas E, R?my P, Zarrouk V, Pillebout E, Jacquot C, Boffa JJ, Karras A, Masse V, Lesavre P, Elie C, Brocheriou I, Knebelmann B, No?l LH, Fakhouri F, Rituximab in severe lupus nephritis: early B-cell depletion affects long-term renal outcome, Clin J Am Soc Nephrol. 2009;4(3):579-87.

[18] Austin HA 3rd, Illei GG, Braun MJ, Balow JE, Randomized, controlled trial of prednisone, cyclophosphamide, and cyclosporine in lupus membranous nephropathy, J Am Soc Nephrol. 2009;20(4):901.

[19] Stone JH, Amend WJ, Criswell LA, Outcome of renal transplantation in ninety-seven cyclosporine-era patients with systemic lupus erythematosus and matched controls, Arthritis Rheum. 1998;41(8):1438.

[20] Stone JH, Millward CL, Olson JL, Amend WJ, Criswell LA, Frequency of recurrent lupus nephritis among ninety-seven renal transplant patients during the cyclosporine era, Arthritis Rheum. 1998;41(4):678.

[21] Kanda H, Kubo K, Tateishi S, Sato K, Yonezumi A, Yamamoto K, Mimura T, Antiproteinuric effect of ARB in lupus nephritis patients with persistent proteinuria despite immunosuppressive therapy, Lupus. 2005;14(4):288.

[22] Teplitsky V, Shoenfeld Y, Tanay A: the rennin-angiotensin system in lupus: physiology,genes and practice,in animals and humans Lupus 15: 319-325, 2006.

12

New Therapeutic Strategies in Lupus Nephritis

Natasha Jordan and Yousuf Karim
Louise Coote Lupus Unit, St Thomas' Hospital, London
United Kingdom

1. Introduction

Lupus nephritis remains a major cause of morbidity and mortality in systemic lupus erythematosus (SLE). Despite overall advances in the clinical management of lupus nephritis in recent decades with earlier recognition of disease and optimization of the currently available immunosuppressive regimens, an estimated 10-15% of patients progress to end-stage renal disease (ESRD) requiring dialysis and/or renal transplantation (Mavragani et al, 2003). Proliferative lupus nephritis (International Society of Nephrology/Renal Pathology Society classes III & IV) is the most aggressive variant of nephritis; figures 1 and 2 illustrate the histology of Class IV nephritis.

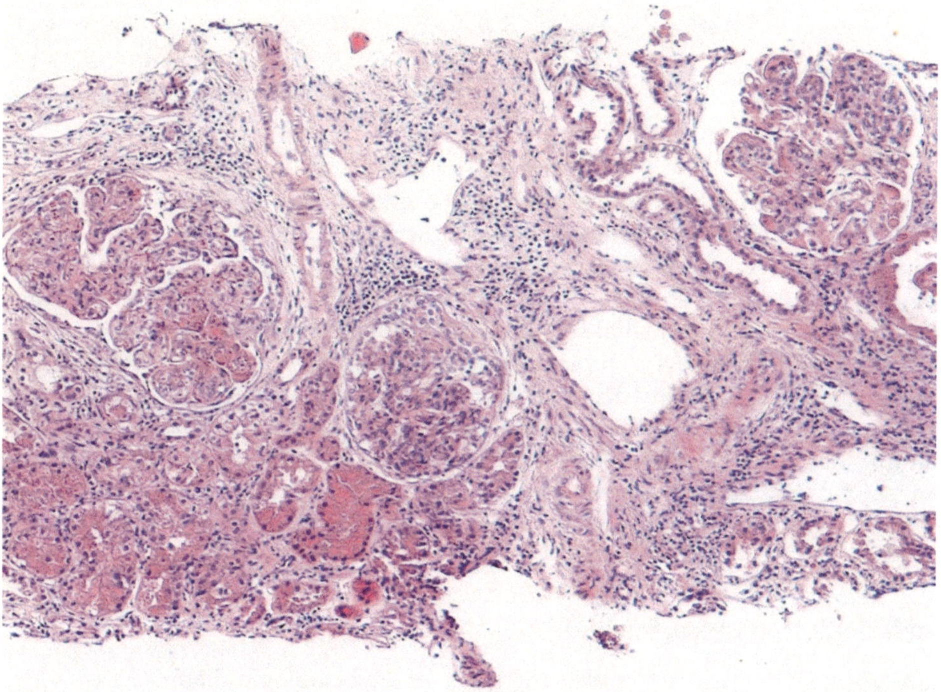

(Courtesy Dr Fahim Tungekar)

Fig. 1. Class IV global proliferative lupus nephritis

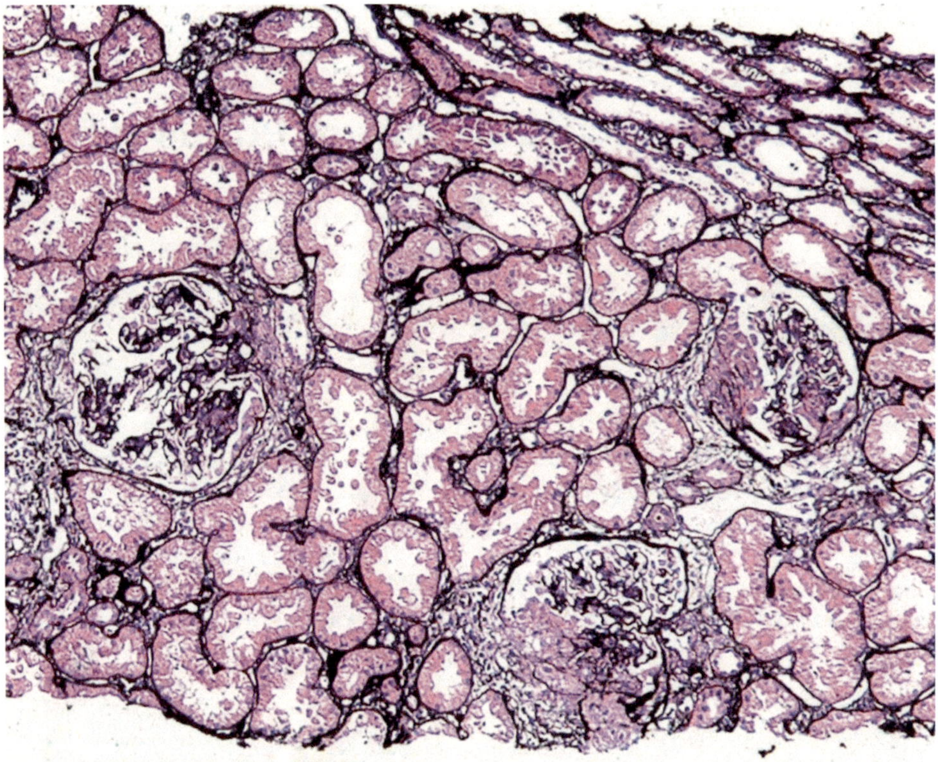

(Courtesy Dr Fahim Tungekar)

Fig. 2. Class IV segmental proliferative lupus nephritis

The rate of progression to ESRD is likely to be even higher patients of Afro-Caribbean descent (Dooley et al, 1997). Commonly used therapeutic agents such as corticosteroids, cyclophosphamide, mycophenolate mofetil and azathioprine have certainly improved clinical outcomes, however a significant proportion of lupus nephritis patients have refractory disease and the potential side effects of these therapies are significant.

A recent retrospective review of lupus nephritis patients over a 30 year period (1975-2005) showed that five year mortality decreased by 60% between the first and second decades but remained unchanged over the third decade. The rate of progression to ESRD also reached a plateau in the third decade. These results suggest that the benefits of conventional immunosuppressive therapies have been maximized and if further improvements in lupus nephritis outcomes are to be achieved, novel therapeutic targets must be developed (Croca et al, 2011).

2. B-cell depletion therapies

Lupus nephritis involves a complex interplay of immunologic disturbances with renal damage resulting from production of pathogenic autoantibodies and immune complexes, which activate complement leading to infiltration of inflammatory cells in the kidney. B lymphocytes play an integral role in this process, they are the precursors of plasma cells that

Class of therapy	*Agent*	*Mechanism of action*	*Clinical Stage*	*Result or Outcome*
B-cell depletion	Rituximab	anti-CD20 chimeric Moab	Phase III	EXPLORER & LUNAR trials failed to meet primary end-points
	Ocrelizumab	anti-CD20 fully humanized Moab	Phase III	Clinical trial suspended
	Epratuzumab	anti-CD22 fully humanized Moab	Phase III	Study ongoing
B-cell survival factors	Belimumab	anti-BLys fully humanized Moab	Phase III	BLISS (52 and 76) FDA approved
	Atacicept	TACI-Ig fusion protein	Phase II/III ongoing	Trial temporarily discontinued, now resumed
T-cell co-stimulation	Abatacept	CTLA-4-Ig fusion protein	Phase II	Failed to meet primary end-point, further trials ongoing
	CD40L	BG9588 IDEC-131	Phase II	Study discontinued due to thromboembolic events Negative trial
Cytokine targets	Tocilizumab	Il-6 fully humanized Moab	Phase I	Well tolerated in phase I trial, further trials pending
	Infliximab Etanercept	anti-TNF-α chimeric Moab TNF-receptor-IgG fusion protein	no controlled trials no controlled trials	
	Medi-546	Interferon-α Moab	Phase I	Trials ongoing
Complement therapies	Eculizumab	anti-C5 fully humanized Moab	Phase I	Safe & well tolerated in phase I trial, no further studies to date

Moab, monoclonal antibody, BLys, B lymphocyte stimulator, TACI-Ig, transmembrane activator and calcium modulator and cyclophylin ligand interactor-immunoglobulin, TNF-receptor-IgG, tumour necrosis factor-receptor-immunoglobulin

Table 1. Summary of emerging biologic therapies in systemic lupus erythematosus

produce these pathogenic autoantibodies and they also function as antigen presenting cells to T lymphocytes. Thus B lymphocytes represent a rational therapeutic target in lupus nephritis. By far the most clinical experience in targeting B-lymphocytes to date has been in the form of B-cell depletion therapy (BCDT). Rituximab, a monoclonal antibody against the cell surface protein, CD20 has been in use clinically for the past decade. Alternative forms of BCDT are under development and in ongoing clinical trials.

2.1 Rituximab (Anti-CD20)

CD20 is a cell surface protein expressed on B lymphocytes from the early pre-B cell until mature B cell stages of development, but is not present on hematopoietic precursor stem cells or plasma cells.The CD20 antigen was first targeted in the immunotherapy of B cell lymphomas (Grillo-Lopez et al, 1999) (Hainsworth et al, 2000) and, subsequently in rheumatoid arthritis (RA) (Edwards et al, 2004). Rituximab is a chimeric mouse/human monoclonal antibody against the B cell-specific antigen CD20, a cell surface protein believed to function in B cell cycle initiation and differentiation. Rituximab induces cell lysis via antibody-dependent cell-mediated cytotoxicity and activation of complement leading to B-cell depletion in the peripheral blood and bone marrow (Reff et al, 1994).

Open trials of rituximab over the past decade have shown encouraging results in active and refractory SLE including lupus nephritis (Leandro et al, 2002) (Looney et al, 2004) (Leandro et al, 2005). However the failure of rituximab to meet its primary and secondary end points in randomized controlled trials of non-renal SLE (EXPLORER) and lupus nephritis (LUNAR) has been disappointing (Merrill et al, 2010). Issues with study design, concomitant use of high dose steroid and other immunosuppressive therapies and the relatively low severity of disease in patients enrolled need to be taken into account when interpreting the results of these trials.

A number of case reports and open-label studies have reported successful treatment of lupus nephritis with rituximab. Vigna-Perez et al reported an open study of 22 LN patients receiving rituximab (0.5 to 1.0 g at Days 1 and 15). This was added to existing treatment consisting of different combinations of azathioprine, mycophenolate, cyclophosphamide and corticosteroids. Significant reduction of disease activity and proteinuria was seen ($P<0.05$). One patient died from invasive histoplasmosis at day 70 (Vigna-Perez et al). Clinical improvements have also been seen using rituximab in membranous lupus nephritis (Jónsdóttir et al, 2010) (Jónsdóttir et al, 2011).

Pepper et al reported the use of rituximab as induction therapy followed by maintenance mycophenolate mofetil in a cohort of eighteen patients with proliferative lupus nephritis. A significant decrease in proteinuria from a mean protein: creatinine ratio (PCR) of 325 mg/mmol at presentation to 132 mg/mmol at 1 year ($p = 0.004$) was demonstrated and this combination of sequential therapy allowed a reduction or total withdrawal of maintenance corticosteroids (Pepper et al, 2009).

The French Autoimmune and Rituximab (AIR) registry reviewed one hundred thirty-six patients who received this treatment for SLE. Articular, cutaneous, renal, and haematologic improvements were noted in 72%, 70%, 74%, and 88% of patients, respectively. Severe infections were noted in 12 patients (9%), with most severe infections occurring within the first 3 months after the last rituximab infusion. Five patients died, three due to severe infection ($n = 3$) and two due to refractory autoimmune disease. Overall response was observed in 71% of patients and among these, 41% experienced a relapse of disease but responded after retreatment with rituximab in 91% of cases (Terrier et al, 2010).

Sangle et al noted progression to ESRD in five patients with severe proliferative, crescentic lupus nephritis (mean activity score 12/24, mean crescents 38%) with raised serum creatinine (mean 278 μmol/l) treated with rituximab, after failure of other immunosuppressive drugs (Sangle et al, 2007). This may reflect that the timing of rituximab therapy in the course of disease may be important for its efficacy.

The degree of B-cell depletion achieved is far more variable in SLE patients treated with rituximab as compared to those with RA or lymphoma (Gunnarson et al, 2007) (Sutter et al, 2008). However the degree and duration of B-cell depletion in SLE patients does correlate to some extent with clinical response and those who fail to deplete tend to have a poorer clinical response (Albert et al, 2008).

The most common adverse effects associated with rituximab therapy are mild to moderate infusion reactions. Two SLE patients treated with rituximab developed progressive multifocal leukoencephalopathy (PML) which should be interpreted in the context of the known 20 patients with SLE reported to have developed PML and had not received rituximab therapy (Calabrese et al, 2007).

The rate of development of human anti-chimeric antibodies (HACAs) is significantly higher in lupus patients treated with rituximab than RA or lymphoma patients who have received this therapy (Smith et al, 2006) (Saito et al, 2005). It is not entirely clear if development of HACAs in rituximab treated lupus patients will lead to reduced efficacy of this medication with repeated use.

A cohort of 76 patients with active SLE refractory to standard immunosuppression have received repeated cycles of rituximab since 2000 with good clinical response and favourable safety profile (Turner-Stokes et al, 2011). The long-term effects of repeated B-cell depletion are unknown, though there is a risk of hypogammglobulinaemia.

Perhaps further randomized controlled trials in moderate to severe lupus patients and a greater understanding from basic science as to why some lupus patients have more profound and long-lasting B-cell depletion will clarify the role of rituximab in SLE and in particular lupus nephritis.

2.2 Ocrelizumab (Anti-CD20)

Ocrelizumab, a fully humanized monoclonal antibody against CD20, is an alternative form of BCDT which entered clinical trials for SLE and rheumatoid arthritis (RA). The potential benefits of this form of BCDT included avoidance of HACA development given its fully humanized structure thus maintaining efficacy and minimizing HACA related side effects. Clinical trials in SLE and RA were suspended in 2010 due to excess deaths due to opportunistic infections and thus no results are currently available for this therapy.

2.3 Epratuzumab (Anti-CD22)

CD22 is a B-cell surface restricted marker and member of a class of adhesion molecules that regulate B-lymphocyte activation and interaction with T lymphocytes. CD22 is expressed in the cytoplasm of pro-B and pre-B cells, and on the surface of maturing B cells (Tedder et al, 1997). CD22 plays a role in inhibition of BCR signaling by controlling calcium efflux in B cells as evidenced by work in CD22-deficient mice (Sato et al, 1998). CD22-deficient mice have reduced numbers of mature B cells in the peripheral blood and bone marrow and these B cells also have a shorter life span and increased apoptosis indicating that CD22 plays a key role in B cell development and survival (Otipoby et al, 1996).

Thus CD22 is an attractive therapeutic target in lupus nephritis. Epratuzumab is a recombinant humanized monoclonal IgG antibody to CD22; it mediates antibody-dependent cellular cytotoxicity and partially depletes B-cells. It is thought that epratuzumab modifies B-cell function without killing them but the precise mechanism of action remains unclear.

Safety of epratuzumab was first demonstrated in clinical trials of non-Hodgkins lymphoma (Leonard et al, 2004). It has also been successfully used in refractory lymphoma in combination with rituximab (Leonard et al, 2005). The main side-effects seen in these studies were infusion reactions.

An open-label non-randomized trial of epratuzumab in mild to moderate SLE showed promising results with consistent improvement observed in all patients enrolled for the 12 week duration of the study, average 35% depletion in B-cell levels, and no evidence of HACA development. The duration of response in this study was very heterogeneous for different BILAG domains, precluding any firm conclusions from being drawn about the specific impact of epratuzumab on lupus nephritis (Dorner et al, 2008). A phase III trial of epratuzumab in patients with moderate to severe SLE is underway.

3. Targeting B-cell survival factors

3.1 Belimumab

BLyS (B lymphocyte stimulator) also known as BAFF is a member of the TNF superfamily and plays an essential role in B-cell survival and development (Stohl et al, 2003). It binds to three different membrane receptors: BCMA (B cell maturation antigen), BAFFR (BR3) and TACI (transmembrane activator and calcium modulator and cyclophylin ligand interactor). Mice deficient in BLyS have reduced levels of mature B cells and immunoglobulins (Schiemann et al, 2001). Overexpansion of BLyS in transgenic mice leads to expansion of B-cells, hypergammaglobulaemia and autoimmune disease (Mackay et al, 1999).

Belimumab is a fully humanized monoclonal antibody against BLyS, which can cause depletion of circulating B cells however less profoundly than anti-CD20 monoclonal antibodies such as rituximab. Belimumab was approved by the FDA for treatment of SLE in March 2011, the first lupus drug to be approved since hydroxychloroquine and corticosteroids were approved in 1955. The safety and effectiveness of belimumab was demonstrated in two clinical trials (BLISS-52, and BLISS-76) that randomized a total of 1684 patients to receive either belimumab or placebo in combination with standard therapy (Wallace et al, 2009) (Jacobi et al, 2010). Treatment with belimumab plus standard therapy reduced disease activity and steroid use.

However, there are reservations regarding the effectiveness of belimumab in the more severe organ manifestations of SLE as patients with active lupus nephritis and central nervous system (CNS) disease were not studied. Study participants of African American descent did not significantly respond well to belimumab, which is also of concern.

Additional studies need to be conducted to definitively determine the safety and efficacy of belimumab in the more severe complications of SLE particularly lupus nephritis.

3.2 Atacicept

An alternative therapeutic approach targeting B cell survival is atacicept, a recombinant fusion protein containing the ligand-binding domain of the transmembrane activator and calcium modulator and cyclophilin-ligand interactor receptor (TACI) and the Fc portion of human immunoglobulin (IgG1). Atacicept inhibits B-cell stimulation by binding to both

BLys and a profileration-inducing ligand (APRIL). Atacicept is believed to selectively impair mature B cells and plasma cells with less impact on progenitor and memory B cells (Nestorov et al, 2008). A phase I study has demonstrated the safety and tolerability of atacicept in patients with mild to moderate SLE (Pena-Rossi et al, 2009). A phase II/III study of atacicept in LN is ongoing and due to be completed in 2012. The study was temporarily discontinued due to decreased immunoglobulin levels in study participants and now has been resumed. Of note, a phase II trial of atacicept in multiple sclerosis was discontinued due to increased disease relapse and new lesions on MRI brain imaging in the study subjects.

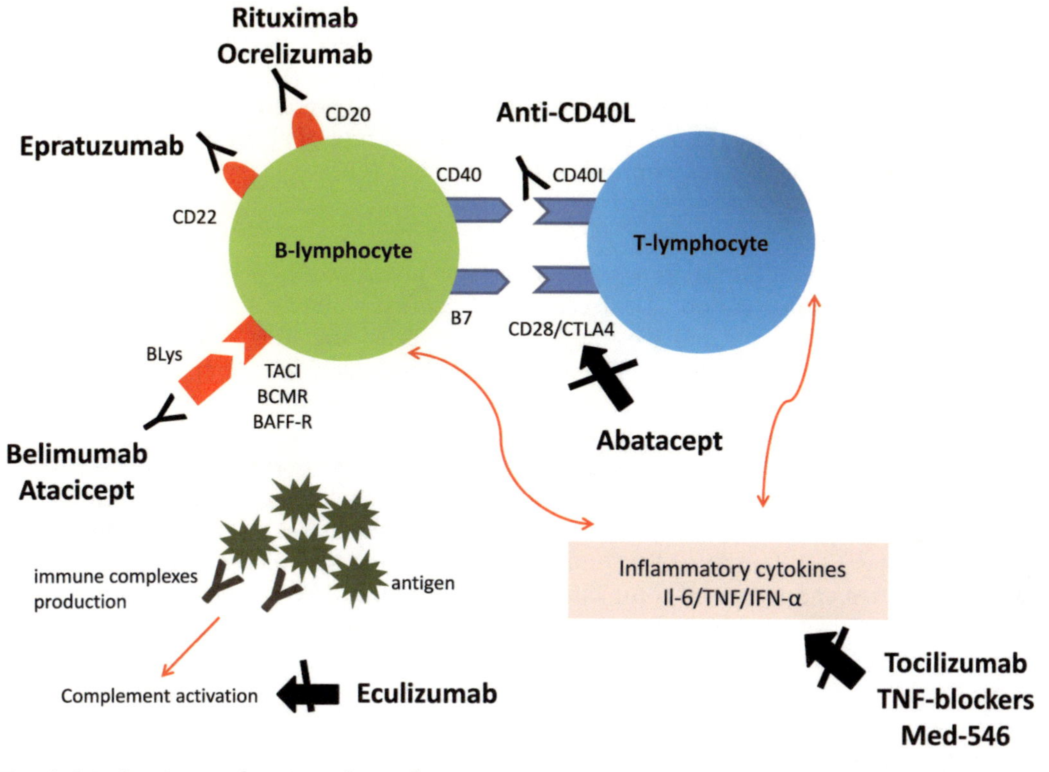

Fig. 3. Mechanisms of action of novel agents

4. Blockade of T-cell co-stimulation

4.1 Abatacept

Immunological tolerance can be induced by blockade of co-stimulatory interactions between T and B lymphocytes. The most well characterized T lymphocyte co-stimulatory ligand is CD28, a glycoprotein which interacts with the co-stimulatory receptors B7-1 (CD80) and B7-2 (CD86). Stimulation of this pathway occurs when naive T cells encounter an antigen presenting cell with the appropriate major histocompatibility complex class II bound antigen, resulting in T lymphocyte proliferation and differentiation (Ledbetter et al, 1990). CTLA4 (cytotoxic T-lymphocyte antigen) is expressed on activated T cells and interacts with B7 with higher affinity than CD28 resulting in a negative feedback mechanism that inhibits T cell activation (Scheipers et al, 1998) (Reiser et al, 1996) (Brunet et al, 1987).

Abatacept is a fusion protein consisting of CTLA-4 combined with the Fc portion of human IgG1 (CTLA-4-Ig). Combination therapy of CTLA-4-Ig and cyclophosphamide has been demonstrated to significantly reduce proteinuria, autoantibody titres and mortality in murine models of lupus nephritis (Daihk et al, 2001), (Finck et al, 1994).
Abatacept has been used successfully in the clinical management of RA and psoriasis (Genovese et al, 2008) (Mease et al, 2011). A randomised double blind placebo controlled trial has evaluated the clinical efficacy and safety of abatacept in 175 lupus patients. These patients had primarily serositis, musculoskeletal and dermatologic features and the trial was not specifically designed to examine the role of CTLA-4-Ig in lupus nephritis. The primary end-point of the study was the proportion of patients with a new flare of SLE (defined as BILAG score of A or B adjudicated as a flare in any organ system). The primary end point was not met. However when reassessed considering only BILAG A flares, 40.7% of patients in the abatacept group experienced a flare after initiation of steroid taper as compared to 54.5% in the placebo group. (Merrill et al, 2010). A clinical trial of abatacept in combination with cyclophosphamide in lupus nephritis is ongoing.

4.2 Anti-CD40 ligand

CD40 ligand (CD40L, CD154) is a transmembrane glycoprotein belonging to the TNF superfamily and is expressed on CD4 T-cells and activated platelets. It binds with CD40 on the surface of B-cells, macrophages and dendritic cells and this interaction between CD40/CD40L plays a pivotal role in B-cell class switching (Davidson et al, 2003). CD40L is overexpressed in murine lupus and monoclonal antibodies against CD40L have successfully treated murine lupus nephritis (Early et al, 1996).
Two humanised anti-CD40L monoclonal antibodies (IDEC-131 and BG9588) have entered clinical trials in SLE patients. Treatment of 85 SLE patients with IDEC-131 failed to demonstrate clinical efficacy over placebo at 20 weeks (Kalunian et al, 2002). An open-label study of 28 patients with proliferative lupus nephritis treated with BG9588 showed reduced anti-dsDNA titres and increased complement levels but was discontinued prematurely due to thromboembolic events (Boumpas et al, 2003). Given the unexpected side effects and lack of efficacy demonstrated in these studies, it is unlikely that anti-CD40L will progress to larger clinical trials in lupus nephritis.

5. Cytokine therapies

5.1 Anti-interleukin-6

Multiple cytokines have been implicated in the pathogenesis of SLE; among these is interleukin-6 (Il-6), a pleiotropic cytokine with both proinflammatory and anti-inflammatory properties. Evidence from murine models of lupus supports the role of Il-6 in the pathogenesis of lupus nephritis. Exogenous IL-6 increases autoantibody production and accelerates progression of nephritis in both the NZB/NZW and BXSB lupus mouse models (Ryffel et al, 1994) (Yang et al, 1998). On the contrary, injection of lupus prone mice with an IL-6 monoclonal antibody decreases anti-dsDNA levels and proteinuria and reduces mortality (Liang et al, 2006) (Mihara et al, 1998). In SLE patients, IL-6 levels have been shown to correlate with disease activity and anti-dsDNA titres. (Chun et al, 2007) (Linker-Israeli et al, 1991). Urinary excretion of IL-6 is increased in those with proliferative forms of lupus nephritis and this excretion is reduced following cyclophosphamide therapy (Peterson et al, 1996) (Tsai et al, 2000).

Tocilizumab is a fully humanized monoclonal antibody against the α-chain of the IL-6 receptor and prevents binding of IL-6 to both membrane bound and soluble IL-6 receptor. A phase I trial over a 12 week period has demonstrated the safety and tolerability of tocilizumab in lupus patients. Five of the twelve patients recruited to this study had renal disease at baseline, all of whom had moderate levels of proteinuria which remained unchanged throughout the duration of the study. There was however a reduction in the number of patients with active urinary sediment and a decrease in anti-dsDNA antibody titres (Illei et al, 2010). The short duration of the study renders it difficult to draw any firm conclusions as to the longer term effects of tocilizumab in lupus nephritis. The principal side effect noted in the study was neutropenia, which was dose related and white cell counts normalized on discontinuation of therapy. Randomized controlled trials of tocilizumab in lupus nephritis are awaited.

5.2 Anti-TNF-α therapies

Anti-TNF therapies (infliximab, adalimumab, etanercept) have become the mainstay of therapy in RA, psoriatic arthritis and ankylosing spondylitis. However the role of anti-TNF blocking agents in the treatment of SLE remains controversial. TNF is overexpressed in the serum, kidneys and skin of SLE patients and high serum levels of TNF correlate with lupus disease activity (Herrera-Esparza et al, 1998) (Aringer et al, 2005) (Zampieri et al, 2006) (Gabay et al, 1997). Murine models provide further evidence of the role of TNF in lupus nephritis. Both MRL/lpr and NZB/NZW lupus mouse models overexpress TNF and this correlates with renal inflammation suggesting potential benefit in TNF blockade in SLE (Boswell et al, 1988) (Yokoyama et al, 1995) (Brennan et al, 1989).

However it is well established that patients treated with anti-TNF therapies develop autoantibodies similar to those seen in clinical lupus and the concern is that these agents when used in SLE patients could induce lupus flares. Anti-nuclear (ANA) antibodies develop in up to 50% of patients treated with anti-TNF agents and anti-dsDNA antibodies in 5-14% (Aringer et al, 2008) (Charles et al, 2000). It should be pointed out that these are mainly IgM antibodies. 0.5-1% develop high affinity IgG antibodies to ds DNA (Charles et al, 2000). The development of clinical lupus-like syndromes in anti-TNF treated patients is rare and in those who do develop this, manifestations are for the main part mild (De Bandt et al, 2005). The development of lupus nephritis as a complication of TNF-induced lupus has been reported but is extremely rare (Mor et al, 2005) (Stokes et al, 2005) (Neradova et al, 2009). New onset anti-phospholipid antibodies have also been noted in individuals treated with TNF blockers and associated vascular events have been documented (Aringer et al, 2008). The development of human anti-chimeric antibodies (HACAs) is also of concern in this patient population and these antibodies are more likely to develop in individuals with SLE given the autoimmune nature of the disease and potentially lead to an increased rate of infusion reactions.

Small cohorts of SLE patients treated with TNF blockers including those with lupus nephritis have been published but as of yet no controlled trials have been conducted (Aringer et al, 2004) (Aringer et al, 2009). In four out of six lupus nephritis patients treated with anti-TNF therapies in an open-labeled study there was a significant sustained reduction in proteinuria following an induction regimen of four infusions of infliximab. Repeated infusions did not confer any additional benefit for these patients (Aringer et al, 2004) (Aringer et al, 2009).

Most lupus patients in these reports were treated with the chimeric monoclonal antibody infliximab, less is known about the clinical impact of the TNF receptor fusion protein, etanercept or the fully humanized TNF monoclonal antibodies adalimumab or golimumab. Overall no firm conclusions can be drawn as regards the use of TNF blockade in lupus nephritis. There may be potential in using these agents, perhaps the fully humanized forms as an induction therapy in lupus nephritis and randomized controlled trials would be needed to clarify the role of anti-TNF therapy in the treatment of SLE.

5.3 Targeting Interferon-α

The concept of interferon-α playing a role in SLE pathogenesis has been noted in the literature since the 1970's. There is a clear association between IFN activity and elevated anti-dsDNA titres and reduction in complement levels, commonly used parameters of clinical lupus activity. Further evidence of the relationship between IFN and lupus stems from the clinical observation that patients receiving recombinant IFN-α for the treatment of hepatitis C or malignancies may develop a lupus-like syndrome and develop autoantibodies. Microarray gene expression analysis has shown wide spread activation of IFN-inducible genes in lupus patients (Baechler et al, 2003) (Crow et al, 2003). IFN pathway activation has been associated with renal disease in lupus (Kirou et al, 2005). IRF5, a lupus susceptibility single nucleotide polymorphism with the highest odds ratio after the MHC plays a pivotal role in IFN pathways and toll-like receptor signaling (Graham et al, 2006). Hence, targeting IFN pathways is a valid therapeutic strategy in lupus patients.

A number of clinical trials of monoclonal antibodies specific for various IFN-α isoforms are ongoing to establish the safety of these agents. An anti-IFN-α monoclonal antibody has been shown to inhibit the IFN signature in peripheral blood mononuclear cells and skin in lupus patients (Yao et al, 2009). This group has proposed a scoring method based on expression of type I IFN-inducible mRNAs, which may divide SLE patients into two distinct subgroups. This might enable type I interferon-inducible genes to be used as biomarkers to identify patients who might respond better to anti-type I IFN treatment (Yao et al, 2011).

Blockade of the IFN receptor is another potential therapeutic target. Given the role of IFN-α in the host defense against viral infection, close clinical monitoring is mandatory in the development of any potential agents targeting this pathway.

6. Complement therapies

6.1 Eculizumab

The importance of the complement system in the pathophysiology of SLE is clear although individual complement components play very different roles in the disease process. Early complement proteins are critical in the clearance of immune complexes and apoptotic material, and their absence predisposes individuals to SLE. Activation of terminal complement is associated with exacerbations of disease, particularly in lupus nephritis. Monoclonal antibodies that specifically inhibit terminal complement activation while preserving early complement function have now been developed. Murine models of lupus nephritis treated with anti-C5 have shown delayed onset proteinuria, improved renal histological findings and longer survival (Wang et al, 1996).

Eculizumab, a monoclonal antibody directed against the complement protein C5, inhibits the cleavage of C5 to C5a and C5b and thus blocks the formation of the terminal membrane attack complex C5b-9 (Cordeiro et al, 2008). Eculizumab has been approved for use in the treatment of paroxysmal nocturnal haemoglobinuria since 2007 (Dmytrijuk et al, 2008). A phase I trial has shown that eculizumab is safe and well tolerated in SLE, but no clear clinical improvements were evident at day 28 and 56 of the study (Rother et al, 2004). To date there have been no further clinical trials to examine the potential efficacy of this therapy.

7. Conclusion

An increased understanding of the immunopathogenesis of SLE during the past decade has lead to the introduction of several new biologic agents into clinical practice. An array of promising new therapies are yet to emerge or are under development. Conventional immunosuppressive therapies have transformed survival in lupus nephritis, but their use is associated with considerable toxic effects and a substantial subset of patients remain refractory to these agents. There is a clear need for new therapeutic agents that overcome these issues, and biologic agents offer exciting opportunities.

An important consideration in the management of lupus nephritis is that patients of different ethnicities have varying clinical outcomes and response to therapy. As alluded to previously, patients of African American descent are more likely to progress to end-stage renal disease (Dooley et al, 1997). Indeed the response to biologic therapy may well vary according to ethnicity. This was well demonstrated in the ALMS study where the efficacy and safety of mycophenolate mofetil (MMF) and intravenous cyclophosphamide (IVC) as induction treatment for lupus nephritis was examined by race, ethnicity and geographical region. This study clearly showed that Black and Hispanic patients responded better to MMF than IVC (Isenberg et al, 2010). The majority of clinical studies in emerging biologic therapies have not addressed the issue of variable clinical response in different ethnic groups. Of note, belimumab was found to be less efficacious in African American patients in phase III clinical trials (Wallace et al, 2009) (Jacobi et al, 2010).

Several of the studies of emerging therapeutic strategies described in this chapter, while encouraging, have targeted SLE disease manifestations in general rather than focusing on outcomes in lupus nephritis. While many of these therapies show promise for their potential use in SLE in general, randomised controlled trials specifically examining their clinical effects in lupus nephritis are needed. In addition to this, the role of new biologic agents to date may have centred on patients who have been refractory to conventional therapies. There are few clinical trials examining their role as first line induction or maintenance therapy. One exception to this has been the successful use of rituximab as first line induction therapy followed by maintenance mycophenolate mofetil in a cohort of eighteen patients with proliferative nephritis (Pepper et al, 2009).

Although so far many biologics e.g. rituximab have been generally well tolerated, (with the exception of rare but important cases of PML), we must not be complacent regarding toxicity, as we do not yet know the long-term effects of these medications on the immune system. Other biologics have had considerable toxicity, such as anti-CD40L (B59588).

A number of key questions remain. How can these therapies be potentially combined with existing proven treatments and indeed with one another to achieve maximum clinical benefit with minimal side effects? It is unlikely that any of these emerging therapies is going to represent a magic therapeutic bullet for all lupus nephritis patients. As is clear to all physicians dealing with the clinical management of SLE this is a heterogeneous disease and there is not one ideal regimen for all. With greater understanding of the pathophysiology of lupus particularly from the genetic perspective, the era of personalized therapy may represent perhaps the greatest advance that is yet to come in the treatment of lupus nephritis.

8. References

Albert D, Dunham J, Khan S, Stansberry J, Kolasinski S, Tsai D, Pullman-Mooar S, Barnack F, Striebich C, Looney RJ, Prak ET, Kimberly R, Zhang Y & Eisenberg R. (2008) Variability in the biological response to anti-CD20 B cell depletion in systemic lupus erythaematosus. *Ann Rheum Dis.* 67(12) Dec 2008:1724-31.

Aringer M, Graninger WB, Steiner G & Smolen JS (2004). Safety and efficacy of tumor necrosis factor alpha blockade in systemic lupus erythematosus: an open-label study. *Arthritis Rheum.* 50(10) Oct 2004:3161-9.

Aringer M & Smolen JS (2005). . Cytokine expression in lupus kidneys. *Lupus.* 14(1) 2005:13-8

Aringer M & Smolen JS (2008). The role of tumor necrosis factor-alpha in systemic lupus erythematosus. *Arthritis Res Ther.* 2008;10(1):202.

Aringer M, Houssiau F, Gordon C, Graninger WB, Voll RE, Rath E, Steiner G & Smolen JS. (2009) Adverse events and efficacy of TNF-alpha blockade with infliximab in patients with systemic lupus erythematosus: long-term follow-up of 13 patients. *Rheumatology (Oxford).* 48(11) Nov 2009:1451-4.

Baechler EC, Batliwalla FM, Karypis G, Gaffney PM, Ortmann WA, Espe KJ, Shark KB, Grande WJ, Hughes KM, Kapur V, Gregersen PK & Behrens TW (2003). Interferon-inducible gene expression signature in peripheral blood cells of patients with severe lupus. *Proc Natl Acad Sci U S A.* 4;100 March 2003(5):2610-5.

Boswell JM, Yui MA, Burt DW & Kelley VE (1988). Increased tumor necrosis factor and IL-1 beta gene expression in the kidneys of mice with lupus nephritis. *J Immunol.* 1;141(9) Nov 1988:3050-4.

Boumpas DT, Furie R, Manzi S, Illei GG, Wallace DJ, Balow JE & Vaishnaw A; BG9588 Lupus Nephritis Trial Group. (2003) A short course of BG9588 (anti-CD40 ligand antibody) improves serologic activity and decreases hematuria in patients with proliferative lupus glomerulonephritis. *Arthritis Rheum.* 48(3) Mar 2003:719-27.

Brennan DC, Yui MA, Wuthrich RP & Kelley VE. (1989). Tumor necrosis factor and IL-1 in New Zealand Black/White mice. Enhanced gene expression and acceleration of renal injury. *J Immunol.* 1;143(11) Dec 1989:3470-5.

Brunet JF, Denizot F, Luciani MF, Roux-Dosseto M, Suzan M, Mattei MG & Golstein P (1987). A new member of the immunoglobulin superfamily-CTLA-4. *Nature.* 16-22;328(6127) Jul 1987:267-70.

Calabrese LH, Molloy ES, Huang D & Ransohoff RM (2007). Progressive multifocal leukoencephalopathy in rheumatic diseases: evolving clinical and pathologic patterns of disease. *Arthritis Rheum.* 56(7):Jul 2007,2116-28.

Charles P.J (2000) Assessment of antibodies to double-stranded DNA induced in rheumatoid arthritisRA patients following treatment with infliximab, a monoclonal antibody to tumor necrosis factor alpha: findings in open-label and randomized placebo-controlled trials. *Arthritis & Rheumatism* 43, 11, Nov 2000;2383–2390.

Chun HY, Chung JW, Kim HA, Yun JM, Jeon JY, Ye YM, Kim SH, Park HS & Suh CH (2007). Cytokine IL-6 and IL-10 as biomarkers in systemic lupus erythematosus. *J Clin Immunol.* 27(5) Sep 2007:461-6.

Cordeiro AC & Isenberg DA (2008). Novel therapies in lupus - focus on nephritis.*Acta Reumatol Port.* 33(2) Apr-Jun 2008:157-69.

Croca SC, Rodrigues T & Isenberg DA (2011). Assessment of a lupus nephritis cohort over a 30-year period. *Rheumatology (Oxford).* 2011 Mar 16.

Crow MK & Kirou KA, Wohlgemuth J (2003). Microarray analysis of interferon-regulated genes in SLE. *Autoimmunity.* 36(8) Dec 2003:481-90.

Daikh DI & Wofsy D.J (2001) Cutting edge: reversal of murine lupus nephritis with CTLA4Ig and cyclophosphamide. *Immunol.* 1;166(5) Mar 2001:2913-6.

Davidson A, Wang X, Mihara M, Ramanujam M, Huang W, Schiffer L & Sinha J (2003). Co-stimulatory blockade in the treatment of murine systemic lupus erythematosus (SLE). *Ann N Y Acad Sci.* 987: Apr 2003; 188-98.

Davis TA, White CA, Grillo-López AJ, Velásquez WS, Link B, Maloney DG, Dillman RO, Williams ME, Mohrbacher A, Weaver R, Dowden S & Levy R (1999). Single-agent monoclonal antibody efficacy in bulky non-Hodgkin's lymphoma: results of a phase II trial of rituximab. *J Clin Oncol.* 17(6) Jun 1999:1851-7.

De Bandt M, Sibilia J, Le Loët X, Prouzeau S, Fautrel B, Marcelli C, Boucquillard E, Siame JL & Mariette X; Club Rhumatismes et Inflammation (2005). Systemic lupus erythematosus induced by anti-tumour necrosis factor alpha therapy: a French national survey. *Arthritis Res Ther.* 7(3) 2005:545-51.

Dmytrijuk A, Robie-Suh K, Cohen MH, Rieves D, Weiss K & Pazdur R (2008). FDA report: eculizumab (Soliris) for the treatment of patients with paroxysmal nocturnal hemoglobinuria. *Oncologist.* 13(9): Sep 2008; 993-1000.

Dooley MA, Hogan S, Jennette C & Falk R (1997). Cyclophosphamide therapy for lupus nephritis: poor renal survival in black Americans. Glomerular Disease Collaborative Network. *Kidney Int.* 51(4): Apr 1997; 1188-95.

Dörner T, Kaufmann J, Wegener WA, Teoh N, Goldenberg DM & Burmester GR (2006). Initial clinical trial of epratuzumab (humanized anti-CD22 antibody) for immunotherapy of systemic lupus erythematosus. *Arthritis Res Ther.* 8(3) 2006:R74.

Early GS, Zhao W & Burns CM (1996). Anti-CD40 ligand antibody treatment prevents the development of lupus-like nephritis in a subset of New Zealand black x New Zealand white mice. Response correlates with the absence of an anti-antibody response. *J Immunol* 157: 1996; 3159-3164.

Edwards JC, Szczepanski L, Szechinski J, Filipowicz-Sosnowska A, Emery P, Close DR, Stevens RM & Shaw T. N (2004) Efficacy of B-cell-targeted therapy with rituximab in patients with rheumatoid arthritis. *Engl J Med.* 17;350(25) Jun 2004 :2572-81.

Finck BK, Linsley PS & Wofsy D (1994). Treatment of murine lupus with CTLA4Ig. *Science.* 26;265(5176) Aug 1994:1225-7.

Gabay C, Cakir N, Moral F, Roux-Lombard P, Meyer O, Dayer JM, Vischer T, Yazici H & Guerne PA (1997). Circulating levels of tumor necrosis factor soluble receptors in systemic lupus erythematosus are significantly higher than in other rheumatic diseases and correlate with disease activity. *J Rheumatol.* 24(2) Feb 1997:303-8.

Genovese MC, Schiff M & Luggen M (2008). Efficacy and safety of the selective co-stimulation modulator abatacept following 2 years of treatment in patients with rheumatoid arthritis and an inadequate response to anti-tumour necrosis factor therapy. *Ann Rheum Dis.* 2008; 67:547–54.

Graham RR, Kozyrev SV, Baechler EC, Reddy MV, Plenge RM, Bauer JW, Ortmann WA, Koeuth T, González Escribano MF; Argentine and Spanish Collaborative Groups, Pons-Estel B, Petri M, Daly M, Gregersen PK, Martín J, Altshuler D, Behrens TW & Alarcón-Riquelme ME (2006). A common haplotype of interferon regulatory factor 5 (IRF5) regulates splicing and expression and is associated with increased risk of systemic lupus erythematosus. *Nat Genet.* 38(5) May 2006:550-5

Gunnarsson I, Sundelin B, Jónsdóttir T, Jacobson SH, Henriksson EW & van Vollenhoven RF (2007). Histopathologic and clinical outcome of rituximab treatment in patients with cyclophosphamide-resistant proliferative lupus nephritis. *Arthritis Rheum.* 56(4): Apr 2007;1263-72.

Hainsworth JD, Burris HA 3rd, Morrissey LH, Litchy S, Scullin DC Jr, Bearden JD 3rd, Richards P & Greco FA (2000). Rituximab monoclonal antibody as initial systemic therapy for patients with low-grade non-Hodgkin lymphoma. *Blood.* 15;95(10) May 2000:3052-6.

Herrera-Esparza R, Barbosa-Cisneros O, Villalobos-Hurtado R & Avalos-Díaz E (1998). Renal expression of IL-6 and TNFalpha genes in lupus nephritis. *Lupus.* 7(3): 1998; 154-8.

Hill GS, Delahousse M, Nochy D & Bariéty J (2005). Class IV-S versus class IV-G lupus nephritis: clinical and morphologic differences suggesting different pathogenesis. *Kidney Int.* 68(5): Nov 2005; 2288-97.

Hillmen P, Young N, Schubert J, Brodsky R, Socié G, Muus P, Röth A, Szer J, Elebute M, Nakamura R, Browne P, Risitano A, Hill A, Schrezenmeier H, Fu C, Maciejewski J, Rollins S, Mojcik C, Rother R & Luzzatto L (2006). "The complement inhibitor eculizumab in paroxysmal nocturnal hemoglobinuria". *N Engl J Med* 355 (12) 2006: 1233–43.

Illei GG, Shirota Y, Yarboro CH, Daruwalla J, Tackey E, Takada K, Fleisher T, Balow JE & Lipsky PE (2010). Tocilizumab in Systemic Lupus Erythematosus - Safety,Preliminary Efficacy, and Impact on Circulating Plasma Cells. *Arthritis Rheum.* 62(2) Feb 2010; 542-52.

Isenberg D, Appel GB, Contreras G, Dooley MA, Ginzler EM, Jayne D, Sánchez-Guerrero J, Wofsy D, Yu X & Solomons N (2010). Influence of race/ethnicity on response to lupus nephritis treatment: the ALMS study. *Rheumatology (Oxford).* 49(1) Jan 2010:128-40.

Jacobi AM, Huang W, Wang T, Freimuth W, Sanz I, Furie R, Mackay M, Aranow C, Diamond B & Davidson A (2010). Effect of long-term belimumab treatment on B cells in systemic lupus erythematosus: extension of a phase II, double-blind, placebo-controlled, dose-ranging study. *Arthritis Rheum.* 62(1):Jan 2010;201-10.

Jónsdóttir T, Gunnarsson I, Mourão AF, Lu TY, van Vollenhoven RF& Isenberg D (2010). Clinical improvements in proliferative vs membranous lupus nephritis following B-cell depletion: pooled data from two cohorts. *Rheumatology (Oxford).* 49(8): 20101502-4.

Jónsdóttir T, Sundelin B, Welin Henriksson E, van Vollenhoven RF& Gunnarsson I (2011). Rituximab-treated membranous lupus nephritis: clinical outcome and effects on electron dense deposits. *Ann Rheum Dis.* 70(6): 2011; 1172-3.

Kalunian KC, Davis JC Jr, Merrill JT, Totoritis MC & Wofsy D; IDEC-131 Lupus Study Group (2002). Treatment of systemic lupus erythematosus by inhibition of T cell costimulation with anti-CD154: a randomized, double-blind, placebo-controlled trial. *Arthritis Rheum.* 46(12): Dec 2002; 3251-8.

Kirou KA, Lee C, George S, Louca K, Peterson MG & Crow MK (2005). Activation of the interferon-alpha pathway identifies a subgroup of systemic lupus erythematosus patients with distinct serologic features and active disease. *Arthritis Rheum.* 52(5): May 2005; 1491-503.

Leandro MJ, Edwards JC, Cambridge G, Ehrenstein MR & Isenberg DA (2002). An open study of B lymphocyte depletion in systemic lupus erythematosus. *Arthritis Rheum.* 46(10): Oct 2002; 2673-7.

Leandro MJ, Cambridge G, Edwards JC, Ehrenstein MR & Isenberg DA (2005). B-cell depletion in the treatment of patients with systemic lupus erythematosus: a longitudinal analysis of 24 patients. *Rheumatology (Oxford).* 44(12): Dec 2005; 1542-5.

Ledbetter JA, Imboden JB, Schieven GL, Grosmaire LS, Rabinovitch PS, Lindsten T, Thompson CB & June CH (1990). CD28 ligation in T-cell activation: evidence for two signal transduction pathways. *Blood.* 75(7): Apr 1990; 1531-9.

Leonard JP, Coleman M, Ketas JC, Chadburn A, Furman R, Schuster MW, Feldman EJ, Ashe M, Schuster SJ, Wegener WA, Hansen HJ, Ziccardi H, Eschenberg M, Gayko U, Fields SZ, Cesano A & Goldenberg DM (2004). Epratuzumab, a humanized anti-CD22 antibody, in aggressive non-Hodgkin's lymphoma: phase I/II clinical trial results. *Clin Cancer Res.* 10(16): Aug 2004; 5327-34.

Leonard JP, Coleman M, Ketas J, Ashe M, Fiore JM, Furman RR, Niesvizky R, Shore T, Chadburn A, Horne H, Kovacs J, Ding CL, Wegener WA, Horak ID & Goldenberg DM (2005). Combination antibody therapy with epratuzumab and rituximab in relapsed or refractory non-Hodgkin's lymphoma. *J Clin Oncol.* 23(22): Aug 2005; 5044-51.

Liang B, Gardner DB, Griswold DE, Bugelski PJ, Song XY (2006). Anti-interleukin-6 monoclonal antibody inhibits autoimmune responses in a murine model of systemic lupus erythematosus. *Immunology.* 119(3): Nov 2006; 296-305.

Linker-Israeli M, Deans RJ, Wallace DJ, Prehn J, Ozeri-Chen T & Klinenberg JR (1991). Elevated levels of endogenous IL-6 in systemic lupus erythematosus. A putative role in pathogenesis. *J Immunol.* 147(1): Jul 1991; 117-23.

Looney RJ, Anolik JH, Campbell D, Felgar RE, Young F, Arend LJ, Sloand JA, Rosenblatt J & Sanz I (2004). B cell depletion as a novel treatment for systemic lupus erythematosus: a phase I/II dose-escalation trial of rituximab. *Arthritis Rheum.* 50(8): Aug 2004; 2580-9.

Mackay F, Woodcock SA, Lawton P, Ambrose C, Baetscher M, Schneider P, Tschopp J & Browning JL (2003). Mice transgenic for BAFF develop lymphocytic disorders along with autoimmune manifestations. *J Exp Med.* 190(11): Dec 1999; 1697-710.

Mavragani CP & Moutsopoulos HM (2003). Lupus nephritis: current issues. *Ann Rheum Dis.* 62(9): Sep 2003; 795-8.

Mease P, Genovese MC, Gladstein G, Kivitz AJ, Ritchlin C, Tak PP, Wollenhaupt J, Bahary O, Becker JC, Kelly S, Sigal L, Teng J & Gladman D (2011). Abatacept in the treatment of patients with psoriatic arthritis: results of a six-month, multicenter, randomized, double-blind, placebo-controlled, phase II trial. *Arthritis Rheum.* 63(4): Apr 2011; 939-48.

Merrill JT, Neuwelt CM, Wallace DJ, Shanahan JC, Latinis KM, Oates JC, Utset TO, Gordon C, Isenberg DA, Hsieh HJ, Zhang D & Brunetta PG (2010) . Efficacy and safety of rituximab in moderately-to-severely active systemic lupus erythematosus: the randomized, double-blind, phase II/III systemic lupus erythematosus evaluation of rituximab trial. *Arthritis Rheum*. 62(1): Jan 2010; 222-33.

Merrill JT, Burgos-Vargas R, Westhovens R, Chalmers A, D'Cruz D, Wallace DJ, Bae SC, Sigal L, Becker JC, Kelly S, Raghupathi K, Li T, Peng Y, Kinaszczuk M & Nash P (2010). The efficacy and safety of abatacept in patients with non-life-threatening manifestations of systemic lupus erythematosus: results of a twelve-month, multicenter, exploratory, phase IIb, randomized, double-blind, placebo-controlled trial. *Arthritis Rheum*. 62(10): Oct 2010; 3077-87.

Mihara M, Takagi N, Takeda Y & Ohsugi Y (1998). IL-6 receptor blockage inhibits the onset of autoimmune kidney disease in NZB/W F1 mice. *Clin Exp Immunol*. 112(3): Jun 1998; 397-402.

Mor A, Bingham C 3rd, Barisoni L, Lydon E & Belmont HM (2005). Proliferative lupus nephritis and leukocytoclastic vasculitis during treatment with etanercept. *J Rheumatol*. 32(4): Apr 2005; 740-3.

Neradová A, Stam F, van den Berg JG & Bax WA (2009). Etanercept-associated SLE with lupus nephritis. *Lupus*. 18(7): Jun 2009; 667-8

Nestorov I, Munafo A, Papasouliotis O & Visich J (2008). Pharmacokinetics and biological activity of atacicept in patients with rheumatoid arthritis. *J Clin Pharmacol*. 48(4): Apr 2008; 406-17.

Otipoby KL, Andersson KB, Draves KE, Klaus SJ, Farr AG, Kerner JD, Perlmutter RM, Law CL & Clark EA (1996). CD22 regulates thymus-independent responses and the lifespan of B cells. *Nature*. 384(6610): Dec 1996; 634-7.

Pena-Rossi C, Nasonov E, Stanislav M, Yakusevich V, Ershova O, Lomareva N, Saunders H, Hill J, & Nestorov I.. An exploratory dose-escalating study investigating the safety, tolerability, pharmacokinetics and pharmacodynamics of intravenous atacicept in patients with systemic lupus erythematosus. *Lupus*. 18(6): May 2009; 547-55

Pepper R, Griffith M, Kirwan C, Levy J, Taube D, Pusey C, Lightstone L & Cairns T (2009). Rituximab is an effective treatment for lupus nephritis and allows a reduction in maintenance steroids. *Nephrol Dial Transplant*. 24(12): Dec 2009; 3717-23.

Peterson E, Robertson AD & Emlen W (1996). Serum and urinary interleukin-6 in systemic lupus erythematosus. *Lupus*. 5(6): Dec 1996; 571-5.

Reiser H & Stadecker MJ (1996). Costimulatory B7 molecules in the pathogenesis of infectious and autoimmune diseases. *N Engl J Med*. 335(18): Oct 1996; 1369-77.

Rother RP, Mojcik CF& McCroskery EW (2004). Inhibition of terminal complement: a novel therapeutic approach for the treatment of systemic lupus erythematosus. *Lupus*. 13(5): 2004; 328-34.

Ryffel B, Car BD, Gunn H, Roman D, Hiestand P & Mihatsch MJ (1994). Interleukin-6 exacerbates glomerulonephritis in (NZB x NZW)F1 mice. *Am J Pathol*. 144(5): May 1994; 927-37.

Saito K, Nawata M, Iwata S, Tokunaga M & Tanaka Y (2005). Extremely high titer of anti-human chimeric antibody following re-treatment with rituximab in a patient with active systemic lupus erythemtosus. *Rheumatology (Oxford)*. 44(11): Nov 2005; 1462-4.

Sangle SR, Davies RJ, Aslam L, Lewis MJ, Wedgwood R & Hughes GRV (2007). Rituximab in the treatment of resistant systemic lupus erythematosus: failure of therapy in rapidly progressive crescentic lupus nephritis. *Rheumatology* 2007; 56: S215

Sato S, Tuscano JM, Inaoki M & Tedder TF (1998). CD22 negatively and positively regulates signal transduction through the B lymphocyte antigen receptor. *Semin Immunol.* 10(4): Aug 1998; 287-97.

Scheipers P & Reiser H (1998). Role of the CTLA-4 receptor in T cell activation and immunity. Physiologic function of the CTLA-4 receptor. *Immunol Res.* 18(2): 1998; 103-15.

Schiemann B, Gommerman JL, Vora K, Cachero TG, Shulga-Morskaya S, Dobles M, Frew E & Scott ML (2001). An essential role for BAFF in the normal development of B cells through a BCMA-independent pathway. *Science.* 293(5537): Sep 2001; 2111-4.

Smith KG, Jones RB, Burns SM & Jayne DR (2006). Long-term comparison of rituximab treatment for refractory systemic lupus erythematosus and vasculitis: Remission, relapse, and re-treatment. *Arthritis Rheum.* 54(9): Sep 2006; 2970-82.

Stohl W (2003). SLE--systemic lupus erythematosus: a BLySful, yet BAFFling, disorder. *Arthritis Res Ther.* 5(3): 2003; 136-8.

Stokes MB, Foster K, Markowitz GS, Ebrahimi F, Hines W, Kaufman D, Moore B, Wolde D & D'Agati VD (2005). Development of glomerulonephritis during anti-TNF-alpha therapy for rheumatoid arthritis. *Nephrol Dial Transplant.* 20(7): Jul 2005; 1400-6.

Sutter JA, Kwan-Morley J, Dunham J, Du YZ, Kamoun M, Albert D, Eisenberg RA & Luning Prak ET (2008). A longitudinal analysis of SLE patients treated with rituximab (anti-CD20): factors associated with B lymphocyte recovery. *Clin Immunol.* 126(3): Mar 2008; 282-90.

Tedder TF, Tuscano J, Sato S & Kehrl JH (1997). CD22, a B lymphocyte-specific adhesion molecule that regulates antigen receptor signaling. *Annu Rev Immunol.* 15: 1997; 481-504.

Terrier B, Amoura Z, Ravaud P, Hachulla E, Jouenne R, Combe B, Bonnet C, Cacoub P, Cantagrel A, de Bandt M, Fain O, Fautrel B, Gaudin P, Godeau B, Harlé JR, Hot A, Kahn JE, Lambotte O, Larroche C, Léone J, Meyer O, Pallot-Prades B, Pertuiset E, Quartier P, Schaerverbeke T, Sibilia J, Somogyi A, Soubrier M, Vignon E, Bader-Meunier B, Mariette X & Gottenberg JE; Club Rhumatismes et Inflammation (2010). Safety and efficacy of rituximab in systemic lupus erythematosus: results from 136 patients from the French AutoImmunity and Rituximab registry. *Arthritis Rheum.* 62(8): Aug 2010; 2458-66.

Tsai CY, Wu TH, Yu CL, Lu JY & Tsai YY (2000). Increased excretions of beta2-microglobulin, IL-6, and IL-8 and decreased excretion of Tamm-Horsfall glycoprotein in urine of patients with active lupus nephritis. *Nephron.* 85(3): Jul 2000; 207-14.

Turner-Stokes T, Lu TY, Ehrenstein MR, Giles I, Rahman A & Isenberg DA (2011). The efficacy of repeated treatment with B-cell depletion therapy in systemic lupus erythematosus: an evaluation. *Rheumatology (Oxford).* 12, 2011 Mar [Epub ahead of print].

Wallace DJ, Stohl W, Furie RA, Lisse JR, McKay JD, Merrill JT, Petri MA, Ginzler EM, Chatham WW, McCune WJ, Fernandez V, Chevrier MR, Zhong ZJ & Freimuth WW (2009). A phase II, randomized, double-blind, placebo-controlled, dose-ranging study of belimumab in patients with active systemic lupus erythematosus. *Arthritis Rheum.* 61(9): Sep 2009; 1168-78.

Wang Y, Hu Q, Madri JA, Rollins SA, Chodera A & Matis LA (1996). Amelioration of lupus-like autoimmune disease in NZB/WF1 mice after treatment with a blocking monoclonal antibody specific for complement component C5. *Proc Natl Acad Sci U S A.* 93(16): Aug 1996; 8563-8.

Yang G, Liu H, Jiang M, Jiang X, Li S, Yuan Y & Ma D (1998). Experimental study on intramuscular injection of eukaryotic expression vector pcDNA3- IL-6 on BXSB mice.*Chin Med J.* 111(1): Jan 1998; 38-42.

Yao Y, Richman L, Higgs BW, Morehouse CA, de los Reyes M, Brohawn P, Zhang J, White B, Coyle AJ, Kiener PA & Jallal B (2009). Neutralization of interferon-alpha/beta-inducible genes and downstream effect in a phase I trial of an anti-interferon-alpha monoclonal antibody in systemic lupus erythematosus. *Arthritis Rheum.* 60(6): Jun 2009; 1785-96.

Yao Y, Higgs BW, Richman L, White B & Jallal B (2011). Use of type I interferon-inducible mRNAs as pharmacodynamic markers and potential diagnostic markers in trials with sifalimumab, an anti-IFNalpha antibody, in systemic lupus erythematosus. *Arthritis Res Ther.*14;12 Apr 2011;Suppl 1:S6. [Epub ahead of print].

Yokoyama H, Kreft B & Kelley VR (1995). Biphasic increase in circulating and renal TNF-alpha in MRL-lpr mice with differing regulatory mechanisms. *Kidney Int.* 47(1): Jan 1995; 122-30.

Zampieri S, Alaibac M, Iaccarino L, Rondinone R, Ghirardello A, Sarzi-Puttini P, Peserico A & Doria A (2006). Tumour necrosis factor alpha is expressed in refractory skin lesions from patients with subacute cutaneous lupus erythematosus. *Ann Rheum Dis.* 65(4): Apr 2006; 545-8.

13

Cardiovascular Involvement in Systemic Lupus Erythematosus

Sultana Abdulaziz[1], Yahya AlGhamdi[2],
Mohammed Samannodi[2] and Mohammed Shabrawishi[2]
[1]*King Fahd Hospital, Jeddah*
[2]*Um AlQura University, Makkah*
Saudi Arabia

1. Introduction

Cardiovascular involvement in systemic lupus erythematosus (SLE) was first reported by Kaposi in 1872 of cardiac irregularity and dyspnea. In 1924, Libman and Sacks reported verrucous endocarditis but ironically did not recognize the association of verrucous endocarditis with SLE. (Petri, 2004) In the last decade, newly recognized clinical entities have been described with the introduction of very sensitive, non-invasive and semi-invasive cardiac imaging techniques.(Turiel, 2005) With the use of very sensitive methods of cardiovascular investigations, it has been found the prevalence of cardiac involvement to be >50%. (Petri, 2004)

Several autoantibodies such as antiDNA, anti-phospholipid antibodies (apl), antiSSA (Ro antibodies) and antiendothelial cell antibodies present in patients with SLE can mediate cardiac damage. These autoantibodies can directly affect the heart tissue or, alternatively, trigger mechanisms able to cause heart damage for example, apl can contribute to cardiac damage enhancing atherosclerosis phenomena, causing thrombosis of coronary arteries or starting an immune-complex mediated reaction and deposition at the valve level. Consequences of autoantibody damage has been reported in several heart structures such as the valves, myocardium, pericardium, conduction tissues and cardiac arteries in patients suffering from SLE, antiphospholipid syndrome (APS), Sjogrens syndrome and other autoimmune rheumatic diseases(ARD). (Tincani et al, 2006)

Overall improvements in medical care including the availability of antibiotics, antihypertensive, and renal replacement therapy coupled with the judicious use of glucocorticoids, antimalarial and immunosuppressive drugs have led to improved survival of SLE patients in the past 50 years. (Nikpou, 2005) In 1976, Urowitz first described the 'bimodal mortality pattern' of SLE. This observation was based on SLE deaths early in the course of the disease were due to active SLE and use of high dose steroids associated with complications such as infection and sepsis. Later in the disease course (›5 years after diagnosis) deaths were frequently associated with inactive SLE, long duration of prednisolone therapy and myocardial infarction (MI) due to atherosclerotic heart disease. (Urowitz, 1976) Cardiac disease has recently been acknowledged as a primary cause of morbidity and mortality in SLE as well as APS, and numerous factors leading to accelerated atherosclerosis has been characterized. Though cardiac involvement is a uncommon cause of flare: it can be forgotten unless a full blown cardiac dysfunction or complication is present. In a prospective study of flares, serositis was present in only 7-9% of the flares. (Petri, 1991) With prolongation of life by modern immunosuppressive therapies, heart lesions develop in all patients at sometime during the course of their disease.

The present chapter:

Emphasizes and describes the cardiac involvement in SLE which may involve all three layers of the heart (pericardium, myocardium and the endocardium).Appreciate the early identification and management of these conditions prevents the late life threatening complications and consequences. Recognize the importance of premature atherosclerosis and that it is the major cause for mortality and premature death in lupus patients. Understand the causation is multifactorial: traditional risk factors as well as SLE related risk factors and inflammatory mediators are involved in the pathogenesis. Early identification and treatment of modifiable risk factors in SLE patients are discussed. There have not yet been any published randomized, controlled trials in patients with SLE in respect to CVD risk factor modifications. Thus treatment and management recommendations are based on published guidelines for other populations at high risk for CVD.

2. Pericarditis

2.1 Clinical features

Pericarditis is the most common cardiac manifestation of active lupus, although often it is not evident clinically. Pericarditis can occur at any time during the course of SLE, it tends to be one of the earlier cardiac manifestations, and can even be the first manifestation of lupus.(Brigden, 1960) Pericarditis was the presenting sign of lupus in 4 of 28 patients who ultimately developed it in one series.(Godeau et al.1981) Pericarditis in SLE presents in the typical way, with precordial pain, usually positional (aggravated by lying down), often with a pleuritic quality, and sometimes with dyspnea. Coexistent pleurisy and/or effusions are common, occurring in 14 of 28 cases in same series. (Godeau et al., 1981) Pericarditis usually appears as an isolated attack or as recurrent episodes, with or without symptoms. Patients may have fever and tachycardia. Friction rubs are rare, perhaps because they are present often for only a few hours and are missed. The "classic" pericardial friction rub has three components, occurring with ventricular contraction, atrial contraction, and at the end of rapid ventricular filling.(Petri, 2004) In a French series, of 28 cases of pericarditis, 23 had pain, 12 had a rub, and 4 required pericardiocentesis because of tamponade.(Godeau et al.,1981) Patients with pericardial effusion (as opposed to thickening) are more likely to have pericardial pain and active lupus elsewhere.(Leung et al, 1990,Cervera et al, 1992) In the study by Cervera et al, only the patients with moderate or severe pericardial effusion had clinical or electrocardiographic evidence of pericarditis.(Cervera et al, 1992) When present, pericardial effusions are usually small and do not cause hemodynamic problems. Pericardial tamponade is rare and has been reported as an initial presentation (Topaloglu, 2006) and even in treated patients. (Shearn, 1959 In a series reported by Rosenbaum, 9 of the 71 patients with pericardial effusion developed pericardial tamponade(21%) of which 5 of the 9 patients required a pericardial window.(Rosenbaum, 2009) Constrictive pericarditis is very rare. Only four cases of constrictive pericarditis have been reported. In two of the four cases constrictive pericarditis developed in spite of corticosteroid therapy. All four known cases have occurred in males. (Petri, 2004)

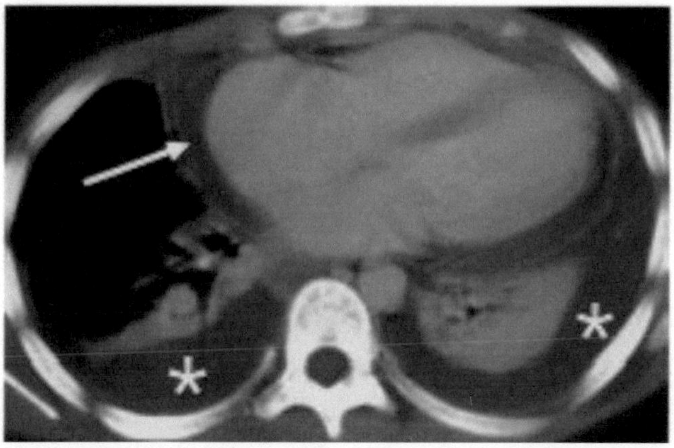

Fig. 1. Serositis in a 13-year-old boy with SLE. Contrast-enhanced CT scan shows bilateral pleural effusions (*), cardiomegaly, and a pericardial effusion (arrow). Bilateral lower lobe atelectasis is also present. (Lalani & Hatieldl, 2004) Copyright permission from RSNA

2.2 Diagnosis

If a patient presents for the first time with pericarditis, it is usually impossible to invoke SLE as the cause until appropriate laboratory tests are available suggesting the diagnosis. However, patients with idiopathic pericarditis more often give a history of recent viral infection, and are more often male. In idiopathic pericarditis there is usually a leukocytosis, whereas a finding of leucopenia would suggest SLE. Pericardial friction rubs may be heard in sicker and untreated patients, but are often absent in milder cases, especially those patients already on corticosteroid and/or NSAID treatment. A significant rise in jugular venous pressure is unusual. (Petri, 2004) In one series, most patients showed electrocardiographic evidence of acute or chronic pericarditis. (Brigden et al, 1960) The diagnosis of pericarditis can be confirmed by ECG findings of elevated ST segments and tall T waves (although slight T-wave changes or transient elevation of ST segments are most characteristic), or by cardiac echocardiogram findings of pericardial effusion or thickened pericardium. Serial electrocardiograms may show a progression of changes in pericarditis. Initially, a diffuse elevation of ST segments (without reciprocal ST segment depression) is found. This is followed by a lowering of ST segments back toward baseline and subsequent T-wave inversion. In most cases, T waves then return to normal. (Petri, 2004) Effusions may be accompanied by a drop in voltage. After severe attacks, the T waves may not recover to their original voltage.(Brigden, 1960) In the series of Godeau *et al.*, of 28 cases, 5 had low voltage, 10 had ST changes, and 20 had depolarization changes.(Godeau et al, 1981) Both effusion and thickening are frequent in echocardiogram studies. Most effusions are mild. Echocardiography (two-dimensional echocardiogram and Doppler echocardiography) is the modality of choice in evaluating pericardial disease, because it is both noninvasive and sensitive. However, echocardiography may be an insensitive technique in diagnosing pericarditis when it is not accompanied by effusion or thickening. (Petri, 2004)

2.3 Prevalence

The frequency of pericarditis depends on the modality of diagnosis.Published series of patients find pericarditis in 12–47% of living SLE patients.(Petri, 2004) In general, the

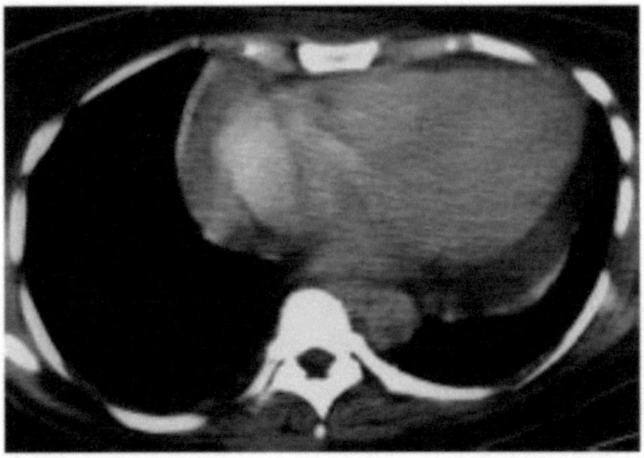

Fig. 2. Lupus pericarditis in a 42-year-old woman. Contrast-enhanced CT scan demonstrates cardiomegaly, a thickened and enhancing pericardium, and a pericardial effusion. . (Lalani & Hatieldl, 2004) Copyright permission from RSNA

echocardiogram is more sensitive than clinical diagnosis, with 19–54% of patients having pericardial effusion or thickening. The echocardiogram is an essential tool in the clinical management of sick patients with cardiac lupus, because clinical diagnosis alone may be faulty. Pericardial abnormalities are the most common echocardiographic finding in SLE patients.(Leung, 1990) However, significant pericardial disease is uncommon, even using echocardiograms, being found in only 7% in one study by Cervera et al. (Cervera et al , 1992) Autopsy studies find a much higher prevalence of pericardial involvement, ranging up to 61–100%. (Petri, 2004)

2.4 Pathology

Pericardial fluid in SLE is usually exudative, the amount of fluid varying from 100 to more than 1000 cc.(Tincani, 2006)White blood counts are in the 30,000 range, primarily neutrophils. Although not helpful in patient management, the fluid may contain anti-DNA and have low complement levels. Complement-fixing material was found in pericardial fluid in patients with SLE, which was felt to be immune complexes. (Petri, 2004) At autopsy, a diffuse or focal fibrinous pericarditis, often with many hematoxylin bodies, with or without effusion, was found. In the series of Brigden *et al.*, the layers of the pericardium were obliterated with occasional deposits of fresh fibrin or effusion. (Brigden, 1960) In another autopsy study, of 11 cases, 6 had acute pericarditis and 5 had chronic obliterative pericarditis (2 of these had pericardiomediastinal adhesions). (Bidani, 1980)

The histopathology in a case of constrictive pericarditis showed fibrosis and mild chronic inflammation, with IgG, IgM, and complement deposition on immunofluorescence. Immunopathogenetic analyses of the pericardium in 2 of 9 patients in an autopsy series demonstrated the vascular deposition of immunoglobulin and complement. (Bidani, 1980) On histopathology, small pericardial blood vessels were surrounded by an infiltrate of lymphocytes, plasma cells, macrophages, and rare polymorphonuclear leukocytes. On immunofluorescence, IgG was present in a predominantly granular pattern around small pericardial vessels.Thus, Bidani and colleagues concluded that immune complex deposition was the cause of pericarditis. (Bidani, 1980)

2.5 Treatment

In early studies, pericarditis usually responded quickly to corticosteroids, with serial chest x-rays showing rapid and radiologic evidence of resorption of fluid.(Brigden,1960) Shearn commented in his review that the "often transient nature of pericarditis makes evaluation of therapy for this condition most difficult.(Shearn, 1959) However, many studies have noted pericardial effusion developing or persisting even with corticosteroid treatment, such as the autopsy study of Kong *et al.*, in which 11 of 12 patients with pericardial effusion had taken corticosteroids.(Kong et al,1962) Occasionally patients progressed to the point of tamponade.(Rosenbaum, 2009) Nonsteroidal anti-inflammatory drugs are helpful for mild cases of pericarditis. Patients presenting with pericardial tamponade may necessitate pericardiocentesis. Refractory cases of large pericardial effusions may benefit from a pericardial window. (Rosenbaum, 2009)

3. Myocarditis

3.1 Clinical features

Myocarditis, as recognized clinically, is rare in SLE. The clinical detection of myocarditis ranges from 3 to 15%, although it appears to be much more common in autopsy studies suggesting the largely subclinical nature of the myocardial pathology. Patients may present in florid congestive heart failure, or more subacutely with tachycardia and dyspnea. Myocardial abnormalities were found in 20% of patients using echocardiograms, but only one patient with an echocardiographic pattern of myocarditis developed myocardial dysfunction clinically.(Cervera, 1992)

Even autopsy studies have shown that myocarditis usually does not lead to cardiac dilatation.(Griffith & Vural, 1951) Brigden *et al.* had no patient in whom congestive heart failure was attributed solely to myocarditis.(Brigden et al, 1960) Shearn had only one patient with heart failure attributable to myocarditis.(Shearn,1959)

However, other series have found myocarditis as a cause of congestive heart failure. (Petri, 2004) Harvey *et al* found that myocarditis was the cause of heart failure in 8 of their 9 patients. (Petri, 2004) Hejtmancik *et al.* found myocarditis to be the major cause in 6 of their 10 cases. (Hejtmancik et al, 1964). Kong *et al.* had 17 patients with cardiomegaly; at autopsy, 15 had myocarditis but of varying degrees of severity.(Kong et al,1962)

The differential diagnosis of congestive heart failure in SLE would include lupus myocarditis, viral myocarditis, toxic myocarditis due to use of antimalarial drugs, anemia, renal failure, pulmonary disease, atherosclerotic heart disease, coronary arteritis, valvular disease, and hypertension.

3.2 Diagnosis

The clinical recognition of myocarditis can easily be missed. In most cases, the patient who had a hematologic and renal flare was not recognized to have myocarditis as well until they presented in congestive heart failure. Myocarditis should be considered in patients with tachycardia not due to fever, in patients with a third heart sound (S3), in patients with abnormal ECGs, in those with new murmurs or conduction disturbances, and in those with congestive heart failure. (Shearn, 1959) Brigden *et al.* suggested that prolongation of the conduction time of either P-R, QRS, or Q-T interval would have been evidence of myocarditis (in the absence of another cause of ventricular hypertrophy), but that they did not encounter these ECG changes in their series.(Brigden, 1960)

Hejtmancik *et al.* made a clinical diagnosis of myocarditis in 21% of their patients (after first excluding hypertension and coronary artery disease), based on (1) cardiac enlargement, (2) ventricular gallop, and (3) electrocardiographic abnormalities.(Hejtmancik et al, 1964) Kong *et al.* found myocarditis at autopsy in 15 of their 16 patients with gallop rhythm.(Kong et al, 1962).The diagnosis of myocarditis can be supported by the finding of global hypokinesia on cardiac echocardiogram and may be confirmed by right ventricular endomyocardial biopsy.(Petri,2004) Although echocardiography cannot diagnose myocarditis with certainty, global hypokinesia, in the absence of other known causes, is strongly suggestive.(Busteed et al, 2004) Other investigations that may help to diagnose myocarditis include a gallium scan18 and magnetic resonance imaging (MRI).(Saremi et al, 2007) Nuclear medicine scans rely on labeling of anti myosin antibodies with radiopharmaceuticals, and may not be available in all clinical settings. Different MRI techniques may support the diagnosis of myocarditis. Contrast enhancement of the myocardium in the setting of acute myocyte membrane rupture results in greater passive diffusion of contrast into the affected intracellular space. A midwall myocardial hyperenhancement pattern is the most frequent finding in both acute and chronic myocarditits, while a subepicardial distribution of lesions is reported only in patients with acute myocarditis.(Saremi et al,2007) However, it is important to note that MRI alone cannot differentiate viral myocarditis from other causes of acute dilated cardiomyopathy. A biopsy is not required in many cases of lupus myocarditis, as the sensitivity and specificity are unknown; but can be useful in some patients to confirm the clinical diagnosis, determine the severity of myocardial involvement, and distinguish this disorder from other causes of myocardial disease like drug induced etc.(Wijetunga & Rockson, 2002) New-onset heart failure of less than 6 days' duration associated with hemodynamic compromise is an American Heart Association/American College of Cardiology/European Society of Cardiology class I indication for endomyocardial biopsy.(Cooper et al,2007)

3.3 Prevalence

In large series of patients, the clinical diagnosis of myocarditis has been made in up to21 %. (Petri, 2004) Autopsy studies, mainly done in the 1950s and 1960s, frequently found myocarditis. More recent postmortem studies,(Bindani, 1980) reflecting the era of corticosteroid treatment, found much lower frequencies, from 0 to 8%. Echocardiographic studies cannot definitively diagnose myocarditis, but global hypokinesia, in the absence of other known causes, is strongly suggestive. (Appenzeller, 2011) Large echo series have found frequencies of global hypokinesis between 5 and 20%. However, segmental areas of hyopkinesis on echocardiogram can also be indicative of myocarditis. Newer imaging modalities, such as magnetic resonance, are largely unstudied. (Appenzeller, 2011)

3.4 Pathology

A common misperception is that myocarditis in SLE is a myositis. CPK levels are usually normal.(Petri, 2004) In fact, only one study found any association with myositis elsewhere.(Borenstein et al, 1978) Myocarditis in SLE is a complicated process, with arteritis or arteriopathy, not primary disease of the myocardial fibers, playing a major role. Kong *et al.* found pathologic evidence of myocarditis (fibrinoid and collagenous degeneration, interstitial edema, necrosis, and/or cellular infiltration) in 15 of 30 autopsies. (Konget al, 1962) The cellular infiltrates of myocarditis consist of foci of interstitial plasma cells and lymphocytes. Immunofluorescence studies confirm that the etiopathogenesis is vascular. In one study, most of the immune deposits were present in the walls of blood vessels of the myocardium.(Bidani, 1980) Immunofluorescence studies of endomyocardial biopsies reveal perivascular deposits of IgG and vascular deposits of C3.(Appenzeller, 2011) A rare and aggressive form is giant cell myocarditis, which is associated with extensive myocytes necrosis, a mixed dense lymphoplasmacytic infiltration, numerous multinucleated giant cells and degranulatd esinophils, leads to rapidly developing progressive congestive heart failure and arrhythmias.(Chung et al, 2005; Martorell et al, 2008) Antimalarial-related myocarditis is often associated with skeletal muscle involvement showing curvilinear and myeloid bodies.(Nord et al,2004)

3.5 Treatment

Myocarditis that comes to clinical attention is usually an urgent situation. Treatment with high-dose intravenous methylprednisolone (such as the "pulse"regimen, 1000 mg daily for 3 days), followed by high dose IV or oral corticosteroid maintenance therapy, is indicated. Intravenous "pulse" cyclophosphamide is added in refractory cases and patients with heart failure. Initial six cycle of monthly pulses of cyclophosphamide 750mg/m2, followed by a repeated cycle if LVEF has not completely normalized, is relatively well tolerated and effective. (Van der Laan Baalbergen et al, 2009) Intravenous immunoglobulin's have been used in one or two case reports with some success.(Sherer et al, 1999)

Supportive therapy for congestive heart failure, including diuresis, digoxin, and afterload reduction (such as with angiotensin converting enzyme (ACE) inhibitors) may be necessary. Anticoagulation should be considered in those patients who have progressed to the stage of cardiomyopathy. Efficacy of therapy can be assessed by serial echocardiographic studies.

One potential therapeutic option in advanced stages of heart failure regardless of the source is cardiac resynchronization therapy (CRT). There have been several reports illustrating the successful use of cardiac resynchronization in patients with SLE and resistant cardiomyopathy. (Reza et al, 2011) Mortality is higher in giant cell myocarditis than other forms of myocarditis. (Cooper et al, 1997)Cardiac transplantation is an option in refractory cases. (Reza et al, 2011)

4. Valvular disease

4.1 Clinical features

Verrucous endocarditis can affect valve leaflets, papillary muscles, and the mural endocardium, as initially described by Libman and Sacks. However, Libman and Sacks and Gross found the tricuspid valve involved most often, whereas more recent studies have found the mitral valve (followed by aortic) to be most affected.(Petri, 2004) In the corticosteroid era, valvular vegetations are found less frequently. Shearn found that none of 11 patients who received corticosteroids had verrucous endocarditis, but 4 patients, who died before corticosteroid therapy was available, did. (Shaern, 1959) In their landmark autopsy study, Bulkley and Roberts also commented on the rarity of vegetations in corticosteroid treated patients. (Bulkley & Roberts, 1975) Occasionally, the presentation may be fulminant, with congestive heart failure due to mitral regurgitation, or brain emboli secondary to valvular vegetations. Verrucous endocarditis (vegetations, "Libman- Sacks") affects the mitral valve most frequently, followed by the aortic valve. (Petri, 2004)

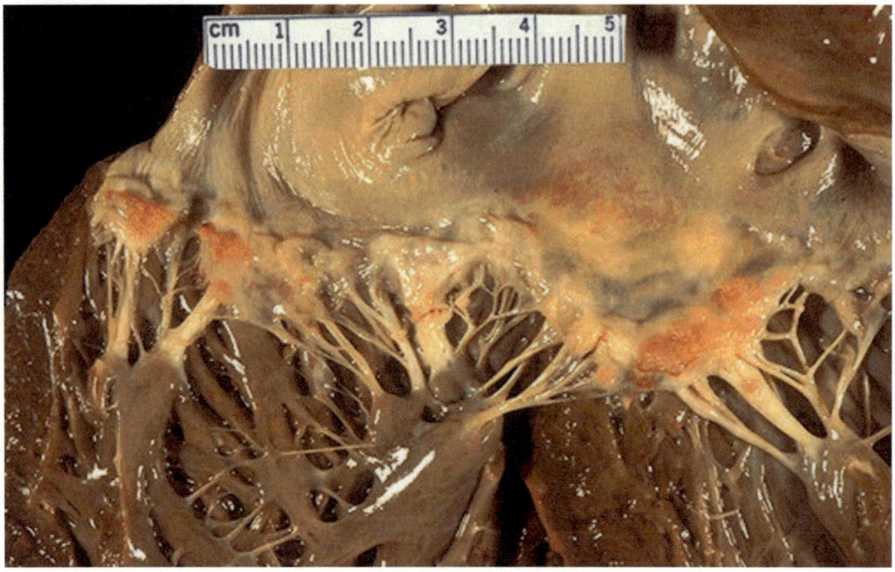

Fig. 3. Libman Sacks Endocarditis.

The presence of vegetations predisposes patients to bacterial endocarditis.(Brigden et al,1960) Although verrucous endocarditis can produce both systolic and diastolic murmurs, these are rarely of sufficient hemodynamic importance to cause congestive heart failure. There is virtually no correlation between the presence of verrucous endocarditis and cardiac murmurs. Shearn found that systolic murmurs occurred in 70% of SLE patients. (Shearn, 1959) Most murmurs were low intensity, and were heard loudest (47%) at the apex. Because murmurs were also associated with fever, infection, tachycardia, and anemia, the differential diagnosis of a new murmur was complex.

Diastolic murmurs occur in only 4% of SLE patients. (Petri, 2004) The differential diagnosis of diastolic murmurs in SLE includes rheumatic or congenital heart disease, bacterial endocarditis, Libman-Sacks endocarditis, and left ventricular dilatation. In general, even when the valvular vegetations of Libman-Sacks endocarditis are large, they do not involve the line of closure, and therefore should not deform the valve. Even involvement of the chordae tendineae should not be sufficient to distort the valve. There are several documented cases, however, in which Libman-Sacks endocarditis appeared to be the only explanation for a diastolic murmur. (Petri, 2004) Two of the four patients with Libman-Sacks endocarditis in Shear's series had a diastolic murmur suggestive of mitral stenosis. However, diastolic murmurs were also heard in two patients without Libman-Sacks endocarditis. (Shearn,1959) It is rare for valvular disease in SLE to be clinically significant. In a series of 421 patients, only 1 to 2% had significant morbidity or mortality. Of the 14 cases with available pathology, only 6 had evidence of SLE valvulopathy, either verrucous vegetations or valvulitis with necrosis and vasculitis. (Straaton et al, 1988)

4.2 Diagnosis

Transesophageal echocardiogram is the modality of choice in terms of sensitivity in detecting valvular disease due to either lupus or anti-phospholipid antibody syndrome.

(Petri, 2004) Most previous series used M-mode echocardiography or two-dimensional Doppler echocardiography and are not completely comparable. Patients with new murmurs or with valvular abnormalities on echocardiogram should have blood cultures to rule out bacterial endocarditis.

4.3 Prevalence

The prevalence of valvular disease in SLE is very high by echocardiography accounting for 54% of the patients.(Maksimowicz-McKinnon & Mandell, 2004) Valvular disease, for the most part, however, is mild and asymptomatic.

4.4 Pathology

Valvular disease occurs predominantly as vegetations (what was termed Libman-Sacks endocarditis in the past), or thickening (that can present as either a regurgitant or stenotic lesion). The mitral valve is affected most often, followed by the aortic valve. Mitral and aortic regurgitation are the most common findings, with stenotic lesions being very rare. Aortic cup sclerosis has been identified as common lesion.The typical valvular and mural endocarditis lesions, which are verrucous, occur as single vegetation or as mulberry-like clusters. When occurring on valves, the vegetations are often on the ventricular surface, near, but not distorting, the line of closure. (Shapiro et al, 1977) The original histologic description of Libman-Sacks endocarditis emphasized the multiplication of endothelial cells, proliferation of Anitschow myocytes, and infiltration of mononuclear cells in the valve ring and valve base, especially the valve pocket. Aggregations of hemosiderin were frequent, along with some fibrosis. Cells underwent karyolysis to form hematoxylin bodies. The mural endothelium was affected, especially near the mitral valve. (Brigden et al, 1960) Histologic studies showed three distinct zones, an outer exudative layer of fibrin, nuclear debris, and hematoxylin-stained bodies; a middle organizing layer of proliferation of capillaries and fibroblasts, and an inner layer of neovascularization. Immunofluorescence showed immunoglobulin and complement deposition in the walls of small junctional vessels in the inner zone of neovascularization, suggesting that circulating immune complexes were critical in the development of the vegetations.(Shapiro et al, 1977) Bidani *et al.* found immunoglobulins and complement deposition in the valve stroma and vegetations in one patient with Libman-Sacks endocarditis. (Bidani, 1980) It is not clear whether Libman-Sacks endocarditis evolves into the valvular thickening that is the second important form of SLE valvulopathy. In modern series, valvular thickening is found more commonly than vegetations (Leung, 1990). Galve *et al.* found that patients with Libman-Sacks endocarditis were younger, had shorter disease duration, and had received less corticosteroid therapy than those with thickened valves. (Galve et al, 1988) The patients with valvular thickening were more likely to have stenotic or regurgitant lesions and to require valve replacement. (Galve et al, 1988) Some authors have expressed concern that corticosteroid treatment might increase the chance that a valve would develop thickening. Changes in valve thickening can occur over time, with valve thickening resolving or new valve thickening appearing. Studies are conflicting on the role of antiphospholipid antibodies playing in the development of the vegetations of Libman-Sacks endocarditis. Valvulopathy is common in the primary anti-phospholipid antibody syndrome, usually found in about a third of patients in large series. (Khamashta et al, 1990) Thrombus formation, usually on the mitral valve, can be massive and require valve replacement.

Mitral and/or aortic valve thrombus (or vegetations) can also be a precipitant of embolic strokes. In SLE patients, some series have shown significantly more valvulopathy in those with anticardiolipin antibody.(Khamashta et al,1990) In patients with the secondary form of anti-phospholipid antibody syndrome and valvulopathy, there is deposition of immunoglobulin and complement, but in addition there is binding of anticardiolipin antibody.(Petri, 2004)

4.5 Treatment

Systemic lupus erythematosus patients with large, sterile vegetations should be anticoagulated to lessen embolic complications. High-dose corticosteroids for 4 to 6 weeks are used to shrunken the vegetations, but this approach is controversial.(Nesher et al, 1997) Some studies have suggested that corticosteroid treatment may contribute to ultimate valve thickening, but this is unproven. In the presence of significant regurgitation, even in the absence of nodules, there is a high risk of bacterial endocarditis particularly in the setting of jet lesions and warrant antibiotic prophylaxis. (Roman & Salmon, 2007)

5. Arrhythmia and conduction defects

5.1 Clinical features

Many autoimmune diseases including systemic lupus erythematosus have a high incidence of autonomic nervous system dysfunction, especially those of cardiac origin. Conduction disturbances and arrhythmias occur in about 10% of patients with SLE. (Mandell, 1987) Conduction defects include AV block, BBB and complete heart block, which is rarely seen in adults. While the most common arrhythmic manifestation include sinus tachycardia, atrial fibrillation, atrial ectopic beat and rarely ventricular arrhythmias. (Eisen et al, 2009) Recently, other anti-SSA/Ro-associated cardiac manifestations have been described in children born to anti-SSA/Ro positive mothers. These include transient fetal first-degree heart block, QTc prolongation, sinus bradycardia, late onset cardiomyopathy, endocardial fibroelastosis and cardiac malformations. Anti-SSA/Ro antibodies are usually not pathogenic to the adult heart, but recently QTc prolongation has been reported in adult lupus patients as well.(Costedoat-Chalumeau et al, 2005)

Sinus tachycardia is the most common cardiac abnormality seen among SLE patients. It is present in about 50% of cases (Hejmancik et al, 1964) and it could be the only manifestation, also it can be correlated to the disease activity. (Guzman et al, 1994) Arrhythmia and conduction defects in SLE patients may be found incidentally or during disease flare, and usually develop with coexisting cardiac manifestation (such as pericarditis, myocarditis and coronary heart disease though, arrhythmia may be the first manifestation of SLE . (Cardoso et al, 2000)Patients with SLE may have prolonged Q-T interval, and this can be a predictor of cardiovascular morbidity and mortality. (Okin et al, 2000)

5.2 Pathogenesis

SLE can lead to arrhythmias and conduction disturbances either as a consequence of pericarditis and myocarditis through direct injury of the conduction system of the heart by inflammatory processes.(Eisen et al, 2009)Supraventricular arrhythmias are usually transient and recedes as soon as the disease is controlled and treated.(Mandell, 1987) They can also be due to myocardial fibrosis as a consequence of occlusive diseases, (ischemia) due to vasculitis and atherosclerosis involvement (Eisen, 2009).These mechanisms will result in collage deposits that accumulate within nodes , causing fibrosis and focal degeneration of the conduction system.(Barati et al, 1975) Autopsy studies have found arteritis of the sinus node, vascular occlusion, vasculopathy, and fibroblastic replacement of the sinuatrial and atrioventricular nodes.(Barati et al, 1975) Q-T interval prolongation is hypothesized to be due to the subclinical atherosclerosis that is known to be augmented in SLE patients , and thus , it can be a marker of silent undetected atherosclerotic vascular disease in SLE patients.(Cardoso et al, 2005) In addition to Q-T interval prolongation, refractory ventricular arrhythmias could be associated with chronic hydroxychloroquine therapy for SLE. (Chen et al, 2006)

5.3 Management

Diagnosis of arrhythmia and conduction defects is by electrocardiograms that are performed usually in patients with an active disease during hospitalization. Those who have had arrhythmias or conduction abnormalities need continuous ECG monitoring. (Petri, 2004) The life threatening conduction defects are treated with permanent pacemaker, while the supra ventricular arrhythmias (unexplained sinus tachycardia) can be controlled with corticosteroids. (Costedoat-Chalumeau, 2005; Guzman et al, 1994)

6. SLE hypertension

6.1 Prevalence

Hypertension has a high prevalence among SLE patients ranging from (35 to 74%) according to different studies (Doria et al, 2003; Petri, 2000) and it is considered as a major risk factor for the progression of renal , vascular and cardiovascular diseases. In addition, it's a major risk factor of severe ischemic stroke, thus reflect the need of regular assessment and strict blood pressure control among SLE patients. (Mikdashi, 2007)

6.2 Pathophysiology

The pathogenesis of hypertension in SLE is multifactorial where alteration of renal function plays a central role; other mechanisms can contribute such as renin angiotensin aldosterone system (RAS), endothelin, oxidative stress, sex steroids and metabolic changes. Involvement of the kidneys in the course of SLE is common and impaired renal function plays a role in development of hypertension by alteration in the renal hemodynamic that leads to reduction in glomerular filtration rate (GFR) and increase in BUN and plasma creatinine levels. (Nakaro et al, 1998) Renal tubular lesions are prevalent in SLE patients, (Daniel et al, 2001) as well as glomerular injury in the form of glomerulonephritis contributes to SLE hypertension that is clinically indicated by the presence of urinary protein in SLE patients. (Ryan, 2009) SLE is usually associated with impaired endothelial function as demonstrated by the high risk of atherosclerosis, and this may also have a role in development of SLE hypertension. (Ryan, 2009)The Renin Angiotensin Aldosterone System (RAS) is activated in SLE (Herlitz et al, 1984) on basis of effectiveness of BP control with ACE Inhibitors and evidence of increase renin, which thus can play a role in developing SLE hypertension. (Ryan, 2009)

Endothelin 1(ET-1) plays a role in the pathophysiology of hypertension through its potent renal vasoconstriction and its ability to cause water and sodium retention.(Miyauchi &

Masaki, 1999) Evidence suggests that ET-1 could have role in the progression of SLE and SLE hypertension as the level of ET-1 are found to be increased in SLE.(Julkunen et al, 1991)
Activated RAS and increased ET 1 levels in SLE could lead to the generation of oxidative stress (Ryan, 2007) that is suggested to be important in pathogenesis of SLE(Alves & Grima, 2003) and it is recognized as a promoter of hypertension through mechanisms such as vascular dysfunction , renal injury and increase sodium reabsorption.(Manning et al, 2003) In addition , metabolic factors can contribute in the pathophysiology of hypertension in SLE and these include: Leptin, which is found to be increased, insulin resistance, and obesity.(Gehi et al 2003)
Inflammatory cytokines (IL-6, TNFα, and CRP) correlate in the mechanism of hypertension. (Bastista, et al, 2005)As these cytokines are increased in SLE, they are suggested to be involved in SLE hypertension through mechanisms such as, promotion of renal vascular endothelial dysfunction, generation of oxidative stress and progression of insulin resistance. (Garcia-Gonzalez et al, 2002)

6.3 Management

(Discussed in the section of management of traditional risk factors 8.6.1.)

7. Coronary arteritis

7.1 Clinical features

Coronary arteritis is extremely rare in SLE. In some cases, it has been found at autopsy, with no clinical correlate during life. The most common clinical presentation is angina and/or myocardial infarction, in a child or young adult who does not have a long history of corticosteroid therapy. (Petri, 2004) There is no clear correlation with extracardiac disease activity, although it has been present in some case. (Korkmaz & Cansu, 2007) Three of eight SLE patients who had a coronary artery aneurysm had no physical or laboratory evidence of active SLE. (Wilson et al, 1992) Aortic aneurysms can also occur in SLE. (Ohara et al, 2000)

7.2 Diagnosis

It is often difficult to distinguish coronary arteritis from accelerated atherosclerosis. Serial coronary angiography has been proposed as the most useful diagnostic modality. Arteritis is suggested when coronary aneurysms are found, if there are smooth focal lesions, or if there are rapidly developing stenoses.(Petri, 2004) However, Wilson *et al*. described a patient with rapidly progressive coronary artery occlusions in whom only advanced atherosclerosis was found at autopsy. (Wilson et al, 1992) Thrombosis or spasm can further confuse the interpretation of coronary angiograms. (Korkmaz & Consu, 2007)

7.3 Prevalence

There are few studies that allow any estimate of the prevalence of coronary arteritis. (Petri, 2004) In one study in the 1960s, 6 of 16 patients were found to have arteritis at autopsy. (Hejmancik et al, 1964)
The cases identified have a predilection for pediatric patients or very young adults, with rare exceptions. Unfortunately, where follow is given, the outcome is usually death.

7.4 Pathology

Histopathology demonstrates transmural vasculitis with both lymphocytic and neutrophilic infiltration of a thrombus. *(Korkmaz & Consu, 2007)*Immunofluorescence studies demonstrate immunoglobulin and complement deposition in coronary arteritis. (Korbet et al, 1984)

7.5 Treatment

The differentiation of coronary arteritis from atherosclerosis is essential for appropriate management. Coronary artery bypasses surgery, angioplasty, or stent placement would be considered in patients with severe atherosclerotic disease, but would be contraindicated in patients with coronary arteritis. Case reports suggest that corticosteroid therapy can have rapid benefit in patients with coronary arteritis. Corticosteroid therapy resulted in relief of angina and angiographic improvement. (Kozkmaz & Cansu, 2007) Not all patients with coronary arteritis do well on corticosteroids, however Heibel *et al.* describe a patient with coronary arteritis who was treated with prednisone and cyclophosphamide, but had new myocardial damage after starting therapy. (Heibel et al, 1976) Angina did not resolve for 3 weeks. (Heibel et al, 1976)

8. Premature atherosclerosis and systemic lupus erythematosus

8.1 Background-premature atherosclerosis and systemic lupus erythematosus

Despite improved life expectancy, patients with systemic lupus erythematosus (SLE) are still at considerable risk for premature death.(Galdman & Urowitz, 2002) This has been related to the high frequency of vascular events (VE) in young to middle-aged SLE patients, in whom atherosclerosis develops at an accelerated pace. (Bruce et al, 2003) Although general, modifiable risk factors for atherosclerosis are also relevant in SLE, they cannot fully explain the increased rate of atheroma formation. (Esdaile et al, 2001) SLE is the prototype of the immune complex mediated systemic inflammatory disorders, and inflammation has a central place in the pathogenesis and growth of atherosclerotic plaques. (Thomas et al, 2002; Becker & Nossent, 2009) Reducing the level of inflammatory activity in SLE would, thus, be a rational way to decrease this VE risk. (Pans-Estel et al, 2009)

Premature atherosclerosis (ATH) has been recognized as a major comorbid condition in systemic lupus erythematosus (SLE). Women with SLE in the 35–44year old age group have an estimated 50-fold increased risk of myocardial infarction (MI) compared to age and sex-matched controls. (Manzi, 1997) Women with SLE also have an increased incidence of subclinical atherosclerosis; in a study using carotid ultrasounds, a 37.1% prevalence of carotid atherosclerosis was found in lupus patients compared to 15.2% of controls.(Szeknanecz & Shoenfeld, 2006) Although traditional risk factors as defined by the Framingham studies (hypertension, hypercholesterolemia, diabetes mellitus, older age, and postmenopausal status) are important in increasing risk for ATH in SLE, they do not adequately explain the increase in cardiovascular disease. In a Canadian cohort, after controlling traditional risk factors, the relative risk attributed to SLE for myocardial infarction (MI) was 10.1 and for stroke 7.9 (Esdaile et al, 2001) It has increasingly become evident that inflammation and immune mechanisms play an important role in the pathogenesis of atherosclerosis in SLE. For many years, the development of atherosclerosis in the general population was regarded as a passive accumulation of lipids in the vessel wall. Recently, however, it has been realized that inflammation plays a role not only in the development of the atherosclerotic lesion but also in the acute rupture of plaques that occurs during acute myocardial ischemic events. (Von Felt, 2008)

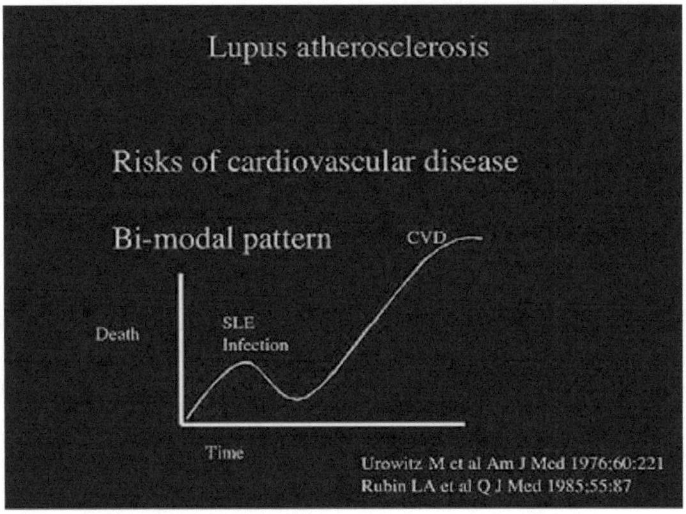

Fig. 4. The bimodal pattern of mortality in SLE patients. (Urowitz et al, 1976; Rubin et al, 1985) Copyright permission from Elsevier

8.2 Etiology of premature CVD in SLE

The pathogenesis of premature atherosclerosis in lupus is multifactorial and includes traditional CV risk factors, lupus -related factors and inflammatory risk factors. Box 1

8.2.1 The role of inflammation in the pathogenesis of atherosclerosis

The recruitment of inflammatory cells to the arterial wall Atherosclerotic lesions begin with the recruitment of inflammatory cells such as monocytes and T cells to the endothelial wall. First, the vascular endothelial cells are stimulated to express leukocyte adhesion molecules, including E-selectin, vascular cell adhesion molecule-1(VCAM-1), and intercellular adhesion molecule-1 (ICAM-1). (Hansson, 2001)These cell-surface proteins are upregulated during periods of inflammation. The expression of adhesion molecules can be induced by proinflammatory cytokines such as tumor necrosis factor-a (TNF-a) and interleukin-1 (IL-1), which upregulate leukocyte adhesion molecules. (Hansson, 2001) VCAM-1 is also induced when endothelial cells are exposed to other inflammatory signals, such as the lipopolysaccharides of Gram-negative bacteria, lysophosphatidylcholine (LPC), and oxidized phospholipids such as oxidized low density lipoprotein (OxLDL). High-density lipoproteins (HDLs) inhibit the expression of adhesion molecules. (Calabresi et al, 1997) After leukocytes adhere to the cell surface, they migrate through the endothelium and into the intima. (Hansson, 2001) This transmigration is influenced by several factors: first, several chemotactic proteins such as monocyte chemotactic protein-1 (MCP-1) are produced by the endothelial and smooth cell layers. The expression of MCP-1 in smooth muscle cells and endothelial cells can be upregulated by cytokines such as TNF-a, IL-1 and by OxLDL. (Hansson, 2001) Conversely, normal HDLs inhibit the expression of MCP-1. The importance of MCP-1 in the development of the atherosclerotic plaque is emphasized by the fact that elevated circulating levels of MCP-1 are positively related to increased carotid artery IMT in humans. (Larson et al, 2005)

Traditional risk factors

- Age
- Smoking
- Hypertension
- Hypercholesterolemia
- Diabetes mellitus
- Family history

Novel cardiovascular disease risk factors

- Cytokines (TNF-α, IFN-α, IL-6 and low IL-10)
- Endothelial (sVCAM-1, VEGF, Ang-2, apoptosis of circulating angiogenic cells/ endothelial progenitor cells and low annexin V binding)
- Elevated C-reactive protein
- Elevated homocysteine
- Metabolic syndrome/insulin resistance

Lupus-specific variables

- Corticosteroids
- SLE disease activity and SLE disease damage
- Antiphospholipid antibodies
- Anti-oxLDL antibodies, reduced antiphosphorylcholine antibodies
- Proinflammatory HDLs
- Lupus dyslipoproteinemia (high VLDL, high triglyceride, low HDL, high lipoprotein A); decreased lipoprotein lipase activity
- Renal disease

Ang-2: Angiopoietin-2; HDL: High-density lipoprotein; oxLDL: Oxidized low-density lipoprotein; SLE: Systemic lupus erythematosus; sVCAM: Soluble vascular cellular adhesion molecule; VLDL: Very low-density lipoprotein.
(Skamra & Ramsey-Goldman, 2010)

Box 1. Risk factors for cardiovascular disease in systemic lupus erythematosus (Elliot JR, Mansi S, 2009. Copyright permission from Elsevier)

8.2.2 Low-density lipoproteins and the development of foam cells

Next, low-density lipoproteins (LDLs) are transported into artery walls, where they become trapped and bound in the extracellular matrix of the subendothelial space.(McMahon & Hahn, 2007) These trapped LDLs are then seeded with reactive oxygen species (ROS) produced by nearby artery wall cells, resulting in the formation of proinflammatory-oxidized LDL . When endothelial cells are exposed to these proinflammatory OxLDL, they release cytokines such as MCP-1, M-CSF, and GRO, resulting in monocyte binding, chemotaxis, and differentiation into macrophages. (Nawab et al, 2000)

The OxLDLs are phagocytized by infiltrating monocytes/ macrophages, which then become the foam cells around which atherosclerotic lesions are built. Elevated levels of circulating OxLDL are strongly associated with documented coronary artery disease in the general population.(Tsimikas et al, 2005) Elevated levels of circulating OxLDL have also been described in SLE patients, especially in those with a history of cardiovascular disease.(Frostegard et al, 2005)

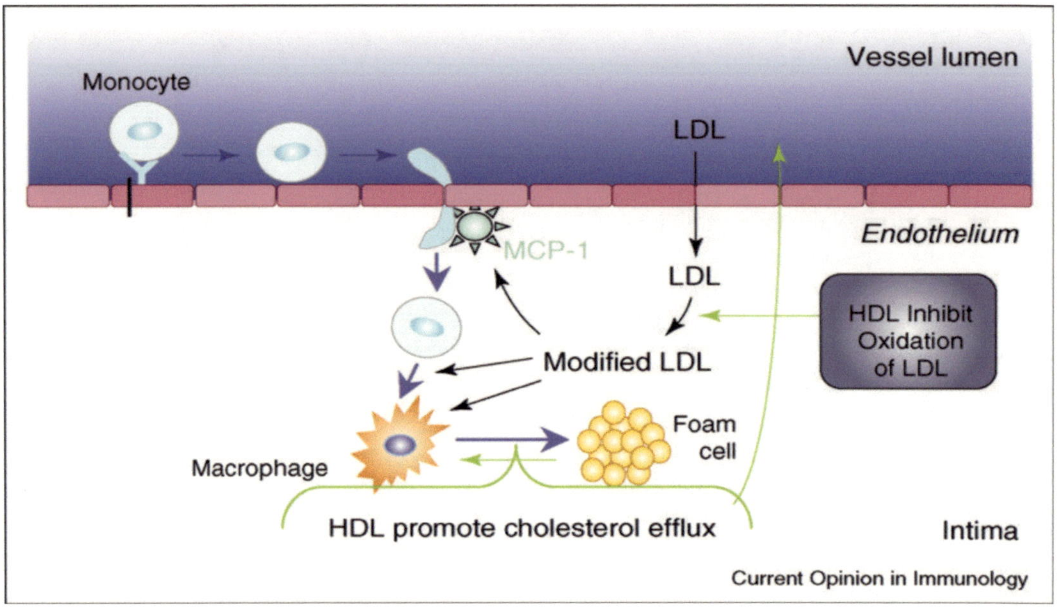

Fig. 5. The interplay of LDL, HDL, and OxLDL with endothelial activation, monocyte migration, foam cell formation, and reverse cholesterol transport. (Macmohan M, Hahn BV,2007.Copyright permission from Elsevier)

Next, monocytes and T cells infiltrate the margin of the plaque formed by foam cells, and muscle cells from the media of the artery are stimulated to grow. These muscle cells encroach on the lumen of the vessel and ultimately lead to fibrosis, which renders the plaques brittle. The occlusion that results in MI can occur when one of these plaques ruptures, or when platelets aggregate in the narrowed area of the artery. (McMahon & Hahn, 2007)

8.2.3 Normal HDL clears OxLDL from the endothelium: Abnormal proinflammatory HDL associate with accelerated atherosclerosis

There are many mechanisms designed to clear OxLDL from the subendothelial space, including macrophage engulfment using scavenger receptors, and enhanced reverse cholesterol transport mediated by lipoprotein transporters in HDL. (McMahon & Hahn, 2007) In addition to reverse cholesterol transport, HDL removes reactive oxygen species from LDL (via anti-oxidant enzymes in the HDL, such as paroxonase), thus preventing the formation of OxLDL and the subsequent recruitment of inflammatory mediators. (Nawab et al, 2000a, Nawab et al, 2004b)

Thus, although quantities of HDL partially determine atherosclerotic risk (low levels are associated with increased risk), HDL function is equally significant. (Barter et al, 2004) During the acute phase response HDL can be converted from their usual anti-inflammatory state to proinflammatory, and can actually cause increased oxidation of LDL. This acute phase response can also become chronic, and may be a mechanism for HDL dysfunction in SLE. It has been found that HDL function is abnormal in many women with SLE, 45% of women with SLE, compared to 20% of rheumatoid arthritis patients and 4% of controls, had proinflammatory HDL (piHDL) that was not only unable to prevent oxidation of LDL but caused increased levels of oxidation.(McMahon et al,2006a)McMahon et al reported 86% of patients with SLE who had plaque on carotid ultrasound had piHDL, compared to 39% who do not have plaque ($p < 0.0001$). (McMahon et al, 2006b) This suggests that detecting piHDL may identify SLE patients at high risk for clinical atherosclerosis. The interplay of LDL, HDL, and OxLDL with endothelial activation, monocyte migration, foam cell formation, and reverse cholesterol transport is illustrated in Figure 9.

8.3 Traditional risk factors

Over the past 15 years, traditional CV risk factors have been described in patients with SLE. Patients from several large lupus cohorts have been reported to have a greater total number of Framingham study and other traditional risk factors, including hypertension, diabetes, dyslipidaemia, tobacco use and sedentary lifestyle than matched control subjects. (Asanuma et al, 2003) Others have discovered a greater occurrence of both insulin resistance and metabolic syndrome. The Toronto Lupus Cohort also reported that SLE patients with CV events have a greater total number of traditional CV risk factors than lupus patients without events. (Bruce et al, 2003) Premature menopause is commonly seen in lupus patients. Compared with age-matched controls, women with lupus are more likely to be post-menopausal (38% vs. 19%) and reach menopause 4 years earlier. (Urowitz et al, 2007) These conventional risk factors of CVD are also associated with sub-clinical measures of atherosclerosis in SLE patients. Older age, hypertension, dyslipidaemia and diabetes are associated with the presence of carotid plaque. Finally, both hypertension and dyslipidaemia are independently predictive of CV events (MI and stroke) in SLE patients. (Elliott et al, 2008)

8.4 Dyslipidaemia in SLE

An atherogenic lipid profile has been described in SLE patients with elevated total cholesterol (TC), triglycerides (TG), low-density lipoprotein (LDL), very low-density lipoprotein (VLDL) and lipoprotein(a) [Lp(a)] concentrations, as well as decreased high-density lipoprotein (HDL) cholesterol levels. (Borba et al, 1994) Patients with lupus may also have altered HDL function. HDL cholesterol is normally an anti-inflammatory molecule that prevents the formation of oxidised LDL (ox-LDL) and foam cells that lead to plaque formation in the vasculature. A pro-inflammatory HDL (piHDL) is less able to prevent oxidation of LDL. piHDL was found in greater frequency in lupus patients with CVD than in those without known coronary disease. (Batuca et al, 2007)Additionally, paraoxonase 1 (PON1) is an anti-oxidant component of HDL that inhibits oxidation of lipoproteins and breaks down ox-LDL. In SLE, PON1 activity is altered, and significant reductions of PON1 are associated with both CV and cerebrovascular events. (Tripi et al, 2006) One possible mechanism for the reduced PON activity seen in SLE may be due to auto-antibody production. In a study by Batuca et al., patients with SLE were noted to have higher titres of antibodies to HDL and apolipoprotein A-1 (a lipoprotein associated with HDL) than healthy controls. (Batuca et al, 2007) PON activity was inversely correlated with the levels of antibodies to apolipoprotein A-1.

8.5 Lupus-related risk factors

Traditional risk factors alone do not fully explain the increased risk of CVD in lupus patients. Esdaile and colleagues reported a 10-fold relative risk of non-fatal MI and 17-fold relative risk of death from CHD, even after controlling for Framingham study risk factors. (Esdaile et al, 2001)These findings suggest that factors related to lupus itself, as well as its therapy, may be independent risk factors for CVD.

8.5.1 Disease activity

Ongoing inflammatory SLE disease activity is associated with CV risk. (Manzi et al 1997, Roman et al, 2003) A six-point increase in the Systemic Lupus Erythematosus Disease Activity Index (SLEDAI) score over 1 year correlated with a 5% increase in a 2-year CV risk. (Karp et al, 2008) This same increase in SLEDAI score was associated with increases of 3.4 mmHg in systolic blood pressure, 1 mg/dl in glucose and 11.6 mg/dl in TG as well as a 2.3- mg/dl decrease in HDL cholesterol. In the study performed by Roman and colleagues, the diagnosis of SLE itself, a longer duration of disease and greater disease damage (measured by SLICC-Damage Index [SLICC-DI]) were independent predictors of carotid plaque. (Roman et al, 2003) Similarly, Manzi et al. demonstrated that duration of lupus and disease damage (measured by SLICC-DI) were significantly associated with a higher carotid plaque index.(Manzi et al, 1999)

8.5.2 Renal disease

Renal disease is one of the most common internal organ manifestations of SLE. Both hypertension and dyslipidaemia are well described with lupus nephritis and renal disease. Lupus renal disease is also associated with increased atherosclerosis. In fact, nearly 50% of deaths in lupus patients with renal disease are attributed to CV or cerebrovascular disease. (Appel et al, 1994)

8.5.3 Autoantibody production

Systemic lupus erythematosus is characterized by autoantibody production. The immune reactions involving antibody production modulate atherosclerosis. Antiphospholipid antibodies and anti-oxLDL have been associated with CAD mortality in the general population. However, the relationship is nonlinear, making antibody status difficult to use as a predictor of individual risk. (Erkkila et al, 2005) Patients with SLE and secondary antiphospholipid antibody syndrome (APS) had a higher prevalence of carotid plaque than patients with primary APS. (Jimenez et al, 2005) In patients with SLE, the prevalence of anticardiolipin antibodies is quoted between 24 and 39% and for lupus anticoagulant it is quoted as 15–30%. However, only 50% of patients with the antiphospholipid antibodies will have a clinical event (defined as arterial or venous thrombosis or pregnancy morbidity), and thus have APS. (Giles & Rahman, 2009) A retrospective analysis carried out by Bessant et al. demonstrated that patients with SLE just prior to a CVD event (MI, angina, cerebrovascular accident [CVA] or peripheral vascular disease) were more likely to have the presence of lupus anticoagulant compared with patients with SLE without CVD, after controlling for disease duration.(Bassant et al,2006) Anti-β-2-glycoprotein I antibody has also been associated with increased risk of acute coronary syndrome in the general population.(Veres et al, 2004). Anti β-2-glycoprotein I antibodies was identified as a significant risk factor for arteriosclerosis obliterans in SLE patients, and was associated strongly with ischemic heart disease in patients with SLE. (Cederholm et al, 2005)

Annexin V plays a role in atherosclerotic lesions since it is believed to form a protective shield over thrombogenic cell surface proteins.(Fig.10) Decreased annexin V binding to the endothelium, caused by anticardiolipin IgG, was found in the sera of patients with SLE and CVD. (Cederholm et al, 2005)

In addition, antibodies against oxLDL have been found in patients with angiographic CAD. The oxidation of LDL may lead to the formation of neoepitopes that bind to scavenger receptors of macrophages and lead to uptake of oxLDL, accelerating foam cell formation in the atherosclerotic plaque. The level of oxLDL was associated with arterial disease (defined as clinically evident MI, angina, peripheral claudication or thrombosis). (Frostegard et al, 2005)

In patients with an established history of hypertension, high levels of IgM antiphosphorylcholine (anti-PC) antibodies were shown to be atheroprotective; they resulted in less progression of IMT on carotid ultrasound (OR: 0.46; 95% CI: 0.25–0.85; p = 0.01) . (Su j et al, 2006) Decreased levels of anti-PC antibodies were observed in both SLE cases with CVD and SLE controls without CVD compared with population controls. (Skamra & Ramsey-Golman, 2010)

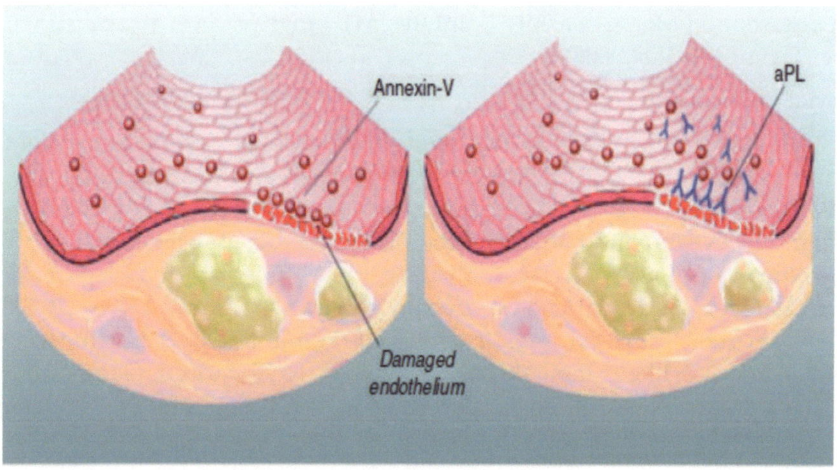

aPL interfere with binding to endothelium of antithrombotic Annexin
V. Frostegard J,J Int Med,2005;257(6)485-495.Copyright permission from John Wiley & Sons.

Fig. 6. Potential mechanism of atherothrombosis in systemic lupus erythematosus (SLE).

8.5.4 SLE therapy

Corticosteroids:

Corticosteroid therapy in SLE patients is often a double-edged sword. While it is still one of the most effective therapies for managing lupus disease activity, it has numerous metabolic side effects on blood pressure, blood glucose, lipids andweight. Petri et al. reported that a change of 10 mg of prednisone leads to an increase of 7.5mg/dl of TC, a 1.1-mmHg increase in mean arterial blood pressure and a 2.5-kg weight gain. (Petri et al, 1994) Additionally, longer duration of corticosteroid therapy is associated with sub-clinical CVD (Manzi et al, 1999) and independently predicts CV events in lupus patients. (Elliott et al, 2008) Lupus patients on corticosteroids are also likely to have greater inflammatory disease burden, placing them at higher CVD risk. MacGregor et al. found a corticosteroid dose-related effect. Above a daily dose of 10 mg of prednisolone, the triglyceride (TG) and Apo B levels were elevated compared with controls without SLE, but below a daily dose of 10 mg prednisolone there was no difference between controls and SLE patients. (Macgregor et al, 1992) Similarly, Petri et al. found that prednisone of over 10 mg daily was associated with hypercholesterolemia, defined as total cholesterol of more than 200 mg/dl. (Petri, 2000) Additionally, Montreal Lupus Clinic researchers reported that SLE patients on 30 mg of corticosteroids have a 60% greater 2-year CV risk than do SLE patients with the same disease activity and traditional risk factors but not on corticosteroids. This finding emphasizes the need for corticosteroid monitoring and the use of steroid-sparing agents in the clinical care of SLE patients. (Thompson et al,2008) Patients with SLE and CVD were more likely than SLE age-matched controls (without CVD) to have taken a mean dosage of prednisone of over 7.5 mg/day ($p = 0.04$) and more likely to have been treated with pulse methylprednisolone ($p = 0.03$) (Bessant et al, 2006) A longer duration of corticosteroid use (11 vs 7 years; $p = 0.002$) was more common in the patients who had an event than in those without an event. (Manzi etal, 1997) Women with SLE who had a longer duration of prednisone use and higher cumulative dose of prednisone are more likely to have carotid plaque on ultrasound (Manzi et al,1999) and the IMT progression is associated with years of steroid use.(Thompson et al,2008)

Anti-malarial medication:

Hydroxychloroquine (HCQ) therapy has been shown to have several beneficial CV effects in SLE patients. HCQ use in SLE patients has been shown to reduce TC, LDL and TG levels. (Wallace et al, 1990)The lipid lowering effect of HCQ is greatest in younger patients (age 16-39 years) and may offset the dyslipidaemia associated with corticosteroid therapy. (Rahman et al, 1999) Lupus patients taking HCQ have had significantly lower mean glucose levels and markers of insulin resistance. (Petri, 1996) HCQ has been postulated to prevent future thrombotic events, (Erkan et al, 2002) and lupus patients on HCQ therapy are less likely than those not on it to have carotid plaque. Its protective effect on the vasculature may be in part due to inhibition of aPL-mediated platelet activation. (Roman et al, 2003)

Immunosuppressant medications:

Roman's study demonstrated that patients with carotid plaque by B-mode ultrasound were less likely to have been treated with prednisone and cyclophosphamide when analyzed by multivariate analysis. (Roman et al, 2003) Mycophenolate mofetil (MMF) has been studied in patients with renal and cardiac transplants and found to reduce allograft vasculopathy and intimal thickening compared with those treated with azathioprine, as reviewed by Gibson and Hayden.(Gibson & Hayden, 2007). While there are no specific studies regarding cardiovascular outcomes in patients with SLE who take MMF, extrapolating the transplant data suggests this may be a useful choice for treating LN. Immunosuppressant medications should be used judiciously and corticosteroid dosage should be minimized, but control of SLE should not be sacrificed to avoid CVD risk. (Skamra &Ramsay-Goldman, 2010)

Estrogens & hormone replacement therapy

Patients with antiphospholipid antibodies are at increased risk of thrombosis. Thus, general recommendations include discontinuing estrogen usage, despite a lack of randomized, controlled trials.(Sammaritano, 2007) A prospective study evaluating patients with SLE who took hormone replacement therapy (HRT) revealed that HRT was not a risk factor for CAD, despite the presence of antiphospholipid antibodies in 74.6% of HRT users.(Hochman et al, 2009) However, the role of hormones in patients with SLE who lack antiphospholipid antibodies has been more clearly defined. Both the Safety of Estrogens in Lupus Erythematosus National Assessment (SELENA) study and the LUMINA study found that exogenous hormones were safe to use in their patient populations as long as SLE was stable, and did not increase the risk of arterial thrombosis in lower risk patients. (Fernandez et al, 2007) Based on risk and needs, oral contraceptive and HRT use are recommended in properly selected patients who do not have antiphospholipid antibodies.(Skamra &Ramsay-Goldman, 2010)

8.5.5 Endothelial dysfunction

Many soluble markers of endothelial dysfunction have been studied in atherosclerosis, including cytokines, chemokines, soluble adhesion molecules and acute phase reactants. Their clinical use is limited by their instability, inadequate laboratory performance and lack of standardization at this time; however, they may prove to be a valuable tool in the future. Biochemical markers of endothelial cell activation, such as soluble thrombomodulin, von Willebrand factor and tissue plasminogen activator, are increased in patients with SLE. (Constans et al, 2003) While soluble vascular cellular adhesion molecule (sVCAM)-1 was elevated only in the patients with SLE and CVD. This is of further interest, since sVCAM-1 is associated with systemic TNF-α. There is positive correlation between TNF-α and plasma TGs, VLDL TGs and VLDL-C]. SLE patients with a higher IMT value using B-mode ultrasound had significantly higher mean plasma VEGF levels compared with controls after adjusting for age, smoking and other Framingham risk factors. (Svenungsson et al, 2003) Thus, these soluble biomarkers may have a future role in identifying SLE patients at risk for CVD.The Tie-2 receptor (a vascular-specific tyrosine kinase receptor), through its interaction with angiopoietin (Ang)-1, maintains vessel integrity, inhibits vascular leakage, suppresses inflammatory gene expression, and prevents recruitment and transmigration of leukocytes. Ang-2 has emerged as a key mediator of endothelial cell activation and facilitates endothelial cell inflammation by counterbalancing the effects of Ang-1 and disrupting these functions. (Skamra &Ramsay-Goldman, 2010) Ang-2 concentrations were elevated in hypertensive patients compared with healthy controls (4.23 ± 3.1 vs 0.88 ± 0.43 ng/ml; $p < 0.0001$); and it was particularly elevated in those patients with atherosclerosis ($p = 0.02$). Furthermore, Ang-2 concentrations correlated with other vascular markers of endothelial cell activation, including VCAM-1 and ICAM-1. Mean serum Ang-2 concentrations were markedly elevated in patients with active SLE compared with inactive SLE (8.6 vs 1.4 ng/ml; $p = 0.010$) and healthy controls (8.6 vs 1.1 ng/ml; $p < 0.001$), and Ang-2 remained significantly elevated in patients with inactive SLE compared with healthy controls. (Skamra &Ramsay-Goldman, 2010) Maintaining vascular integrity after damage is a role played by endothelial progenitor cells (EPCs) and myelomonocytic circulating angiogenic cells. Decreased levels or abnormal function of those cells is an established atherosclerotic risk factor. (Hill et al, 2003) SLE patients possess significantly fewer numbers of circulating EPCs as well as impaired differentiation of EPCs and circulating angiogenic cells into mature endothelial cells that are capable of producing VEGF. These abnormalities are triggered by IFN-α, which induces EPC and circulating angiogenic cell apoptosis. SLE EPCs/circulating angiogenic cells have increased IFN-α expression, which might promote accelerated atherosclerosis. (Hill et al, 2003)

8.5.6 Cytokines

In addition to the relationship between TNF-α and IFN-α, other cytokines and their associated polymorphisms (IL-10 and IL-6) have also been implicated in the relationship between CVD and SLE. IL-10 has an atheroprotective role compared with TNF-α, which is atherogenic. Both IL-10 and TNF-α are seen increased in SLE patients with CVD compared with SLE patients without CVD or controls. IL-6 overproduction has been associated with SLE, CVD and C-reactive protein (CRP) elevations. Measurement of individual cytokines is laborious and may be difficult to interpret without an overall cytokine profile. The role of IL-10 and IL-6 and many other cytokines in SLE and CVD remains to be fully elucidated. (Skamra &Ramsay-Goldman, 2010)

8.5.7 CRP

In addition to its relationship with arterial stiffness, an elevated level of serum CRP has been associated with MI and stroke in the general population. Its role in risk stratification remains unclear because it might improve risk prediction beyond the traditional Framingham calculation; however, further study will be required before it can be accepted as a standard CVD risk factor. (Lloyd-Jones et al, 2006) In patients with SLE, an elevated serum CRP has been associated with the presence of carotid plaque. Elevated CRP has also been associated with the highest quartile of IMT on carotid ultrasound in SLE patients. (Manzi et al, 1999) CRP is also found to have association with cardiovascular events and SLE disease activity as measured by the Systemic Lupus Activity Measure, but not with overall damage accrual as measured by the SLICC-DI. (Szalai et al, 2005; Bertoli et al, 2008)

8.5.8 Homocysteine

Homocysteine is believed to be a toxin that results in endothelial injury and dysfunction in patients with CVD, but its exact role remains to be defined. Homocysteine may have a role in differentiating between patients with SLE and CVD and those with CVD without SLE. Patients with SLE from the Toronto Lupus Cohort had higher mean homocysteine levels compared with age-matched controls, despite having higher folate levels. Studies found that a homocysteine level above 14.1 mmol/l was an independent risk factor for development of CAD in patients with SLE after controlling for established risk factors (Svenungsson et al, 2001, Petri, 2009) Homocysteine concentration was found to be significantly higher among patients with progressive plaque compared with patients without carotid plaque. (Roman et al, 2007) In addition to SLE, renal failure is a known cause of hyperhomocysteinemia. While the role of homocysteine is not completely defined, Von Feldt suggests that it may be a useful initial test in the evaluation of SLE patients in order to determine the presence and extent of subclinical atherosclerotic disease. (Von Feldt et al, 2008)

8.6 Assessment and management

8.6.1 Assessment and management of traditional risk factors (table 1.)

Obesity

Assessment

The National Heart, Lung, and Blood Institute (NHLBI), (National Institute of Health,1998) American Heart Association (AHA) (Smith et al, 2006) and the American College of Cardiology (ACC) recommends checking weight and height to calculate BMI, as well as waist circumference, at each visit. Waist circumference is a marker of visceral or intra-abdominal fat and should be assessed at the iliac crest. Goal BMI is recommended from 18.5 to 24.6 kg/m2 and waist circumference should be <40 inches in men and <36 inches in women. (Smith et al, 2006)

Management

Preventing obesity is the first line of defense. Physicians should educate patients to avoid weight gain by promoting healthy eating and physical activity. Specific to lupus itself, aggressive control of joint and fatigue symptoms and global lupus disease activity could help facilitate physical exercise. As corticosteroid use can lead to weight gain and other metabolic risks, minimizing the corticosteroid dose by adding a steroid-sparing agent, such as HCQ, or an immunosuppressive agent may be needed. For those patients with a BMI >25 kg/m^2 or whose waist circumference is >40 inches in men or >35 inches in women, a combined dietary and physical exercise programs is indicated. These dietary and exercise recommendations can also be applied to patients with dyslipidaemia, hypertension and diabetes (see below).

Diet: AHA Diet and Lifestyle recommendations (Lichtenstein et al, 2006) advocate the following: a diet rich in fruits, vegetables and whole-grain, high-fiber foods, consuming fish (specifically oily fish) twice a week, limiting saturated fat to <7% (trans fat to <1%) and cholesterol to <300 mg /day by choosing lean meats and fat-free or low-fat dairy products, minimizing beverages and foods with added sugars, low or no salt diet and consuming alcohol in moderation.

Consultation with a nutritionist or dietitian is strongly encouraged. An individualized dietary plan, taking into account specific health concerns and medications, will be a powerful tool for lupus patients and their CV health. (Elliott &Manzi, 2009)

Exercise. Physicians should take every office visit as an opportunity to encourage patients to exercise. The AHA recommends 30 min of moderate-intensity (brisk walking) aerobic activity 5 days per week or 20 min of vigorous-intensity (jogging) 3 days a week for healthy adults. Haskell et al, 2007) Resistance training (weight lifting) to improve muscle strength and endurance is advocated twice per week and should include all 10 major muscle groups. Patients should be encouraged to increase their daily lifestyle activities, such as walking to the store and using stairs instead of elevators. For those with cardiac history or recent vascular surgery, physicians should provide a medically supervised exercise program. (Smith et al, 2006)

In addition to CV benefits, physical exercise may improve conditions related specifically to SLE disease. SLE patients can improve their aerobic capacity and exercise tolerance and fatigue after following an exercise program, without aggravating their SLE disease. (Clarke-Jenssen et al, 2005) Aerobic exercise can also improve quality of life in patients with SLE by improving both depression levels and global sense of well-being. (Avan & Martin, 2007)

Risk factors	Monitoring strategies	Management strategies
Obesity	Check weight, height, and waist circumference at each visit Goal BMI <25 kg/m2 Goal waist circumference <35 inches for women or <40 inches for men	Regular exercise Dietary counseling Referral to nutritionist and exercise therapist Referral to hospital- or community-based weight loss programs Lowest possible dose of corticosteroids
Dyslipidemia	Check fasting lipid panel at initial visit, then yearly If dyslipidemic, check lipids every 6 months or 6 weeks after medication changes Goal LDL <100 mg/dl Goal LDL <70 mg/dl for those with known CVD or PVD or diabetes	Encourage lifestyle modification with diet, exercise, and weight loss counseling Lowest possible dose of corticosteroids Consider hydroxychloroquine therapy Consider lipid lowering therapy for those not at LDL goal Consider ASA therapy Consider preventive cardiology evaluation
Hypertension	Check blood pressure at each visit and between visits for those on corticosteroids or NSAIDs Goal BP <130/80 mmHg	Aggressive blood pressure control Encourage lifestyle modification with diet, exercise, and weight loss counseling Addition of ACE inhibitor for those with diabetes or renal disease Lowest possible dose of corticosteroids Consider ASA therapy
Diabetes Mellitus/Insulin Resistance	Check fasting glucose yearly Consider checking fasting insulin and calculate insulin resistance Oral glucose tolerance test if needed. Goal fasting glucose <126 mg/dl Goal HbA1c <7%	Endocrinology evaluation Early aggressive therapy to maintain HbA1c<7% Encourage lifestyle modification with diet,exercise, and weight loss counseling Consider hydroxychloroquine therapy Consider ASA therapy Aggressive management of blood pressure, lipids, and other CV risk factors
Tobacco Use	Ask patient about tobacco use at each visit Goal of complete tobacco cessation	Discuss importance of tobacco cessation Assess willingness to quit Referral to tobacco cessation program Suggest pharmacotherapy Consider ASA therapy

BMI: body mass index. LDL: low-density lipoprotein. HDL: high-density lipoprotein. CVD: cardiovascular disease. PVD:peripheral vascular disease. BP: blood pressure. NSAIDs: nonsteroidal anti-inflammatory drugs. HbA1c: glycosylated hemoglobin.ASA: aspirin.

Table 1. Assessment and Management strategies of traditional risk factors in patients with SLE. (Elliot JR, Mansi S, 2009. Copyright permission from Elsevier)

Given these data, physicians should consider referring patients to an exercise physiologist or specialists in physical exercise. An individualized exercise plan that takes into account patients specific needs and limitations may help to assure their long-term commitment to being physically fit. (Elliott &Manzi, 2009)

Dyslipidaemia:

Assessment At baseline and yearly, a fasting lipid panel (TC, LDL, HDL and TG levels) should be performed on patients with SLE. It is proposed that lupus patients be considered CHD risk equivalents, similar to patients with diabetes. Accordingly, based on the National Cholesterol Education Program Adult Treatment Panel (ATP III), (National Cholesterol Education Program [NCEP], 2001) the goal cholesterol levels in lupus patients should be: TC <200 mg/dl, LDL <100 mg/dl, TG <150 mg/dl and HDL >40 mg/dl.

Management

Lifestyle modifications should be considered as first-line approach, with an emphasis on reducing saturated and transunsaturated fat and cholesterol intake and weight loss. The American Diabetes Association (ADA) and the ACC issued a consensus statement recommending both lifestyle modifications and lipid pharmacological therapy, regardless of LDL level, for all patients with known CVD or for high-risk groups, such as patients with diabetes .(Brunzell et al, 2008) They further recommended a tighter LDL goal of <70 mg/dl. There is a scarcity of lipid-lowering therapy clinical trials in SLE. Petri et al. reported an improvement in carotid IMT in SLE patients treated with atorvastatin.(Petri et al, 2006) Most do not advocate the wide-spread use of statins in all SLE patients, (Toloza et al, 2007 but reserve its use for those with established vascular disease or diabetes.
Based on the available literature, Elliott & Manzi propose the following management of dyslipidaemia in SLE patients:

- Regardless of LDL level, corticosteroid therapy should be minimized, HCQ be considered and lifestyle modifications be initiated.
- LDL goal of <100 mg/dl or <70 mg/dl for those with sub-clinical CVD, known CV or peripheral vascular disease (PVD), or diabetes
- Consideration of lipid-lowering therapy for LDL >100 mg/dl or >70 mg/dl for those with subclinical CVD, known CVD or PVD, or diabetes

Hypertension

Assessment

The Joint National Committee on Prevention, Detection, Evaluation, and Treatment of High Blood Pressure (JNC 7) continues to define hypertension as exceeding 140/90 mmHg. (Chobanian et al, 2003) However, the report recommends for the first time, a more stringent goal of <130/80 mmHg for patients with high-risk conditions, such as diabetes or chronic kidney disease. Based on this literature, Elliott & Manzi recommended a goal blood pressure of <130/80 mmHg for patients with SLE. Additionally, a blood pressure reading should be obtained at each physician visit and between visits for lupus patients on corticosteroids and non-steroidal anti-inflammatory drugs.

Management

Lifestyle modifications regarding diet, specifically salt restriction, exercise, weight control and alcohol moderation, is recommended for all patients with a blood pressure >140/90 mmHg. Except for those with known ischaemic heart disease or diabetes, lowering of blood pressure is more important than the choice of anti-hypertensive agent. Anti-hypertensive therapy should also be initiated when blood pressure readings are >140/90 mmHg. Aggressive combination therapy is often needed to obtain blood pressure goals, and the JNC 7 recommends starting combination therapy when SBP >150 mmHg or DBP >90 mmHg.(Chobanian et al, 2003) Angiotensin-converting enzyme (ACE) inhibitors, angiotensin receptor blockers (ARBs), calcium channel blockers or thiazide diuretics are typically first-line therapy for hypertension. However, a beta-blocker should be used in patients with known CAD and an ACE or ARB is recommended in those with diabetes or renal disease. Corticosteroid therapy should also continue to be minimized given its relationship with blood pressure elevation. (Elliott & Manzi, 2009)

Diabetes mellitus

Assessment

All lupus patients should have a fasting glucose checked yearly. The American Diabetic Association (ADA) defines diabetes with either a fasting plasma glucose of >126 mg/dl or a glucose tolerance test of >200 mg dl. (Nathan et al, 2006) Goals of therapy should be near-normal glucose levels and a haemoglobin A1C level of <7%.

Management

Lupus patients with diabetes should undergo structured diabetic education programs that emphasize aggressive lifestyle changes in diet, exercise and weight management. The ADA also recommends metformin therapy in addition to lifestyle changes for all patients newly diagnosed with diabetes. (Nathan et al, 2006) If this regimen is not effective in reaching glucose or haemoglobin A1C goals, then another oral diabetic agent or insulin should be started. Endocrinology referral should be strongly encouraged for these patients.
Other risk factors: Other CV risk factors must also be evaluated and aggressively treated. As described above, blood pressure therapy is recommended at >140/90 mmHg and statin therapy at LDL >100 mg /dl. All patients should be counseled on tobacco cessation and considered for aspirin therapy.HCQ should also be considered for all lupus patients with impaired glucose function and diabetes. Similarly, corticosteroid therapy should be minimized to avoid exacerbations of hyperglycaemia.

8.6.2 SLE-specific and inflammatory risk factor assessment and management

A summary of the assessment and management strategies for lupus-specific and inflammatory CV risk factors is outlined in Table 2.

8.7 Conclusion

Cardiovascular involvement in SLE may easily be overlooked until a full blown cardiac dysfunction or complication occurs.

- Cardiac involvement in SLE involves all the three layers of the heart (pericardium, myocardium, endocardium)
- Pericarditis is a common cardiac manifestation of SLE and can present rarely with cardiac tamponade being the initial presentation. Diagnosis is based on ECG and echocardiography findings. Pericarditis responds well to steroid therapy, and rarely may progress to cardiac tamponade necessitating pericardiocentesis.Refractory cases may require pericardial window.

Risk factors	Monitoring strategies	Management strategies
SLE Disease activity	Assess disease activity and medications at each visit	Lowest possible dose of corticosteroids Add steroid sparing agent if unable to lower corticosteroid dose Consider hydroxychloroquine therapy Consider ASA therap
SLE Renal disease	Assess renal parameters at each visit: BP, serum albumin, creatinine, and urinalysis Goal BP <130/80 mmHg Goal to normalize creatinine and albumin Goal proteinuria <300 mg/dl	Aggressive blood pressure control Addition of ACE inhibitor Consider ASA therapy
Antiphospholipids or Lupus Anticoagulant positivity	Check antiphospholipids, Lupus Anticoagulant, and beta 2 glycoprotein antibody status initially and as needed	Consider hydroxychloroquine therapy Consider ASA therapy
Inflammatory CV risk factors In SLE		
C-reactive protein	Consider checking as an additive predictive factor	Unclear at this time
Homocysteine	Check initially and as needed	Unclear at this time, but consider folic acid supplementation for hyperhomocysteinemia

Table 2. Summary of SLE-specific CV risk factors in patients with SLE (Elliot JR, Mansi S, 2009. Copyright permission from Elsevier)

- Myocarditis presents in 3-15% of the SLE patients clinically,but a common finding in autopsy studies. It may present with florid heart failure or subacutely as tachycardia and dyspnea.Myocarditis should be considered in patient with tachycardia and fever, with a 3rd heart sound with abnormal ECG in those with a new murmurs or conduction disturbances and those with congestive heart failure.Treatment is with high dose steroid and with IV cyclophosphamide in refractory cases in addition to antifailure therapy.Anticoagugation should be considered in those with cardiomyopathy.
- Valvular heart disease due to Libman Sacks endocarditis is found less frequently in the era of corticosteroids.The mitral valve is the most common valve involved followed by the the aortic valve.Echocardiography is the modality of choice for diagnosis.Use of steroids to shinken the vegetation is controversial and as may led to fibrosis. Bacterial prophylaxis is indicated in patients with significant regurtitation with jet lesions even in the absence of nodules.

- Arrhythmia and conduction defects occour in 10% of the patients with SLE either as a consequence of pericarditis or myocarditis or involment of the conduction system by fibrosis or atherosclerosis. AntiSSA/RO associated cardiac manifestations include transient fetal heart block, QTc prolongation, sinus bradycardis, late on-set cardiomyopathy, endocardial fibroelastosis and cardiac malformations.In the adult heart may cause QTc prolongation in lupus patients.
- Coronary arteritis presents with angina or myocardial infarction in a child or a young adult who do not have a long history of corticosteroid therapy.Serial coronary angiography is the proposed diagnostic modality.Corticosteroids may have rapid relief of the angina and may need cyclophosphamide.
- Premature atherosclerosis, cardiovascular risk factors and cardiovascular events all occur at a younger age in patients with SLE compared with the general population.
- After controlling for traditional Framingham risk factors, patients with SLE still have a 7.5-fold (95% CI: 5.1–10.4) excess risk of overall coronary heart disease.This suggests that SLE itself carries an independent risk for CVD and exposes the failure of the Framingham risk calculator to capture a younger at-risk population.
- Traditional risk factors, lupus related, and novel inflammatory CV risk factors are implicated in the pathogenesis of premature atherosclerosis.
- Treatment recommendations for patients with SLE are based on other high-risk populations since there are no randomized, controlled trials that demonstrate the efficacy of interventions on cardiovascular events in SLE.
- Lifestyle modifications and/or statins should be used to lower LDL-cholesterol below 100 mg/dl as suggested in the National Cholesterol Education Program (NCEP) Adult Treatment Panel III guidelines.
- Hypertension should be treated to maintain a blood pressure less than 130/80 mmHg. First-choice medication for patients with SLE should probably be angiotensin-converting enzyme inhibitors (or angiotensin receptor blockers), especially in patients with concomitant lupus nephritis or diabetes mellitus.
- Low-dose daily aspirin therapy is recommended in patients with SLE barring an absolute contraindication.
- Use of antimalarial medications in all patients with SLE is recommended.
- Use of corticosteroids should be minimized and immunosuppressant medications should be used judiciously, but control of SLE should not be sacrificed to minimize CVD risk.
- Smoking cessation, regular aerobic exercise and maintaining a normal BMI are recommended in all patients with SLE.

9. Acknowledgments

The work to produce this chapter was supported by Alzaidi's Chair of research in rheumatic diseases- Umm Alqura University.

10. References

Alves, J. D., & Grima, B. (2003). Oxidative stress in systemic lupus erythematosus and antiphospholipid syndrome: a gateway to atherosclerosis. *Curr Rheumatol Rep, 5*(5), 383-390.

Appel, G. B., Pirani, C. L., & D'Agati, V. (1994). Renal vascular complications of systemic lupus erythematosus. *J Am Soc Nephrol, 4*(8), 1499-1515.

Appenzeller, S., Pineau, C., & Clarke, A. (2011). Acute lupus myocarditis: Clinical features and outcome. *Lupus, 20*(9), 981-988.

Asanuma, Y., Oeser, A., Shintani, A. K., Turner, E., Olsen, N., Fazio, S., Linton, M. F., Raggi, P., & Stein, C. M. (2003). Premature coronary-artery atherosclerosis in systemic lupus erythematosus. *N Engl J Med, 349*(25), 2407-2415.

Ashrafi, R., Garg, P., McKay, E., Gosney, J., Chuah, S., & Davis, G. (2011). Aggressive cardiac involvement in systemic lupus erythematosus: a case report and a comprehensive literature review. *Cardiol Res Pract, 2011*, 578390.

Ayan, C., & Martin, V. (2007). Systemic lupus erythematosus and exercise. *Lupus, 16*(1), 5-9.

Batuca, J. R., Ames, P. R., Isenberg, D. A., & Alves, J. D. (2007). Antibodies toward high-density lipoprotein components inhibit paraoxonase activity in patients with systemic lupus erythematosus. *Ann N Y Acad Sci, 1108*, 137-146.

Bautista, L. E., Vera, L. M., Arenas, I. A., & Gamarra, G. (2005). Independent association between inflammatory markers (C-reactive protein, interleukin-6, and TNF-alpha) and essential hypertension. *J Hum Hypertens, 19*(2), 149-154.

Becker-Merok, A., & Nossent, J. (2009). Prevalence, predictors and outcome of vascular damage in systemic lupus erythematosus. *Lupus, 18*(6), 508-515.

Berg, G., Bodet, J., Webb, K., Williams, G., Palmer, D., Ruoff, B., & Pearson, A. (1985). Systemic lupus erythematosis presenting as isolated congestive heart failure. *J Rheumatol, 12*(6), 1182-1185.

Bernatsky, S., Boivin, J. F., Joseph, L., Manzi, S., Ginzler, E., Gladman, D. D., Urowitz, M., Fortin, P. R., Petri, M., Barr, S., Gordon, C., Bae, S. C., Isenberg, D., Zoma, A., Aranow, C., Dooley, M. A., Nived, O., Sturfelt, G., Steinsson, K., Alarcon, G., Senecal, J. L., Zummer, M., Hanly, J., Ensworth, S., Pope, J., Edworthy, S., Rahman, A., Sibley, J., El-Gabalawy, H., McCarthy, T., St Pierre, Y., Clarke, A., & Ramsey-Goldman, R. (2006). Mortality in systemic lupus erythematosus. *Arthritis Rheum, 54*(8), 2550-2557.

Bertoli, A. M., Vila, L. M., Reveille, J. D., & Alarcon, G. S. (2008). Systemic lupus erythematosus in a multiethnic US cohort (LUMINA): LXI. Value of C-reactive protein as a marker of disease activity and damage. *J Rheumatol, 35*(12), 2355-2358.

Bessant, R., Duncan, R., Ambler, G., Swanton, J., Isenberg, D. A., Gordon, C., & Rahman, A. (2006). Prevalence of conventional and lupus-specific risk factors for cardiovascular disease in patients with systemic lupus erythematosus: A case-control study. *Arthritis Rheum, 55*(6), 892-899.

Bharati, S., de la Fuente, D. J., Kallen, R. J., Freij, Y., & Lev, M. (1975). Conduction system in systemic lupus erythematosus with atrioventricular block. *Am J Cardiol, 35*(2), 299-304.

Bidani, A. K., Roberts, J. L., Schwartz, M. M., & Lewis, E. J. (1980). Immunopathology of cardiac lesions in fatal systemic lupus erythematosus. *Am J Med, 69*(6), 849-858.

Borba, E. F., Santos, R. D., Bonfa, E., Vinagre, C. G., Pileggi, F. J., Cossermelli, W., & Maranhao, R. C. (1994). Lipoprotein(a) levels in systemic lupus erythematosus. *J Rheumatol, 21*(2), 220-223.

Borba, E. F., & Bonfa, E. (1997). Dyslipoproteinemias in systemic lupus erythematosus: influence of disease, activity, and anticardiolipin antibodies. *Lupus, 6*(6), 533-539.

Borenstein, D. G., Fye, W. B., Arnett, F. C., & Stevens, M. B. (1978). The myocarditis of systemic lupus erythematosus: association with myositis. *Ann Intern Med, 89*(5 Pt 1), 619-624.

Brigden, W., Bywaters, E. G., Lessof, M. H., & Ross, I. P. (1960). The heart in systemic lupus erythematosus. *Br Heart J, 22*, 1-16.

Bruce, I. N., Urowitz, M. B., Gladman, D. D., Ibanez, D., & Steiner, G. (2003). Risk factors for coronary heart disease in women with systemic lupus erythematosus: the Toronto Risk Factor Study. *Arthritis Rheum, 48*(11), 3159-3167.

Brunzell, J. D., Davidson, M., Furberg, C. D., Goldberg, R. B., Howard, B. V., Stein, J. H., & Witztum, J. L. (2008). Lipoprotein management in patients with cardiometabolic risk: consensus conference report from the American Diabetes Association and the American College of Cardiology Foundation. *J Am Coll Cardiol, 51*(15), 1512-1524.

Bulkley, B. H., & Roberts, W. C. (1975). The heart in systemic lupus erythematosus and the changes induced in it by corticosteroid therapy. A study of 36 necropsy patients. *Am J Med, 58*(2), 243-264.

Busteed, S., Sparrow, P., Molloy, C., & Molloy, M. G. (2004). Myocarditis as a prognostic indicator in systemic lupus erythematosus. *Postgrad Med J, 80*(944), 366-367.

Calabresi, L., Franceschini, G., Sirtori, C. R., De Palma, A., Saresella, M., Ferrante, P., & Taramelli, D. (1997). Inhibition of VCAM-1 expression in endothelial cells by reconstituted high density lipoproteins. *Biochem Biophys Res Commun, 238*(1), 61-65.

Cardoso, C. R., Sales, M. A., Papi, J. A., & Salles, G. F. (2005). QT-interval parameters are increased in systemic lupus erythematosus patients. *Lupus, 14*(10), 846-852.

Cederholm, A., Svenungsson, E., Jensen-Urstad, K., Trollmo, C., Ulfgren, A. K., Swedenborg, J., Fei, G. Z., & Frostegard, J. (2005). Decreased binding of annexin v to endothelial cells: a potential mechanism in atherothrombosis of patients with systemic lupus erythematosus. *Arterioscler Thromb Vasc Biol, 25*(1), 198-203.

Cervera, R., Khamashta, M. A., Font, J., Reyes, P. A., Vianna, J. L., Lopez-Soto, A., Amigo, M. C., Asherson, R. A., Azqueta, M., Pare, C., & et al. (1991). High prevalence of significant heart valve lesions in patients with the 'primary' antiphospholipid syndrome. *Lupus, 1*(1), 43-47.

Cervera, R., Font, J., Pare, C., Azqueta, M., Perez-Villa, F., Lopez-Soto, A., & Ingelmo, M. (1992). Cardiac disease in systemic lupus erythematosus: prospective study of 70 patients. *Ann Rheum Dis, 51*(2), 156-159.

Chen, C. Y., Wang, F. L., & Lin, C. C. (2006). Chronic hydroxychloroquine use associated with QT prolongation and refractory ventricular arrhythmia. *Clin Toxicol (Phila), 44*(2), 173-175.

Chobanian, A. V., Bakris, G. L., Black, H. R., Cushman, W. C., Green, L. A., Izzo, J. L., Jr., Jones, D. W., Materson, B. J., Oparil, S., Wright, J. T., Jr., & Roccella, E. J. (2003). The

Seventh Report of the Joint National Committee on Prevention, Detection, Evaluation, and Treatment of High Blood Pressure: the JNC 7 report. *JAMA, 289*(19), 2560-2572.

Chung, L., Berry, G. J., & Chakravarty, E. F. (2005). Giant cell myocarditis: a rare cardiovascular manifestation in a patient with systemic lupus erythematosus. *Lupus, 14*(2), 166-169.

Clarke-Jenssen, A. C., Fredriksen, P. M., Lilleby, V., & Mengshoel, A. M. (2005). Effects of supervised aerobic exercise in patients with systemic lupus erythematosus: a pilot study. *Arthritis Rheum, 53*(2), 308-312.

Clinical guidelines on the identification, evaluation, and treatment of overweight and obesity in adults–the evidence report. In. (1998), vol. 6 (pp. 51S–209S): National Institutes of Health.

Constans, J., Dupuy, R., Blann, A. D., Resplandy, F., Seigneur, M., Renard, M., Longy-Boursier, M., Schaeverbeke, T., Guerin, V., Boisseau, M. R., & Conri, C. (2003). Anti-endothelial cell autoantibodies and soluble markers of endothelial cell dysfunction in systemic lupus erythematosus. *J Rheumatol, 30*(9), 1963-1966.

Cooper, L. T., Jr., Berry, G. J., & Shabetai, R. (1997). Idiopathic giant-cell myocarditis--natural history and treatment. Multicenter Giant Cell Myocarditis Study Group Investigators. *N Engl J Med, 336*(26), 1860-1866.

Cooper, L. T., Baughman, K. L., Feldman, A. M., Frustaci, A., Jessup, M., Kuhl, U., Levine, G. N., Narula, J., Starling, R. C., Towbin, J., & Virmani, R. (2007). The role of endomyocardial biopsy in the management of cardiovascular disease: a scientific statement from the American Heart Association, the American College of Cardiology, and the European Society of Cardiology. Endorsed by the Heart Failure Society of America and the Heart Failure Association of the European Society of Cardiology. *J Am Coll Cardiol, 50*(19), 1914-1931.

Costedoat-Chalumeau, N., Georgin-Lavialle, S., Amoura, Z., & Piette, J. C. (2005). Anti-SSA/Ro and anti-SSB/La antibody-mediated congenital heart block. *Lupus, 14*(9), 660-664.

Daniel, L., Sichez, H., Giorgi, R., Dussol, B., Figarella-Branger, D., Pellissier, J. F., & Berland, Y. (2001). Tubular lesions and tubular cell adhesion molecules for the prognosis of lupus nephritis. *Kidney Int, 60*(6), 2215-2221.

Doria, A., Shoenfeld, Y., Wu, R., Gambari, P. F., Puato, M., Ghirardello, A., Gilburd, B., Corbanese, S., Patnaik, M., Zampieri, S., Peter, J. B., Favaretto, E., Iaccarino, L., Sherer, Y., Todesco, S., & Pauletto, P. (2003). Risk factors for subclinical atherosclerosis in a prospective cohort of patients with systemic lupus erythematosus. *Ann Rheum Dis, 62*(11), 1071-1077.

Edwards, M. H., Pierangeli, S., Liu, X., Barker, J. H., Anderson, G., & Harris, E. N. (1997). Hydroxychloroquine reverses thrombogenic properties of antiphospholipid antibodies in mice. *Circulation, 96*(12), 4380-4384.

Eisen, A., Arnson, Y., Dovrish, Z., Hadary, R., & Amital, H. (2009). Arrhythmias and conduction defects in rheumatological diseases--a comprehensive review. *Semin Arthritis Rheum, 39*(3), 145-156.

Elliott J.R., Manzi, S., Sattar A, et al. (2008). Carotid intima-media thickness and plaque predict future cardiovascular events in women with systemic lupus erythematosus. Arthritis Rheum, 58(9 Suppl), Abstract 669

Elliott, J. R., & Manzi, S. (2009). Cardiovascular risk assessment and treatment in systemic lupus erythematosus. *Best Pract Res Clin Rheumatol, 23*(4), 481-494.

Erkan, D., Yazici, Y., Peterson, M. G., Sammaritano, L., & Lockshin, M. D. (2002). A cross-sectional study of clinical thrombotic risk factors and preventive treatments in antiphospholipid syndrome. *Rheumatology (Oxford), 41*(8), 924-929.

Erkkila, A. T., Narvanen, O., Lehto, S., Uusitupa, M. I., & Yla-Herttuala, S. (2005). Antibodies against oxidized LDL and cardiolipin and mortality in patients with coronary heart disease. *Atherosclerosis, 183*(1), 157-162.

Esdaile, J. M., Abrahamowicz, M., Grodzicky, T., Li, Y., Panaritis, C., du Berger, R., Cote, R., Grover, S. A., Fortin, P. R., Clarke, A. E., & Senecal, J. L. (2001). Traditional Framingham risk factors fail to fully account for accelerated atherosclerosis in systemic lupus erythematosus. *Arthritis Rheum, 44*(10), 2331-2337.

Fernandez, M., Calvo-Alen, J., Alarcon, G. S., Roseman, J. M., Bastian, H. M., Fessler, B. J., McGwin, G., Jr., Vila, L. M., Sanchez, M. L., & Reveille, J. D. (2005). Systemic lupus erythematosus in a multiethnic US cohort (LUMINA): XXI. Disease activity, damage accrual, and vascular events in pre- and postmenopausal women. *Arthritis Rheum, 52*(6), 1655-1664.

Fernandez, M., Calvo-Alen, J., Bertoli, A. M., Bastian, H. M., Fessler, B. J., McGwin, G., Jr., Reveille, J. D., Vila, L. M., & Alarcon, G. S. (2007). Systemic lupus erythematosus in a multiethnic US cohort (LUMINA L II): relationship between vascular events and the use of hormone replacement therapy in postmenopausal women. *J Clin Rheumatol, 13*(5), 261-265.

Frostegard, J., Svenungsson, E., Wu, R., Gunnarsson, I., Lundberg, I. E., Klareskog, L., Horkko, S., & Witztum, J. L. (2005). Lipid peroxidation is enhanced in patients with systemic lupus erythematosus and is associated with arterial and renal disease manifestations. *Arthritis Rheum, 52*(1), 192-200.

Galve, E., Candell-Riera, J., Pigrau, C., Permanyer-Miralda, G., Garcia-Del-Castillo, H., & Soler-Soler, J. (1988). Prevalence, morphologic types, and evolution of cardiac valvular disease in systemic lupus erythematosus. *N Engl J Med, 319*(13), 817-823.

Garcia-Gonzalez, A., Gonzalez-Lopez, L., Valera-Gonzalez, I. C., Cardona-Munoz, E. G., Salazar-Paramo, M., Gonzalez-Ortiz, M., Martinez-Abundis, E., & Gamez-Nava, J. I. (2002). Serum leptin levels in women with systemic lupus erythematosus. *Rheumatol Int, 22*(4), 138-141.

Gardner, S. Y., McGee, J. K., Kodavanti, U. P., Ledbetter, A., Everitt, J. I., Winsett, D. W., Doerfler, D. L., & Costa, D. L. (2004). Emission-particle-induced ventilatory abnormalities in a rat model of pulmonary hypertension. *Environ Health Perspect, 112*(8), 872-878.

Gehi, A., Webb, A., Nolte, M., & Davis, J., Jr. (2003). Treatment of systemic lupus erythematosus-associated type B insulin resistance syndrome with cyclophosphamide and mycophenolate mofetil. *Arthritis Rheum, 48*(4), 1067-1070.

Gibson, W. T., & Hayden, M. R. (2007). Mycophenolate mofetil and atherosclerosis: results of animal and human studies. *Ann N Y Acad Sci, 1110*, 209-221.

Giles, I., & Rahman, A. (2009). How to manage patients with systemic lupus erythematosus who are also antiphospholipid antibody positive. *Best Pract Res Clin Rheumatol, 23*(4), 525-537.

Gladman, D. D., Hussain, F., Ibanez, D., & Urowitz, M. B. (2002). The nature and outcome of infection in systemic lupus erythematosus. *Lupus, 11*(4), 234-239.

Gladman DD,Urowitz MB.(2002) Prognosis, mortality, and morbidity in systemic lupus erythematosus.In: *Dubois' Lupus Erythematosus,*Wallace DJ, Hahn BH,(ed), 1255-1273, Lippincott Willams & Wilkins, ISBN 978-0-7897-9394, Philadelphia, USA

Godeau, P., Guillevin, L., Fechner, J., Herreman, G., & Wechsler, B. (1981). Cardiac involvement in systemic lupus erythematosus. 103 cases (author's transl). *Nouv Presse Med, 10*(26), 2175-2178.

Graham, I., A. D., Borch-Johnsen K, Boysen G, Burell G, Cifkova R, et al. (2007). European guidelines on cardiovascular disease prevention in clinical practice: executive summary. Atherosclerosis, 149(1), 1-45.

Griffith, G. C., & Vural, I. L. (1951). Acute and subacute disseminated lupus erythematosus; a correlation of clinical and postmortem findings in eighteen cases. *Circulation, 3*(4), 492-500.

Guzman, J., Cardiel, M. H., Arce-Salinas, A., & Alarcon-Segovia, D. (1994). The contribution of resting heart rate and routine blood tests to the clinical assessment of disease activity in systemic lupus erythematosus. *J Rheumatol, 21*(10), 1845-1848.

Hansson, G. K. (2005). Inflammation, atherosclerosis, and coronary artery disease. *N Engl J Med, 352*(16), 1685-1695.

Haskell, W. L., Lee, I. M., Pate, R. R., Powell, K. E., Blair, S. N., Franklin, B. A., Macera, C. A., Heath, G. W., Thompson, P. D., & Bauman, A. (2007). Physical activity and public health: updated recommendation for adults from the American College of Sports Medicine and the American Heart Association. *Circulation, 116*(9), 1081-1093.

Heibel, R. H., O'Toole, J. D., Curtiss, E. I., Medsger, T. A., Jr., Reddy, S. P., & Shaver, J. A. (1976). Coronary arteritis in systemic lupus erythematosus. *Chest, 69*(5), 700-703.

Hejtmancik, M. R., Wright, J. C., Quint, R., & Jennings, F. L. (1964). The Cardiovascular Manifestations of Systemic Lupus Erythematosus. *Am Heart J, 68*, 119-130.

Herlitz, H., Edeno, C., Mulec, H., Westberg, G., & Aurell, M. (1984). Captopril treatment of hypertension and renal failure in systemic lupus erythematosus. *Nephron, 38*(4), 253-256.

Hill, J. M., Zalos, G., Halcox, J. P., Schenke, W. H., Waclawiw, M. A., Quyyumi, A. A., & Finkel, T. (2003). Circulating endothelial progenitor cells, vascular function, and cardiovascular risk. *N Engl J Med, 348*(7), 593-600.

Hochman, J., Urowitz, M. B., Ibanez, D., & Gladman, D. D. (2009). Hormone replacement therapy in women with systemic lupus erythematosus and risk of cardiovascular disease. *Lupus, 18*(4), 313-317.

Jimenez, S., Garcia-Criado, M. A., Tassies, D., Reverter, J. C., Cervera, R., Gilabert, M. R., Zambon, D., Ros, E., Bru, C., & Font, J. (2005). Preclinical vascular disease in systemic lupus erythematosus and primary antiphospholipid syndrome. *Rheumatology (Oxford), 44*(6), 756-761.

Karp, I., Abrahamowicz, M., Fortin, P. R., Pilote, L., Neville, C., Pineau, C. A., & Esdaile, J. M. (2008). Recent corticosteroid use and recent disease activity: independent determinants of coronary heart disease risk factors in systemic lupus erythematosus? *Arthritis Rheum, 59*(2), 169-175.

Khamashta, M. A., Cervera, R., Asherson, R. A., Font, J., Gil, A., Coltart, D. J., Vazquez, J. J., Pare, C., Ingelmo, M., Oliver, J., & et al. (1990). Association of antibodies against phospholipids with heart valve disease in systemic lupus erythematosus. *Lancet, 335*(8705), 1541-1544.

Kong, T. Q., Kellum, R. E., & Haserick, J. R. (1962). Clinical diagnosis of cardiac involvement in systemic lupus erythematosus. A correlation of clinical and autopsy findings in thirty patients. *Circulation, 26*, 7-11.

Korbet, S. M., Schwartz, M. M., & Lewis, E. J. (1984). Immune complex deposition and coronary vasculitis in systemic lupus erythematosus. Report of two cases. *Am J Med, 77*(1), 141-146.

Korkmaz, C., Cansu, D. U., & Kasifoglu, T. (2007). Myocardial infarction in young patients (< or =35 years of age) with systemic lupus erythematosus: a case report and clinical analysis of the literature. *Lupus, 16*(4), 289-297.

Larsson, P. T., Hallerstam, S., Rosfors, S., & Wallen, N. H. (2005). Circulating markers of inflammation are related to carotid artery atherosclerosis. *Int Angiol, 24*(1), 43-51.

Lalani, A.L,Hatfield G. A.(2004)Imaging Finding in Systemic Lupus Erythematosus. *RadioGraphics*, 24:1069-1086

Leung, W. H., Wong, K. L., Lau, C. P., Wong, C. K., & Cheng, C. H. (1990). Cardiac abnormalities in systemic lupus erythematosus: a prospective M-mode, cross-sectional and Doppler echocardiographic study. *Int J Cardiol, 27*(3), 367-375.

Leung, W. H., Wong, K. L., Lau, C. P., Wong, C. K., & Liu, H. W. (1990). Association between antiphospholipid antibodies and cardiac abnormalities in patients with systemic lupus erythematosus. *Am J Med, 89*(4), 411-419.

Lichtenstein, A. H., Appel, L. J., Brands, M., Carnethon, M., Daniels, S., Franch, H. A., Franklin, B., Kris-Etherton, P., Harris, W. S., Howard, B., Karanja, N., Lefevre, M., Rudel, L., Sacks, F., Van Horn, L., Winston, M., & Wylie-Rosett, J. (2006). Diet and lifestyle recommendations revision 2006: a scientific statement from the American Heart Association Nutrition Committee. *Circulation, 114*(1), 82-96.

Lloyd-Jones, D. M., Liu, K., Tian, L., & Greenland, P. (2006). Narrative review: Assessment of C-reactive protein in risk prediction for cardiovascular disease. *Ann Intern Med, 145*(1), 35-42.

MacGregor, A. J., Dhillon, V. B., Binder, A., Forte, C. A., Knight, B. C., Betteridge, D. J., & Isenberg, D. A. (1992). Fasting lipids and anticardiolipin antibodies as risk factors for vascular disease in systemic lupus erythematosus. *Ann Rheum Dis, 51*(2), 152-155.

Mandell, B. F. (1987). Cardiovascular involvement in systemic lupus erythematosus. *Semin Arthritis Rheum, 17*(2), 126-141.

Manzi, S., Meilahn, E. N., Rairie, J. E., Conte, C. G., Medsger, T. A., Jr., Jansen-McWilliams, L., D'Agostino, R. B., & Kuller, L. H. (1997). Age-specific incidence rates of myocardial infarction and angina in women with systemic lupus erythematosus: comparison with the Framingham Study. *Am J Epidemiol, 145*(5), 408-415.

Manzi, S., Selzer, F., Sutton-Tyrrell, K., Fitzgerald, S. G., Rairie, J. E., Tracy, R. P., & Kuller, L. H. (1999). Prevalence and risk factors of carotid plaque in women with systemic lupus erythematosus. *Arthritis Rheum, 42*(1), 51-60.

Martorell, E. A., Hong, C., Rust, D. W., Salomon, R. N., Krishnamani, R., Patel, A. R., & Kalish, R. A. (2008). A 32-year-old woman with arthralgias and severe hypotension. *Arthritis Rheum, 59*(11), 1670-1675.

McMahon, M., Grossman, J., FitzGerald, J., Dahlin-Lee, E., Wallace, D. J., Thong, B. Y., Badsha, H., Kalunian, K., Charles, C., Navab, M., Fogelman, A. M., & Hahn, B. H. (2006). Proinflammatory high-density lipoprotein as a biomarker for atherosclerosis in patients with systemic lupus erythematosus and rheumatoid arthritis. Arthritis Rheum, 54(8), 2541-2549.

McMahon, M., Grossman, J., FitzGerald, Ragavendra, N., Charles, C., Chen, W., Watson, K., Hahn, B. (2006). The novel biomarker proinflammatory HDL is associated wtih carotid artery plaque in women with SLE. Arthritis Rheum, (Abstract).

McMahon, M.,Hahn BV.(2007)Atherosclerosis and systemic lupius erythematosus-mechanistic basis of association.*Current Opinion in Immunology,*19:633-639.

Mikdashi, J., Handwerger, B., Langenberg, P., Miller, M., & Kittner, S. (2007). Baseline disease activity, hyperlipidemia, and hypertension are predictive factors for ischemic stroke and stroke severity in systemic lupus erythematosus. *Stroke, 38*(2), 281-285.

Miyauchi, T., & Masaki, T. (1999). Pathophysiology of endothelin in the cardiovascular system. *Annu Rev Physiol, 61*, 391-415.

Nagore, E., Requena, C., Sevila, A., Coll, J., Costa, D., Botella-Estrada, R., Sanmartin, O., Serra-Guillen, C., & Guillen, C. (2004). Thickness of healthy and affected skin of children with port wine stains: potential repercussions on response to pulsed dye laser treatment. *Dermatol Surg, 30*(12 Pt 1), 1457-1461.

Nakano, M., Ueno, M., Hasegawa, H., Watanabe, T., Kuroda, T., Ito, S., & Arakawa, M. (1998). Renal haemodynamic characteristics in patients with lupus nephritis. *Ann Rheum Dis, 57*(4), 226-230.

Nathan, D. M., Buse, J. B., Davidson, M. B., Heine, R. J., Holman, R. R., Sherwin, R., & Zinman, B. (2006). Management of hyperglycemia in type 2 diabetes: A consensus algorithm for the initiation and adjustment of therapy: a consensus statement from the American Diabetes Association and the European Association for the Study of Diabetes. *Diabetes Care, 29*(8), 1963-1972.

Navab, M., Berliner, J. A., Watson, A. D., Hama, S. Y., Territo, M. C., Lusis, A. J., Shih, D. M., Van Lenten, B. J., Frank, J. S., Demer, L. L., Edwards, P. A., & Fogelman, A. M. (1996). The Yin and Yang of oxidation in the development of the fatty streak. A review based on the 1994 George Lyman Duff Memorial Lecture. *Arterioscler Thromb Vasc Biol, 16*(7), 831-842.

Navab, M., Hama, S. Y., Anantharamaiah, G. M., Hassan, K., Hough, G. P., Watson, A. D., Reddy, S. T., Sevanian, A., Fonarow, G. C., & Fogelman, A. M. (2000). Normal high density lipoprotein inhibits three steps in the formation of mildly oxidized low density lipoprotein: steps 2 and 3. *J Lipid Res, 41*(9), 1495-1508.

Nesher, G., Ilany, J., Rosenmann, D., & Abraham, A. S. (1997). Valvular dysfunction in antiphospholipid syndrome: prevalence, clinical features, and treatment. *Semin Arthritis Rheum, 27*(1), 27-35.

Nikpour, M., Urowitz, M. B., & Gladman, D. D. (2005). Premature atherosclerosis in systemic lupus erythematosus. *Rheum Dis Clin North Am, 31*(2), 329-354, vii-viii.

Nord, J. E., Shah, P. K., Rinaldi, R. Z., & Weisman, M. H. (2004). Hydroxychloroquine cardiotoxicity in systemic lupus erythematosus: a report of 2 cases and review of the literature. *Semin Arthritis Rheum, 33*(5), 336-351.

Ohara, N., Miyata, T., Kurata, A., Oshiro, H., Sato, O., & Shigematsu, H. (2000). Ten years' experience of aortic aneurysm associated with systemic lupus erythematosus. *Eur J Vasc Endovasc Surg, 19*(3), 288-293.

Okin, P. M., Devereux, R. B., Howard, B. V., Fabsitz, R. R., Lee, E. T., & Welty, T. K. (2000). Assessment of QT interval and QT dispersion for prediction of all-cause and cardiovascular mortality in American Indians: The Strong Heart Study. *Circulation, 101*(1), 61-66.

Petri, M. (1996). Hydroxychloroquine use in the Baltimore Lupus Cohort: effects on lipids, glucose and thrombosis. *Lupus, 5 Suppl 1*, S16-22.

Petri, M. (2000). Detection of coronary artery disease and the role of traditional risk factors in the Hopkins Lupus Cohort. *Lupus, 9*(3), 170-175.

Petri, M., Genovese, M., Engle, E., & Hochberg, M. (1991). Definition, incidence, and clinical description of flare in systemic lupus erythematosus. A prospective cohort study. *Arthritis Rheum, 34*(8), 937-944.

Petri, M., Perez-Gutthann, S., Spence, D., & Hochberg, M. C. (1992). Risk factors for coronary artery disease in patients with systemic lupus erythematosus. *Am J Med, 93*(5), 513-519.

Petri, M., Lakatta, C., Magder, L., & Goldman, D. (1994). Effect of prednisone and hydroxychloroquine on coronary artery disease risk factors in systemic lupus erythematosus: a longitudinal data analysis. *Am J Med, 96*(3), 254-259.

Petri, M,(2004).Cardiovascular Systemic Lupus Erythematosus, *Systemic Lupus Erythematosus,* Robert G. Lahita, (Ed) 913-941, Elsevier, ISBN 0-12-433901-8, USA

Petri, M., Kim, M. Y., Kalunian, K. C., Grossman, J., Hahn, B. H., Sammaritano, L. R., Lockshin, M., Merrill, J. T., Belmont, H. M., Askanase, A. D., McCune, W. J., Hearth-Holmes, M., Dooley, M. A., Von Feldt, J., Friedman, A., Tan, M., Davis, J., Cronin, M., Diamond, B., Mackay, M., Sigler, L., Fillius, M., Rupel, A., Licciardi, F., & Buyon, J. P. (2005). Combined oral contraceptives in women with systemic lupus erythematosus. *N Engl J Med, 353*(24), 2550-2558.

Petri, M. A., Kiani, A. N., Post, W., Christopher-Stine, L., & Magder, L. S. (2011). Lupus Atherosclerosis Prevention Study (LAPS). *Ann Rheum Dis, 70*(5), 760-765.

Pons-Estel, G. J., Gonzalez, L. A., Zhang, J., Burgos, P. I., Reveille, J. D., Vila, L. M., & Alarcon, G. S. (2009). Predictors of cardiovascular damage in patients with systemic lupus erythematosus: data from LUMINA (LXVIII), a multiethnic US cohort. *Rheumatology (Oxford), 48*(7), 817-822.

Rahman, P., Gladman, D. D., Urowitz, M. B., Yuen, K., Hallett, D., & Bruce, I. N. (1999). The cholesterol lowering effect of antimalarial drugs is enhanced in patients with lupus taking corticosteroid drugs. *J Rheumatol, 26*(2), 325-330.

Roman, M. J., Shanker, B. A., Davis, A., Lockshin, M. D., Sammaritano, L., Simantov, R., Crow, M. K., Schwartz, J. E., Paget, S. A., Devereux, R. B., & Salmon, J. E. (2003). Prevalence and correlates of accelerated atherosclerosis in systemic lupus erythematosus. *N Engl J Med, 349*(25), 2399-2406.

Roman, M. J., Devereux, R. B., Schwartz, J. E., Lockshin, M. D., Paget, S. A., Davis, A., Crow, M. K., Sammaritano, L., Levine, D. M., Shankar, B. A., Moeller, E., & Salmon, J. E. (2005). Arterial stiffness in chronic inflammatory diseases. *Hypertension, 46*(1), 194-199

Roman, M. J., Crow, M. K., Lockshin, M. D., Devereux, R. B., Paget, S. A., Sammaritano, L., Levine, D. M., Davis, A., & Salmon, J. E. (2007). Rate and determinants of progression of atherosclerosis in systemic lupus erythematosus. *Arthritis Rheum, 56*(10), 3412-3419.

Roman, M. J., & Salmon, J. E. (2007). Cardiovascular manifestations of rheumatologic diseases. *Circulation, 116*(20), 2346-2355.

Rosenbaum, E., Krebs, E., Cohen, M., Tiliakos, A., & Derk, C. T. (2009). The spectrum of clinical manifestations, outcome and treatment of pericardial tamponade in patients with systemic lupus erythematosus: a retrospective study and literature review. *Lupus, 18*(7), 608-612.

Ryan, M. J. (2009). The pathophysiology of hypertension in systemic lupus erythematosus. *Am J Physiol Regul Integr Comp Physiol, 296*(4), R1258-1267.

Sammaritano, L. R. (2007). Therapy insight: guidelines for selection of contraception in women with rheumatic diseases. *Nat Clin Pract Rheumatol, 3*(5), 273-281; quiz 305-276.

Saremi, F., Ashikyan, O., Saggar, R., Vu, J., & Nunez, M. E. (2007). Utility of cardiac MRI for diagnosis and post-treatment follow-up of lupus myocarditis. *Int J Cardiovasc Imaging, 23*(3), 347-352.

Selzer, F., Sutton-Tyrrell, K., Fitzgerald, S. G., Pratt, J. E., Tracy, R. P., Kuller, L. H., & Manzi, S. (2004). Comparison of risk factors for vascular disease in the carotid artery and aorta in women with systemic lupus erythematosus. *Arthritis Rheum, 50*(1), 151-159.

Shapiro, R. F., Gamble, C. N., Wiesner, K. B., Castles, J. J., Wolf, A. W., Hurley, E. J., & Salel, A. F. (1977). Immunopathogenesis of Libman-Sacks endocarditis. Assessment by light and immunofluorescent microscopy in two patients. *Ann Rheum Dis, 36*(6), 508-516.

Shearn, M. A. (1959). The heart in systemic lupus erythematosus. *Am Heart J, 58*, 452-466.

Sherer, Y., Levy, Y., & Shoenfeld, Y. (1999). Marked improvement of severe cardiac dysfunction after one course of intravenous immunoglobulin in a patient with systemic lupus erythematosus. *Clin Rheumatol, 18*(3), 238-240.

Skamra, C., & Ramsey-Goldman, R. (2010). Management of cardiovascular complications in systemic lupus erythematosus. *Int J Clin Rheumtol, 5*(1), 75-100.

Smith, S. C., Jr., Allen, J., Blair, S. N., Bonow, R. O., Brass, L. M., Fonarow, G. C., Grundy, S. M., Hiratzka, L., Jones, D., Krumholz, H. M., Mosca, L., Pasternak, R. C., Pearson, T., Pfeffer, M. A., & Taubert, K. A. (2006). AHA/ACC guidelines for secondary prevention for patients with coronary and other atherosclerotic vascular disease: 2006 update: endorsed by the National Heart, Lung, and Blood Institute. *Circulation, 113*(19), 2363-2372.

Straaton, K. V., Chatham, W. W., Reveille, J. D., Koopman, W. J., & Smith, S. H. (1988). Clinically significant valvular heart disease in systemic lupus erythematosus. *Am J Med, 85*(5), 645-650.

Su, J., Georgiades, A., Wu, R., Thulin, T., de Faire, U., & Frostegard, J. (2006). Antibodies of IgM subclass to phosphorylcholine and oxidized LDL are protective factors for atherosclerosis in patients with hypertension. *Atherosclerosis, 188*(1), 160-166.

Svenungsson, E., Jensen-Urstad, K., Heimburger, M., Silveira, A., Hamsten, A., de Faire, U., Witztum, J. L., & Frostegard, J. (2001). Risk factors for cardiovascular disease in systemic lupus erythematosus. *Circulation, 104*(16), 1887-1893.

Svenungsson, E., Fei, G. Z., Jensen-Urstad, K., de Faire, U., Hamsten, A., & Frostegard, J. (2003). TNF-alpha: a link between hypertriglyceridaemia and inflammation in SLE patients with cardiovascular disease. *Lupus, 12*(6), 454-461.

Svenungsson, E., Cederholm, A., Jensen-Urstad, K., Fei, G. Z., de Faire, U., & Frostegard, J. (2008). Endothelial function and markers of endothelial activation in relation to cardiovascular disease in systemic lupus erythematosus. *Scand J Rheumatol, 37*(5), 352-359.

Szalai, A. J., Alarcon, G. S., Calvo-Alen, J., Toloza, S. M., McCrory, M. A., Edberg, J. C., McGwin, G., Jr., Bastian, H. M., Fessler, B. J., Vila, L. M., Kimberly, R. P., & Reveille, J. D. (2005). Systemic lupus erythematosus in a multiethnic US Cohort (LUMINA). XXX: association between C-reactive protein (CRP) gene polymorphisms and vascular events. *Rheumatology (Oxford), 44*(7), 864-868.

Szekanecz Z.,Shoenfeld Y.(2004) Lupus and cardiovascular disease: the facts *Lupus,*15:3-10

Szekanecz, Z., Szucs, G., Szanto, S., & Koch, A. E. (2006). Chemokines in rheumatic diseases. *Curr Drug Targets, 7*(1), 91-102.

Thomas, G. N., Tam, L. S., Tomlinson, B., & Li, E. K. (2002). Accelerated atherosclerosis in patients with systemic lupus erythematosus: a review of the causes and possible prevention. *Hong Kong Med J, 8*(1), 26-32.

Thompson, T., Sutton-Tyrrell, K., Wildman, R. P., Kao, A., Fitzgerald, S. G., Shook, B., Tracy, R. P., Kuller, L. H., Brockwell, S., & Manzi, S. (2008). Progression of carotid intima-media thickness and plaque in women with systemic lupus erythematosus. *Arthritis Rheum, 58*(3), 835-842.

Tincani, A., Rebaioli, C. B., Taglietti, M., & Shoenfeld, Y. (2006). Heart involvement in systemic lupus erythematosus, anti-phospholipid syndrome and neonatal lupus. *Rheumatology (Oxford), 45 Suppl 4*, iv8-13.

Toloza, S., Urowitz, M. B., & Gladman, D. D. (2007). Should all patients with systemic lupus erythematosus receive cardioprotection with statins? *Nat Clin Pract Rheumatol, 3*(10), 536-537.

Topaloglu, S., Aras, D., Ergun, K., Altay, H., Alyan, O., & Akgul, A. (2006). Systemic lupus erythematosus: an unusual cause of cardiac tamponade in a young man. *Eur J Echocardiogr, 7*(6), 460-462.

Tripi, L. M., Manzi, S., Chen, Q., Kenney, M., Shaw, P., Kao, A., Bontempo, F., Kammerer, C., & Kamboh, M. I. (2006). Relationship of serum paraoxonase 1 activity and paraoxonase 1 genotype to risk of systemic lupus erythematosus. *Arthritis Rheum, 54*(6), 1928-1939.

Tsimikas, S., Brilakis, E. S., Miller, E. R., McConnell, J. P., Lennon, R. J., Kornman, K. S., Witztum, J. L., & Berger, P. B. (2005). Oxidized phospholipids, Lp(a) lipoprotein, and coronary artery disease. *N Engl J Med, 353*(1), 46-57.

Turiel, M., Peretti, R., Sarzi-Puttini, P., Atzeni, F., & Doria, A. (2005). Cardiac imaging techniques in systemic autoimmune diseases. *Lupus, 14*(9), 727-731.

Uchida, T., Inoue, T., Kamishirado, H., Nakata, T., Sakai, Y., Takayanagi, K., & Morooka, S. (2001). Unusual coronary artery aneurysm and acute myocardial infarction in a middle-aged man with systemic lupus erythematosus. *Am J Med Sci, 322*(3), 163-165.

Urowitz, M. B., Bookman, A. A., Koehler, B. E., Gordon, D. A., Smythe, H. A., & Ogryzlo, M. A. (1976). The bimodal mortality pattern of systemic lupus erythematosus. *Am J Med, 60*(2), 221-225.

Urowitz, M. B., Kagal, A., Rahman, P., & Gladman, D. D. (2002). Role of specialty care in the management of patients with systemic lupus erythematosus. *J Rheumatol, 29*(6), 1207-1210.

Urowitz, M. B., Ibanez, D., & Gladman, D. D. (2007). Atherosclerotic vascular events in a single large lupus cohort: prevalence and risk factors. *J Rheumatol, 34*(1), 70-75.

van der Laan-Baalbergen, N. E., Mollema, S. A., Kritikos, H., Schoe, A., Huizinga, T. W., Bax, J. J., Boumpas, D. T., & van Laar, J. M. (2009). Heart failure as presenting manifestation of cardiac involvement in systemic lupus erythematosus. *Neth J Med, 67*(9), 295-301.

Veres, K., Lakos, G., Kerenyi, A., Szekanecz, Z., Szegedi, G., Shoenfeld, Y., & Soltesz, P. (2004). Antiphospholipid antibodies in acute coronary syndrome. *Lupus, 13*(6), 423-427.

Von Feldt, J. M. (2008). Premature atherosclerotic cardiovascular disease and systemic lupus erythematosus from bedside to bench. *Bull NYU Hosp Jt Dis, 66*(3), 184-187.

Wallace, D. J. (1987). Does hydroxychloroquine sulfate prevent clot formation in systemic lupus erythematosus? *Arthritis Rheum, 30*(12), 1435-1436.

Wallace, D. J., Metzger, A. L., Stecher, V. J., Turnbull, B. A., & Kern, P. A. (1990). Cholesterol-lowering effect of hydroxychloroquine in patients with rheumatic disease: reversal of deleterious effects of steroids on lipids. *Am J Med, 89*(3), 322-326.

Wijetunga, M., & Rockson, S. (2002). Myocarditis in systemic lupus erythematosus. *Am J Med, 113*(5), 419-423.

Wilson, V. E., Eck, S. L., & Bates, E. R. (1992). Evaluation and treatment of acute myocardial infarction complicating systemic lupus erythematosus. *Chest, 101*(2), 420-424.

14

Pulmonary Manifestations of Systemic Lupus Erythematosus

Abdul Ghafoor Gari, Amr Telmesani and Raad Alwithenani
Umm Al-Qura University
Saudi Arabia

1. Introduction

Systemic lupus erythematosus (SLE) is an autoimmune disease that primarily affects women of childbearing age with 10:1 female to male ratio.(Siegel & Lee, 1973) Any organ can be affected by SLE; pulmonary involvement is usually in the latter course of the disease.(Haupt *et al.*, 1981; Orens *et al.*, 1994; Quadrelli *et al.*, 2009) It is important to note that lung involvement is proportionately more common in men.(Kamen & Strange, 2010) Any part of the pulmonary system can be affected including airways, lung parenchyma, pulmonary vasculature, pleura and diaphragm.(Gross *et al.*, 1972; Haupt *et al.*, 1981; Kamen & Strange, 2010; Orens *et al.*, 1994; Quadrelli *et al.*, 2009; Weinrib *et al.*, 1990) If SLE develops after age 49 years, it has a higher incidence of serositis, pulmonary involvement and mortality.(Boddaert *et al.*, 2004) It is difficult to find out the true prevalence of pulmonary complications of SLE since many cases are due to infections.(Kamen & Strange, 2010) A recent autopsy study of 90 patients diagnosed with SLE, according to the American College of Rheumatology, pleuropulmonary involvement occurred in 98% of the autopsies. (Quadrelli *et al.*, 2009) The most frequent findings were pleuritis (78%), bacterial infections (58%), alveolar hemorrhage (26%), followed by distal airway alterations (21%), opportunistic infections (14%) and pulmonary thromboembolism (8%), both acute and chronic.(Quadrelli *et al.*, 2009) In a larger series, 25% of patients with SLE had clinical and/or radiographic evidence of pulmonary involvement.(Pego-Reigosa *et al.*, 2009)

2. Clinical features

SLE can affect the lungs in many ways. In the next section we will review the pulmonary diseases associated with SLE according to the anatomic involvement.

2.1 Pleural diseases

Pleuritis is the most common pleuropulmonary manifestation of SLE.(Orens *et al.*, 1994) It is the initial manifestation in 5% to 10%.(Winslow *et al.*, 1958) Symptoms of pleuritis are present in 45% to 60% of patients with SLE and may be associated with pleural effusion.(Good *et al.*, 1983; Orens *et al.*, 1994; Pines *et al.*, 1985) Pleural effusion in SLE tends to be bilateral, small to moderate in size; however, large effusions may occur.(Bouros *et al.*, 2008) Typical presentation of pleural involvement is pleuritic chest pain (pain that increases with inspiration), dyspnea, and fever. Physical examination may reveal pleural friction rub and signs of pleural effusion. Chest X-ray shows blunting of the costophrenic angle. Some patients may have asymptomatic pleural effusion. Other causes of pleural effusion such as parapneumonic effusion, pulmonary embolism, and heart failure need to be ruled out. Pleural fluid analysis is needed to rule out other etiologies and to confirm the diagnosis of lupus pleuritis. Pleural fluid is exudative (elevated pleural fluid protein and lactate dehydrogenase levels) when analyzed. Cell counts are elevated with predominance of lymphocytes or neutrophils. Pleural fluid glucose level is low, but not as low as in patients with rheumatoid arthritis. Special tests reveal low pleural complement level and positive anti-nuclear antibody (ANA). These tests are not sensitive enough to rule out lupus pleuritis when tests are negative. (Hunder *et al.*, 1972; Small *et al.*, 1982) Pleural fluid ANA titer ≥ 1:160 and pleural fluid / serum ANA ratio of ≥ 1 strongly support the diagnosis.(Good *et al.*, 1983) The finding of lupus erythematosus cells in pleural fluid confirms the diagnosis; however this test is rarely performed.(Kamen & Strange, 2010) Pleural biopsy is rarely needed, if done it will show a peculiar immunofluorescent pattern characterized by staining of nuclei with anti-IgG, anti-IgM and anti-C3.(Pertschuk *et al.*, 1977) Patients with pleural disease usually respond to nonsteriodal anti-inflammatory drugs (NSAIDs). Low doses of oral glucocorticoids hasten the resolution. Small asymptomatic effusions usually resolve without treatment.(Winslow *et al.*, 1958) NSAIDs are sufficient for mild cases; for severe cases or for patients on steroids, giving higher doses of steroid is required.(Orens *et al.*, 1994; Wiedemann & Matthay, 1989) In refractory pleural effusions tetracycline or talc pleurodesis can be an alternative option.(Gilleece *et al.*, 1988; Kaine, 1985; McKnight *et al.*, 1991)

2.2 Parenchymal lung disease

2.2.1 Acute lupus pneumonitis

Acute lupus pneumonitis (ALP) is an uncommon but well recognized complication of SLE. There is some controversy over the definition ALP.(Swigris *et al.*, 2008) In two recent series, the prevalence of ALP in patients with SLE was 2% to 8%.(Kim *et al.*, 2000; Mochizuki *et al.*, 1999) It is difficult to estimate the exact prevalence given the significant clinical and radiological overlap between ALP, bacterial pneumonia and alveolar hemorrhage. ALP tends to affect younger patients and those with recent diagnosis of SLE. In 50% of patients with SLE who develop ALP, the pulmonary complication is the initial presentation of lupus.(Matthay *et al.*, 1975) Clinical presentation includes abrupt onset of fever, cough, dyspnea, pleuritic chest pain and occasionally hemoptysis.(Matthay *et al.*, 1975) Physical examination usually reveals signs of hypoxia and bibasilar crackles. Radiographic findings include bilateral alveolar infiltrates with predominance in lower lung fields (figure 1). Pleural effusion occurs in half of the cases.(Matthay *et al.*, 1975) Rarely the initial chest radiograph may be normal or may show pulmonary nodules.(Susanto & Peters, 1997) CT scan of the chest may show diffuse ground glass opacities and areas of consolidation.(Swigris *et al.*, 2008) A fulminant form of ALP may occur during pregnancy.(Comer *et al.*, 1996) The clinical and radiographic features are not specific. Other causes of alveolar infiltrates like infectious pneumonia, alveolar hemorrhage, pulmonary edema, and organizing pneumonia should be considered. It is important to rule out infectious complications. Many of these patients are on systemic steroids and other immunosuppressive medications and are at increased risk of opportunistic infections. Early bronchoscopy and bronchoalveolar lavage (BAL) with or without transbronchial biopsy is mandatory in most cases. BAL should be sent for cell count and differential, bacterial, fungal and viral culture, cytology and for Pneumocystis jiroveci stain. Occasionally a thoracoscopic lung biopsy may be needed. The pathological findings are not specific. The most common findings include diffuse alveolar damage (DAD) with or without alveolar hemorrhage and capillaritis.(Harvey *et al.*, 1954; Keane & Lynch, 2000) Other pathologic features include alveolar wall injury, alveolar edema, hyaline membrane formation, immunoglobulin and complement deposition. There seems to be some association between ALP and anti-Ro/SSa antibodies. One study showed that patients with SLE and pulmonary complications had an 81% positive result for anti-Ro/SSa antibodies, while patients without pulmonary involvement had a 38% positive antibody.(Boulware & Hedgpeth, 1989) A more recent review confirmed this association (Mochizuki *et al.*, 1999) The high frequency of anti-Ro/SSa antibodies raises the possibility of their role in the pathogenesis of ALP.(Cheema & Quismorio, 2000) Prognosis is poor, with mortality reaching up to 50% as reported in an old study.(Matthay *et al.*, 1975) The outcome is worse if ALP occurs postpartum.(Matthay *et al.*, 1975) Eosinophilia or neutrophilia on BAL carries worse prognosis than lymphocytosis.(Witt *et al.*, 1996) Because infectious causes can't be ruled out, empiric broad spectrum antibiotics should be started immediately and continued until infection is excluded. There are no randomized clinical trials for the treatment of ALP, however it is agreed on that the main treatment is systemic corticosteroids (prednisone 1-1.5 mg/kg/day). If no adequate response within 72 hours, treatment should be with intravenous pulse steroids (1g methylprednisolone daily for three days).(Kamen & Strange, 2010) Additional immunosuppresants such as cyclophosphamide should also be considered. In patients refractory to corticosteroids, intravenous immunoglobulin, plasma exchange or rituximab can be of some help with very little evidence (Eiser & Shanies, 1994; Lim *et al.*, 2006; Pego-Reigosa *et al.*, 2009; Winder *et al.*, 1993)

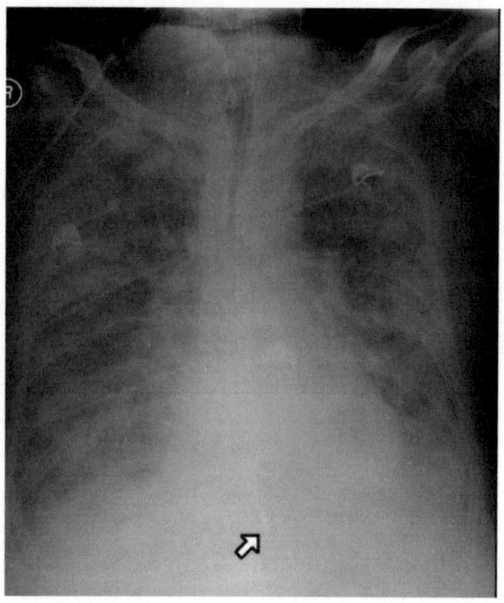

Fig. 1. Chest X-ray showing diffuse alveolar infiltrates in a patient with acute lupus pneumonitis

2.2.2 Diffuse alveolar hemorrhage

Diffuse alveolar hemorrhage (DAH) is a rare complication of SLE. (Badsha *et al.*, 2004; Eagen *et al.*, 1978; Zamora *et al.*, 1997) Its prevalence among SLE patients ranges between

<2% and 5.4 % (Santos-Ocampo *et al.*, 2000; Zamora *et al.*, 1997), and the mortality rate ranges between 50% to 90%.(Erickson *et al.*, 1994; Schwab *et al.*, 1993) Usually it occurs in established disease, especially with lupus nephritis.(Zamora *et al.*, 1997) Other extrapulmonary manifestations occur with variable degree.(Abud-Mendoza *et al.*, 1985; Barile *et al.*, 1997; Koh *et al.*, 1997; Liu *et al.*, 1998; Myers & Katzenstein, 1986; Schwab *et al.*, 1993; Zamora *et al.*, 1997) However it can occasionally be the initial presentation of SLE.(Zamora *et al.*, 1997) Risk factors thought to be contributing to the development of DAH are higher titer of circulating anti-DNA antibody, active extra-pulmonary disease, and established SLE diagnosis.(Orens *et al.*, 1994)

Clinical presentation of patients with DAH is not specific; symptoms include acute shortness of breath, cough, hemoptysis and fever. The absence of hemoptysis doesn't rule out DAH. In fact hemoptysis is only present in 54% of patients.(Santos-Ocampo *et al.*, 2000) Fever is present in more than 80% of patients.(Santos-Ocampo *et al.*, 2000) Signs of respiratory distress and hypoxia are noted upon physical examination. Chest radiograph shows bilateral alveolar infiltrates. Unilateral pulmonary infiltrates is noted in up to 18%.(Santos-Ocampo *et al.*, 2000) CT imaging demonstrates new bilateral ground glass opacities and consolidation. Acute drop in hemoglobin is frequently encountered. In most series anemia was noted >90 of all episodes of DAH. (Abud-Mendoza *et al.*, 1985; Barile *et al.*, 1997; Koh *et al.*, 1997; Liu *et al.*, 1998; Myers & Katzenstein, 1986; Schwab *et al.*, 1993; Zamora *et al.*, 1997) If diffusion capacity for carbon monoxide (DLCO) is measured it will be elevated due to the excess hemoglobin in the alveolar spaces. An increase of DLCO by 30% or a value of >130% predicted suggest DAH in the right clinical setting.(Carette *et al.*, 1984; Dweik *et al.*, 1997; Ewan *et al.*, 1976; Harmon & Leatherman, 1988; Leatherman *et al.*, 1984; Young, 1989) Low complement level is found in more than 70% of all episodes of DAH.(Koh *et al.*, 1997; Liu *et al.*, 1998; Myers & Katzenstein, 1986; Santos-Ocampo *et al.*, 2000; Schwab *et al.*, 1993;) Magnetic resonant imaging (MRI) is another imaging study that can suggest the presence of blood in the alveoli given the paramagnetic effect of iron.(Hsu *et al.*, 1992) BAL is mandatory to rule out infection and help in the diagnosis of DAH. BAL can confirm the diagnosis if bloody return increases with serial aliquots. BAL should be evaluated for the presence of hemosiderin-laden macrophages, their presence indicate alveolar hemorrhage. Transbronchial biopsy (TBBx) may be attempted in stable patients. Unfortunately many of these patients require ventilatory support and may not be able to sustain the complication of TBBx. Thoracoscopic lung biopsy is rarely needed. Two pathological patterns have been described. Bland hemorrhage is more common and occurs in 72% while capillaritis occurs in 14% of the times. Both pathological patterns are associated with intra-alveolar hemorrhage and hemosiderin–laden macrophages.(Myers & Katzenstein, 1986; Schwab *et al.*, 1993b; Zamora *et al.*, 1997) IgG , C3 or immune complexes deposition occurs in 50% of the cases.(Myers & Katzenstein, 1986) There are no randomized control trials addressing treatment options for DAH. Supportive care is highly valued since many of these patients end up in the intensive care unit requiring mechanical ventilation. The most acceptable regimen include pulse intravenous steroids (methylprednisolone 1gm per day for three days) followed by 1mg/kg of oral prednisone plus intravenous cyclophosphamide every four weeks.(Schwab *et al.*, 1993a; Swigris *et al.*, 2008) DAH is one of the few indications where plasmapharesis has been shown to be effective, especially in refractory cases. (Erickson *et al.*, 1994; Santos-Ocampo *et al.*, 2000) Plasmapharesis may improve survival in patients who failed treatment with high dose steroids and cyclophosphamide.(Erickson *et al.*, 1994) More recently rituximab has been used in refractory cases with promising results.(Pottier *et al.*, 2011) The mean duration of alveolar hemorrhage from onset to radiographic resolution is 7.8 days.(Santos-Ocampo *et al.*, 2000) DAH is known to recur within the same subject. In one study, recurrence occurred in more than 40% of patients.(Santos-Ocampo *et al.*, 2000)

2.2.3 Chronic interstitial lung disease

Chronic interstitial lung disease (ILD) is a well-recognized pulmonary manifestation of SLE. The prevalence of chronic ILD in symptomatic patients with lupus is 3%.(Haupt *et al.*, 1981; Weinrib *et al.*, 1990) The prevalence increases with an increase in the duration of SLE.(Jacobsen *et al.*, 1998) It may present as a chronic and insidious disease or it may follow the development of ALP (Boulware & Hedgpeth, 1989; Weinrib *et al.*, 1990) Chronic ILD occurs more commonly in men and older patients. Pulmonary fibrosis affects 18% of patients above 50 years compared to 2% of patients under 18 years.(Cheema & Quismorio, 2000) Clinically, patients usually present with gradually progressive shortness of breath. Chronic dry cough can be the initial presentation in some patients. Physical examination may show fine bibasilar inspiratory crackles, however finger clubbing is rare.(Renzoni *et al.*, 1997) Spirometry shows restrictive pattern with proportionate reduction in forced expiratory volume in one second (FEV1) and forced vital capacity (FVC) with normal or increased FEV1/FVC ratio. Lung volumes and DLCO are typically reduced. Early on, the only abnormality in pulmonary function test is an isolated reduction in DLCO. Chest radiographs may be normal at the beginning. As the disease progresses it may show irregular linear opacities and marked interstitial markings. Reduced lung volume is a late finding. High resolution CT (HRCT) of the chest may show diffuse ground glass opacities. Other features include diffuse interstitial infiltrates, sepal thickening, honeycombing and traction bronchiectasis (figure2). The pattern of ILD mimics that of idiopathic interstitial pneumonia (IIP). The presence of pleural disease is common in patients with SLE while it is rare in IIP. One study attempted to correlate HRCT findings with clinical and pulmonary function tests (PFTs). There was no correlation between abnormal HRCT, pulmonary symptoms, disease activity and drug therapy.(Fenlon *et al.*, 1996) The PFT findings did not correlate with the presence or the severity of ILD on HRCT.(Fenlon *et al.*, 1996) This lack of correlation was confirmed in another study.(Sant *et al.*, 1997) The rate of abnormal CT findings in asymptomatic patients is high, reaching 30%.(Bankier *et al.*, 1995; Fenlon *et al.*, 1996; Haupt *et al.*, 1981) There is no current recommendation to screen asymptomatic SLE patients with HRCT. Bronchoscopy with BAL is done to rule out infections. Thoracoscopic lung biopsy is needed to identify the underlying pathology. Several histopathological patterns are known to occur. The most common pattern is non-specific interstitial pneumonia (NSIP), cellular, fibrotic or mixed.(Tansey *et al.*, 2004) This pattern is characterized by homogeneous infiltration of alveolar walls with large number of lymphocytes and plasma cells. Organizing pneumonia, which used to be called bronchiolitis obliterans organizing pneumonia (BOOP) has also been reported.(Gammon *et al.*, 1992) Lymphoid interstitial pneumonia (LIP) and usual interstitial pneumonia (UIP) are found more commonly in patients with secondary Sjögren's syndrome or overlap syndrome.(Schattner *et al.*, 2003; Tansey *et al.*, 2004) There are no placebo control trials to guide the treatment of ILD in SLE. Systemic corticosteroids (Prednisone 60mg/d for at least four weeks) improved respiratory symptoms and DLCO in the majority of patients when followed up for a mean of 7.3 years. (Weinrib *et al.*, 1990) In patients who don't respond to corticosteroids, treatment with cyclophosphamide, azathioprine, or mycophenolate should be considered. Another approach is to start combination therapy; cyclophosphamide and oral glucocorticoids for severe cases and oral steroids with azathioprine for less severe cases.(Swigris *et al.*, 2008) The prognosis of ILD associated with SLE is better than the idiopathic forms.(Renzoni *et al.*, 1997) The course is usually slow and tends to stabilize or improve with time.

2.3 Pulmonary vascular diseases

2.3.1 Thromboembolic disease

Patients with SLE are at increased risk of venous thromboembolism (VTE) with a prevalence of 9%.(Gladman & Urowitz, 1980) It is usually related to disease activity. Patients with antiphospholipid antibodies have an even more increased risk reaching up to 35% to 42%. (Love & Santoro, 1990) Antiphospholipid antibodies (aPL) maybe present in up to two thirds of patients with lupus.(Ruiz-Irastorza *et al.*, 2004; Somers *et al.*, 2002) The two major antibodies that constitute aPL are lupus anticoagulant and anticardiolipin antibodies (IgG or IgM). Criteria of diagnosing antiphospholipid syndrome are discussed elsewhere. In addition to VTE, patients with antiphospholipid syndrome are at increased risk of recurrent abortions, pulmonary hypertension (PH), DAH, acute respiratory distress syndrome (ARDS), and cardiac valvular lesions. (Kamen & Strange, 2010; Swigris *et al.*, 2008) If small-vessel occlusion occurs in three or more organs the condition is known as catastrophic antiphospholipid syndrome (CAPS). (Asherson & Cervera, 1995; Asherson *et al.*, 2001; Cervera *et al.*, 2007; Cervera & Asherson, 2008) Cardiopulmonary involvement is common with this syndrome and it usually results in ARDS (Asherson *et al.*, 2008; Bucciarelli *et al.*, 2006) VTE can occur either acutely (deep vein thrombosis or acute pulmonary embolism) or chronically resulting in chronic thromboembolic pulmonary hypertension (CTEPH). Clinical features and diagnosis of VTE are similar to unprovoked situations. Once VTE develops,

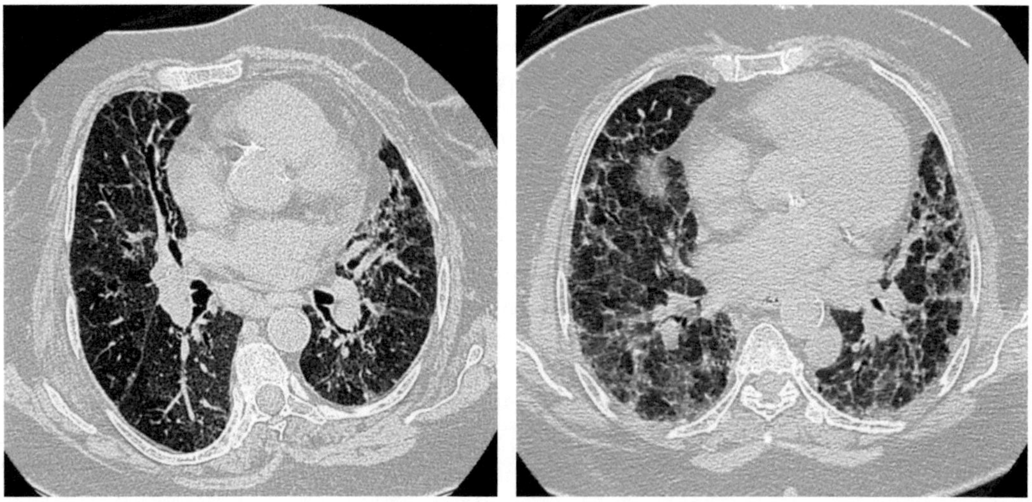

Fig. 2. (Left) HRCT chest showing areas of ground glass opacities and traction bronchiectasis. Surgical lung biopsy confirmed the diagnosis of non-specific interstitial pneumonia (cellular type). (Right) HRCT chest showing interstitial thickening and areas of honeycombing. Fibrotic form of non-specific interstitial pneumonia was evident on lung biopsy

long term anticoagulation with warfarin and a target INR of 2.0 to 3.0 is highly recommended. It used to be recommended to achieve a higher target INR, but in one study, high intensity warfarin (target INR 3.0-4.0) was found not superior to moderate intensity warfarin (target INR 2.0-3.0). Moderate intensity warfarin had lower rate of major bleeding.(Crowther *et al.*, 2003) Recommendation for primary prevention is lacking. Some authors use long term low dose aspirin.(Swigris *et al.*, 2008) Patients with CAPS usually require systemic glucocorticoids, immunosuppressants, plasmapharesis and intravenous immunoglobulin in addition to anticoagulation.(Swigris *et al.*, 2008) Mortality rate can reach up to 50%.(Asherson & Cervera, 1995; Asherson *et al.*, 2001, 2008)

2.3.2 Pulmonary hypertension

Pulmonary Hypertension (PH) is defined as a mean pulmonary artery pressure (PAP) ≥ 25mmHg at rest. (McLaughlin *et al.*, 2009) The prevalence of PH in SLE patients varies between 0.5% to 15%. (Asherson & Oakley, 1986; Asherson *et al.*, 1990) In one study, 50 consecutive patients with SLE were carefully tested by transthoracic echocardiogram to look particularly for PH, none was found to have any echocardiographic evidence of PH. In that cohort almost one third were found to have an isolated reduction in DLCO, which could be a marker of early pulmonary vascular involvement.(Hodson *et al.*, 1983; Gari *et al.*, 2009) The prevalence is definitely lower than those with scleroderma. Raynaud's phenomenon occurs in 75% of SLE associated pulmonary arterial hypertension (PAH) compared to only 20% of patients with SLE and no PH.(Matthay *et al.*, 1975) The duration of SLE doesn't correlate with the development of PAH.(Asherson & Oakley, 1986; Asherson & Cervera, 2007) Clinical presentations of SLE associated PAH is similar to idiopathic pulmonary arterial pulmonary hypertension (IPAH). Symptoms include dyspnea, fatigue, chest pain and lower limb swelling. Physical examination includes jugular venous distension with a large v wave, loud pulmonic component with wide splitting of the second heart sound, murmur of tricuspid regurgitation and/or pulmonic insufficiency, and lower limb edema. Physical findings may be minimal in mild PH. In patients with suspected PH, transthoracic echocardiogram is the best initial diagnostic test. Right ventricular systolic pressure (RVSP) which is an approximation of systolic PAP can only be measured if a tricuspid regurgitation (TR) signal is detected. TR signal is only available in 30% of population. Although PH is more common in SLE patients than general population, other causes of PH need to be ruled out. Tests to evaluate for other causes include HIV, hepatitis B and hepatitis C serology, aPL antibodies, HRCT chest to evaluate for interstitial lung disease, ventilation perfusion scan (V/Q) to look for any evidence of chronic pulmonary emboli leading to CTEPH, and polysomnogram if obstructive sleep apnea is suspected. Eventually right heart catheterization is required to confirm the diagnosis of PAH and to rule out PH secondary to left heart disease. The pathogenesis of SLE associated PAH is not clear; the high prevalence of aPL antibodies suggests that thrombosis may play a role. (Prabu *et al.*, 2009) Histopathologic changes are identical to IPAH and include plexiform lesions, intimal fibrosis, and thickening of the media. In addition, complement and immunoglobulin deposits are found in some patients suggesting that immune deposits may be involved in the pathogenesis.(Quismorio *et al.*, 1984) Several aspects need to be considered when it comes to treating SLE associated PAH. All patients should receive long term anticoagulation especially those with aPL antibodies. Oxygen, diuretics and digoxin should be considered in all patients. PH specific therapies used to treat IPAH are also effective in treating SLE associated PAH. Epoprostenol, bosentan, sildenafil, ambrisentan and tadalafil have all been shown to be effective in treating PAH.(Barst RJ *et al.*,1996; Galie *et al.*, 2005, 2008, 2009; Rubin *et al.*, 2004) PAH specific therapies were found to improve 6-minute walk distance (6MWD) and functional class.

Adding immunosuppressants may provide further improvement. Intravenous cyclophosphamide (monthly for six months) was shown to be effective. It reduced the systolic PAP when measured by transthoracic echocardiogram, and improved 6MWD.(Gonzalez-Lopez *et al.*, 2004; Jais *et al.*, 2008) Oral glucocorticoids in conjunction with immunosuppressants lowered PAP and improved 6MWD.(Tanaka *et al.*, 2002; Sanchez *et al.*, 2006) It is not very clear when to use immunosuppressants in SLE associated PAH. Patients with mild PH may benefit from immunosuppressive therapy while patients with moderate to severe PH need PH specific therapy with or without immunosuppressants.(Swigris *et al.*, 2008) The prognosis of SLE associated PAH is worse than IPAH, with a 5-year survival of only 17% compared to 68% in patients with IPAH.(Chung *et al.*, 2006) Given the rarity of PH in patients with SLE, there is no recommendation to screen asymptomatic patients with echocardiogram. On the other hand, patients with scleroderma should have annual transthoracic echocardiogram to evaluate for the presence of PH.

2.3.3 Acute reversible hypoxia

This is a rare complication of lupus. In one series 27% of hospitalized patients had this condition.(Abramson *et al.*, 1991) It is characterized by an abrupt onset of unexplained hypoxia and hypocapnea. Radiographic chest imaging is normal. Ventilation perfusion (V/Q) scan doesn't show any evidence of thromboembolism. Arterial blood gases demonstrates an increase in Alveolar-arterial (A-a) PO2 gradient. The pathogenesis of this syndrome is not clear, but it is believed to be due to complement activation leading to leukoaggregation within pulmonary capillaries.(Abramson *et al.*, 1991; Belmont *et al.*, 1994) Plasma C3a level is markedly elevated if measured during the episode.(Abramson *et al.*, 1991) Most cases respond quickly to high dose of systemic corticosteroids.(Abramson *et al.*, 1991; Martinez-Taboada *et al.*, 1995)

2.4 Airway disease

2.4.1 Upper airway involvement

Involvement of the upper airways can occur in up to 30% of patients with SLE. A variety of disorders have been described including laryngeal mucosal inflammation or ulceration, cricoarytenoiditis, vocal cord paralysis, and necrotizing vasculitis.(Langford & Van Waes, 1997; Teitel *et al.*, 1992) Patients present with hoarseness and or dyspnea. Severe upper airway obstruction due to angioedema requiring mechanical ventilation has also been reported.(Thong *et al.*, 2001) Angioedema usually present with lips and mouth swelling, dysphagia, odynophagia and breathing difficulty, it could be due to SLE or medications used in SLE like angiotensin-converting enzyme inhibitors.(Agah *et al.*, 1997) Routine chest imaging with Chest x-ray and chest CT is usually normal in patients with upper airway obstruction. Spirometry may show flattening of the inspiratory or expiratory loop or both depending on the location of the obstruction. Specialized imaging of the upper airways with 3-D reconstruction is important to demonstrate the site of obstruction. Direct visualization with fibro-optic laryngoscopy or bronchoscopy is needed to assess for vocal cord mobility. Generally, corticosteroid therapy will be effective in case of laryngeal mucosal inflammation or ulceration, and vocal cord paralysis.(Smith *et al.*, 1977; Teitel *et al.*, 1992). In those who don't respond to glucocorticoids, infectious causes should be considered. Typical pathogens are Haemophilus influenzae and streptococcus, other rare infections include Histoplasma, coccidioides, cryptococus, blastomycosis and candida.(Toomey *et al.*, 1974)

2.4.2 Lower airway involvement

Diseases involving the lower airways in patient with SLE include bronchial wall thickening, bronchiectasias and bronchiolitis obliterans (BO). In a prospective study of 34 subjects with SLE, HRCT chest showed bronchial wall thickening and bronchiectasias in 21% of patients. These changes were predominantly asymptomatic.(Fenlon *et al.*, 1996) Bronchiolar disorders are rare.(Pego-Reigosa *et al.*, 2009) Abnormalities in PFTs have been reported in up to two thirds of patient with SLE.(Andonopoulos *et al.*, 1988) In one study of 57 consecutive lupus patients, mild to moderate airflow obstruction was noted in 16%.(Groen *et al.*, 1992) BO has been rarely reported.(Beylot-Barry *et al.*, 1994; Godeau *et al.*, 1991; Kawahata *et al.*, 2008) The disease is characterized by severe airflow obstruction that's mostly irreversible. Patients usually have progressive dyspnea. PFTs show reduction in FEV1/FVC ratio. If obstruction is severe, gas trapping (elevated residual volume) and hyperinflation (elevated total lung capacity) may be noted. HRCT chest shows mosaic attenuation pattern that gets accentuated in the expiratory images (figure 3). Histopathologic confirmation is rarely required. Disease is usually progressive. Systemic corticosteroids and immunosuppressive therapies have been tried with little success.(Beylot-Barry *et al.*, 1994; Kawahata *et al.*, 2008) More recently anticholinergics were reported to have a favorable outcome.(Kawahata *et al.*, 2008)

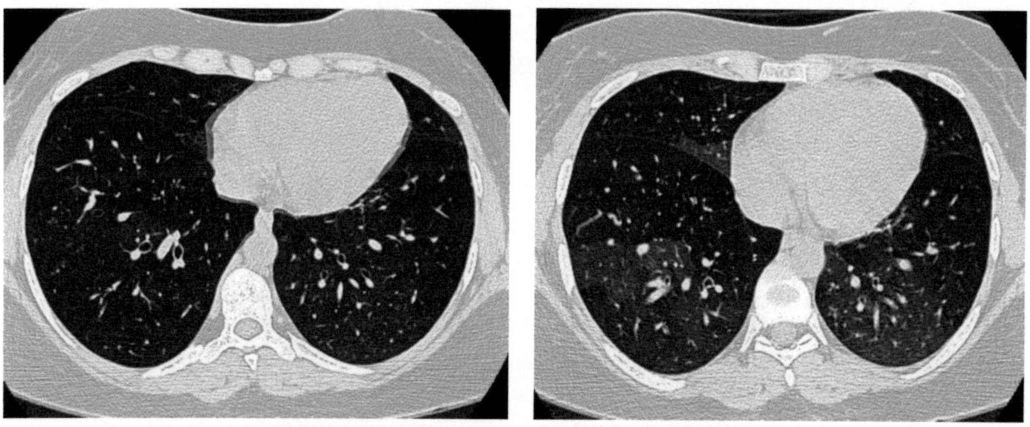

Fig. 3. (Left) Inspiratory HRCT scan of a 35 year old woman with SLE and bronchiolitis obliterans showing mosaic attenuation. (Right) Expiratory HRCT scan in the same subject showing an increase in mosaic pattern indicating small airways disease.

2.5 Muscular involvement

Shrinking lung syndrome (SLS) is a rare manifestation of SLE. 77 patients with SLS have been reported in the literature, with a prevalence of 0.6% to 0.9%.(Pego-Reigosa *et al.*, 2009; Toya & Tzelepis, 2009) It was first described in patients with lupus who presented with unexplained dyspnea, decreased lung volumes and elevation of the diaphragm on radiographic imaging and restriction on pulmonary function tests in the absence of any parenchymal disease.(Hoffbrand & Beck, 1965; Karim *et al.*, 2002; Warrington *et al.*, 2000) It can rarely be the presenting feature of SLE.(Stevens *et al.*, 1990) The pathogenesis is still unclear with conflicting results. One hypothesis is myositis of the diaphragm or phrenic neuropathy.(Hardy *et al.*, 2001; Rubin & Urowitz, 1983;) In one study, patients with elevated diaphragms had an abnormal transdiaphragmatic pressure, indicating diaphragmatic weakness.(Gibson *et al.*, 1977) However normal muscle strength of the diaphragm in patients with SLS has been reported.(Hawkins *et al.*, 2001; Laroche *et al.*, 1989) Clinically, patients present with dyspnea that is particularly worse when supine. Pleuritic chest pain is present in 65% of patients.(Toya & Tzelepis, 2009) Physical examination reveals diminished breath sounds at the lung bases with or without basilar crackles. Chest radiographs and CT show elevation of both diaphragms with basal linear atelectasis and without any evidence of parenchymal lung disease (figure 4). PFT's show restriction with preserved DLCO corrected for alveolar volume (DL/VA). Assessment of respiratory muscles show reduced maximal inspiratory pressure (MIP) and stable maximal expiratory pressure (MEP). Diaphragmatic weakness can be established by measuring the transdiaphragmatic pressure or by doing electromyography of the diaphragms. Autopsy findings include diffuse fibrosis and atrophy of the diaphragms. (Rubin & Urowitz, 1983) There are no randomized clinical trials for the treatment of SLS. Several agents have been tried with variable effects. Oral glucocorticoids with or without immunosuppressive medications have been shown effective. (Soubrier *et al.*, 1995; Walz-Leblanc *et al.*, 1992) Other treatment options for SLS include theophylline, azathioprine, methotrexate, cyclophosphamide and rituximab.(Benham *et al.*, 2010; Karim *et al.*, 2002; Soubrier *et al.*, 1995; Toya & Tzelepis, 2009; Van Veen *et al.*, 1993; Walz-Leblanc *et al.*, 1992) Disease usually stabilizes or improves with treatment with good overall prognosis.(Martens *et al.*, 1983) Respiratory failure rarely occurs.(Ernest & Leung, 2010)

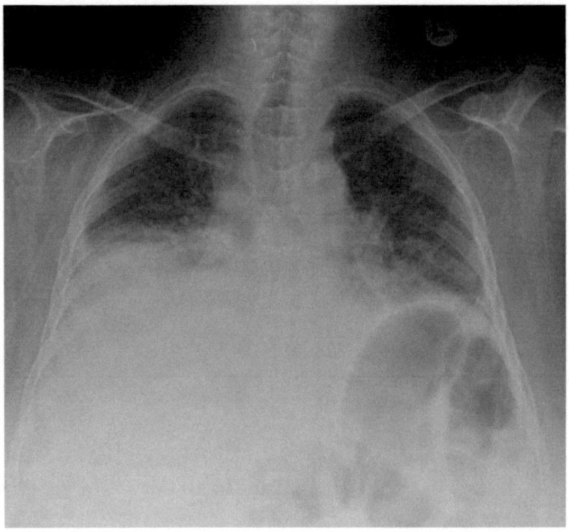

Fig. 4. Chest X-ray showing gross elevation of both diaphragms in a patient with SLE and shrinking lung syndrome

2.6 Associated lung disorders

2.6.1 Adult respiratory distress syndrome (ARDS)

The prevalence of ARDS is 4% to 15% in patients with lupus.(Andonopoulos, 1991; Kim *et al.*, 1999) If it develops the mortality rate can reach up to 70%.(Kim *et al.*, 1999) ARDS related mortality contributes to 30% of all Lupus deaths. The most frequent cause of ARDS is sepsis; other causes include ALP, DAH, and CAPS. In lupus patients, ARDS tend to occur at a younger age and is more progressive than ARDS in non-SLE patients. (Andonopoulos, 1991; Kim *et al.*, 1999; Pego-Reigosa *et al.*, 2009) It is important to identify the underlying cause. Treatment of ARDS is supportive.

2.6.2 Infectious complications

SLE can impair the immune system at multiple levels.(Orens *et al.*, 1994; Rudd *et al.*, 1981) The clinical significance of this is unknown since the risk of infection in the absence of immunosuppression is negligible. Most patients with infectious complications are on immunosuppressive drugs. Infections account for 30% to 50% of all deaths of SLE.(Bernatsky *et al.*, 2006; Zandman-Goddard & Shoenfeld, 2005;) Bacterial pathogens account for 75% of all infections, mycobacteria 12%, fungal infections 7%, and viruses 5%.(Kinder *et al.*, 2007) Opportunistic infections such as Pneumocystis jiroveci, Nocardia, Aspergillus and Cytomegalovirus have been reported.(Fessler, 2002; Petri, 1998; Zandman-Goddard & Shoenfeld, 2005) Clinical picture is indistinguishable from non-infectious complications such as ALP and DAH, hence aggressive diagnostic approach is recommended with chest imaging, bronchoscopy and BAL. Empiric broad-spectrum antibiotics should be started awaiting identification of an organism. Once a pathogen is isolated treatment should be tailored accordingly. Risk of infection can be reduced by influenza and pneumococcal vaccination.(O'Neill & Isenberg, 2006) Since many patients with SLE require systemic glucocorticoids and immunosuppresants at some point, screening for latent Tuberculosis (TB) is important, especially in high prevalence areas. This can be done via skin testing or interferon gamma release assay (IGRA). For those taking glucocorticoids, induration of 5mm or greater is considered a positive tuberculin skin test. If latent TB is identified treatment is recommended with a nine month course of Isoniazid. The role of Pneumocystis jiroveci pneumonia (PCP) prophylaxis is less clear. It is suggested for those who are on heavy immunosuppression.(Li *et al.*, 2006)

2.6.3 Lung cancer

Studies have shown an increased risk of lung cancer in patients with SLE.(Bernatsky *et al.*, 2006; Pego-Reigosa *et al.*, 2009) Histological pattern is similar to that in general population, adenocarcinoma being most common. However there is tendency for uncommon thoracic malignancies such as carcinoids and bronchoalveolar carcinoma.(Bin *et al.*, 2007; Pego-Reigosa *et al.*, 2009)

2.7 Drug reactions

In this section we will cover two aspects of drugs and SLE. First we will briefly discuss drugs that can cause SLE and the associated pulmonary manifestations. After that we will elaborate on pulmonary drug toxicity associated with commonly used medications to treat SLE.

Pulmonary manifestations of drug induced lupus are similar to idiopathic SLE.(Cush & Goldings, 1985; Yung & Richardson, 1994) Most commonly it presents with pleurisy and pleural effusion.(Wiedemann & Matthay, 1989) Common drugs include Procainamide and hydralazine. Newer biologic agents such as entanercept have been reported to cause drug induced lupus.(Abunasser *et al.*, 2008)

Common drugs used to treat lupus and are known to cause pulmonary complications include Methotrexate and Cyclophosphamide.

Pulmonary complications related to methotrexate are rare, estimated less than 1%.(Lateef *et al.*, 2005) Methotrexate can cause acute, subacute or chronic lung toxicity. It is usually not dose dependent but rather idiosyncratic.(Imokawa *et al.*, 2000; Ohosone *et al.*, 1997) Subacute pneumonitis is most common and presents with fever, cough and dyspnea. Crackles are usually noted on physical examination. It usually presents within the first year of starting the drug. If left unrecognized it can progress into pulmonary fibrosis in up to 10%. Radiologic findings are not specific. Ground glass opacities and diffuse interstitial infiltrates are frequently noted on HRCT. BAL is needed to rule out infections. Histologic findings include varying degree of inflammation and fibrosis. Ill-defined granulomas, and increased tissue eosinophils have been observed. (Malik *et al.*, 1996; Sostman *et al.*, 1976) Once diagnosis is made methotrexate needs to be stooped and systemic steroids should be started. Prognosis is usually favorable.

Cyclophosphamide lung toxicity is also idiosyncratic. It can present as early onset or late onset pneumonitis.(Malik *et al.*, 1996) Early onset disease appears within the first six months of starting treatment. It presents with non-productive cough, fever and dyspnea. (Pego-Reigosa *et al.*, 2009) CT chest shows bilateral upper lobe predominant ground glass opacities. PFT shows reduction in lung volumes and DLCO. BAL is needed to rule out infections. Discontinuing the drug along with systemic glucocorticoids usually improve symptoms and lung function. Late onset pneumonitis usually occurs after several years of exposure to cyclophosphamide. It is a slowly progressive disease. It presents with progressive dyspnea and dry cough. Chest imaging shows interstitial fibrosis affecting the upper lobes. This condition usually does not respond to steroids. Lung transplantation is an option in appropriate candidates.

3. Assessment of patients with dyspnea

3.1 Assessment of patients with chronic dyspnea

The work up of patients with SLE and chronic dyspnea can be lengthy (Figure 5). Chronic dyspnea can be due to a variety of conditions such as interstitial lung disease related to SLE or drugs used to treat lupus, pleural disease, pulmonary hypertension, systolic heart failure, upper airway disease, obliterative bronchiolitis, shrinking lung syndrome or chronic infections. Certain clues on history can be helpful; for example dyspnea increasing in the supine position suggests diaphragmatic involvement due to SLS, dyspnea and hoarseness suggest upper airway involvement, Dyspnea with pleuritic chest pain suggests pleuritis related to SLE. All patients require CXR, HRCT chest and full PFT. If chest imaging is normal with or without isolated reduction in DLCO, then transthoracic echocardiogram should be done to assess for the presence of PH. If PH is detected, patients should not be labeled to have SLE associated PAH until other causes have been ruled out. So hepatitis B and C serology, HIV testing, and V/Q scan should be done. All patients should have right heart catheterization to confirm the presence of PH and to rule out left heart disease. If SLE-PAH is diagnosed PH specific therapies should be started. If chest imaging shows elevation of the diaphragms, especially in the presence of normal DLCO adjusted for alveolar volume, shrinking lung syndrome should be suspected. Electromyography or transdiaphragmatic pressure measurement should be obtained. Either of these two tests may show evidence of diaphragmatic weakness. If confirmed, trial of systemic steroids is advised. The presence of pleural effusion on CXR or CT chest suggests pleural disease associated with SLE. The pleural fluid should be analyzed to rule out other causes. In situations where chest imaging is normal but there is flattening of the inspiratory loop, expiratory loop or both, upper airway obstruction needs to be ruled out. Special imaging of the upper airways is recommended. If interstitial changes are the predominant features on chest imaging, interstitial lung diseases related to lupus or drugs are the main differential. Bronchoscopy with BAL should be done to rule out chronic infections. Thoracoscopic lung biopsy is helpful to identify the pathological pattern of involvement.

3.2 Assessment of patients with acute dyspnea

Several conditions can predispose patients to episodes of acute dyspnea. Pulmonary infections, ALP, DAH, PE, and acute reversible hypoxia are the major culprits. Assessment starts with clinical evaluation. (Figure 6) is a proposed algorithm for work up of patients with SLE presenting with acute dyspnea. Most conditions are indistinguishable on clinical bases. The presence of hemoptysis should raise the suspicion of DAH or PE. After clinical evaluation and stabilization of the patient it is important to get a CXR. If CXR is normal then it is more likely that dyspnea is due to either acute reversible hypoxia or PE. V/Q scan will differentiate between the two. V/Q scan will be normal in the former and it will show mismatched perfusion defects in the latter. If CXR shows pleural effusion or wedge shaped

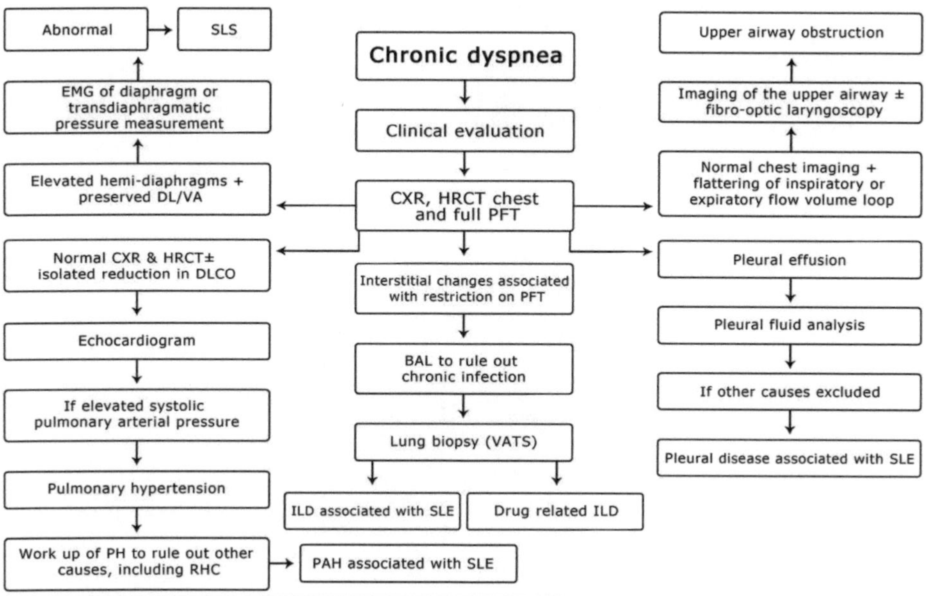

Fig. 5. Work-up of patients with SLE presenting with chronic dyspnea.
bronchoalveolar lavage (BAL); chest x-ray (CXR); diffusion capacity for carbon monoxide (DLCO); diffusion capacity for carbon monoxide adjusted for alveolar volume (DL/VA); high resolution computed tomography (HRCT); interstitial lung disease (ILD); pulmonary arterial hypertension (PAH); pulmonary function test (PFT); pulmonary hypertension (PH); right heart catheterization (RHC); shrinking lung syndrome (SLS); systematic lupus erythematosus (SLE); video-assisted thoracoscopic surgery (VATS).

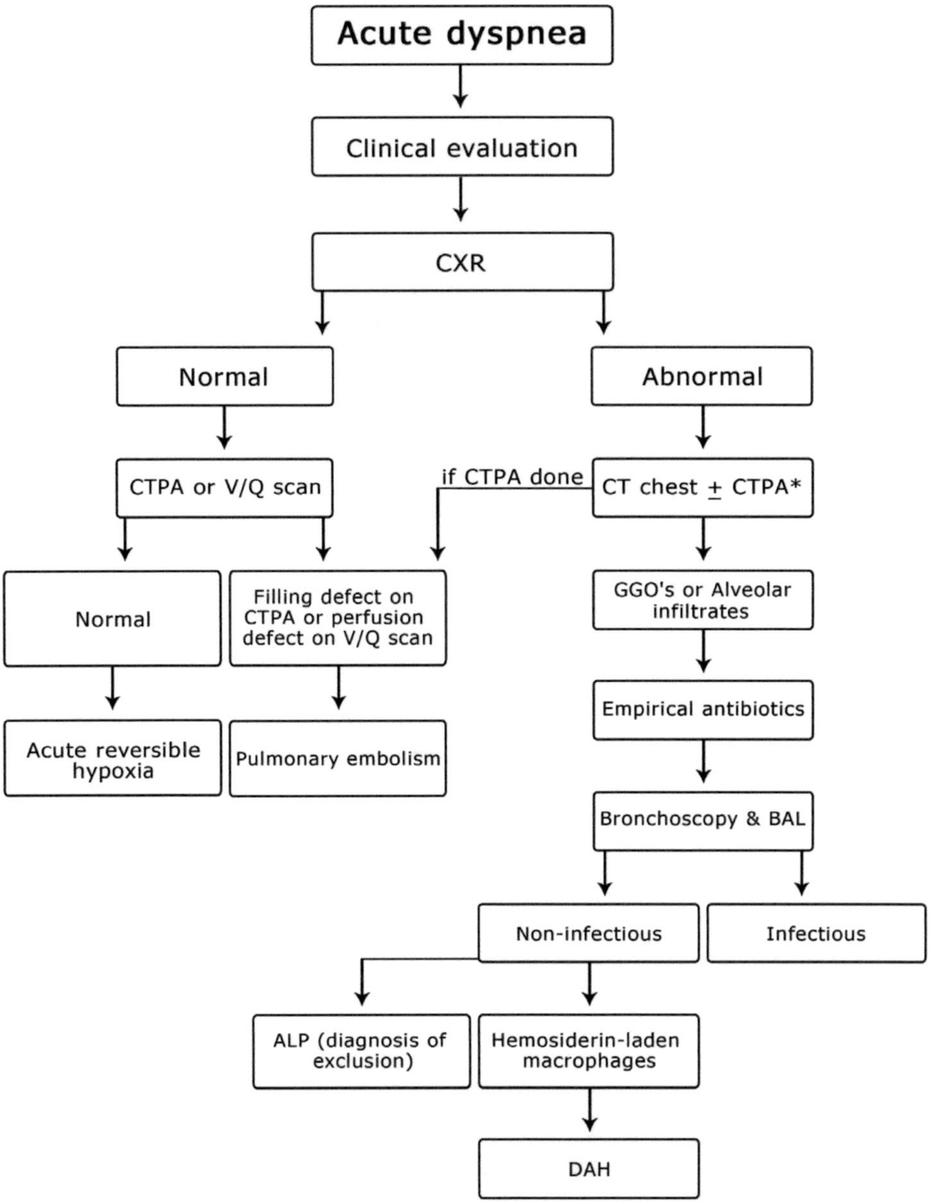

Fig. 6. Work-up of patients with SLE presenting with acute dyspnea.
acute lupus pneumonitis (ALP); bronchoalveolar lavage (BAL); chest x-ray (CXR); computed tomography (CT); computed tomography pulmonary angiogram (CTPA); diffuse alveolar hemorrhage (DAH); ground-glass opacities (GGO's); ventilation/perfusion lung scan (V/Q Scan)
* CTPA is done if pulmonary embolism suspected

opacities it is important to get CT pulmonary angiogram to look for evidence of PE. If CXR shows mainly alveolar infiltrates, CT chest should be considered. In these situations bronchoscopy with BAL, with or without TBBX, is highly recommended. The presence of hemosiderin laden macrophages confirms the diagnosis of DAH. If TBBX is performed and it showed features of DAD, then the likely diagnosis is ALP. BAL should be routinely sent for cultures. Empiric antibiotics should be started immediately until the results of cultures are known. It is not unusual to start patients on both broad spectrum antibiotics and systemic corticosteroids while the work up is being actively pursued.

4. Conclusion

SLE can affect many aspects of the pulmonary system. There is significant overlap in the clinical presentation of many SLE associated pulmonary conditions. Aggressive work up is needed early on to identify the underlying etiology.

5. Acknowledgment

The work to produce this chapter was supported by Alzaidi's Chair of research in rheumatic diseases- Umm Alqura University.

6. References

Abramson, S. B., Dobro, J., Eberle, M. A., Benton, M., Reibman, J., Epstein, H. et al. (1991) Acute reversible hypoxemia in systemic lupus erythematosus. *Ann Intern Med* 114: 941-947.

Abud-Mendoza, C., Diaz-Jouanen, E., & Alarcon-Segovia, D. (1985) Fatal pulmonary hemorrhage in systemic lupus erythematosus. Occurrence without hemoptysis. *J Rheumatol* 12: 558-561.

Abunasser, J., Forouhar, F. A., & Metersky, M. L. (2008) Etanercept-induced lupus erythematosus presenting as a unilateral pleural effusion. *Chest* 134: 850-853.

Agah, R., Bandi, V., & Guntupalli, K. K. (1997) Angioedema: the role of ACE inhibitors and factors associated with poor clinical outcome. *Intensive Care Med* 23: 793-796.

Andonopoulos, A. P., Constantopoulos, S. H., Galanopoulou, V., Drosos, A. A., Acritidis, N. C., & Moutsopoulos, H. M. (1988) Pulmonary function of nonsmoking patients with systemic lupus erythematosus. *Chest* 94: 312-315.

Andonopoulos, A. P. (1991) Adult respiratory distress syndrome: an unrecognized premortem event in systemic lupus erythematosus. *Br J Rheumatol* 30: 346-348.

Asherson, R. A., & Oakley, C. M. (1986) Pulmonary hypertension and systemic lupus erythematosus. *J Rheumatol* 13: 1-5.

Asherson, R. A., Higenbottam, T. W., Dinh Xuan, A. T., Khamashta, M. A., & Hughes, G. R. (1990) Pulmonary hypertension in a lupus clinic: experience with twenty-four patients. *J Rheumatol* 17: 1292-1298.

Asherson, R. A., & Cervera, R. (1995) Review: antiphospholipid antibodies and the lung. *J Rheumatol* 22: 62-66.

Asherson, R. A., Cervera, R., Piette, J. C., Shoenfeld, Y., Espinosa, G., Petri, M. A. et al. (2001) Catastrophic antiphospholipid syndrome: clues to the pathogenesis from a series of 80 patients. *Medicine (Baltimore)* 80: 355-377.

Asherson, R. A., & Cervera, R. (2007) Pulmonary hypertension, antiphospholipid antibodies, and syndromes. *Clin Rev Allergy Immunol* 32: 153-158.

Asherson, R. A., Cervera, R., Merrill, J. T., & Erkan, D. (2008) Antiphospholipid antibodies and the antiphospholipid syndrome: clinical significance and treatment. *Semin Thromb Hemost* 34: 256-266.

Badsha, H., Teh, C. L., Kong, K. O., Lian, T. Y., & Chng, H. H. (2004) Pulmonary hemorrhage in systemic lupus erythematosus. *Semin Arthritis Rheum* 33: 414-421.

Bankier, A. A., Kiener, H. P., Wiesmayr, M. N., Fleischmann, D., Kontrus, M., Herold, C. J. et al. (1995) Discrete lung involvement in systemic lupus erythematosus: CT assessment. *Radiology* 196: 835-840.

Barile, L. A., Jara, L. J., Medina-Rodriguez, F., Garcia-Figueroa, J. L., & Miranda-Limon, J. M. (1997) Pulmonary hemorrhage in systemic lupus erythematosus. *Lupus* 6: 445-448.

Barst RJ, FAU - Rubin, L. J., Rubin LJ, FAU - Long, W. A., Long WA, FAU - McGoon, M. D. et al. A comparison of continuous intravenous epoprostenol (prostacyclin) with conventional therapy for primary pulmonary hypertension. The Primary Pulmonary Hypertension Study Group. - *N Engl J Med.1996 Feb 1;334(5):296-302.*

Belmont, H. M., Buyon, J., Giorno, R., & Abramson, S. (1994) Up-regulation of endothelial cell adhesion molecules characterizes disease activity in systemic lupus erythematosus. The Shwartzman phenomenon revisited. *Arthritis Rheum* 37: 376-383.

Benham, H., Garske, L., Vecchio, P., & Eckert, B. W. (2010) Successful treatment of shrinking lung syndrome with rituximab in a patient with systemic lupus erythematosus. *J Clin Rheumatol* 16: 68-70.

Bernatsky, S., Boivin, J. F., Joseph, L., Manzi, S., Ginzler, E., Gladman, D. D. et al. (2006) Mortality in systemic lupus erythematosus. *Arthritis Rheum* 54: 2550-2557.

Beylot-Barry, M., Doutre, M. S., Bletry, O., & Beylot, C. (1994) Lupus bronchiolitis obliterans: diagnostic difficulties. *Rev Med Interne* 15: 332-335.

Bin, J., Bernatsky, S., Gordon, C., Boivin, J. F., Ginzler, E., Gladman, D. et al. (2007) Lung cancer in systemic lupus erythematosus. *Lung Cancer* 56: 303-306.

Boddaert, J., Huong, D. L., Amoura, Z., Wechsler, B., Godeau, P., & Piette, J. C. (2004) Late-onset systemic lupus erythematosus: a personal series of 47 patients and pooled analysis of 714 cases in the literature. *Medicine (Baltimore)* 83: 348-359.

Boulware, D. W., & Hedgpeth, M. T. (1989) Lupus pneumonitis and anti-SSA(Ro) antibodies. *J Rheumatol* 16: 479-481.

Bouros, D., Pneumatikos, I., & Tzouvelekis, A. (2008) Pleural involvement in systemic autoimmune disorders. *Respiration* 75: 361-371.

Bucciarelli, S., Espinosa, G., Asherson, R. A., Cervera, R., Claver, G., Gomez-Puerta, J. A. et al. (2006) The acute respiratory distress syndrome in catastrophic antiphospholipid syndrome: analysis of a series of 47 patients. *Ann Rheum Dis* 65: 81-86.

Carette, S., Macher, A. M., Nussbaum, A., & Plotz, P. H. (1984) Severe, acute pulmonary disease in patients with systemic lupus erythematosus: ten years of experience at the National Institutes of Health. *Semin Arthritis Rheum* 14: 52-59.

Cervera, R., Bucciarelli, S., Espinosa, G., Gomez-Puerta, J. A., Ramos-Casals, M., Shoenfeld, Y. et al. (2007) Catastrophic antiphospholipid syndrome: lessons from the "CAPS Registry"--a tribute to the late Josep Font. *Ann N Y Acad Sci* 1108: 448-456.

Cervera, R., & Asherson, R. A. (2008) Catastrophic antiphospholipid (Asherson's) syndrome. *Br J Hosp Med (Lond)* 69: 384-387.

Cheema, G. S., & Quismorio, F. P.,Jr. (2000) Interstitial lung disease in systemic lupus erythematosus. *Curr Opin Pulm Med* 6: 424-429.

Chung, S. M., Lee, C. K., Lee, E. Y., Yoo, B., Lee, S. D., & Moon, H. B. (2006) Clinical aspects of pulmonary hypertension in patients with systemic lupus erythematosus and in patients with idiopathic pulmonary arterial hypertension. *Clin Rheumatol* 25: 866-872.

Comer, M., D'Cruz, D., Thompson, I., Erskine, K., & Dacre, J. (1996) Pneumonitis in a lupus twin pregnancy: a case report. *Lupus* 5: 146-148.

Crowther, M. A., Ginsberg, J. S., Julian, J., Denburg, J., Hirsh, J., Douketis, J. et al. (2003) A comparison of two intensities of warfarin for the prevention of recurrent thrombosis in patients with the antiphospholipid antibody syndrome. *N Engl J Med* 349: 1133-1138.

Cush, J. J., & Goldings, E. A. (1985) Drug-induced lupus: clinical spectrum and pathogenesis. *Am J Med Sci* 290: 36-45.

Dweik, R. A., Arroliga, A. C., & Cash, J. M. (1997) Alveolar hemorrhage in patients with rheumatic disease. *Rheum Dis Clin North Am* 23: 395-410.

Eagen, J. W., Memoli, V. A., Roberts, J. L., Matthew, G. R., Schwartz, M. M., & Lewis, E. J. (1978) Pulmonary hemorrhage in systemic lupus erythematosus. *Medicine (Baltimore)* 57: 545-560.

Eiser, A. R., & Shanies, H. M. (1994) Treatment of lupus interstitial lung disease with intravenous cyclophosphamide. *Arthritis Rheum* 37: 428-431.

Erickson, R. W., Franklin, W. A., & Emlen, W. (1994) Treatment of hemorrhagic lupus pneumonitis with plasmapheresis. *Semin Arthritis Rheum* 24: 114-123.

Ernest, D., & Leung, A. (2010) Ventilatory failure in shrinking lung syndrome is associated with reduced chest compliance. *Intern Med J* 40: 66-68.

Ewan, P. W., Jones, H. A., Rhodes, C. G., & Hughes, J. M. (1976) Detection of intrapulmonary hemorrhage with carbon monoxide uptake. Application in goodpasture's syndrome. *N Engl J Med* 295: 1391-1396.

Fenlon, H. M., Doran, M., Sant, S. M., & Breatnach, E. (1996) High-resolution chest CT in systemic lupus erythematosus. AJR Am J Roentgenol 166: 301-307.

Fessler, B. J. (2002) Infectious diseases in systemic lupus erythematosus: risk factors, management and prophylaxis. *Best Pract Res Clin Rheumatol* 16: 281-291.

Galie, N., Ghofrani, H. A., Torbicki, A., Barst, R. J., Rubin, L. J., Badesch, D. et al. (2005) Sildenafil citrate therapy for pulmonary arterial hypertension. *N Engl J Med* 353: 2148-2157.

Galie, N., Olschewski, H., Oudiz, R. J., Torres, F., Frost, A., Ghofrani, H. A. et al. (2008) Ambrisentan for the treatment of pulmonary arterial hypertension: results of the ambrisentan in pulmonary arterial hypertension, randomized, double-blind, placebo-controlled, multicenter, efficacy (ARIES) study 1 and 2. *Circulation* 117: 3010-3019.

Galie, N., Brundage, B. H., Ghofrani, H. A., Oudiz, R. J., Simonneau, G., Safdar, Z. et al. (2009) Tadalafil therapy for pulmonary arterial hypertension. *Circulation* 119: 2894-2903.

Gammon, R. B., Bridges, T. A., al-Nezir, H., Alexander, C. B., & Kennedy, J. I.,Jr. (1992) Bronchiolitis obliterans organizing pneumonia associated with systemic lupus erythematosus. *Chest* 102: 1171-1174.

Gari A, Dias B, Khan F, Pope J, Mehta S. (2009) Prevalence of Pulmonary Hypertension in Unselected Patients With Systemic Lupus Erythematosus in an Academic Tertiary Care Centre. *Chest* 136: 55S.

Gibson, C. J., Edmonds, J. P., & Hughes, G. R. (1977) Diaphragm function and lung involvement in systemic lupus erythematosus. *Am J Med* 63: 926-932.

Gilleece, M. H., Evans, C. C., & Bucknall, R. C. (1988) Steroid resistant pleural effusion in systemic lupus erythematosus treated with tetracycline pleurodesis. *Ann Rheum Dis* 47: 1031-1032.

Gladman, D. D., & Urowitz, M. B. (1980) Venous syndromes and pulmonary embolism in systemic lupus erythematosus. *Ann Rheum Dis* 39: 340-343.

Godeau, B., Cormier, C., & Menkes, C. J. (1991) Bronchiolitis obliterans in systemic lupus erythematosus: beneficial effect of intravenous cyclophosphamide. *Ann Rheum Dis* 50: 956-958.

Gonzalez-Lopez, L., Cardona-Munoz, E. G., Celis, A., Garcia-de la Torre, I., Orozco-Barocio, G., Salazar-Paramo, M. et al. (2004) Therapy with intermittent pulse cyclophosphamide for pulmonary hypertension associated with systemic lupus erythematosus. *Lupus* 13: 105-112.

Good, J. T.,Jr, King, T. E., Antony, V. B., & Sahn, S. A. (1983) Lupus pleuritis. Clinical features and pleural fluid characteristics with special reference to pleural fluid antinuclear antibodies. *Chest* 84: 714-718.

Groen, H., ter Borg, E. J., Postma, D. S., Wouda, A. A., van der Mark, T. W., & Kallenberg, C. G. (1992) Pulmonary function in systemic lupus erythematosus is related to distinct clinical, serologic, and nailfold capillary patterns. *Am J Med* 93: 619-627.

Gross, M., Esterly, J. R., & Earle, R. H. (1972) Pulmonary alterations in systemic lupus erythematosus. *Am Rev Respir Dis* 105: 572-577.

Hardy, K., Herry, I., Attali, V., Cadranel, J., & Similowski, T. (2001) Bilateral phrenic paralysis in a patient with systemic lupus erythematosus. *Chest* 119: 1274-1277.

Harmon, K. R., & Leatherman, J. W. (1988) Respiratory manifestations of connective tissue disease. *Semin Respir Infect* 3: 258-273.

Harvey, A. M., Shuman, L. E., Tumulty, P. A., Conley, C. L., & Schoenrich, E. H. (1954) Systemic lupus erythematosus: review of the literature and clinical analysis of 138 cases. *Medicine (Baltimore)* 33: 291-437.

Haupt, H. M., Moore, G. W., & Hutchins, G. M. (1981) The lung in systemic lupus erythematosus. Analysis of the pathologic changes in 120 patients. *Am J Med* 71: 791-798.

Hawkins, P., Davison, A. G., Dasgupta, B., & Moxham, J. (2001) Diaphragm strength in acute systemic lupus erythematosus in a patient with paradoxical abdominal motion and reduced lung volumes. *Thorax* 56: 329-330.

Hodson, P., Klemp, P., & Meyers, O. L. (1983) Pulmonary hypertension in systemic lupus erythematosus: a report of four cases. *Clin Exp Rheumatol* 1: 241-245.

Hoffbrand, B. I., & Beck, E. R. (1965) "Unexplained" Dyspnoea and Shrinking Lungs in Systemic Lupus Erythematosus. *Br Med J* 1: 1273-1277.

Hsu, B. Y., Edwards, D. K.,3rd, & Trambert, M. A. (1992) Pulmonary hemorrhage complicating systemic lupus erythematosus: role of MR imaging in diagnosis. *AJR Am J Roentgenol* 158: 519-520.

Hunder, G. G., McDuffie, F. C., & Hepper, N. G. (1972) Pleural fluid complement in systemic lupus erythematosus and rheumatoid arthritis. *Ann Intern Med* 76: 357-363.

Imokawa, S., Colby, T. V., Leslie, K. O., & Helmers, R. A. (2000) Methotrexate pneumonitis: review of the literature and histopathological findings in nine patients. *Eur Respir J* 15: 373-381.

Jacobsen, S., Petersen, J., Ullman, S., Junker, P., Voss, A., Rasmussen, J. M. et al. (1998) A multicentre study of 513 Danish patients with systemic lupus erythematosus. II. Disease mortality and clinical factors of prognostic value. *Clin Rheumatol* 17: 478-484.

Jais, X., Launay, D., Yaici, A., Le Pavec, J., Tcherakian, C., Sitbon, O. et al. (2008) Immunosuppressive therapy in lupus- and mixed connective tissue disease-associated pulmonary arterial hypertension: a retrospective analysis of twenty-three cases. *Arthritis Rheum* 58: 521-531.

Kaine, J. L. (1985) Refractory massive pleural effusion in systemic lupus erythematosus treated with talc poudrage. *Ann Rheum Dis* 44: 61-64.

Kamen, D. L., & Strange, C. (2010) Pulmonary manifestations of systemic lupus erythematosus. *Clin Chest Med* 31: 479-488.

Karim, M. Y., Miranda, L. C., Tench, C. M., Gordon, P. A., D'cruz, D. P., Khamashta, M. A., & Hughes, G. R. (2002) Presentation and prognosis of the shrinking lung syndrome in systemic lupus erythematosus. *Semin Arthritis Rheum* 31: 289-298.

Kawahata, K., Yamaguchi, M., Kanda, H., Komiya, A., Tanaka, R., Dohi, M. et al. (2008) Severe airflow limitation in two patients with systemic lupus erythematosus: effect of inhalation of anticholinergics. *Mod Rheumatol* 18: 52-56.

Keane, M. P., & Lynch, J. P.,3rd. (2000) Pleuropulmonary manifestations of systemic lupus erythematosus. *Thorax* 55: 159-166.

Kim, J. S., Lee, K. S., Koh, E. M., Kim, S. Y., Chung, M. P., & Han, J. (2000) Thoracic involvement of systemic lupus erythematosus: clinical, pathologic, and radiologic findings. *J Comput Assist Tomogr* 24: 9-18.

Kim, W. U., Kim, S. I., Yoo, W. H., Park, J. H., Min, J. K., Kim, S. C. et al. (1999) Adult respiratory distress syndrome in systemic lupus erythematosus: causes and prognostic factors: a single center, retrospective study. *Lupus* 8: 552-557.

Kinder, B. W., Freemer, M. M., King, T. E.,Jr, Lum, R. F., Nititham, J., Taylor, K. et al. (2007) Clinical and genetic risk factors for pneumonia in systemic lupus erythematosus. *Arthritis Rheum* 56: 2679-2686.

Koh, W. H., Thumboo, J., & Boey, M. L. (1997) Pulmonary haemorrhage in Oriental patients with systemic lupus erythematosus. *Lupus* 6: 713-716.

Langford, C. A., & Van Waes, C. (1997) Upper airway obstruction in the rheumatic diseases. *Rheum Dis Clin North Am* 23: 345-363.

Laroche, C. M., Mulvey, D. A., Hawkins, P. N., Walport, M. J., Strickland, B., Moxham, J., & Green, M. (1989) Diaphragm strength in the shrinking lung syndrome of systemic lupus erythematosus. *Q J Med* 71: 429-439.

Lateef, O., Shakoor, N., & Balk, R. A. (2005) Methotrexate pulmonary toxicity. *Expert Opin Drug Saf* 4: 723-730.

Leatherman, J. W., Davies, S. F., & Hoidal, J. R. (1984) Alveolar hemorrhage syndromes: diffuse microvascular lung hemorrhage in immune and idiopathic disorders. *Medicine (Baltimore)* 63: 343-361.

Li, J., Huang, X. M., Fang, W. G., & Zeng, X. J. (2006) Pneumocystis carinii pneumonia in patients with connective tissue disease. *J Clin Rheumatol* 12: 114-117.

Lim, S. W., Gillis, D., Smith, W., Hissaria, P., Greville, H., & Peh, C. A. (2006) Rituximab use in systemic lupus erythematosus pneumonitis and a review of current reports. *Intern Med J* 36: 260-262.

Liu, M. F., Lee, J. H., Weng, T. H., & Lee, Y. Y. (1998) Clinical experience of 13 cases with severe pulmonary hemorrhage in systemic lupus erythematosus with active nephritis. *Scand J Rheumatol* 27: 291-295.

Love, P. E., & Santoro, S. A. (1990) Antiphospholipid antibodies: anticardiolipin and the lupus anticoagulant in systemic lupus erythematosus (SLE) and in non-SLE disorders. Prevalence and clinical significance. *Ann Intern Med* 112: 682-698.

Malik, S. W., Myers, J. L., DeRemee, R. A., & Specks, U. (1996) Lung toxicity associated with cyclophosphamide use. Two distinct patterns. *Am J Respir Crit Care Med* 154: 1851-1856.

Martens, J., Demedts, M., Vanmeenen, M. T., & Dequeker, J. (1983) Respiratory muscle dysfunction in systemic lupus erythematosus. *Chest* 84: 170-175.

Martinez-Taboada, V. M., Blanco, R., Armona, J., Fernandez-Sueiro, J. L., & Rodriguez-Valverde, V. (1995) Acute reversible hypoxemia in systemic lupus erythematosus: a new syndrome or an index of disease activity? *Lupus* 4: 259-262.

Matthay, R. A., Schwarz, M. I., Petty, T. L., Stanford, R. E., Gupta, R. C., Sahn, S. A., & Steigerwald, J. C. (1975) Pulmonary manifestations of systemic lupus erythematosus: review of twelve cases of acute lupus pneumonitis. *Medicine (Baltimore)* 54: 397-409.

McKnight, K. M., Adair, N. E., & Agudelo, C. A. (1991) Successful use of tetracycline pleurodesis to treat massive pleural effusion secondary to systemic lupus erythematosus. *Arthritis Rheum* 34: 1483-1484.

McLaughlin, V. V., Archer, S. L., Badesch, D. B., Barst, R. J., Farber, H. W., Lindner, J. R. et al. (2009) ACCF/AHA 2009 expert consensus document on pulmonary hypertension a report of the American College of Cardiology Foundation Task

Force on Expert Consensus Documents and the American Heart Association developed in collaboration with the American College of Chest Physicians; American Thoracic Society, Inc.; and the Pulmonary Hypertension Association. *J Am Coll Cardiol* 53: 1573-1619.

Mochizuki, T., Aotsuka, S., & Satoh, T. (1999) Clinical and laboratory features of lupus patients with complicating pulmonary disease. *Respir Med* 93: 95-101.

Myers, J. L., & Katzenstein, A. A. (1986) Microangiitis in lupus-induced pulmonary hemorrhage. *Am J Clin Pathol* 85: 552-556.

Ohosone, Y., Okano, Y., Kameda, H., Fujii, T., Hama, N., Hirakata, M. et al. (1997) Clinical characteristics of patients with rheumatoid arthritis and methotrexate induced pneumonitis. *J Rheumatol* 24: 2299-2303.

O'Neill, S. G., & Isenberg, D. A. (2006) Immunizing patients with systemic lupus erythematosus: a review of effectiveness and safety. *Lupus* 15: 778-783.

Orens, J. B., Martinez, F. J., & Lynch, J. P.,3rd. (1994) Pleuropulmonary manifestations of systemic lupus erythematosus. *Rheum Dis Clin North Am* 20: 159-193.

Pego-Reigosa, J. M., Medeiros, D. A., & Isenberg, D. A. (2009) Respiratory manifestations of systemic lupus erythematosus: old and new concepts. *Best Pract Res Clin Rheumatol* 23: 469-480.

Pertschuk, L. P., Moccia, L. F., Rosen, Y., Lyons, H., Marino, C. M., Rashford, A. A., & Wollschlager, C. M. (1977) Acute pulmonary complications in systemic lupus erythematosus. Immunofluorescence and light microscopic study. *Am J Clin Pathol* 68: 553-557.

Petri, M. (1998) Infection in systemic lupus erythematosus. *Rheum Dis Clin North Am* 24: 423-456.

Pines, A., Kaplinsky, N., Olchovsky, D., Rozenman, J., & Frankl, O. (1985) Pleuro-pulmonary manifestations of systemic lupus erythematosus: clinical features of its subgroups. Prognostic and therapeutic implications. *Chest* 88: 129-135.

Pottier, V., Pierrot, M., Subra, J. F., Mercat, A., Kouatchet, A., Parrot, A., & Augusto, J. F. (2011) Successful rituximab therapy in a lupus patient with diffuse alveolar haemorrhage. *Lupus* 20: 656-659.

Prabu, A., Patel, K., Yee, C. S., Nightingale, P., Situnayake, R. D., Thickett, D. R. et al. (2009) Prevalence and risk factors for pulmonary arterial hypertension in patients with lupus. *Rheumatology (Oxford)* 48: 1506-1511.

Quadrelli, S. A., Alvarez, C., Arce, S. C., Paz, L., Sarano, J., Sobrino, E. M., & Manni, J. (2009) Pulmonary involvement of systemic lupus erythematosus: analysis of 90 necropsies. *Lupus* 18: 1053-1060.

Quismorio, F. P.,Jr, Sharma, O., Koss, M., Boylen, T., Edmiston, A. W., Thornton, P. J., & Tatter, D. (1984) Immunopathologic and clinical studies in pulmonary hypertension associated with systemic lupus erythematosus. *Semin Arthritis Rheum* 13: 349-359.

Renzoni, E., Rottoli, P., Coviello, G., Perari, M. G., Galeazzi, M., & Vagliasindi, M. (1997) Clinical, laboratory and radiological findings in pulmonary fibrosis with and without connective tissue disease. *Clin Rheumatol* 16: 570-577.

Rubin, L. A., & Urowitz, M. B. (1983) Shrinking lung syndrome in SLE--a clinical pathologic study. *J Rheumatol* 10: 973-976.

Rubin, L. J., & American College of Chest Physicians. (2004) Diagnosis and management of pulmonary arterial hypertension: ACCP evidence-based clinical practice guidelines. *Chest* 126: 7S-10S.

Rudd, R. M., Haslam, P. L., & Turner-Warwick, M. (1981) Cryptogenic fibrosing alveolitis. Relationships of pulmonary physiology and bronchoalveolar lavage to response to treatment and prognosis. *Am Rev Respir Dis* 124: 1-8.

Ruiz-Irastorza, G., Egurbide, M. V., Ugalde, J., & Aguirre, C. (2004) High impact of antiphospholipid syndrome on irreversible organ damage and survival of patients with systemic lupus erythematosus. *Arch Intern Med* 164: 77-82.

Sanchez, O., Sitbon, O., Jais, X., Simonneau, G., & Humbert, M. (2006) Immunosuppressive therapy in connective tissue diseases-associated pulmonary arterial hypertension. *Chest* 130: 182-189.

Sant, S. M., Doran, M., Fenelon, H. M., & Breatnach, E. S. (1997) Pleuropulmonary abnormalities in patients with systemic lupus erythematosus: assessment with high resolution computed tomography, chest radiography and pulmonary function tests. *Clin Exp Rheumatol* 15: 507-513.

Santos-Ocampo, A. S., Mandell, B. F., & Fessler, B. J. (2000) Alveolar hemorrhage in systemic lupus erythematosus: presentation and management. *Chest* 118: 1083-1090.

Schattner, A., Aviel-Ronen, S., & Mark, E. J. (2003) Accelerated usual interstitial pneumonitis, anti-DNA antibodies and hypocomplementemia. *J Intern Med* 254: 193-196.

Schwab, E. P., Schumacher, H. R.,Jr, Freundlich, B., & Callegari, P. E. (1993) Pulmonary alveolar hemorrhage in systemic lupus erythematosus. *Semin Arthritis Rheum* 23: 8-15.

Siegel, M., & Lee, S. L. (1973) The epidemiology of systemic lupus erythematosus. *Semin Arthritis Rheum* 3: 1-54.

Small, P., Frank, H., Kreisman, H., & Wolkove, N. (1982) An immunological evaluation of pleural effusions in systemic lupus erythematosus. *Ann Allergy* 49: 101-103.

Smith, G. A., Ward, P. H., & Berci, G. (1977) Laryngeal involvement by systemic lupus erythematosus. *Trans Sect Otolaryngol Am Acad Ophthalmol Otolaryngol* 84: 124-128.

Somers, E., Magder, L. S., & Petri, M. (2002) Antiphospholipid antibodies and incidence of venous thrombosis in a cohort of patients with systemic lupus erythematosus. *J Rheumatol* 29: 2531-2536.

Sostman, H. D., Matthay, R. A., Putman, C. E., & Smith, G. J. (1976) Methotrexate-induced pneumonitis. *Medicine (Baltimore)* 55: 371-388.

Soubrier, M., Dubost, J. J., Piette, J. C., Urosevic, Z., Rami, S., Oualid, T. et al. (1995) Shrinking lung syndrome in systemic lupus erythematosus. A report of three cases. *Rev Rhum Engl Ed* 62: 395-398.

Stevens, W. M., Burdon, J. G., Clemens, L. E., & Webb, J. (1990) The 'shrinking lungs syndrome'--an infrequently recognised feature of systemic lupus erythematosus. *Aust N Z J Med* 20: 67-70.

Susanto, I., & Peters, J. I. (1997) Acute lupus pneumonitis with normal chest radiograph. *Chest* 111: 1781-1783.

Swigris, J. J., Fischer, A., Gillis, J., Meehan, R. T., & Brown, K. K. (2008) Pulmonary and thrombotic manifestations of systemic lupus erythematosus. *Chest* 133: 271-280.

Tanaka, E., Harigai, M., Tanaka, M., Kawaguchi, Y., Hara, M., & Kamatani, N. (2002) Pulmonary hypertension in systemic lupus erythematosus: evaluation of clinical characteristics and response to immunosuppressive treatment. *J Rheumatol* 29: 282-287.

Tansey, D., Wells, A. U., Colby, T. V., Ip, S., Nikolakoupolou, A., du Bois, R. M. et al. (2004) Variations in histological patterns of interstitial pneumonia between connective tissue disorders and their relationship to prognosis. *Histopathology* 44: 585-596.

Teitel, A. D., MacKenzie, C. R., Stern, R., & Paget, S. A. (1992) Laryngeal involvement in systemic lupus erythematosus. *Semin Arthritis Rheum* 22: 203-214.

Thong, B. Y., Thumboo, J., Howe, H. S., & Feng, P. H. (2001) Life-threatening angioedema in systemic lupus erythematosus. *Lupus* 10: 304-308.

Toomey, J. M., Snyder, G. G.,3rd, Maenza, R. M., & Rothfield, N. F. (1974) Acute epiglottitis due to systemic lupus erythematosus. *Laryngoscope* 84: 522-527.

Toya, S. P., & Tzelepis, G. E. (2009) Association of the shrinking lung syndrome in systemic lupus erythematosus with pleurisy: a systematic review. *Semin Arthritis Rheum* 39: 30-37.

Van Veen, S., Peeters, A. J., Sterk, P. J., & Breedveld, F. C. (1993) The "shrinking lung syndrome" in SLE, treatment with theophylline. *Clin Rheumatol* 12: 462-465.

Walz-Leblanc, B. A., Urowitz, M. B., Gladman, D. D., & Hanly, P. J. (1992) The "shrinking lungs syndrome" in systemic lupus erythematosus--improvement with corticosteroid therapy. *J Rheumatol* 19: 1970-1972.

Warrington, K. J., Moder, K. G., & Brutinel, W. M. (2000) The shrinking lungs syndrome in systemic lupus erythematosus. *Mayo Clin Proc* 75: 467-472.

Weinrib, L., Sharma, O. P., & Quismorio, F. P.,Jr. (1990) A long-term study of interstitial lung disease in systemic lupus erythematosus. *Semin Arthritis Rheum* 20: 48-56.

Wiedemann, H. P., & Matthay, R. A. (1989) Pulmonary manifestations of the collagen vascular diseases. *Clin Chest Med* 10: 677-722.

Winder, A., Molad, Y., Ostfeld, I., Kenet, G., Pinkhas, J., & Sidi, Y. (1993) Treatment of systemic lupus erythematosus by prolonged administration of high dose intravenous immunoglobulin: report of 2 cases. *J Rheumatol* 20: 495-498.

Winslow, W. A., Ploss, L. N., & Loitman, B. (1958) Pleuritis in systemic lupus erythematosus: its importance as an early manifestation in diagnosis. *Ann Intern Med* 49: 70-88.

Witt, C., Dorner, T., Hiepe, F., Borges, A. C., Fietze, I., & Baumann, G. (1996) Diagnosis of alveolitis in interstitial lung manifestation in connective tissue diseases: importance of late inspiratory crackles, 67 gallium scan and bronchoalveolar lavage. *Lupus* 5: 606-612.

Young, K. R.,Jr. (1989) Pulmonary-renal syndromes. *Clin Chest Med* 10: 655-675.

Yung, R. L., & Richardson, B. C. (1994) Drug-induced lupus. *Rheum Dis Clin North Am* 20: 61-86.

Zamora, M. R., Warner, M. L., Tuder, R., & Schwarz, M. I. (1997) Diffuse alveolar hemorrhage and systemic lupus erythematosus. Clinical presentation, histology, survival, and outcome. *Medicine (Baltimore)* 76: 192-202.

Zandman-Goddard, G., & Shoenfeld, Y. (2005) Infections and SLE. *Autoimmunity* 38: 473-485.

15

Approach to Patients with SLE Presenting with Neurological Findings

Alkhotani Amal
Umm AlQura University
Saudi Arabia

1. Introduction

The nervous system is commonly involved by SLE. Its involvement classified as primary when it is related to the disease process and secondary when it is related to other factors like medication side effect or infection. The nervous system involvement by lupus was described by Hebra and Kaposi in 1875 who described a patient with lupus and coma (Appenzeller et al.,2006). Shortly after Bowen report case of psychosis and mood disturbance (Appenzeller et al., 2006).

The nervous system involvement rang from overt presentation to more subtle finding. In spite the advances in SLE diagnosis and managements, the neuropsychiatric syndromes remain one of the major causes of morbidity and mortality in SLE patients. Still they remain poorly understood and under recognised. The aim of this chapter is provide an overview of neurological presentation in SLE patients.

2. Definition

As there is wide Varity of different neurological and psychiatric presentations among SLE patient, the American college of Rheumatology (ACR) established in 1999 19 different neuropsychiatric SLE (NPSLE) syndromes (table-1). Either central or peripheral nervous system can be affected by the disease process. Their involvement can be generalized e.g headache, cognitive dysfunction or focal e.g. cerebrovascular disease and demyelinating syndromes.

Before attributing any of the neuropsychiatric (NP) manifestation to SLE secondary causes should be ruled out. As most of SLE patient are immunocompromised either by the disease process or secondary to immunocompressive therapy infection is a common problem in this patients. Other secondary causes can be metabolic impairments or complication from hypertension e.g posterior reversible leukoencephalopathy.

3. Epidemiology

The reported prevalence of NPSLE is varied from 37- 95 %(Muscal & Brey,2010) depending on the case definition used and the inclusion criteria. Most of NPSLE affect central nervous system(91.6%) and out of those 79% are diffuse in nature and 21% focal(Hanly et al.,2008).The peripheral nervous system involvement is much less than CNS involvement.

NPSLE Associated with Central Nervous System	NPSL Associated with Peripheral Nervous System
- Aseptic Meningitis - Cerebrovascular disease - Demyelinating syndromes - Headaches - Movement Disorders (Chorea) - Myelopathy - Seizure Disorders - Acute Confusional State - Anxiety Disorders - Cognitive Dysfunction - Mood Disorders - Psychosis	- Acute Inflammatory Demyelinating Syndromes (Gulliain -Barre Syndrome) - Autonomic Neuropathy - Mononeuropathy, single or multiplex - Myasthenia Gravis - Cranial Neuropathy - Plexopathy - Polyneuropathy

Table 1. Neuropsychiatric Syndromes Associated with SLE

The most frequently reported PNS involvement is peripheral neuropathy between 2.4to 7% (Hanly et al.,2010)(Ainiala et al.,2001). Recently Hanly and his colleague conducted a large cohort of SLE patients. They reported around 40.3% of SLE patient had at least one NP event and 17.4% had recurrent events (Hanly et al.,2010). The most frequent NP was headache 47.1% followed by mood disorders in 16.5%, Seizure in this cohort reported in 7.5% and cognitive dysfunction in 5.1%.

In other studies when a mild cognitive impairment and mild mood disorders were included higher prevalence of NPSLE is 80-91% (Ainiala et al.,2001)(Brey et al.,2002). When formal neuropsychiatric evaluation is used cognitive dysfunction is reported in 80% of the patient (Ainiala et al.,2001)(Brey et al.,2002). In 70% of those are classified as mild cognitive impairment with impairment of one or two cognitive domains (Ainiala et al.,2001).

The reported prevalence of cerebrovascular accident range between 4.7 to 15% (Hanly et al., 2010) (Ainiala et al.,2001).

The prevalence of other NPSLE syndromes is much less with reported prevalence of demyelinating syndrome and movement disorder of 1%.

CNS manifestations present as an initial feature of SLE in 24% of cases (Joseph et al.,2007). In general around 50-60% of NPSLE occurred at disease onset or within the first year after SLE onset.

3.1 Risk factors

Risk factors associated with CNS involvements are:-

1. Generalized disease activity.
2. Prior history or concurrent NPSLE.
3. Presence of antiphospholipid antibodies especially for focal CNS lesions and seizure (The European League Aganist Rheumatism EULAR, 2010).It was also noted that patients with APS who had a history of two or more abortion are six times more likely to have CNS events(Karassa et al.,2000).

In term of SLE disease activity two studies have shown that skin lesions are the most frequent lesions associated with CNS disease (EULAR, 2010)(Karassa et al.,2000). Two studies have shown a protective effect of arthritis to CNS disease ((EULAR, 2010). This was not consistent in other study were arthritis was a second common manifestation after skin disease (Joseph et al.,2007).

4. Pathogenesis

The neuropsychatric lupus has different manifestations. As the manifestations can be generalized or focal no single pathophysilogical mechanism has been implicated in its pathogenesis. Different mechanisms are thought to affect the nervous system and caused the development of NPSLE. Those different mechanisms include vasculopathy, autoantibodie and cytokines.

4.1 Vasculopathy

Vascular occlusion is universally reported in autopsy cases in patient with lupus. Although vasculitis is thought to be the cause of small vessels disease in lupus patient, its occurrence is rare. The most frequent cause is found to be a non inflammatory vasculopathy.

On pathology multiple microinfracts, cortical atrophy, gross infracts were seen on the brain. Microhemorrhages are common in NPSLE . Larger haemorrhages like intracerebral are rare. The most common vascular pathology is noninflammatory lesions characterized by endothelial proliferation, intimal fibrosis and lymphocytic infiltration. It may associated by thrombosis (Ellison et al.,1993).

The pathogenesis of the vascular injury initially thought to be secondary to immune complex deposition but now it thought to be secondary to complement activation (Muscal & Brey, 2010).

4.2 Autoantibodies

Autoantibodies play a major role for the development of different manifestations of SLE. Different antibodies have been reported in association with NPSLE. Among those the most frequent antibodies are antiphospholipid (API) and antiribosomal abs.

Antiphospholipid antibodies that includes lupus anticoagulant, anti cardiolipin and anti-beta2 glycoprotein I antibodies are groups of antibodies which target the phospholipid binding plasma proteins such as beta 2 glycoprotein I and prothrombin. As they alter the expression and secretion of procoagulant on the cell surface they subsequently prompt thrombosis.

Their presences were associated with recurrent thrombosis and fatal losses. Multiple neurological presentations are linked to their presence in patient with and without SLE. It associated in particular with focal neurological events like stroke. They also have linked to seizure, movement disorders, cognitive impairment and myelitis.

A subset of anti- DNA antibodies were found to react with NR2 glutamate receptors.Glutamate is an exiatatory neurotransmitter in the brain. It react with NMDA(N-methyl-D-aspartate) receptors which is present throughout the brain tissue. NMDARS that containing NR2A andNR2B are more expressed in CA1 region of the hippocampus and the amygdale. Excessive stimulation of NMDARS results into excessive influx of calcium into the neuronal tissue causing mitochondrial stress and subsequent neuronal death (Aranow et al, 2010).

In animal models anti NR2 receptors antibodies did not cause brain damage in the presence of intact blood brain barrier (BBB). When BBB compromised using bacterial lipolysaccharide (LPS) damage to hippocampal neurons took place with no evidence of inflammation. Those mice performed badly on memory function (Kowal et al,2004). When epinephrine is used to compromise the BBB the hippocampus of those mice was normal but the antibodies react with neurons of the amygdale. Those mice had impaired fear response (Huerta et al.,2006).

Studies have shown a correlation between the CSF anti- NR2 level with diffuse NPSLE not with focal NPSLE (Arinuma et al, 2008) and no relation to serum anti-NR2 level. This may implicate intrathecal production of anti-NR2 antibodies or migration of antibodies through compromised BBB.

Anti- ribosomal P antibodies was reported in association with SLE. Their presence was linked to lupus related Psychosis and depression.

4.3 Cytokine effects

Elevated level of interleukin (IL-1),IL2, IL-6, IL-8, and interferon gamma (IFNϒ) were found in the CSF of patient with NPSLE (Rhiannon, 2007)(Chandy et al.,2008). Also elevated level of tumour necrosis factor (TNF) family ligands BAFF (B- cell activating factor of TNF family) and APRIL (a proliferation- inducing ligand) were seen in CSF of SLE patients. However the level of APRIL was higher in NPSLE patients when compared to SLE patient without NP (Chandy et al,2008).

The cytokines are thought to be produced locally by the infiltrating immune cells or by the glial cells or the neurons. Different cytokines had different effects. Their role in the pathogenesis of NPSLE is related to stimulating antibodies productions, effecting neurotransmitter release and the release of corticotrophin releasing hormone (CRH). The stimulation of glucocorticoid production results in persistent elevation of glucocorticoid that plays a role in hippocampal atrophy.

5. Approach

A careful evaluation of SLE patients presenting with new neurological symptoms and signs is needed to rule out secondary causes before attributing it to SLE. Different secondary causes can be a cause for neurological symptoms in SLE patients. The management will be different if the presentation related to lupus or to other causes.

The evaluation of SLE patients presenting with neurological symptoms and signs will be the same as non SLE patients. This includes careful clinical, laboratory and imaging studies. The diagnosis of NPSLE is a diagnosis by exclusion. No single laboratory or imaging study will confirm that the neurological presentation is caused by SLE itself. The presence of other lupus related activity could support the diagnosis of NPSLE.

5.1 History

Detailed history is mandatory when evaluating lupus patient presenting with new neurological presentation. Detailed description of the neurological symptoms is necessary to assist for localization and identifying a potential cause for the problem. The onset of the symptoms will help identifying problems with acute versus more chronic disorder. The severity of the presentation and associated other neurological symptoms will help in determine the nature and will assist further regarding the management plan. The presence of fever may suggest the presence of infection.

Detailed SLE history regarding time of diagnosis, disease course, previous neurological presentation and complications related to disease are particular important. Most of NPSLE present at time of generalized disease activity. Patients with prior neurological involvement are also at higher risk to have recurrence or development of other neurological disorders. Neurological complications can be also developed secondary to other organ involvement by lupus for example acute stroke can be a presentation of libman Sacks endocarditis , or in other example patient may develop posterior reversible leukoencephalopathy (PRES) secondary to hypertension which can be secondary to renal disease in lupus patient. Detailed drug history is important as patient may develop complication related to therapy like psychosis from steroid therapy. Patient on immunosuppressive treatment are immunocompromised so they are at high risk of development of bacterial, viral and fungal infections. Subacute neurological symptom in SLE patient may represent JC virus infection that causes progressive multifocal leukoencephalopathy (PML). PML is a demylinating disease that mainly reported with HIV patients. Multiple cases of PML also reported in SLE patient either on or not on immunosuppressive therapy (Molloy &Calbrese, 2009).The possibility of infection should be ruled out before attributing a neurological presentation to SLE and starting aggressive immunosuppressive therapy.

Other medication history might be the cause for the neurological presentation. In particular antipsychotic therapy as they can induce movement disorders. The management in that instance will necessitate medication changes rather than immunosuppression.

Detailed family history of same problem or other neurological disorders may point to genetically related neurological diagnosis not necessary attributing it to SLE.

When patient present acutely with symptoms and signs suggestive of acute stroke a quick assessment is necessary not to delay thrombolytic therapy if indicated (further discussion regarding cerbrovascular disease is discussed below).

In patient presenting with seizure careful history to characterize the seizure whether it is generalized or focal. The presence of focal seizure could represent structural lesion as a cause of the seizure. Careful medication and systemic review is mandatory as the seizure can be secondary to metabolic abnormalities e.g. uremia or medication induced seizure. The presence of other associated neurological symptoms could point to other possible causes of seizure. In particular the presence of headache, disturb conscious level could be related to posterior reversible leukoencephalopathy, limbic encephalitis or viral encephalitis. The presence of other focal neurological deficit can point to structural lesions such as stroke. One should exclude other non lupus related causes of seizure such as head trauma or genetically determent epilepsy.

5.2 Examination

The aim of the examination is to localize the neurological presentation and reach a possible diagnosis which will be supported by the laboratory investigations.

Careful systemic as well neurological examinations are required when dealing with SLE patients with neurological presentation. In particularly patient need to checked for fever, and had blood pressure measurements. The presence of other area of vascular occlusion could point to vascular cause of the neurological events.

In patient presenting with cognitive problem full neuropsychological assessment should be carried out. That will include assessing simple attention, complex attention, memory, visuospatial processing, language, reasoning/problem solving, psychomotor speed and executive functions.

5.3 Laboratory examination

Full laboratory assessment to rule out infection and metabolic abnormality that could be the cause for the neurological events. That will include complete blood count, electrolytes, kidney and liver function test.

Cerebrospinal fluid assessment is necessary in certain cases to rule out infection or other unrelated condition. In patient with subacute presentation and demylination on imaging the CSF should be sent for JC virus PCR. The CSF level of autoantibodies and inflammatory mediators are not recommended now as it still a research interest.

5.4 Supplementary tests

EEG is indicated in patient presenting with seizure or in patient with acute confusional state. For patient with seizure the EEG will help in determine the subset of patients who are at high risk of seizure recurrence. The most frequent EEG abnormalities reported in SLE patient is bitemporal slowing in 65% of patients (Lampropoulos et al., 2005).

Nerve conduction study and electromyography is indicated in patient presenting with peripheral nervous system related complaints.

5.5 Imaging

In acute setting in patient presenting with acute onset neurological events computerized tomography (CT) brain is the imaging modality of choice to rule out haemorrhage. It is also an easily accessible and widely available. The use of CT brain initially will be important to identify a subset of patients who may need thrombolytic therapy.

MRI (magnetic resonance imaging)is a preferred imaging modality to evaluate lupus patients with neurological symptoms. It is more sensitive than CT in detecting anatomical abnormalities and determines the extent of disease process. The most frequent abnormalities in MRI is hyperintense white matter lesions which is seen in 70% of patients (Appenzeller et al.,2007).Their presence have been linked to the presence of Apl . Cerebral atrophy is seen in 6-12% in SLE patients (Huizinga et al.,2001)(Appenzeller et al.,2005-2007).

Other advanced imaging technique may be of value in assessing patients with NPSLE although there clinical uses are not widely available. Those includes MTR (magnetization transfer ratio), diffusion weighted images, MRS (magnetic resonance spectroscopy), functional MRI and single photon emission computed tomography.

Investigation	
Laboratory	CBC, Electrolytes, Kidney and liver function
CSF	WBC, Glucose, protein,
	Gram stain and culture
	Viral PCR
Imaging	CT brain
	MRI brain and spinal cord
Electrophysiology	EEG
	EMG

CBC, complete blood count; WBC, white blood cell; CT computerized tomography; MRI , magnetic resonance imaging; EEG, electroencephalogram

Table 2. Recommended investigation in SLE patient with neurological presentation

6. Management

Once the diagnosis of NPSLE is confirmed the treatment will include treatment of potential aggravating factors, symptomatic treatment for the events and more specific treatment related to SLE itself.

In some condition symptomatic treatment will be required first before specific therapy is indicated. For example in patient presenting with seizure after excluding secondary causes starting antiepileptic is required before the decision on specific treatment is made(Hanly & Harrison, 2005).

The severity and the nature of neurological events will also play a role in the decision on treatment. For example patient with non serious headache will require only symptomatic treatment.

In the presence of severe neurological disease the Europan League Aganist Rheumatism (EULAR, 2010) recommends the use corticosteroid alone or with cyclophosphamide. A Cochrane review of cyclophosphamid versus methylprednisolone in treatment of NPSLE did not find a randomised clinical trial comparing the two.

When patient failed to respond to conventional treatment or in the presence of severe disease multiple reports suggested the addition of other treatment modalities can be effective. Those include plasma exchange, rituximab or intravenous immunoglobulin.

The combination of the treatment modalities (cyclophosmaide/corticosteroid/ plasma exchange(Bartolucci et al.,2007) or plasmapheresis alone or with cyclophosphamide (Neuwelt,2003)) was evaluated in small series of refractory disease. Results from those showed favourable outcome with combination modalities.

Rituximab is an anti-CD20 antibody that directly target B cells. Rituximab was studied in refractory cases of NPSLE and showed a rapid improvement of clinical as well radiological finding in those patients (Takunaga et al.,2006).

In the presence of thrombotic disease the management will depend whether patient had arterial versus venous thrombosis and the presence of antiphospholipid. Anticoagulation is recommended for venous thrombosis as well in the presence of arterial thrombosis with antiphospholipid antibodies. In absence of antiphospholipid antibodies and the presence of arterial thrombosis careful evaluation and management for secondary risk factors with the use of antiplatelets are indicated.

7. Common neurological disorders associated with SLE

7.1 Headache

Headache is one of the most commonly reported neurological symptoms associated with SLE. There is no specific type of headache found to have increase prevalence in patient with SLE (Mitsikostas,2004).

When patient with SLE patient present with acute headache, special attention is warranted to rule out infection, aseptic meningitis and venous sinus thrombosis. On examination special attention is required looking for fever, meningeal signs and examination for the fundi to rule papilledema. In the presence for focal finding, papilldema or altered mental status brain imaging is required. Brain MRI with venogram is preferred to rule out venous sinus thrombosis. In presence of fever or signs of infection CSF examination is mandatory.

No specific treatment is required for nonspecific headache.

7.2 Cognitive dysfunction

It is one of the most commonly reported NPSLE syndromes. Most of the patient had mild to moderate impairment, only around 3-5% had severe impairment (EULAR, 2010). The most commonly reported abnormality is overall slowing, decrease memory, impaired working memory and executive dysfunction (Hanly,2005).

Different report linked cognitive impairment to the presence of Apl (McLurin et al.,2005)(Denburg et al, 1997). It is also reported in patient who suffered from stroke and with Apl microinfracts although the pattern is different between the two. Cognitive dysfunction from stroke develops acutely and remains the same in contrast to those with microinfract as it shows stepwise deterioration. Different studies have showed a contradicting results regarding the association between global disease activity and the presence of cognitive impairment (Kozora et al.,1996)(Hay et al.,1992)(Carbotte etal.,1995). Some of the studies found an association and other did not found any association. The use of glucocorticoid associated with cognitive impairment in middle age patients irrespective of disease activity (McLurin et al.,2005). The effect of prednisone use was not significant for young and old patients.

Other causes can alter the cognitive function. Of those the development of mood disorders are particularly important. It is very well known that depression worsen cognitive function and even cause a pseudodementia. Patients with SLE also under psychological stress from the disease itself or from medications and that also can alter cognitive function even in absence of psychiatric disease (Hanly,2005).

Formal neuropsychological testing is required to diagnose cognitive dysfunction. The main limitation of formal neuropsychological testing is time consuming and it need to be administered by an expert. The minimental test is not a good tool for screening for cognitive impairment.

MRI is indicated if the patient is less than 60 years, rapid and unexplained moderate to severe impairment, recent and significant head trauma, presence of other neurological symptoms or signs and the development of it in the setting of immunosuppressive therapy or antiplatelets (EULAR, 2010).

Patient should be screened and treated for potential precipitating factors such as metabolic and endocrine abnormalities. Associated psychiatric disorders should be treated. Control of cardiovascular risk factors also is recommended. Mclaurine in 2005 reported a beneficial effect of regular aspirin use on cognitive function in elderly patient with other vascular risk factors particularly in diabetics (McLurin et al.,2005).

The use of glucocorticoid with or without immunosuppressive will be considered in the presence of SLE disease activity or other NPSLE events.

Memantine is a drug used to treat dementia. One randomized clinical trial looked at the use of memantine to treat patient with SLE and cognitive impairment. No significant improvement in cognitive function in the treated group. At current the use of memantine for SLE patient with cognitive impairment is not recommended. Further clinical trial is needed (Petri et al.,2011).

7.3 Cerbrovascular disease

SLE patients are at high risk of developing vascular complications. Among those are stroke and transit ischemic attacks. Multiple causes can lead to strokes in SLE patients. The most frequent cause is atherosclerotic diseases. Other rare causes include embolic strokes from libman Sacks endocarditis and cerebral vasculitis.

In study of carotid ultrasound in asymptomatic SLE patients carotid plaques were seen in 25-40% of patients. Different risk factors were associated with the development of strokes in SLE patients. Those includes high disease activity, moderate to high titres of antiphospholipid antibodies, heart valve disease, hypertension, age and smoking (EULAR, 2010) (Toloza et al,2004)(Bessantbet al.,2004)(Futrell & Millikan,1988).
Evaluation of stroke/TIA patient will be the same as non SLE patient. Thrombolytic therapy can be given unless there are contraindications. Patient should be screened for cardiovascular risk factors and have aggressive measures to control them. Further managements will include the use of antiplatelet and carotid endartectomy if indicated. Patients who fill full the criteria of antiphospholipid syndromes chronic anticoagulant therapy is indicated with a target INR of 2-3 (EULAR,2010)(Crowther et al,2003)(Finazzi et al.,2005).

7.4 Seizure

Seizure in SLE patient can be attributed to the disease activity or it could be related to secondary causes. The secondary causes of seizure in SLE patients are:- infection, electrolytes abnormalities, uremia, hypertension, medication side effect or hypoxia. It also can be a presentation of unrelated condition such as brain tumours.
The reported prevalence of seizure is between 7.5% to 14% (Hanly et al.,2010)(Mikdashi et al.,2005)(Appenzeller et al.,2004). Seizure present at disease onset in 31.7% of patients (Mucal & Brey,2010), and most frequently occurred within 5 years from diagnosis. Most of the patient 88.3% had single events and around 11.7% had epilepsy. The most frequently reported seizure type is generalized tonic clonic seizure followed by complex partial seizure. Seizure can present as the only NP syndrome or accompany other neurological events mainly ischemic or hemorrhagic strokes and psychosis.
Multiple studies confirmed the relation between seizure and the presence of Apl(Mikdashi et al.,2005)(Appenzeller et al.,2004)(Gibbs & Husain,2002)(Herranza et al.,1994)(Liou et al.,1996). Also the presence of Apl were associated with shorter time to seizure occurrence (Andrade et al.,2008). Seizure occurrence is related to high diasese activity, severe organ damage in particular nephritis and the presence of Apl. Factors associated with epilepsy are the same as those associated with seizure. Patients who had epilepsy are more likely to be men (Mikdashi et al.,2005) and more likely to have abnormal MRI and EEG.
The most frequent abnormality reported in brain MRI in patient with seizure is global atrophy and the presence of multiple subcortical hyperintense lesions. The most frequent EEG finding is diffuse slowing. The presence of interictal epileptic activity is associated with high recurrence rate of epileptic seizure.
As most of the patients will have only one seizure, treatment with antiepileptic is not recommended. The patient should be investigated with EEG, brain MRI and have Apl antibody screening. Patient who had positive test for Apl should be monitored carefully as they have high recurrence rate. In the presence of other SLE activity or flare treatment with glucocorticoid with or without immunosuppressive is recommended (EULAR, 2010).

7.5 Acute confusional state

It is a condition characterized by acute onset of altered mental state with decrease attention. A carful exclusion of secondary causes such as metabolic, infection and side effect of medications is mandatory. CSF examination is required to exclude infection. Brain imaging is indicated to rule out structural lesions. EEG is also indicated to rule out seizure disorders.

Treatment includes symptomatic treatment with antipsychotics to control agitation, glucocorticoid and immunosuppressive agents.

7.6 Myelopathy

Patient with SLE may present with symptoms and signs of spinal cord dysfunction which may indicate the presence of myelitis. Myelitis is less commonly reported than other NPSLE syndromes (1-3% of patient) (Lukjanowicz & Brzosko,2009). Most commonly patient will present with acute transverse myelitis and less commonly will have longitudinal myelitis.

Acute transverse myelitis involves less than 4 segments of the spinal cord in contrast to longitudinal myelitis which involve more than 4 segments of the cord. The thoracic cord is the most commonly affected followed by the cervical cord (D'Cruz et al.,2004).

Around 73% of SLE patient presenting with myelitis were positive for apl (D'Cruz et al.,2004).

Patient with myeliitis present acutely with motor weakness and sensory symptoms. The extent of the symptoms depends on the level of the lesion and the extent of the inflammatory changes. Bladder and bowel dysfunction is seen in all patients with myelitis.

Lupus myelitis is usually developed in the first 5 years after disease onset (Kovacs et al.,2000)(Chan & Boey, 1996). One third of the cases have another major NPSLE (EULAR,2010). In 21-48% of patients will have associated optic neuritis (Kovacs et al.,2000) (Chan & Boey, 1996) . The recurrence rate for myelitis is seen in 21-55% of patients (Kovacs et al.,2000)(Chan & Boey, 1996)(Lehnhardt et al.,2006).

When patient with SLE present with feature of myleopathy a careful exclusion of other causes of myeolpathy is necessary before attributing the presentation to SLE. A contrast enhanced MRI of spinal cord is mandatory to rule out mass lesions as a cause for myelopathy. The most frequently reported abnoramlites is T2 hyperintensities which become more pronounced after contrast (Lukjanowicz &Brzosko,2009)(Provenzale et al.,1994)(Boumpas et al.,1990)(Salmaggi et al,1994). In a group of patients the intial MRI can be normal especially if it was done early. If the initial MRI is normal repeat study in 2-7 days after onset is recommended (Lukjanowicz &Brzosko,2009). Brain MRI is indicated when there is associated neurological symptoms and to help differentiating it from multiple sclerosis.

Cerbrospinal fluid examination is recommended to rule out infectious aetiology (EULAR,2010). In 50-70% of cases mild CSF abnormalities are seen including mild lymphocytosis and elevated protein with normal glucose.

An inflammatory CSF with granulocytes pleocytosis, elevated protein and low glucose is reported with lupus myelitis especially with longitudinal myelitis. In the presence of this finding a carful exclusion of infectious cause is mandatory.

In the presence of longitudinal myelitis and associated optic neuritis serum should be send for anti neuromyelitis antibodies(anti- NMO IgG) to rule out the presence of neuromyelitis optica. Anti NMO IgG is a highly sensitive and specific antibody that target aquaporin 4 the main water channel in the CNS.

An aggressive treatment with immunosuppressive is recommended in a setting of ATM. The presence of inflammatory CSF should not delay the start of immunosuppressive. In that case a combined treatment of antimicrobial with immunosuppressive is recommended waiting for the culture results. Antimicrobial should be discontinued once infection is ruled out.

Treatment with intravenous steroid should be initiated followed by cyclophosphamide with oral steroid.
The treatment should be initiated early in the disease course.
Plasmapheresis has been used with immunosuppressive medication in severe cases in particular in patient with of longitudinal myelitis ((D'Cruz et al.,2004). Although an earlier reports by Kovacs showed patients who had combined treatment of steroid, immunosuppressive and plasmapheresis did worse than patient who had only steroid with or without imunnosupressive (Kovacs et al.,2000). This is may be because patients who had aggressive treatments with three modalities had higher disease activity at the onset of myelitis.
In the presence of Apl anticoagulant therapy is recommended with the immunosuppressive therapy. Patients with apl and Transverse myelitis who had combination therapy of immunosuppressive and anticoagulant have good functional outcome (D'Cruz et al.,2004).
The functional outcome is good for patient who had early treatment. The presence of longitudinal transverse myelitis is associated with poor functional prognosis (Gertner,2007)(Kimura et al.,2002).

7.7 Movement's disorders

The most frequently reported movement disorder with SLE patient is chorea. It has been linked to antiphospholipid antibodies. Other causes of chorea such as hereditary, metabolic, endocrine causes should be excluded. Brain imaging is indicated to rule out structural causes in the presence of focal neurological signs.
Patient need to be treated symptomatically with dopamine antagonist and in severe cases the use of glucocoticoid and immunosuppressive therapy is recommended. In the presence of antiphospholipid antibodies patient need to be on antiplatelets or anticoagulants depending on the presence of other APS related symptoms.
Parkinsonism is also reported in association with SLE in multiple cases. Usually it is associated with severe multisystem CNS involvements. The good response of the reported cases to immunosuppressive therapy suggests that it is a manifestation of the disease not a coincidence of Parkinson disease and SLE.

7.8 Peripheral nervous system Involvements

Peripheral neuropathy is the most frequent reported peripheral nervous system (PNS) involvement with SLE. The most frequent type is sensory neuropathy followed by sensorimotor neuropathy then pure motor neuropathy (Goransson et al.,2006).A subset of SLE patients may present with sensory symptoms and still have normal NCS. This is because the NCS evaluate the large myelinated fibers and the presence of normal study does not rule out small fiber neuropathy. In studies when symptomatic patients with negative NCS had skin biopsy an evidence of small fiber nruropathy was found (Goransson et al.,2006)(Omdal et al.,2002). This indicates that small fiber neuropathy is the cause of the symptomatic patients with normal NCS. Managements of peripheral neuropathy include symptomatic treatments for neuropathic pain as well glucocorticoid with or without immunosuppressive therapy depending on the severity of the disease. In the presence of severe cases, or failure of conventional treatments other modalities such as plasmaphersis, intravenous immunoglobulin and rituximab can be used.
Other PNS involvements by SLE are much less. Patient may present with mononeuritis multiplex, acute demylenating polyradiculopathy, chronic demylinating polyradiculopathy

and myasthenia gravis also reported. The managements of those patients will be the same as non SLE patients.

8. Prognosis

In spite of recent advances in diagnosis and management, NPSLE remain one of the major causes of disease related morbidity. Swedish study of SLE patients did not find difference in mortality in SLE patients with or without NP. However patients with NPSLE have more functional impairments when compared to non NPSLE patients (Jonsen, 2002). Prompt diagnosis and management may played a role in reducing mortality but significant morbidity and functional incapacity still a major problem in SLE patients with neuropsychiatric symptoms.

9. Acknowledgment

The work to produce this chapter was supported by Alzaidi's Chair of research in rheumatic diseases- Umm Alqura University.

10. References

H.Ainiala, J. Lukkola, J.Peltola, et al. The Prevalaence of Neuropsychiatric Syndromes in Systemic Lupus Erythrematosus. Neurology 200157: 496-500.

Andrade, Alarcon,et al. Seizure in Patients with Systemic Lupus Erythematosus: data from LUMINA, a multiethnic Cohort. Ann Rheum Dis 2008;67(6):829-834

Antonella, Garzia, et al. Neuropsychatric Lupus Syndromes: Relationship With Antiphospholipid Antibodies. Neurology 2003;61:108-110.

Appenzeller, Cendes, Costallat. Epileptic Seizure in Systemic Lupus Erythematosus. Neurology 2004;63:1808-1812

Appenzeller, Bonilha, et al. Longitudinal Analysis of Gray and white Matter Loss in Patients with Systemic Lupus Erythematosus. Neuroimage 34;694-701.

Appenzeller, Rondina, Costallat, Cendes. Cerebral and Corpus Callosum Atrophy in Systemic Lupus Erythematosus.Arthritis Rheum 2005; 52: 2783-2789.

Appenzeller, Costallat, Cendes. Neurolupus. Arch Neur 2006;63:458-460. Appenzeller, Pike, Clarke.Magnetic Resonance Imaging in the Evaluation of Central Nervous System Manifestation in Systemic Lupus Erythematosus. Clin Rev Allerg immunol 2007.

Aranow, Diamond, Mackey. Glutamate Receptor Biology and its Clinical Significance in Neuropsychiatric SLE. Rheum Dis Clin North Am. 2010 February;36(1):187-201

Arinum et al. Association of Cerebrospinal Fluid Anti-NR2 Glutamate Receptor Antibodies with Diffuse Neuropsychiatric Systemic Lupus Erythematosus. Arthritis and Rheumatism. 2008 Apri;58(4):1130-1135.

Barile-fabris, et al. Controlled Clinical Trial Of IV Cyclophosphamide versus IV Methylprednisolone in Severe Neurological Manifestation in Systemic Lupus Erythematosus. Ann Rheum Dis 2005:64:620-625.

Bartolucci, Brechignac,et al. Adjunctive Plasma Excahnge to Treat Neuropsychiatric Lupus: a Retrospective Study on 10 Patients. Lupus 2007:16(10):871-822.

Bertsias et al,EULAR recommendations for the management of Systemic Lupus Erythematosus with neuropsychiatric manifestation: report of task force of the EULAR standing committe for clinical affairs. Ann Rheum Dis, 2010: 69: 2074-2082 Bosma, Huizinga, et al. Abnormal Brain Diffusivity in Patient with Neuropsychiatric Systemic Lupus Erythematosus. AJNR 2003; 24:850-854.

Bosma, Steens, et al. Multisequence magnetic Resonance Imaging Study of Neuropsychiatric Systemic Lupus Erythematosus. Arthritis & Rheumatism 2004; 50(10):3195-3201

Boumpass, et al.Acute Transverse Myelities in Systemic Lupus Erythematosus: magnatic Resonance Imaging and review of Literature. J Rheumatol 1990;17:89-92.

Brey, Holliday, et al.Neuropsychiatric Syndromes in Lupus. Neurology 2002;58:1214-1220

Brey. Neuropsychiatric Lupus Clinical and Imaging Aspects. Bulletin of the NYU Hospital for Joint Diseases 2007;65(30:194-199.

Briani, lucchetta, et al. Neurolupus is Associated with Anti-ribosomal P protein Antibodies; an Inception Cohort Study. J Autoimmun 2009 Mar; 32(2):79-84. Carbott, Denburg. Cognitive Dysfunction in Systemic Lupus Erythematosus is independent of active disease. Journal of Rheumatology 1995;22:863-867.

Castellino, Padovan, et al. Single Photon Emission Computed Tomography and Magnetic Resonance Imaging Evaluation in SLE Patients with and without Neuropsychiatric Involvement. Rheumatology 2008; 4:319-323.

Chan,Boey. Transverse myelopathy in SLE: clinical and Functional outcomes. Lupus1996;5:294-299.

Chandy, Trysberg, Eriksson. Intrathecal Levels of APRIL and BAFF in Patients with Systemic Lupus Erythematosus: relationship to Neuropsychiatric Syndromes. Arthritis Research & Therapy2008:10 (4).

Crowther,et al.A Comprison of two intensities of Warfarin for the Prevention of Recurrent Thrombosis in Patient with Antiphospholipid Antibodies Syndromes. N Eng J Med 2003;349:1133-1138.

D'cruz, Mellor-Pita,et al. Transverse Myelitis as the First Manifestation Systemic Lupus Erythematosus or Lupus Like Disaes: Good Functional Outcome and relevance of Antiphospholipid Antibodies. The J of Rheumatology 2204;31:280-285.

Denburg, Carbotte, et al. The Relationship of Antiphospholipid Antibodies to Cognitive Function in Patients with Systemic Lupus Erythematosus. J int neuropschol soc 1997;3(4):377-386.

Elliso.n, Gatter, Heryet, Esiri. Intramural Platelet Deposition in Cerebral Vasculopathy of Systemic Lupus Erythematosus. J Cli Pathol 1993; 46:37-40

Eyal Muscal, Brey. Neurological Manifestation Of Systemic upus Erythematosus in Children and adult. Neurol Clin.2010 Feb: 28(1);61-73

Fady Joseph, Lammie, Scolding. CNS Lupus A study of 41 Patients. Neurology 2007; 69:644-654.

Finazzi, et al. A Randomized Clinical Trial of High Intensity Warfarin vs Conventional Antithrombotic Therapy for the Prevention of recurrent Thrombosis in Patient with Antiphospholipid Syndrome. J Throm Haemost 2005;3:848-853.

Furtrell. Millikan. Frequency , Etiology, and Prevention of Stroke in Patients with Systemic Lupus Erythematosus. Stroke 1989;20(5):583-590.

Gibbis &Husain. Epilepsy Associated with Lupus Anticoagulant. Seizure 2002;11(3):207-209

Goransson, et al. Small Diameter Nerve Fiber Neuropathy in Systemic Lupus Erythematosus. Arch neurol 2006;63:401-404.

Hammad,Tsukada, Torre. Cerebral Occlusive Vasculopathy in Systemic Lupus Erythematosus and speculation on the part palyed by complement. Annals of the Rheumatic Diseases 1992;51:550-552

Hanly, Harrison. Management of Neuropsychiatric Lupus. Best Practice 7 Research Clinical Rheumatology 2005:19(5):799-821).

Hanly, Urowitz, Siannis, et al. Autoantibodies and Neuropsychiatric Events at the Time of Systemic upus Erythematosus Diagnosis. Arthritis & Rheumatism. March 2008 (58): 843-853.

Hanly, urowitz, L. Su et al. Prospective Analysis of neuropsychiatric Events In An International Disease Inception Cohort of SLE Patients. ann Rheum Dis. 2010 March; 69(3): 529-535.

Hay, et al. Psychiatric disorder and cognitive Impairment in Systemic Lupus Erythematosus. Arthritis and Rheumatism 1992;35(40:411-416.

Heinlein, Gertner. Marked Inflammation in Catastrophic Longitudinal Myelitis Associated With Systemic Lupus Erythematosus. Lupus 2007;16:823-826.

Herranz, Rivier, et al. Association between Antiphospholipid Antibodies and Epilepsy in Patients with Systemic Lupus Erythematosus. Arthritis Rheum 1994;37(4):568-571

Hingorani, MacGregor, Isenberg, A.Rahman. Risk of Coronary Heart Disease and Stroke in a Large British Cohort Of Patients with Systemic Lupus Erythematosus. Rheumatology 2004;43:924-929.

Huerta, et al. Immunity and Behavior, antibody alter emotion. Proc Natl Acad Sci USA 2006;103(3):678-683.

Huizinga, Steens, Van Buchem. Imaging Modalities in Central Nervous System Systemic Lupus Erythematosus. Curr Opin Rheumatol 13:383-388.

Jonsen, Bengtsson, et al. Outcome of Neuropsychiatric Systemic Lupus Erythematosus within a defined Swedish Population :increased Morbidity but Low Mortality. Rheumatology 2002:41:1308-1312

Kato, et al. Systemic Lupus Erythematosus Related Transverse myelitis Presenting Longitudinal Involvement of The Spinal Cord. Internal Medicine 2002;41(2):156-160.

Katsumata, Harigai, et al. Diagnostic Reliability of Magnetic Resonance Imaging for Central Nervous System Syndromes in Systemic Lupus Erythematosus: a prospective Cohort study. BMC Musculoskeletal Disorders 2010:11.

Kovacs, Lafferty, et al. Transverse myelopathy in Systemic Lupus Erythematosus; an analysis of 14 cases and Review of the literature. Ann rheuma dis 2000;59;120-124

Kowal, et al. Cognition and Immunity, antibody impairs memory. Immunity 2004; 21(2):179-188

Kozora, et al. Analysis of Cognitive and Psychological Defecits in Systemic Lupus Erythematosus patients without overt Central Nervous System Disease. Arthritis and Rheumatism 1996;39(12):2035-2045

Lampropoulos, Koutroumandis, et al. Electroencephalography in The assessment of Neuropsychiatric Manifestations in Antiphospholipid Syndrome and Systemic Lupus Erythematosus. Arthritis & rheumatism 2005; 52(3):841-846

Lehnhardt,et al.Autologous Blood stem Cell Transplantation in refractory Systemic Lupus Erythematosus with Recurrent Longitudinal Myelitis and Cerbral Infraction. Lupus 2006;15:240-243.

Levy, Uziel, et al. Intravenous immunoglobulins in Peripheral Neuropathy associated with vasculitis. Ann Rheum Dis 2003;62:1221-1223.

Liou, Wang, et al. Elevated Levels of Anticardiolipin Antibodies and Epilepsy in Lupus Patients. Lupus 1996;5(4):307-312.

Lukjanowicz, Brzosko. Myelitis in The Course of Systemic Lupus Erythematosus. POl Arch MedWewn2009;119:67-73.

McLaurin, Holliday, Williams, Brey. Predictors of Cognitive Dysfunction in Patients with Systemic Lupus Erythematosus. Neurology 2005;64:297-303.

Mikadashi, Krumholz,Handwerger. Factors at Diagnosis Predict Subsequent Occurrence of Seizure in Systemic Lupus Erythematosus. Neurology 2005;64:2102-2107.

Mitsikostas, Sfikakis, Goadsby. A meta analysis for Headache in Systemic Lupus Erythematosus: the Evidence and the Myth. Brain 2004;127:1200-1209.

Molloy, Calbrese. Progressive Multifocal Leukoencephalopathy. Arthritis & Rheumatism 2009;60(12):3761-3765

Nasir, Kerr, Birnbaum. Nineteen Episodes of Recurrent Myelitis in a Woman With Neuromyelitis Optica and Systemic Lupus Erythematosus. Arch neurol 2009; 66(90:1160-1163.

Neuwelt. The Role of Plasmapheresis in the Treatment of Severe Central Nervous System Neuropsychiatric Systemic Lupus Erythematosus. Ther Apher Dial 2003:7(20):173-182.

Okamoto, kobayashi, Yamanaka. Cytokines and Chemokines in neuropsychiatric Syndromes of Systemic Lupus Erythematosus. J of biomedicine and biotechnology 2010.

Okuma, et al. Comparison between Single antiplatelet therapy and Combination of Antiplatelet and Anticoagulation Therapy for Secondery Prevention in Ischemic Stroke Patients with Antiphospholipid Syndrome. Int J Med Sci 2010;7:15-18

Omdal, et al. Peripheral Neuropathy in Systemic Lupus Erythematosus. Neurology 1991;41:808-811.

Omdal, et al. Small Nerve Fiber Involvment in Systemic Lupus Erythematosus. Arthritis & Rheumatisim 2002;46(5):1228-1232.

Petri, Nagibuddin, et al. Memantine in Systemic Lupus Erythematosus: A Randomized Double Blind Placebo Controlled Trial. Semin Arthritis Rheum 2011(pubmed)

Provenzale, et al. Lupus Related Myelitis:serial MRI findings.AJNR Am J Neuroradio 1994;15:1911-1917

Takunaga, Saito, et al. Efficacy of Rituximab (anti- CD20) for Refractory Systemic Lupus Erythematosus Involving The Centeral Nervous System. Ann Rheum Dis 2007:66:470-475.

Toloza, et al. Systemic Lupus Erythematosus in Multiethnic US Cohort(LUMINA). Arthritis and Rheumatism 2004;50(12):3947-3957.

Rhiannon J, Systemic Lupus Erthematosus involving the nervous system: presentation, pathogenesis, and management. Clinic Rev allerg Immunol.

Salmaggi, et al.spinal Cord Involvment and Systemic Lupus Erythematosus: Clinical and Magnatic Resonance Finding in 5 Patients. clin Exp Rheumatol 1994:12:389-394.

Syuto, shimizu, et al. Association of antiphosphatidylserine/prothrombin antibodies with Neuropsychiatric Systemic Lupus Erythematosus. Clin rheumatol. 2009 july; 28(7):841-845.

16

The Pathophysiology of Systemic Lupus Erythematosus and the Nervous System

Joel M. Oster
Assistant Clinical Professor of Neurology
Tufts University and Lahey Clinic
Boston and Burlington Massachusetts
USA

1. Introduction

The pathophysiology of Neuropsychiatric SLE (NPSLE) will be described in this chapter. Systemic Lupus Erythematosis (SLE) is a multiorgan and multisystem autoimmune disorder and its pathophysiology may have protean effects on all components of the nervous system. The central (CNS) and peripheral nervous systems (PNS) may be involved in SLE. About 25 % of SLE may begin in childhood and SLE may present both steadily chronic and more episodic neurologic symptoms as well throughout the life span. The presentation of symptoms and clinical signs is a reflection of the location and type of pathophysiology of the disease in which there is chronic inflammation of varied degrees that may wax and wane. The chronic disease process is responsible for making the CNS for example more vulnerable to lowered seizure threshold and episodic seizures despite the ongoing more chronic pathophysiology involving the inflammation of the blood vessels. The disease may exert effects on peripheral nerves and over time accumulated lesions or immune mediated damage may make tissues more susceptible to damage. Chronic inflammation or immune mediated damage or vasculitis of blood vessels or the vascular supply of the nerves may predispose to neuropathy and lead to progressive deterioration in function over time as lesion burden accumulates in the PNS. Similarly, SLE may also damage various end organs that may impact the nervous system once affected. For example, SLE may impact the heart and cardiovascular system or be associated with antiphospholipid antibodies that may contribute to embolic strokes. Other end organs may be affected for example kidney dysfunction or renal failure that may lead to uremic encephalopathy. Having a rash present or palpable purpura and multiorgan involvement may present clinical clues that SLE is the diagnosis along with clinical evidence of multisystem involvement. Other pathophysiology exists as noted below. In these regards, this chapter seeks to characterize the pathophysiology of the major categories of disease and syndromes on the nervous system in SLE. The categorization of the signs and symptoms and overall disease state and pathophysiology and structures involved will relate to how these conditions are ultimately diagnosed and treated.

Neurologists need to be aware of the varied presentations of SLE as neurologic symptoms may be the first signs or symptoms that come to medical attention for evaluation. Unfortunately since SLE results from chronic and indolently progressive pathophysiology, often only subtle neurologic signs develop insidiously over years and therefore often the diagnosis of SLE may be only possible retrospectively in these regards in some cases.

2. The proposed autoimmune mechanism of SLE on the nervous system and resultant effects

While the definitive mechanisms are unknown, the general principle is that antibodies or immune complexes may attack the blood supply to the neural structures. HLA type may regulate the susceptibility to SLE. Studies of twins seem to indicate that many other factors may work in conjunction with HLA typing to produce clinical disease. Although antineuronal antibodies exist, it is unclear how they exert their effects. Over time, it is thought that progressive inflammation may lead to progressive decline and dysfunction. Recent articles or case reports that delineate that antithyroglobulin antibodies, antimicrosomal antibodies, anti cardiolipin antibodies, B2Glycoprotein I antibodies, antinuclear antibodies, the presence of lupus anticoagulant, and other antibodies may be some of the proposed mediators of immune damage of the CNS. Arguably, much research is needed in this area and complete mechanisms are not understood. SLE mediated attack on tissues is a diverse one including varied mechanisms of deposition of immune complexes, cytokines, and numerous modulators of these activities are postulated to be involved. Studies indicate that there may be attack of neural elements or tissues through the autoantibodies and activated leukocytes.

Medications (such as phenytoin) may produce drug induced lupus, which often spares the kidneys and CNS. The antibody profile of this entity and general immunology however may also differ from non-medication induced SLE. Over time, SLE in the CNS may cause demyelination and various demyelinating syndromes or multiple sclerosis like illness that may seemingly relapse and remit. Similarly a vasculitis may progress either fulminantly or indolently. Multiple yet to be described pathophysiologies may account for the varied syndromes noted below. Varied preponderances or ratios of antibody types in local tissues may also explain somehow whether or nor there is more central or more peripherally mediated neural damage. While the above observations are noted, the mechanism of CNS involvement remains unknown since neither the presence of antineuronal and antiastrocyte antibodies correlate with any CNS pathology or level of involvement. The literature and clinical experience notes that neurological complications may be fulminant or fatal. In general, diagnosis is made on a clinical basis although laboratory confirmation of positive antinuclear antibodies, anti-DNA, anti-RNA, and low complements are supportive in many cases along with identifying other systemic or multiorgan involvement.

3. The importance of the physical and neurological examination: A clinical key to pathophysiology

If SLE or NPSLE is suspected, a careful and detailed meticulous history and physical is mandatory. Specific attention to nearly every organ system in the general medical examination may yield clues about the presence of an underlying autoimmune or infiltrative or inflammatory disorder. From the moment the patient enters the office, one may notice the malar rash or the anterior tibial vasculitic infiltrative leucocytoclastic mediated rash. Specifically with regards to the neurologic system, a systematic approach should be used in gathering history and examination of mental status, cranial nerves, motor function, reflexes, coordination/cerebellar function, as well as sensory function and gait. Auscultation of the carotid and vertebral arteries, the heart, and looking for Lhermitte's sign and stigmata of emboli are mandatory. Because of the infiltrative nature of SLE, CNS manifestations of the disease include cognitive dysfunction, headaches, confusion, fatigue, depression, mood disorders, demyelinating syndromes, seizures, movement disorders, and strokes. Headaches, depression, fatigue, mood disorders, and cognitive disorders are associated with SLE but the mechanisms of the pathophysiology producing these exact symptoms or syndromes is poorly understood. It is postulated that various degrees of lesion burden in various locations on the CNS may be associated with these symptoms.

In the peripheral nervous system, peripheral nerve damage causing peripheral neuropathy, facial pain, tingling, burning, or numbness may occur. Chronic inflammatory diseases may cause dysfunction of individual named nerves, usually by interfering with their blood supply, thereby causing a mononeuritis or if multiple nerves are involved, a more confluent and diffuse or regionalized mononeuritis multiplex may result over time. Of note, SLE itself or associated treatments such as with corticosteroids that can cause papilledema or pseudotumor.

4. Diagnosing CNS lupus and ancillary testing- a window into the pathophysiology of neuropsychiatric SLE

Laboratory testing may give clues about the pathophysiology of NPSLE. Abnormal CSF is identified in about 50 % of cases with increased mononuclear cells along with oligoclonal bands, and antineuronal antibodies. CT scans and angiograms and MRI scans collectively may be unhelpful when there are no focal findings or if there is mild and diffuse disease, although MRI is the most sensitive radiologic tool to detect virtually any inflammatory, demyelinating, or infiltrative pathology relating to NPSLE. Laboratory markers often do not correlate with neurologic disability although high IgG titers of antineuronal antibodies in CSF may correlate with diffuse disease or high lesion burden on the nervous system. Although 70% of patients may have abnormal electroencephalograms, the findings on the EEG are not necessarily diagnostic of NPSLE by these EEG abnormalities themselves. NPSLE may mimic demyelinating disease and most often the patient may need evidence of multisystem or multiorgan involvement to make the diagnosis. The multiorgan or multisystem manifestations according to previously published guidelines include the presence of malar rash, a discoid rash, the presence of photosensitivity, oral ulcers, arthritis, serositis, renal disease or neurologic or hematologic disorders, or immunologic disorders or the presence of antinuclear antibodies. According to these guidelines if four such clinical criteria are present at any time during the course of the disease, a diagnosis of SLE may be made with 98 % specificity and 97 % sensitivity.

5. CNS disease: General principles

NPSLE may involve as many as 75% of SLE cases according to Johnson and Richardson. Impaired mentation, consciousness, seizures, cranial neuropathies and derangements of

CNS functions may either occur transiently, mildly, or late in the disease as lesion burden accumulates. CSF analysis may be basically normal or show only a mild lymphocytic pleocytosis with an increased protein. According to some sources, most of the central nervous system manifestations can be accounted for the pathophysiology of numerous micro infarcts due to the accumulation of lesions in arterioles and capillaries. The literature postulates that deposition of immune complexes in the vascular endothelium mediates vascular injury and since many patients also have concomitant hypertension, this also affects cerebral blood vessels predisposing them to hemorrhage. As mentioned above, cardiac injury can predispose to embolic complications of endocarditis. Visual complaints are common, especially in children and may include retinal artery occlusion, retinal hemorrhage, cotton wool exudates, papilledema and optic neuritis. Complications of SLE may lead to hypertensive encephalopathy, cerebral vein thrombosis, cranial neuropathies, brainstem dysfunction, and rarely myelopathy. SLE may predispose to bacterial or fungal meningitis or opportunistic infection or cause an aseptic meningitis.

6. Pathophysiology of encephalopathy

Encephalopathy is a general term indicating impaired brain function and this may occur with any amount of brain or CNS involvement in NPSLE. Clinically encephalopathies may present with confusion, lethargy or coma. Encephalopathies may also present more chronically as "brain failure" in which a patient may exhibit dementia or cognitive dysfunction. There are both acute and chronic presentations involving psychiatric symptoms. The literature notes that in general, patients with neuropsychiatric manifestations of SLE in the CNS may have abnormalities on functional neuroimaging and MRI suggesting either a disruption of normal blood flow or a dysregulation of normal metabolic function. Encephalopathies may be due to cerebritis. NSAIDS or nonsteroidal anti-inflammatory drugs may also contribute to encephalopathy by producing aseptic meningitis.

Since many patients with SLE are on chronic immunosupression, the CNS may be infected with opportunistic organisms and result in meningitis, encephalitis, or abscess. Medications used for treatment of these entities may also contribute or cause encephalopathy.

Posterior Reversible Encephalopathy Syndrome (PRES) generally occurs in patients with uncontrolled hypertension who are on immunosupression therapy. Renal involvement of SLE is common with PRES. This syndrome may present as a fulminant encephalopathy involving bi-occipital patchy swelling on MRI neuroimaging which has been described in the literature. Fortunately with control of the hypertension, clinical and radiologic reversibility may occur. The pathophysiology of this condition in NPSLE is unknown but is thought to be due to abnormal permeability of blood vessles.

Brain biopsy may be needed to clarify the pathophysiology when MRI findings cannot distinguish cerebritis from another process such as neoplasm like changes or those of opportunistic infection. Meningeal biopsy may be needed to diagnose chronic meningitis when other methods fail in cases of idiopathic chronic encephalopathies.

Focal neurological deficits may result from strokes due to either cardioembolic valvular disease or fulminant vasculitic changes of the cerebrovasculature, or thrombosis associated with the antiphospholipid antibodies. Dyskinesias may occur and the pathophysiology is thought to be due to the effects of the antiphospholipid antibodies.

7. Pathophysiology of demyelinating disease

SLE may cause changes in both CNS and PNS myelin. The changes may relapse and remit, thereby mimicking attacks of Multiple Sclerosis(MS) like illnesses radiologically and clinically. It should be noted that the neuroimmunology of these conditions may differ substantially, and that the pathophysiology of both entities and the differences are not fully understood. The spectrum of radiological involvement can identify minor and non specific white matter changes to more confluent appearing lesions throughout the neuraxis. NPSLE pathophysiology may therefore mimic what are termed the clinically isolated syndromes of MS such as optic neuritis, transverse myelitis, and more wide spread pathology. A Devic-like syndrome in which there is optic neuritis and changes in the spinal cord is possible, and Devic's disease or Neuromyelitis Optica may be differentiated by the occurrence of NMO antibodies or the presence of antibodies to aquaporin 4 which are noted in Devic's disease.

8. The pathophysiology of seizures in NPSLE

Seizures occur in up to about 25% of patients with NPSLE compared with about 1% in the general population. Seizures may present early in the course of NPSLE. While focal seizures are postulated to be caused from microinfarcts that damage the cortex, systemic derangements and metabolic disturbances and certain medications may cause generalized seizures. Seizures are thought to result from cortical injury from cerebral vascultis, cardioembolism, or any lesion that may develop within the brain. The presence of cortical location and the presence of cortical hemorrhage or blood products generally increase the likelihood of seizures. The literature indicates that high dose steroid therapy given in pulses is associated with the development of status epilepticus by an unknown mechanism. Focal seizures may also become generalized seizures, and virtually any seizure type may be seen in SLE. Generalized or multifocal onset seizures are common in children with SLE and occur about 10 % of cases. While antiepileptic therapy is often prescribed, these medications do not generally treat what is thought to represent the underlying pathophysiology as the seizures may relate to ongoing inflammation that is somehow contributing to cortical irritability. Nonetheless, many patients are often managed in the short term with anti-seizure medications. Some authors suggest that anti-epileptic medication should be continued until a normal or benign EEG pattern is observed. No study on this however has been performed, and guidelines on how long anti-epileptic medication should continue are lacking. It should be noted that a benign or normal EEG may be seen in patients who have seizure disorders. EEG or EEG monitoring may be useful in patients who may be at risk or have ongoing subclinical status epilepticus during a fulminant NPSLE related encephalopathy but it is unknown if persistence of status epilepticus correlates with a certain type or subset of ongoing pathophsyiology of NPSLE in that circumstance. Treatment using antiseizure medications may be useful in an acute setting but these medications do not alter the direct pathophysiology of NPSLE. Since multiorgan failure may contribute to encephalopathy, electrolyte disturbances, or hypertension, treatment of these entities are necessary to gain control of the seizures that are provoked through those pathophysiologies in NPSLE. The author advises caution in diagnosing patients with first time seizures as idiopathic and in general such patients ought to be seen in follow up to ensure no other systemic or multiorgan involvement may be developing. It may be only in retrospective analysis that these patients might be diagnosed with NPSLE. The epidemiology and pathophysiology of these cases is unknown although the author has noted the subsequent onset of SLE or at least the fulfillment of SLE by clinical criteria over time in several such patients. Since NPSLE is a chronic disease, there may also be a need for lifetime prophylaxis with anti-seizure medications but trials and definitive guidelines on this are lacking, and anecdotally patients with epilepsy and NPSLE may be noted to be best controlled in general when the systemic SLE is controlled.

9. Psychiatric symptoms

Psychosis is common with NPSLE and steroids may accentuate clinical psychiatric features, although an although an associated cognitive disorder may be temporary or progressive. It may be difficult to distinguish corticosteroid induced encephalopathies with psychiatric symptoms from those of SLE. Since psychiatric symptoms may occur with numerous disease states, these symptoms combined with multisystem involvement of SLE are especially characteristic and may lead to diagnosis. The pathophysiology is unknown although depression and anxiety and psychiatric symptoms may be the initial symptoms of NPSLE. Combinations of depression, anxiety, progressive cognitive dysfunction, and encephalopathy are thought to be mediated by the previously noted mechanisms of chronic inflammation.

10. Vasculitis

Vasculitis in NPSLE often becomes a consideration in patient with autoimmune disease and in young patients with ischemic or hemorrhagic strokes. Patients often have an accompanying encephalopathy, fever, headaches, seizures, and cognitive changes. If there are multifocal levels of neurologic dysfunction, malar rash or palpable purpura present, or an abnormal urine sediment, then SLE as a clinical diagnosis may be likely.

Since angiography typically shows irregular beading and caliber changes of large and medium branches of the anterior, middle, and posterior cerebral arteries, it is believed that the major pathophysiolgy of vasculitis in NPSLE is due to this finding. While angiography may be positive, histology often shows degeneration within the walls of the smallest blood vessels, while more inflammatory mediators and infiltrates of such are noted in the medium and large vessels. Complete understanding of these mechanisms are being studied. There may ultimately be both inflammatory and non inflammatory processes involved. Aggressive treatment with intravenous steroids and immune modulators are required to treat this often fulminantly presenting, fatal or devastating process.

11. Pathophysiology of ischemic stroke in NPSLE

Ischemic stroke may result from cardiogenic embolism that is due to nonbacterial or from Libman-Sachs endocarditis which occurs on the ventricular or atrial surface of the mitral valve. The presence of antiphospholipid antibodies may also predispose to strokes and venous thrombosis as previously noted. Ischemic stroke in NPSLE occurs in children and is usually caused by small vessel vascultits. The literature indicates that stroke may occur in up to 10 % of pediatric series of NPSLE and occur by mechanisms noted above. Thrombotic strokes may present in a more evolving or subacute pattern often with premonitory symptoms, and ischemic ones generally present abruptly with deficits maximally present at onset.

Stroke should be clinically distinguished from hemorrhage and other CNS pathologies and hemorrhage may be likely in association with cardiac emboli or with cerebral venous thrombosis which can also present with seizures.

12. Pathophysiology of chorea in NPSLE

Chorea in NPSLE may precede systemic symptoms of SLE by about 1 year as some articles indicate and can resolve prior to the evolution of other symptoms or signs. The mechanism is unknown. In children, distinguishing this from Sydenham's chorea may be quite difficult since NPSLE may also falsely elevate serum antistreptococcal antibody titres which are characteristically seen in Sydenham's disease. Dopamine blockers such as haloperidol or chlorpromazine may be useful as well as aspirin or corticosteroids. The diagnosis may be made by finding the presence of lupus anticoagulant or with recurrent vascular thrombosis or spontaneous abortions in patients not meeting full criteria for diagnosis of SLE. Chorea in pregnancy (Chorea gravidarum) may also be a manifestation of NPSLE. A pattern of relapsing and remitting chorea of different intensities may suggest NPSLE.

13. Pathophysiology of fatigue in NPSLE

This has been described in the literature and it is suggested that many of such patients do not have evidence of muscle disease or myopathy. Therefore the mechanism is postulated to be due to brain or CNS dysfunction however further details about the pathophysiology is unknown. Depression, myopathy, sleep disorder, and systemic disease may need to be excluded. The literature indicates that chronic orthostatic hypotension should be excluded since this condition also may present with fatigue, although it is not known if infiltration of autonomic nerves in NPSLE is the causative pathophysiology which may actually predispose to orthostatic hypotension.

14. Cranial nerve involvement

Cranial nerve involvement is thought to be rare and transient, generally affecting cranial nerve III. Other cranial nerve involvement has been reported and although the mechanism of cranial neuropathy in NPSLE in general is not fully understood, the pathophysiology is thought to be due to vasculitic changes in the blood supply of the cranial nerves similar to that of a mononeuritis multiplex. While involvement of the nuclei or fasicles of the various cranial nerves is possible within the brain or brainstem, case series and pathologic correlates on this are lacking.

15. Pathophysiology of vision and migraine in NPSLE

The literature indicates that visual and migrainous disturbances occur bilaterally and late in the course of SLE. NPSLE is associated with retinal disease, optic neuritis, and migraine headaches. While the presence of an acute headache in NPSLE could ultimately simply be migraine, it is recommended that one should only make this diagnosis as a diagnosis of exclusion since other encephalopathies, opportunistic infections, meningitis or cerebritis, or venous thromboses or stroke may also present with headache and may occur in SLE.

16. Spinal cord involvement/myelopathy

While this is noted to occur, it is thought to occur rarely. Little literature is available. The author notes experience with patients who have had a fulminant course of CNS disease either from vasculitis or encephalopathy who may also have evidence of myelopathy develop. The mechanism on this and its relative rarity is not well understood. The literature indicates that spinal involvement and pathophysiology in NPSLE is often functionally devastating and may occur acutely, subacutely, or chronically. Syndromes involving a transverse myelitis type presentation, infarction, or the identification of a rapidly expanding type lesion have been described.

17. Peripheral nervous system involvement and neuromuscular disease

Peripheral manifestations of NPSLE involve progressive neropathy, myopathy, and diseases of the neuromuscular junction(NMJ). NPSLE affecting the NMJ may appear clinically similar to myasthenia gravis. Peripheral neuropathy is postulated to be caused by vasculitic injury to the blood supply of the nerves- the vasa nervorum - which as noted previously produces either a mononeuritis multiplex or a regionalized or more confluent, generalized apparent polyneuropathy. SLE may produc peripheral demyelination. Chronic demyelination can result in a chronic sensory or sensorimotor polyneuropathy. SLE acutely may exhibit pathophysiology present resembling acute inflammatory demyelinating polyradiculoneuropathy or (AIDP) and may mimic Guillian-Barre syndrome. Patients may present with burning or numbness sensations, usually starting distally and as disease progresses and as lesion burden accumulates on the peripheral nerves, more proximal involvement may become evident over time.

Myopathy may result from the inflammatory cascade and may mimic dermatomyositis or polymyositis. One also has to keep in mind that patients diagnosed with SLE may be on chronic steroid regimens. The pathophysiology of steroid regimens may contribute to muscle fiber atrophy without inflammatory infiltrates. Various medications may also contribute to pathophysiology of myopathy in NPSLE.

Distinguishing between neuromuscular disease and polyradiculopathy may be difficult, and EMG, CPK and aldolase testing, and muscle biopsies may be required. CPK/Creatine kinase and aldolase may be mildly elevated in SLE myopathy and may not be able to exclude other causes of myopathy for example from medications.

EMG and Nerve conduction studies(NCS) may provide useful clinical data. In an inflammatory myopathy which would be expected in cases of NPSLE, the EMG may be very active with fibrillations and positive sharp waves and simply may be a marker of muscle irritability. There may be increased insertional activity and myopathic motor units and recruitment abnormalities noted along with complex repetitive discharges. Caution is advised in evaluating patients on treatment for SLE with chronic immunosupression or steroids since a normal needle examination on EMG may be obtained despite the presence of disease and it is not known how much disease burden is required for this testing to be positive. Repetitive stimulation may be useful in evaluating neuromuscular junction failure or pathology which is rare but described in NPSLE. NCS may identify multiple nerves involved from mononeuritis multiplex, sensory or sensorimotor symmetric distal polyneuropathy, or AIDP (Acute Immune-mediated Demyelinating Polyradiculopathy). Abnormal F waves and H response abnormalities may indicate more proximal root dysfunction.

Nerve biopsy may be useful in identifying active vasculitis as pathology early in the clinical course this may be positive. In more indolent confluent polyneuropathies, there may simply be noted nonspecific demyelination. Muscle biopsy may be used to differentiate inflammatory from other causes of myopathy.

Nerve biopsies may identify inflammatory infiltrates, necrotizing vasculitis in epineurial arterioles or perivascular infiltrates. Immunoflorescence may be useful in identifying immune complexes or complement deposition onto vessel walls. Demyelination or nerve fiber count reduction may be noted.

In Summary, the pathophysiology of NPSLE is complex and mechanisms are at best only partly understood. Hopefully in the future, new developments along multiple lines will lead to a better understanding of the disease state which could lead to additional treatments.

18. References

[1] Adams and Victor's Principles of Neurology. Ropper AH et al. 7th-9th editions. McGraw-Hill.

[2] Merritt's Neurology- 12th Edition, Rowland and Pedley Editors. Lippincott Williams and Wilkins. Philadelphia, 2010.

[3] Harrison's Principles of Internal Medicine, 17th Edition. Kasper DL, Braunwald E, Fauci AS et al. New York:McGraw-Hill, 2008

[4] Neurology in Clinical Practice 5-6th editions. Bradley et al. Butterworth-Heinemann, 2007-2008.

[5] Johnson RT, Richardson EP. The neurological manifestations of systemic lupus erythematosus. Medicine (Baltimore) 1968 Jul;47(4):337–369.

[6] Richardson J. Systemic Lupus Erythematosus. Ulster Med J. 1969 Summer' 38(2): 157-66

[7] Joseph FG, Scolding NJ. Neurolupus. Practical Neurology 2010;10:4-15.

[8] Ellis SG, Verity MA. Central nervous system involvement in systemic lupus erythematosus: a review of neuropathologic findings in 57 cases, 1955–1977. *Semin Arthritis Rheum* 1979;8:212–21

[9] Joseph FG, Lammie GA, Scolding NJ. CNS lupus: a study of 41 patients. *Neurology* 2007;69:644–54.

17

Haematological Manifestations in Systemic Lupus Erythematosus

Nahid Janoudi and Ekhlas Samir Bardisi
KFSH&RC Jeddah
Saudi Arabia

1. Introduction

Systemic lupus erythematosus (SLE) is the most common multisystem connective tissue disease. It is characterised by a wide variety of clinical features and presence of numerous auto-antibodies, circulating immune complexes and widespread immunologically determined tissue damage [1]. Hematological abnormalities are common in SLE. All the cellular elements of the blood & coagulation pathway can be affected in SLE patients.

The major hematological manifestations of SLE are anemia, leucopenia, thrombocytopenia, and antiphospholipid syndrome (APS). Hematological abnormalities in patients with this disease require careful long-term monitoring and prompt therapeutic intervention.

Throughout the chapter we will analyze each abnormality, enumerate and explain the causes of each one and discuss an approach to the management.

2. Anemia in systemic lupus erythematosus

Anemia is found in about 50% of SLE patients, many mechanisms contribute to the development of anemia, including inflammation, renal insufficiency, blood loss, dietary insufficiency, medications, haemolysis, infection, hypersplenism, myelofibrosis, myelodysplasia, and aplastic anemia that is suspected to have an autoimmune pathogenesis [2-9] table 1.

2.1 Anemia of chronic disease

A frequent cause of anemia in SLE is suppressed erythropoiesis from chronic inflammation (anemia of chronic disease or anemia of chronic inflammation), being the most common form (60 to 80 %) [5]. this type of anemia is normocytic and normochromic with a relatively low reticulocyte count. Although serum iron levels may be reduced, bone marrow iron stores are adequate and the serum ferritin concentration is elevated. In the absence of either symptoms attributable to anemia (eg: dyspnea on exertion, easy fatigability) or renal insufficiency, anemia of chronic inflammation does not require specific treatment.

Patients with symptoms due to anemia of chronic inflammation, who have no other definite indication for glucocorticoid or other immunosuppressive therapy, may be given a trial of an agent that promotes erythropoiesis. The following two agents are an example:

Anemia of chronic disease
Blood loss
Gastrointestinal loss, menorrhagias
Nutritional deficiencies
Iron, folate, B12
Immune mediated
Haemolysis, red cell aplasia, haemophagocytosis, aplastic anaemia, pernicious anaemia
Myelofibrosis
Uremia
Treatment induced
Microangiopathic haemolysis
Disseminated intravascular coagulation, thrombotic thrombocytopenic purpura, drugs
Hypersplenism
Infection
Myelodysplasia

Table 1. Causes of anemia in patients with SLE

- Epoetin alfa (recombinant human erythropoietin)
- Darbepoetin alfa, a unique molecule that stimulates erythropoiesis with a longer half-life than recombinant human erythropoietin.

In one study that assessed the response to erythropoietin in patients with SLE and anemia of chronic inflammation, 58 percent had an adequate response to erythropoietin supplementation [7].

Patients who are symptomatically anemic, having signs of active inflammations, and do not respond to an agent that promotes erythropoiesis, often improve when glucocorticoids are used in high doses(1 mg/kg per day of prednisone or its equivalent in divided doses). If, after approximately one month of treatment, the response is unsatisfactory (eg, hemoglobin still <11 g/dL) the dose of glucocorticoids should be rapidly reduced, and discontinued if there is no other indication for their use. If there is a response, the dose should be tapered as rapidly as to possible to the lowest dose that maintains the improvement. Immunosuppressive agents also may help, but carry a risk of further bone marrow suppression.

2.2 Renal insufficiency

An inappropriately low level of erythropoietin is a hallmark of anemia due to renal insufficiency. The primary cause of anemia in this setting is typically deficient production of erythropoietin by the diseased kidneys. In the patient with SLE, anemia, and renal insufficiency who does not have other evidence of active inflammation, administration of erythropoiesis-stimulating agents may be indicated when the anemia is causing symptoms or the hemoglobin concentration is <11 gm/dL.

2.3 Iron deficiency anemia

Anemia may reflect acute or chronic blood loss from the gastrointestinal tract, usually secondary to medications (nonsteroidal antiinflammatory drugs or steroids), or may be due to excessive menstrual bleeding. Iron deficiency anemia is not uncommon, especially among teenagers or young women. Long-term anemia of chronic inflammation can also lead to iron deficiency, since, hepcidin, the key inducer of the anemia of chronic inflammation, inhibits iron absorption from the gastrointestinal tract.

Pulmonary hemorrhage is a rare cause of anemia in SLE. Not all patients have hemoptysis. Other symptoms of alveolar hemorrhage are dyspnea and cough. The presence of alveolar infiltrates on a chest radiograph or ground-glass opacities on chest CT are suggestive of alveolar hemorrhage.

2.4 Red cell aplasia

Red cell aplasia, probably due to antibodies directed against either erythropoietin or bone marrow erythroblasts, has been observed, although it is rare [5,6,10]. This form of anemia usually responds to steroids, although cyclophosphamide and cyclosporine have been successfully employed.

Even rarer are isolated case reports of aplastic anemia, presumably mediated by auto antibodies against bone marrow precursors; immunosuppressive therapy also may be effective in this setting [11-13].

In addition, bone marrow suppression can also be induced by medications, including antimalarials and immunosuppressive drugs.

2.5 Autoimmune hemolytic anemia

Overt autoimmune hemolytic anemia (AIHA), characterized by an elevated reticulocyte count, low haptoglobin levels, increased indirect bilirubin concentration, and a positive direct Coombs' test, has been noted in up to 10 percent of patients with SLE [2-4,8,14]. The presence of hemolytic anemia may be associated with other manifestations of severe disease such as renal disease, seizures, and serositis [14].

Other patients have a positive Coombs' test without evidence of overt hemolysis. The presence of both immunoglobulin and complement on the red cell is usually associated with some degree of hemolysis, while the presence of complement alone (eg, C3 and/or C4) is often not associated with hemolysis [1-4].

AIHA responds to steroids (1 mg/kg per day of prednisone or its equivalent in divided doses) in 75 to 96 percent of patients [15, 16]. Once the hematocrit begins to rise and the reticulocyte count falls, steroids can be rapidly tapered. If there is no response, we can consider pulse steroids (eg,1000 mg methylprednisolone intravenously daily for three days) [15], azathioprine (up to 2 mg/kg per day) [17], cyclophosphamide (up to 2 mg/kg) [18], or splenectomy. Success rates for splenectomy as high as 60 percent have been reported [19], although others have found no benefit [20].

Other described approaches to patients with refractory AIHA include intravenous immune globulin [18], danazol [21-23], mycophenolate mofetil [24], and rituximab [25].

2.6 Microangiopathic hemolytic anemia

Lupus has also been associated with a thrombotic microangiopathic hemolytic anemia [26] as manifested by a peripheral blood smear showing schistocytes and elevated serum levels of lactate dehydrogenase (LDH) and bilirubin. Many affected patients also have thrombocytopenia, kidney involvement, fever, and neurologic symptoms. This pentad of features is compatible with a diagnosis of thrombotic thrombocytopenic purpura (TTP). However, the pathogenesis of TTP in these patients is likely heterogeneous, as it may reflect vasculitis or antiphospholipid syndrome as well [27, 28].

Whether the occurrence of both SLE and TTP in an individual patient is a coincidence or represents a true association is an unsettled question.

Other patients with microangiopathic red cell destruction do not have fever or neurologic disease, producing a pattern of hemolytic-uremic syndrome. The pathogenesis of this syndrome is not completely understood. In one report of 4 patients plus 24 others identified from a literature review, antiphospholipid antibodies (aPL) were searched for in eight and found in five [26].

The presence of aPL in SLE patients with severe hemolytic anemia, renal dysfunction, and central nervous system involvement has also been reported [31].

In a review of 28 reported patients, those treated with plasma infusions or plasmapheresis, glucocorticoids alone, or no therapy had mortality rates of 25, 50, and 100 percent, respectively [26]. However, in another series of 15 patients with SLE and microangiopathic hemolytic anemia, all responded to treatment with high-dose glucocorticoids and none were treated with plasmapheresis [32]. In a retrospective study [27] in which 70 percent of patients with SLE and TTP underwent plasma exchange, the response rate of 74 percent was comparable to that observed in patients with idiopathic TTP.

Patients with SLE, severe microangiopathic hemolytic anemia, and other major organ dysfunction should be treated with plasmapheresis and plasma infusion as in other cases of thrombotic thrombocytopenic purpura or the hemolytic-uremic syndrome. Those with less severe disease may be treated with high-dose glucocorticoids and observed carefully with the addition of plasmapheresis should they deteriorate or fail to improve with steroid treatment alone.

3. An approach to lupus patient with anaemia

After the detailed analysis and discussion of each type of anemia associated with SLE, here is a simple approach to anemic SLE patient with an easy mechanism to the diagnosis.

Anaemia can be divided into those conditions with impaired red cell production (marrow suppression, nutrient deficiency) and those with increased red cell destruction (haemolysis, hypersplenism) or blood loss. Measurement of reticulocyte production (reticulocyte index) usually used to make this distinction and it is the major step for determination of causes of anaemia. IDA is defined by serum ferritin level below: 20 µg/dl. Pernicious anemia (PA) is defined by serum vitamin B12 of less than: 180 pmol/l together with one or more of the following: an abnormal Schilling test result or the presence of anti-intrinsic factor antibody in the blood.

It is also important to mention that the examination of the peripheral blood smear is a mandatory step in the initial evaluation of all SLE patients with hematologic disorders. The examination of blood films stained with Wright's stain frequently provides important clues in the diagnosis of anemias and various disorders of leukocytes and platelets and we can discover a life threatening conditions like TTP early on. For example, some of the abnormalities suspicious for the presence of hemolysis in blood smear include the following:

- Spherocytes (microspherocytes and elliptocytes) indicate autoimmune hemolytic anemia
- Fragmented RBC (schistocytes, helmet cells) indicating the presence of microangiopathic hemolytic anemia (thrombotic thrombocytopenic purpura-hemolytic uremic syndrome)
- Acanthocytes (spur cells) in patients with liver disease.
- Blister or "bite" cells due to the presence of oxidant-induced damage to the red cell and its membrane (G-6-PD).
- RBCs with inclusions, as in malaria, babesiosis, and Bartonella infections (" non-immune hemolytic anemia due to systemic disease", ").
- Teardrop RBCs with circulating nucleated RBC and early white blood cell forms, indicating the presence of marrow involvement, as in primary myelofibrosis or tumor infiltration.

So at a practical level, when you are faced with SLE anaemia, it will be easy to differentiate among the possible mechanisms with only a few tests. If the reticulocytes are increased, a haemolytic process or acute bleeding should be the probable cause. If the reticulocytes are inadequate, you should rule out a nutritional deficiency of iron, vitamin B12, or folate. Ferritin determination suffices for diagnosing IDA. If the ferritin concentration is greater than 20 µg/dl, IDA is virtually never present and a bone marrow examination may be considered, but we have to mention that ferritin is an acute phase reactant and it can be elevated in any patients with inflammatory process due to any cause, although the diagnostic yield may be very low and anaemia of chronic disease is the most common diagnosis of exclusion (figure 1).

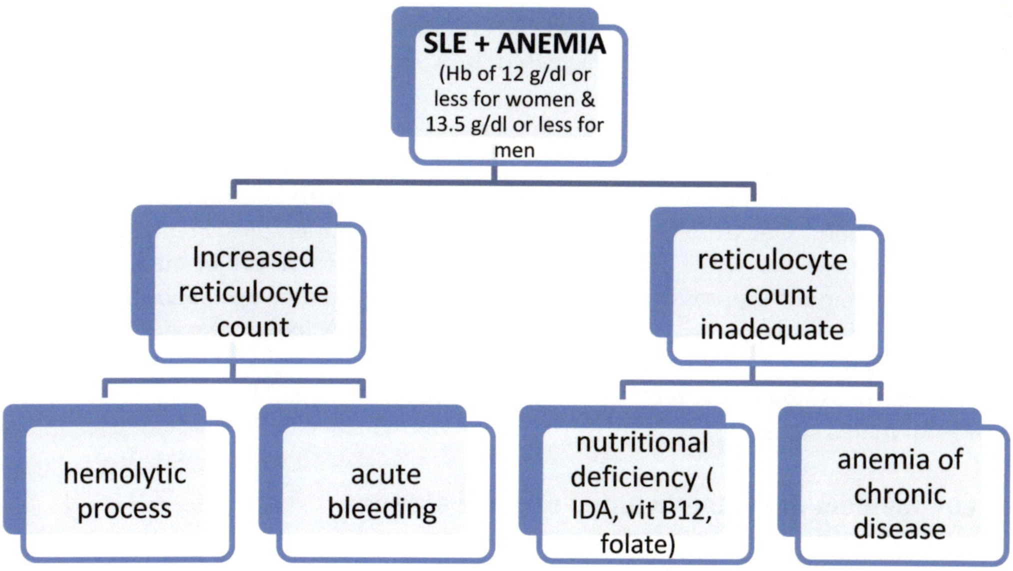

Fig. 1.

4. Leukopenia in systemic lupus erythematosus

Leukopenia is common in SLE and usually reflects disease activity. A white blood cell count of less than 4500/microL has been noted in approximately 50 percent of patients, especially those with active disease [3, 4], while lymphocytopenia occurs in approximately 20 percent [3]. In comparison, a white blood cell count below 4000/microL (an American College of Rheumatology criterion for SLE) occurs in only 15 to 20 percent of patients [3, 33]. Neutropenia, lymphocytopenia, and decreased circulating eosinophils and basophils may all contribute to leukopenia.

4.1 Neutropenia

Neutropenia in patients with SLE can result from: immune mechanisms, medications (eg, cyclophosphamide or azathioprine), bone marrow dysfunction, or hypersplenism [3,4,33,34]. Other clinical features that may be associated with moderate to severe neutropenia (absolute neutrophils <1000/microL) include infection, anemia, thrombocytopenia, and a history of neuropsychiatric involvement [34].

4.2 Lymphocytopenia

Lymphocytopenia (lymphocytes less than 1500/microL), especially involving suppressor T cells, has been observed in 20 to 75 percent of patients, particularly during active disease [1-3, 37, 38]. This finding is strongly associated with IgM, cold reactive, complement fixing, and presumably cytotoxic antilymphocyte antibodies; such antibodies were noted in 26 of 29 patients with SLE and the antibody titer correlated directly with the degree of lymphopenia [39].

4.3 Decreased eosinophils and basophils

Steroid therapy may result in low absolute eosinophil and monocyte counts [41]. The number of basophils may also be decreased in SLE, particularly during active disease [42].

4.4 Leukopenia

In SLE rarely needs treatment. An exception is the patient with neutropenia and recurrent pyogenic infections. One problem is the toxicity of the usual therapies. Prednisone (10 to 60 mg/day) can raise the white blood cell count but can also result in an increased risk of infections; immunosuppressive agents such as azathioprine or cyclophosphamide have the potential to cause worsening of the leukopenia via bone marrow suppression, respectively [43].

Cautious use of azathioprine, with careful monitoring of the white blood cell count, may be considered in this setting.

5. Leukocytosis in systemic lupus erythematosus

Leukocytosis (mostly granulocytes) can occur in SLE. When present, it is usually due to infection or the use of high doses of glucocorticoids [43], but may occur during acute exacerbations of SLE. A shift of granulocytes to more immature forms (a "left" shift) suggests infection.

6. Thrombocytopenia in systemic lupus erythematosus

Mild thrombocytopenia (platelet counts between 100,000 and 150,000/microL) has been noted in 25 to 50 percent of patients; while counts of less than 50,000/microL occur in only 10 percent [1, 3,4,33]. There are several potential causes of thrombocytopenia in patients with SLE. Immune mediated platelet destruction is most often the cause, but platelet consumption may also occur in association with microangiopathic hemolytic anemia (see 'Microangiopathic hemolytic anemia' above) or could be due to impaired platelet production as a result of the use of cytotoxic, immunosuppressive, or other drugs.

The major mechanism is immunoglobulin binding to platelets followed by phagocytosis in the spleen, as in idiopathic thrombocytopenic purpura (ITP) [47]. Membrane glycoproteins (GP) are most often the target of such antibodies (eg, GP IIb/IIIa) but anti-HLA specificity also occurs [48].

Antigen-dependent B cell development in lymphoid tissues is influenced by binding of CD40 on B cells to CD40-ligand on activated T cells. The finding of autoantibodies to CD40-ligand in patients with SLE, APS, and ITP, but not in the serum of healthy blood donors suggests that interference with T cell and B cell interaction may play a role in the development of thrombocytopenia [49].

Other important mechanisms in selected patients include bone marrow suppression by immunosuppressive drugs (other than corticosteroids), increased consumption due to a thrombotic thrombocytopenic purpura [TTP] [26], the antiphospholipid syndrome, or antibodies that block the thrombopoietin receptor on megakaryocytes or their precursors.

ITP may be the first sign of SLE, followed by other symptoms as long as many years later. It has been estimated that 3 to 15 percent of patients with apparently isolated ITP go on to develop SLE [50].

Evans syndrome (ie, both autoimmune thrombocytopenia and autoimmune hemolytic anemia) also may precede the onset of SLE. Severe bleeding from thrombocytopenia is only experienced by a minority of patients; however, SLE patients with thrombocytopenia are more likely to have associated significant organ damage, such as heart and kidneys and the CNS [51].

6.1 Medical therapy

Platelet counts between 50,000/microL and 20,000/microL rarely cause more than a prolonged bleeding time, while counts of less than 20,000/microL may be associated with petechiae, purpura, ecchymoses, epistaxis, gingival, and other clinical bleeding.

Treatment of thrombocytopenia is usually recommended for symptomatic patients with counts of less than 50,000/microL and for all patients with counts of less than 20,000/microL.

The treatment of ITP in SLE is the same as that in patients without lupus.

Briefly, the mainstay of treatment is glucocorticoid therapy. Older studies used prednisone (1 mg/kg per day in divided doses) [54, 55]. However, treatment with four to eight cycles of oral high dose dexamethasone (40 mg per day for four days) at intervals of two weeks to four weeks may result in similar remission rates and better long-term responses than those observed in historical controls treated with daily prednisone [56].

Most patients respond to glucocorticoid therapy within one to eight weeks [57]. If there is no significant increase in the platelet count within one to three weeks or side effects are intolerable, the following options may be considered and used depends upon the severity of the thrombocytopenia and the presence or absence of other manifestations of SLE:

- Azathioprine
- Cyclophosphamide [58].
- Intravenous immune globulin is very effective and may be preferred to azathioprine or cyclophosphamide when a rapid rise in platelet count is necessary (as in the patient who is actively bleeding or requires emergent surgery) [59].
- Mycophenolate mofetil may be useful in the patient refractory to other medical therapy [60].
- Rituximab has been used to treat ITP in patients without SLE who were refractory to other treatments and this B lymphocyte depleting approach may be beneficial for other manifestations of lupus [25].

6.2 Splenectomy

Splenectomy can raise the platelet count but it does not reliably produce a durable remission of thrombocytopenia. Relapse following splenectomy may occur and has been noted at varying times from 1 to 54 months after surgery [62].

6.3 Thrombocytopenia following splenectomy

Patients with persistent thrombocytopenia after splenectomy may subsequently respond to azathioprine, cyclophosphamide, rituximab, intravenous immunoglobulin, or danazol [23,63,64]. If possible, splenectomy should be preceded by immunization with pneumococcal vaccine to reduce the risk of pneumococcal sepsis.

7. Thrombocytosis in systemic lupus erythematosus

Thrombocytosis is a less frequent finding in patients with SLE and it might be occurring as an acute phase reactant and a sign of active disease.

8. Pancytopenia in systemic lupus erythematosus

Although peripheral destruction of red cells, leukocytes, and platelets may occur together and lead to clinically significant pancytopenia, depression of all three cell lines also suggests bone marrow failure, as in the case in aplastic anemia. Thus, bone marrow examination is the most important diagnostic test to perform.

Causes of marrow failure include drugs and coincidental diseases including: the acute leukemias, large granular lymphocyte leukemia, the myelodysplastic syndromes, marrow replacement by fibrosis or tumor, severe megaloblastic anemia, paroxysmal nocturnal hemoglobinuria (PNH), and overwhelming infection. In addition, unexplained cytopenia can be associated with bone marrow necrosis, dysplasia, and distortion of the bone marrow architecture [70].

Among patients with SLE an unusual cause of pancytopenia is the **macrophage activation syndrome**. The clinical characteristics of 12 patients with SLE-associated macrophage activation syndrome included [71]:

Fever (100%), weight loss (80%), arthritis (50%), pericarditis (42%), rash (66%) myocarditis (33%), nephritis (33%), splenomegaly (27%), hepatomegaly (13%), lymphadenopathy(73%), anemia (100%), leukopenia (87%), hyperferritinemia (100%), anti-DNA antibodies (80%),low CRP (<30 mg/L) (90%), hypocomplementemia (60%).

The demonstration of hemophagocytosis in the bone marrow or in material obtained from peripheral lymph nodes is a characteristic finding.
The few reported cases of macrophage activation syndrome in patients with SLE have usually responded to treatment with glucocorticoids and immunosuppressive agents. Optimal treatment is uncertain.

9. Lymphadenopathy and splenomegaly in systemic lupus erythematosus

Enlargement of lymph nodes occurs in approximately 50 percent of patients with SLE. The nodes are typically soft, nontender, discrete, varying in size from 0.5 to several centimeters, and usually detected in the cervical, axillary, and inguinal areas. Lymphadenopathy is more frequently noted at the onset of disease or in association with an exacerbation. Biopsies reveal areas of follicular hyperplasia and necrosis, the appearance of hematoxylin bodies is highly suggestive of SLE, although unusual [1].
Lymph node enlargement can also be due to infection or a lymphoproliferative disease in SLE. When infections are present, the enlarged nodes are more likely to be tender.
Prominent lymphadenopathy may also be a manifestation of **angioimmunoblastic T cell lymphoma**. This disorder has other clinical features (arthritis, Coombs-positive hemolytic anemia, skin rash, fever, and weight loss) that are suggestive of systemic lupus erythematosus or systemic onset juvenile rheumatoid arthritis (Still's disease). Enlargement of the spleen occurs in 10 to 46 percent of patients, particularly during active disease. Splenomegaly is not necessarily associated with a cytopenia. Pathologic examination of spleen reveals an onion skin appearance of the splenic arteries, a lesion that is thought to represent healed vasculitis.
In view of the frequent presence of lymphadenopathy and splenomegaly in SLE, the possibility of a **lymphoproliferative malignancy** may be considered. The risk of non-Hodgkin lymphoma appears to be increased four- to five fold in patients with lupus.
A lymph node biopsy may be warranted when the degree of lymphadenopathy is out of proportion to the activity of the lupus.
One of the rare diseases that reported to be associated with SLE is:

9.1 Kikuchi-Fujimoto's disease (KFD)

Also called histiocytic necrotizing lymphadenitis which is a rare benign and self limited disease, of unknown etiology, affects mainly young women [77]. It presents with localized lymphadenopathy, predominantly in the cervical region, less commonly include axillary and mesenteric lymphadenopathy accompanied by fever and leucopenia in up to 50% of the cases [78, 79]. KFD has been reported in association with systemic lupus erythematosus (SLE), the relation between Kikuchi's disease and SLE is not yet completely understood and remains complex. The reports imply that SLE may be present before, at the same time, or after the clinical appearance of KFD [77-79].
KFD can be a complication of prolonged and multiple immunosuppressant use in SLE patients, There is a published case report in 2011 of KFD that diagnosed based on a lymph node biopsy in a 31 year old Saudi female patient with an established diagnosis of stage IV lupus nephritis. She presented with fever, axillary lymphadenopathy and neutropenia. The patient is known to have SLE for 16 years prior to the presentation with history of prolonged use of many immunosuppressive medications. The patient treated with intravenous antibiotic as a case of febrile neutropenia and recovered spontaneously. They

concluded that in most of the cases the diagnosis of KFD was made before or at the same time of the diagnosis of SLE. In this case report the diagnosis of KFD was made years after the diagnosis of SLE. They also noted that the patient received prolonged courses of immunosuppressant medications including mycophenolate mofetil, and then 6 cycles of cyclophosphamide, she was placed then on azothioprine and hydroxychloroquine. So they consider the prolonged use of immunosuppressant medications a risk factor for KFD in a well established SLE with lupus nephritis.

10. Antibodies to clotting factors and anti-phospholipids syndrome in systemic lupus erythematosus

Antibodies to a number of clotting factors, including VIII, IX, XI, XII, and XIII have been noted in patients with SLE [1,2,33]. These antibodies may not only cause abnormalities of in vitro coagulation tests but may also cause bleeding.

Much more common are aPL (antiphospholipid antibodies), the presence of which has been associated with a prolongation of the partial thromboplastin time (PTT) (lupus anticoagulant activity) and an increased risk of arterial and venous thrombosis, thrombocytopenia, and fetal loss [72, 73]. Antibodies to other phospholipids and to phospholipid binding proteins (eg, anticardiolipin antibodies) in moderate or high levels may also be associated with these clinical phenomena. When aPL occurs in association with one or more of these clinical features in a patient with SLE it suggests the presence of the APS.

10.1 Antiphospholipid syndrome

The antiphospholipid syndrome (APS) is defined by two major components:

1. The occurrence of at least one clinical feature: vascular event or pregnancy morbidity AND
2. The presence of at least one type of autoantibody known as an antiphospholipid antibody (aPL).

In addition, there are aPL-related clinical manifestations that are not part of the APS Classification Criteria, such as livedo reticularis, thrombocytopenia, cardiac valve disease, or aPL-nephropathy.

APL is directed against serum proteins bound to anionic phospholipids and may be detected by a: Lupus anticoagulant tests, Anticardiolipin antibody ELISA and Anti-ß2 glycoprotein-I ELISA.

The full clinical significance of other autoantibodies, including those directed against prothrombin, annexin V, phosphatidylserine, and phosphatidylinositol, remain unclear.

APS occurs as a primary condition or in the setting of an underlying systemic autoimmune disease, particularly SLE [72].

- **Classification criteria** have been developed for research purposes. They may be helpful to clinicians, but not all the classification criteria need to be met to make a clinical diagnosis of APS.

Definite APS is considered present if at least one of the following clinical criteria and at least one of the following laboratory criteria are satisfied:

- Clinical: one or more episodes of venous, arterial, or small vessel thrombosis and/or morbidity with pregnancy.

- Thrombosis: unequivocal imaging or histological evidence of thrombosis in any tissue or organ, OR
- Pregnancy morbidity : otherwise unexplained death at ≥10 weeks gestation of a morphologically normal fetus, OR
- One or more premature births before 34 weeks of gestation because of eclampsia, preeclampsia, or placental insufficiency, OR
- Three or more embryonic (<10 week gestation) pregnancy losses unexplained by maternal or paternal chromosomal abnormalities or maternal anatomic or hormonal causes.
- Laboratory : the presence of aPL, on two or more occasions at least 12 weeks apart and no more than five years prior to clinical manifestations, as demonstrated by one or more of the following: IgG and/or IgM aCL in moderate or high titer), antibodies to ß2-GP-I of IgG or IgM isotype at a high titer. LA activity detected according to published guidelines [72, 75].

10.1.1 Pathology

The characteristic pathologic finding in the APS is a bland thrombosis with minimal vascular or perivascular inflammation. This change is not specific for the APS, as it also occurs in the kidney in a variety of other disorders including the hemolytic-uremic syndrome/thrombotic thrombocytopenic purpura, systemic sclerosis (scleroderma), and malignant hypertension. Larger vessels, both arteries and veins, may develop in situ thrombosis or be sites from or into which emboli originate or lodge.

10.1.2 Clinically

- The APS is characterized by venous or arterial thromboses, morbidity occurring in the setting of pregnancy, and/or aPL-related clinical manifestations that are not part of the APS Classification Criteria, such as livedo reticularis, thrombocytopenia, cardiac valve disease, or aPL-nephropathy [73, 74].

In a series of 1000 patients with either primary or secondary APS, the various disease features were [74]:

Deep vein thrombosis (32%), Thrombocytopenia (22%), Livedo reticularis (20%), Stroke (13%), Superficial thrombophlebitis (9%), Pulmonary embolism (9%), Fetal loss (8 %), TIA (7%), Hemolytic anemia (7%).

In rare patients, APS results in multi-organ failure because of multiple blood vessel occlusions, a condition referred to as "catastrophic antiphospholipid syndrome".

In addition to those already mentioned above, other possible aPL-related clinical manifestations include migraine headache, Reynaud phenomenon, pulmonary hypertension, avascular necrosis, cutaneous ulcers that resemble pyoderma gangrenosum, adrenal insufficiency due to hemorrhagic infarction, and cognitive deficits [72-75].

- **Thrombosis**: the risk of both venous and arterial thrombosis and/or thromboembolism is increased in individuals with positive tests for LA activity or medium or high levels of aCL. The risk of recurrent thrombosis or thromboembolism may be further enhanced in those with positivity to three aPL activities (LA, aCL, and ß2-glycoprotein-I) upon repeated testing [74].

Initial site: venous thromboses are more common than arterial thromboses in the APS [73, 74]. The most common site of DVT is the calf, but the renal veins, the hepatic, axillary, subclavian, and retinal veins, the cerebral sinuses, and the vena cava may also be involved. The most common site of arterial thrombosis is the cerebral vessels, but coronary, renal, and mesenteric arteries and arterial bypass graft occlusions have also been noted.

To some degree, the site of thrombosis may be related to the type of aPL present. This was illustrated in a retrospective study of 637 patients with APS in which DVT and PE were more frequent among patients with LA, while coronary, cerebrovascular, and peripheral arterial events were more likely in those with elevated levels of IgG or IgM aCL.

- **Deep venous thrombosis**: APL can be detected in approximately 5 to 21 percent of all patients with DVT [72]. The incidence of DVT may correlate with the level of aCL. As an example, one study found that DVT occurred in 44% of patients with high titers of aCL, in 29% with low titers, and in only 10% of those without these antibodies [73].

Stroke: the APS is strongly linked to ischemic stroke [74, 80]. The occurrence of livedo reticularis in association with a stroke is known as **Sneddon's syndrome** [73]. In the great majority of cases, Sneddon's syndrome is associated with detectable aPL.

A thrombotic stroke occurring in a young patient with no overt risk factors for cerebrovascular disease is the classic setting to suspect the APS. In one study, aPL was found in 25% of patients younger than 45 years of age who presented with a stroke of unclear etiology [81]. In another report, 20 percent of stroke victims under the age of 50 had aPL [74]. Ischemic stroke may be a manifestation in situ thrombosis or due to embolism arising from a valvular heart disease. If routine transthoracic echocardiography is normal, transesophageal echo may be indicated to assess for vegetations due to nonbacterial endocarditis.

Several studies have evaluated the risk of stroke associated with the presence of aPL:

In a review of 2000 healthy male subjects, the relative risk of stroke at 15 years of follow-up was 2.2 in subjects with aPL []. Events were observed primarily in subjects who had both ß2-GP-I and IgG aCL (ie, ß2-GP-I dependent aCL).

In the Stroke Prevention in Young Women study, the presence of LAs and aCL was evaluated in 160 cases and 340 controls [74]. After adjustment for potential confounders, the relative odds of stroke for women with an aCL of any isotype or an LA was 1.87 (95% CI 1.2 to 2.8). Similar findings of an increased risk of ischemic stroke associated with aCL limited to women were noted in a report from the Framingham Cohort and Offspring Study (hazard ratio for women 2.6; 95% CI 1.3 to 5.4) [73].

Neurologic syndromes besides stroke: strong associations are now recognized between the presence of aPL and the occurrence of cognitive deficits and/or white matter lesions. However, the link with the APS is less strong for other neurological associations.

White matter lesions: see chapter of neurology in SLE.

Other neurological associations: epilepsy, depression, psychosis, chorea and hemiballismus, transverse myelopathy, sensorineural hearing loss, orthostatic hypotension, migraine.

Recurrent thrombotic events: are common in APS. Most but not all observers have noted that an initial arterial thrombosis tends to be followed by an arterial event, and that an initial venous thrombosis is usually followed by a venous event [72].

Pregnancy loss and preeclampsia: the presence of APS may be related to several types of morbidity during pregnancy. These include fetal death after 10 weeks gestation, premature birth due to severe preeclampsia or placental insufficiency, or multiple embryonic losses (<10 weeks gestation).

In patients with preeclampsia or HELLP syndrome, the possibility of the catastrophic APS must be considered, particularly in patients with histories of thrombosis or spontaneous abortions [73].

Hematologic manifestations: prominent hematologic manifestations of APS include thrombocytopenia, microangiopathic hemolytic anemia and, in rare cases, bleeding:

Thrombocytopenia: a review of 13 studies of 869 patients with SLE, found that thrombocytopenia was more common in those with LA (55 percent) and aCL (29 PERCENT) than in those without these antibodies [50]. Conversely, patients with thrombocytopenia associated with autoimmune disorders frequently have aPL (eg, 70 to 82 percent of patients with SLE and thrombocytopenia, and 30 to 40 percent of those with ITP [26, 49, 50].

Thrombotic microangiopathy: APL has been implicated in some cases of TTP/HUS that occur in SLE. See hematological manifestations in SLE.

Bleeding episodes: the presence of antibodies to prothrombin should be suspected when a patient with a known LA also has a low prothrombin level and develops bleeding complications rather than thrombosis.

Pulmonary disease: pulmonary embolism occurs in approximately one-third of patients with the APS who develop DVT. Other recognized pulmonary complications of the APS include [26, 48-50]: Pulmonary arterial thrombosis with or without thromboembolic pulmonary hypertension and alveolar hemorrhage.

In addition, fibrosing alveolitis, adult respiratory distress syndrome, and nonthromboembolic pulmonary hypertension have been reported in association with aPL [50, 72]. However, the relationship to these disorders to aPL is unclear

Cardiovascular disease: patients with aPL commonly have cardiac disease, including valvular thickening, mitral valve nodules, and nonbacterial vegetations. Involvement of the mitral and aortic valves can lead to valvular regurgitation and rarely to stenosis.

APL have also been incriminated in intracardiac thrombi, pericardial effusion, cardiomyopathy, emboli in those with or without infective endocarditis, premature restenosis of vein grafts for coronary bypass, and peripheral vascular disease [50].

Cutaneous: APL has been associated with many cutaneous abnormalities including splinter hemorrhages, livedo reticularis, cutaneous necrosis and infarction, [49, 50].

Gastrointestinal disease: patients with aPL may have ischemia involving the esophagus, stomach, duodenum, jejunum, ileum, or colon resulting in gastrointestinal bleeding, abdominal pain, an acute abdomen, esophageal necrosis with perforation, or giant gastric or atypical duodenal ulceration [73]. Splenic or pancreatic infarction may also occur. In addition, the liver may involved; hepatic or portal venous thrombosis may result in the Budd-Chiari syndrome, hepatic-veno-occlusive disease, hepatic infarction, portal hypertension, and cirrhosis. [72].

Ocular manifestations: amaurosis fugax, retinal venous and arterial occlusion, and anterior ischemic optic neuropathy have occurred in patients with aPL [72].

Catastrophic APS: a small subset of patients with APS has widespread thrombotic disease with multiorgan failure, which is called "catastrophic APS." Preliminary criteria proposed for classification .purposes have been published and validated (Among 1000 patients with the APS followed for a mean of seven years, only 8 (0.8 percent) developed catastrophic APS [73, 74]. In the majority of these patients, multiorgan involvement was present at the time of diagnosis of APS.

Patients with catastrophic APS may have laboratory features such as elevated fibrin degradation products, depressed fibrinogen levels, or elevated D-dimer concentrations that are more typically found with disseminated intravascular coagulation (DIC).

Catastrophic APS is frequently fatal, with a reported mortality rate approaching 50 percent despite anticoagulant and immunosuppressive treatment [74].

10.1.3 Primary APS versus SLE

The antiphospholipid syndrome was first described as a complication of the disease 'SLE'. However, in many cases - indeed probably the vast majority did **NOT** have any evidence of lupus. This gave rise to the term 'Primary Antiphospholipid Syndrome' (PAPS). For those patients where the clotting tendency is secondary to another disease such as lupus, the condition is often called 'Secondary Anitphospholipid Syndrome'. It should be stressed that the majority of patients with 'Primary' APS (Hughes Syndrome) do **NOT** go on to develop lupus in later life. The inter-relationship between lupus and APS (Hughes Syndrome) is highlighted in this diagram below:

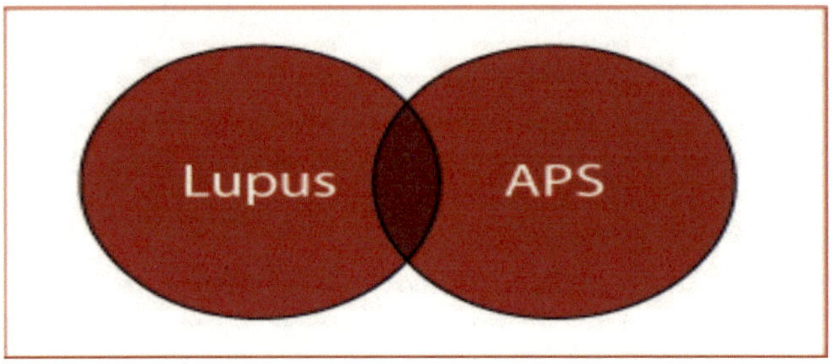

some data suggest that the clinical manifestations of primary APS and APS associated with SLE are similar [73]. In contrast, a subsequent study of 122 patients noted that the frequency of arterial thromboses, venous thromboses, and fetal loss was greater in patients with APS and SLE than in those with primary APS [72].

A separate issue is the frequency of evolution of APS into SLE or lupus-like disease. Three studies involving 70 to 128 patients with APS found a variable rate of development of SLE over time:

Zero percent at five years, 4 percent at 6.5 years, 13 percent at nine years.

10.1.4 Mortality

The presence of aPL in the serum of patients with SLE has been identified as an independent risk factor for premature death. There was an increased risk of premature death in patients with aPL, thrombocytopenia, and arterial occlusion. Other factors associated with premature death were the intensity of anticoagulation treatment, renal involvement, pleuritis, and disease activity.

10.1.5 Management and recommendation

Current therapies for the APS include the following medications: low molecular weight heparin , unfractionated heparin, warfarin, antiplatelet agents, aspirin , clopidogrel, hydroxychloroquine **(see below).**

Initial approach to thrombosis:

treatment for venous thromboembolic disease is part of the American Colleuge of Chest Physicians (ACCP) Evidence-Based Clinical Practice Guidelines (8th Edition), as the following: for patients with objectively confirmed deep vein thrombosis (DVT) or pulmonary embolism (PE), we recommend anticoagulant therapy with subcutaneous (SC) low-molecular-weight heparin (LMWH), monitored IV, or SC unfractionated heparin (UFH), unmonitored weight-based SC UFH, or SC fondaparinux (all Grade 1A). For patients with a high clinical suspicion of DVT or PE, we recommend treatment with anticoagulants while awaiting the outcome of diagnostic tests (Grade 1C).

For patients with confirmed PE, we recommend early evaluation of the risks to benefits of thrombolytic therapy (Grade 1C); for those with hemodynamic compromise, we recommend short-course thrombolytic therapy (Grade 1B); and for those with nonmassive PE, we recommend against the use of thrombolytic therapy (Grade 1B).

In acute DVT or PE, we recommend initial treatment with LMWH, UFH or fondaparinux for at least 5 days rather than a shorter period (Grade 1C); and initiation of vitamin K antagonists (VKAs) together with LMWH, UFH, or fondaparinux on the first treatment day, and discontinuation of these heparin preparations when the international normalized ratio (INR) is > or = 2.0 for at least 24 h (Grade 1A).

For patients with DVT or PE secondary to a transient (reversible) risk factor, we recommend treatment with a VKA for 3 months over treatment for shorter periods (Grade 1A). For patients with unprovoked DVT or PE, we recommend treatment with a VKA for at least 3 months (Grade 1A), and that all patients are then evaluated for the risks to benefits of indefinite therapy (Grade 1C).

We recommend indefinite anticoagulant therapy for patients with a first unprovoked proximal DVT or PE and a low risk of bleeding when this is consistent with the patient's preference (Grade 1A), and for most patients with a second unprovoked DVT (Grade 1A). We recommend that the dose of VKA be adjusted to maintain a target INR of 2.5 (INR range, 2.0 to 3.0) for all treatment durations (Grade 1A).

For prevention of post-thrombotic syndrome (PTS) after proximal DVT, we recommend use of an elastic compression stocking (Grade 1A). For DVT of the upper extremity, we recommend similar treatment as for DVT of the leg (Grade 1C). Selected patients with lower-extremity (Grade 2B) and upper-extremity (Grade 2C). DVT may be considered for thrombus removal, generally using catheter-based thrombolytic techniques. For extensive superficial vein thrombosis, we recommend treatment with prophylactic or intermediate doses of LMWH or intermediate doses of UFH for 4 weeks (Grade 1B).

The optimal duration of anticoagulation for venous thromboembolic disease following a first event is uncertain. However, given the high likelihood of recurrence in the untreated patient and the potentially devastating nature of recurrent thromboembolic events, we recommend lifelong anticoagulation for patients with the APS (**Grade 1B**) [86-89].

Prophylaxis of the asymptomatic patient

In the absence of symptoms or a history of symptoms attributable to the APS, we do not recommend the use of aspirin as prophylaxis (**Grade 2B**). For patients with SLE and aPL but no APS manifestations, the combination of low-dose aspirin and hydroxychloroquine may be considered (**Grade 2C**)[80-89].

11. Acknowledgments

The work to produce this chapter was supported by Alzaidi's Chair of research in rheumatic diseases - Umm Alqura University.

12. References

Laurence, J, Wong, JE, Nachman, R. The cellular hematology of systemic lupus erythematosus. In: Systemic Lupus Erythematosus, 2d ed, Lahita, RG (Ed), Churchill Livingstone, New York 1992.

Shoenfeld, Y, Ehrenfeld, M. Hematologic manifestations. In: The Clinical Management of Systemic Lupus Erythematosus, 2d ed, Schur, PH (Ed), Lippincott, Philadelphia 1996.

Nossent JC, Swaak AJ. Prevalence and significance of haematological abnormalities in patients with systemic lupus erythematosus. Q J Med 1991; 80:605.

Keeling DM, Isenberg DA. Haematological manifestations of systemic lupus erythematosus. Blood Rev 1993; 7:199.

Liu H, Ozaki K, Matsuzaki Y, et al. Suppression of haematopoiesis by IgG autoantibodies from patients with systemic lupus erythematosus (SLE). Clin Exp Immunol 1995; 100:480.

Habib GS, Saliba WR, Froom P. Pure red cell aplasia and lupus. Semin Arthritis Rheum 2002; 31:279.

Voulgarelis M, Kokori SI, Ioannidis JP, et al. Anaemia in systemic lupus erythematosus: aetiological profile and the role of erythropoietin. Ann Rheum Dis 2000; 59:217.

Giannouli S, Voulgarelis M, Ziakas PD, Tzioufas AG. Anaemia in systemic lupus erythematosus: from pathophysiology to clinical assessment. Ann Rheum Dis 2006; 65:144.

Schett G, Firbas U, Füreder W, et al. Decreased serum erythropoietin and its relation to anti-erythropoietin antibodies in anaemia of systemic lupus erythematosus. Rheumatology (Oxford) 2001; 40:424.

Hara A, Wada T, Kitajima S, et al. Combined pure red cell aplasia and autoimmune hemolytic anemia in systemic lupus erythematosus with anti-erythropoietin autoantibodies. Am J Hematol 2008; 83:750.

Winkler A, Jackson RW, Kay DS, et al. High-dose intravenous cyclophosphamide treatment of systemic lupus erythematosus-associated aplastic anemia. Arthritis Rheum 1988; 31:693.

Brooks BJ Jr, Broxmeyer HE, Bryan CF, Leech SH. Serum inhibitor in systemic lupus erythematosus associated with aplastic anemia. Arch Intern Med 1984; 144:1474.

Roffe C, Cahill MR, Samanta A, et al. Aplastic anaemia in systemic lupus erythematosus: a cellular immune mechanism? Br J Rheumatol 1991; 30:301.

Jeffries M, Hamadeh F, Aberle T, et al. Haemolytic anaemia in a multi-ethnic cohort of lupus patients: a clinical and serological perspective. Lupus 2008; 17:739.

Jacob HS. Pulse steroids in hematologic diseases. Hosp Pract (Off Ed) 1985; 20:87.

Gomard-Mennesson E, Ruivard M, Koenig M, et al. Treatment of isolated severe immune hemolytic anaemia associated with systemic lupus erythematosus: 26 cases. Lupus 2006; 15:223.

Corley CC Jr, Lessner HE, Larsen WE. Azathioprine therapy of "autoimmune" diseases. Am J Med 1966; 41:404.

Murphy S, LoBuglio AF. Drug therapy of autoimmune hemolytic anemia. Semin Hematol 1976; 13:323.

Coon WW. Splenectomy for cytopenias associated with systemic lupus erythematosus. Am J Surg 1988; 155:391.

Rivero SJ, Alger M, Alarcón-Segovia D. Splenectomy for hemocytopenia in systemic lupus erythematosus. A controlled appraisal. Arch Intern Med 1979; 139:773.

Chan AC, Sack K. Danazol therapy in autoimmune hemolytic anemia associated with systemic lupus erythematosus. J Rheumatol 1991; 18:280.

Ahn YS, Harrington WJ, Mylvaganam R, et al. Danazol therapy for autoimmune hemolytic anemia. Ann Intern Med 1985; 102:298.

Letchumanan P, Thumboo J. Danazol in the treatment of systemic lupus erythematosus: a qualitative systematic review. Semin Arthritis Rheum 2011; 40:298.

Alba P, Karim MY, Hunt BJ. Mycophenolate mofetil as a treatment for autoimmune haemolytic anaemia in patients with systemic lupus erythematosus and antiphospholipid syndrome. Lupus 2003; 12:633.

Looney RJ. B cell-targeted therapy in diseases other than rheumatoid arthritis. J Rheumatol Suppl 2005; 73:25.

Nesher G, Hanna VE, Moore TL, et al. Thrombotic microangiographic hemolytic anemia in systemic lupus erythematosus. Semin Arthritis Rheum 1994; 24:165.

Matsuyama T, Kuwana M, Matsumoto M, et al. Heterogeneous pathogenic processes of thrombotic microangiopathies in patients with connective tissue diseases. Thromb Haemost 2009; 102:371.

George JN, Vesely SK, James JA. Overlapping features of thrombotic thrombocytopenic purpura and systemic lupus erythematosus. South Med J 2007; 100:512.

Musio F, Bohen EM, Yuan CM, Welch PG. Review of thrombotic thrombocytopenic purpura in the setting of systemic lupus erythematosus. Semin Arthritis Rheum 1998; 28:1.

Manadan AM, Harris C, Schwartz MM, Block JA. The frequency of thrombotic thrombocytopenic purpura in patients with systemic lupus erythematosus undergoing kidney biopsy. J Rheumatol 2003; 30:1227.

Sultan SM, Begum S, Isenberg DA. Prevalence, patterns of disease and outcome in patients with systemic lupus erythematosus who develop severe haematological problems. Rheumatology (Oxford) 2003; 42:230.

Dold S, Singh R, Sarwar H, et al. Frequency of microangiopathic hemolytic anemia in patients with systemic lupus erythematosus exacerbation: Distinction from thrombotic thrombocytopenic purpura, prognosis, and outcome. Arthritis Rheum 2005; 53:982.

Budman DR, Steinberg AD. Hematologic aspects of systemic lupus erythematosus. Current concepts. Ann Intern Med 1977; 86:220.

Martínez-Baños D, Crispín JC, Lazo-Langner A, Sánchez-Guerrero J. Moderate and severe neutropenia in patients with systemic lupus erythematosus. Rheumatology (Oxford) 2006; 45:994.

Perez HD, Lipton M, Goldstein IM. A specific inhibitor of complement (C5)-derived chemotactic activity in serum from patients with systemic lupus erythematosus. J Clin Invest 1978; 62:29.

Abramson SB, Given WP, Edelson HS, Weissmann G. Neutrophil aggregation induced by sera from patients with active systemic lupus erythematosus. Arthritis Rheum 1983; 26:630.

Rivero SJ, Díaz-Jouanen E, Alarcón-Segovia D. Lymphopenia in systemic lupus erythematosus. Clinical, diagnostic, and prognostic significance. Arthritis Rheum 1978; 21:295.

Vilá LM, Alarcón GS, McGwin G Jr, et al. Systemic lupus erythematosus in a multiethnic US cohort, XXXVII: association of lymphopenia with clinical manifestations, serologic abnormalities, disease activity, and damage accrual. Arthritis Rheum 2006; 55:799.

Winfield JB, Winchester RJ, Kunkel HG. Association of cold-reactive antilymphocyte antibodies with lymphopenia in systemic lupus erythematosus. Arthritis Rheum 1975; 18:587.

Amasaki Y, Kobayashi S, Takeda T, et al. Up-regulated expression of Fas antigen (CD95) by peripheral naive and memory T cell subsets in patients with systemic lupus erythematosus (SLE): a possible mechanism for lymphopenia. Clin Exp Immunol 1995; 99:245.

Isenberg DA, Patterson KG, Todd-Pokropek A, et al. Haematological aspects of systemic lupus erythematosus: a reappraisal using automated methods. Acta Haematol 1982; 67:242.

Camussi G, Tetta C, Coda R, Benveniste J. Release of platelet-activating factor in human pathology. I. Evidence for the occurrence of basophil degranulation and release of platelet-activating factor in systemic lupus erythematosus. Lab Invest 1981; 44:241.

Boumpas DT, Chrousos GP, Wilder RL, et al. Glucocorticoid therapy for immune-mediated diseases: basic and clinical correlates. Ann Intern Med 1993; 119:1198.

Euler HH, Harten P, Zeuner RA, Schwab UM. Recombinant human granulocyte colony stimulating factor in patients with systemic lupus erythematosus associated neutropenia and refractory infections. J Rheumatol 1997; 24:2153.

Hellmich B, Schnabel A, Gross WL. Treatment of severe neutropenia due to Felty's syndrome or systemic lupus erythematosus with granulocyte colony-stimulating factor. Semin Arthritis Rheum 1999; 29:82.

Starkebaum G. Chronic neutropenia associated with autoimmune disease. Semin Hematol 2002; 39:121.

Pujol M, Ribera A, Vilardell M, et al. High prevalence of platelet autoantibodies in patients with systemic lupus erythematosus. Br J Haematol 1995; 89:137.

Michel M, Lee K, Piette JC, et al. Platelet autoantibodies and lupus-associated thrombocytopenia. Br J Haematol 2002; 119:354.

Nakamura M, Tanaka Y, Satoh T, et al. Autoantibody to CD40 ligand in systemic lupus erythematosus: association with thrombocytopenia but not thromboembolism. Rheumatology (Oxford) 2006; 45:150.

Karpatkin S. Autoimmune thrombocytopenic purpura. Blood 1980; 56:329.

Ziakas PD, Giannouli S, Zintzaras E, et al. Lupus thrombocytopenia: clinical implications and prognostic significance. Ann Rheum Dis 2005; 64:1366.

DAMESHEK W, REEVES WH. Exacerbation of lupus erythematosus following splenectomy in idiopathic thrombocytopenic purpura and autoimmune hemolytic anemia. Am J Med 1956; 21:560.

BEST WR, DARLING DR. A critical look at the splenectomy-S.L.E. controversy. Med Clin North Am 1962; 46:19.

George JN, Woolf SH, Raskob GE, et al. Idiopathic thrombocytopenic purpura: a practice guideline developed by explicit methods for the American Society of Hematology. Blood 1996; 88:3.

Blanchette V, Freedman J, Garvey B. Management of chronic immune thrombocytopenic purpura in children and adults. Semin Hematol 1998; 35:36.

Mazzucconi MG, Fazi P, Bernasconi S, et al. Therapy with high-dose dexamethasone (HD-DXM) in previously untreated patients affected by idiopathic thrombocytopenic purpura: a GIMEMA experience. Blood 2007; 109:1401.

Goebel KM, Gassel WD, Goebel FD. Evaluation of azathioprine in autoimmune thrombocytopenia and lupus erythematosus. Scand J Haematol 1973; 10:28.

Boumpas DT, Barez S, Klippel JH, Balow JE. Intermittent cyclophosphamide for the treatment of autoimmune thrombocytopenia in systemic lupus erythematosus. Ann Intern Med 1990; 112:674.

Maier WP, Gordon DS, Howard RF, et al. Intravenous immunoglobulin therapy in systemic lupus erythematosus-associated thrombocytopenia. Arthritis Rheum 1990; 33:1233.

Vasoo S, Thumboo J, Fong KY. Refractory immune thrombocytopenia in systemic lupus erythematosus: response to mycophenolate mofetil. Lupus 2003; 12:630.

Braendstrup P, Bjerrum OW, Nielsen OJ, et al. Rituximab chimeric anti-CD20 monoclonal antibody treatment for adult refractory idiopathic thrombocytopenic purpura. Am J Hematol 2005; 78:275.

Hall S, McCormick JL Jr, Greipp PR, et al. Splenectomy does not cure the thrombocytopenia of systemic lupus erythematosus. Ann Intern Med 1985; 102:325.

You YN, Tefferi A, Nagorney DM. Outcome of splenectomy for thrombocytopenia associated with systemic lupus erythematosus. Ann Surg 2004; 240:286.

Vesely SK, Perdue JJ, Rizvi MA, et al. Management of adult patients with persistent idiopathic thrombocytopenic purpura following splenectomy: a systematic review. Ann Intern Med 2004; 140:112.

West SG, Johnson SC. Danazol for the treatment of refractory autoimmune thrombocytopenia in systemic lupus erythematosus. Ann Intern Med 1988; 108:703.

Cervera H, Jara LJ, Pizarro S, et al. Danazol for systemic lupus erythematosus with refractory autoimmune thrombocytopenia or Evans' syndrome. J Rheumatol 1995; 22:1867.

Aviña-Zubieta JA, Galindo-Rodrìguez G, Robledo I, et al. Long-term effectiveness of danazol corticosteroids and cytotoxic drugs in the treatment of hematologic manifestations of systemic lupus erythematosus. Lupus 2003; 12:52.

Ahn YS, Harrington WJ, Seelman RC, Eytel CS. Vincristine therapy of idiopathic and secondary thrombocytopenias. N Engl J Med 1974; 291:376.

Castellino G, Govoni M, Prandini N, et al. Thrombocytosis in systemic lupus erythematosus: a possible clue to autosplenectomy? J Rheumatol 2007; 34:1497.

Voulgarelis M, Giannouli S, Tasidou A, et al. Bone marrow histological findings in systemic lupus erythematosus with hematologic abnormalities: a clinicopathological study. Am J Hematol 2006; 81:590.

Lambotte O, Khellaf M, Harmouche H, et al. Characteristics and long-term outcome of 15 episodes of systemic lupus erythematosus-associated hemophagocytic syndrome. Medicine (Baltimore) 2006; 85:169.

Somers E, Magder LS, Petri M. Antiphospholipid antibodies and incidence of venous thrombosis in a cohort of patients with systemic lupus erythematosus. J Rheumatol 2002; 29:2531.

Shah NM, Khamashta MA, Atsumi T, Hughes GR. Outcome of patients with anticardiolipin antibodies: a 10 year follow-up of 52 patients. Lupus 1998; 7:3.

Vlachoyiannopoulos PG, Toya SP, Katsifis G, et al. Upregulation of antiphospholipid antibodies following cyclophosphamide therapy in patients with systemic lupus erythematosus. J Rheumatol 2008; 35:1768.

Esdaile JM, Abrahamowicz M, Joseph L, et al. Laboratory tests as predictors of disease exacerbations in systemic lupus erythematosus. Why some tests fail. Arthritis Rheum 1996; 39:370.

Vilá LM, Alarcón GS, McGwin G Jr, et al. Systemic lupus erythematosus in a multiethnic cohort (LUMINA): XXIX. Elevation of erythrocyte sedimentation rate is associated with disease activity and damage accrual. J Rheumatol 2005; 32:2150.

Charalabopoulos K, Papalimneou V, Charalabopoulos A, Chaidos A, Bai M, Bourantas K, Agnantis N Kikuchi-Fujimoto disease in Greece. A study of four cases and review ofthe literature. In vivo2002;16:311–316

Yasar Kucukardali, Emrullah Solmazgul, Erdogan Kunter, Oral Oncul, Sukru Yildirim,Mustafa Kaplan.Kikuchi–Fujimoto Disease: analysis of 244 cases Clin.Rheumatol 2007;26: 50–54

15. Alex Santana, Bruno Lessa, Liliana Galra˜ oIsabella Lima, Mittermayer Santiago Kikuchi-Fujimoto's disease associated with systemic lupus erythematosus: case report and review of the literature .Clin Rheumatol 2005;24: 60–63

Ansell J, Hirsh J, Poller L, et al. The pharmacology and management of the vitamin K antagonists: the Seventh ACCP Conference on Antithrombotic and Thrombolytic Therapy. Chest 2004; 126:204S.

Weitz JI. Low-molecular-weight heparins. N Engl J Med 1997; 337:688.

Segal JB, Streiff MB, Hofmann LV, et al. Management of venous thromboembolism: a systematic review for a practice guideline. Ann Intern Med 2007; 146:211.

Koopman, MM, Prandoni, P, Piovella, F, et al. Treatment of venous thrombosis with intravenous unfractionated heparin administered in the hospital as compared wit subcutaneous low-molecular-weight heparin administered at home. N Engl J Med 1996; 334:682.

Levine M, Gent M, Hirsh J, et al. A comparison of low-molecular-weight heparin administered primarily at home with unfractionated heparin administered in the hospital for proximal deep-vein thrombosis. N Engl J Med 1996; 334:677.

Boccalon H, Elias A, Chalé JJ, et al. Clinical outcome and cost of hospital vs home treatment of proximal deep vein thrombosis with a low-molecular-weight heparin: the Vascular Midi-Pyrenees study. Arch Intern Med 2000; 160:1769.

O'Shaughnessy D, Miles J, Wimperis J. UK patients with deep-vein thrombosis can be safely treated as out-patients. QJM 2000; 93:663.

Grau E, Tenias JM, Real E, et al. Home treatment of deep venous thrombosis with low molecular weight heparin: Long-term incidence of recurrent venous thromboembolism. Am J Hematol 2001; 67:10.

Dunn A, Bioh D, Beran M, et al. Effect of intravenous heparin administration on duration of hospitalization. Mayo Clin Proc 2004; 79:159.

Douketis JD. Treatment of deep vein thrombosis: what factors determine appropriate treatment? Can Fam Physician 2005; 51:217.

18

Lymphoproliferative Disorders in Patients with Systemic Lupus Erythematosus

Carlos Panizo[1] and Ricardo García-Muñoz[2]
[1]Hematology Service, Clínica Universidad de Navarra, Pamplona, Navarra
[2]Hematology Service, Hospital San Pedro, Logroño, La Rioja
Spain

1. Introduction

Lymphoproliferative disorders can develop in the setting of many immunosupressive conditions, and they have been well established following solid organ transplantation or allogeneic bone marrow transplantation (Blaes & Morrison, 2010). The incidence varies, depending on the type of organ transplanted, the degree of immunosuppression, the number of episodes of acute rejection and the patient's immune status to Epstein-Barr virus. The 2008 World Health Organization Classification of Tumours of Haematopoietic and Lymphoid Tissues defines monomorphic posttransplant lymphoproliferative disorders (PTLD) as lymphoid or plasmacytic proliferations that fulfill the criteria for one of the B-cell or T/NK-cell neoplasms recognized in immunocompetent patients. However, indolent B-cell lymphomas, such as extranodal marginal zone lymphoma of mucosa-associated lymphoid tissue (MALT lymphoma), are specifically excluded from this category. Autoimmune and chronic inflammatory disorders are also associated with increased risks of non-Hodgkin lymphoma (NHL). Concretely in rheumatoid arthritis and systemic lupus erythematosus (SLE), an increased risk of malignant lymphomas has been described repeatedly, whereas the evidence is less consistent for other inflammatory disorders that display autoimmune phenomena, such as psoriasis, inflammatory bowel disorders and sarcoidosis. The risk of NHL in SLE patients is estimated to be 3- to 4-fold higher (Smedby et al., 2008a). Although the incidence of PTLD is thought to be bimodal and typically related to Epstein-Barr virus in the first year after solid-organ transplantation, the relationship between Epstein-Barr virus and NHL in SLE and other autoimmune diseases is not yet well established.

Because different NHL subtypes develop at different stages of lymphocyte differentiation, the incidence of specific NHL subtypes varies based on the type of autoimmune and inflammatory disorder as well as on the type and amount of autoimmune therapy. Data regarding the histology of the NHL that develops in patients with SLE suggest that these lesions derive from lymphocytes that have been exposed to antigen (Bernatsky et al., 2005a). Lymphoma development after the antigen-exposure stages of differentiation might suggest that chronic antigenic stimulation has a role in auto immunity-related lymphomas. From the lymphoma perspective, diffuse large B-cell lymphomas seem to display the most pronounced and general association with autoimmunity and inflammation, although certain specific T-cell lymphomas have been linked to distinct autoimmune conditions (e.g.

enteropathy-type T-cell lymphoma to coeliac disease) (Smedby et al., 2008b). Studies of lymphoproliferative disorders occurring in patients with SLE have shown an increased risk of marginal zone lymphoma, predominantly of the MALT type, and of diffuse large B-cell lymphoma (DLBCL) (Bernatsky et al., 2005b).
The mechanisms responsible for the association between lymphoma and SLE remain unknown. Exposure to immunosuppressive agents has been blamed for the elevated risk of lymphoma, but cases of lymphoma in patients with no history of having received immunosuppressive drugs have also been reported. The study of Bernatsky et al looking for the incidence of cancer in patients with SLE, reports that the highest relative risk of hematological malignancy occurred in the first year after diagnosis of SLE which indicates that cancer risk is not completely explained by cumulative doses of immunosuppressive drugs (Bernatsky et al., 2005b).

2. Objective

SLE is an autoimmune disease characterized by immune mediated attacks against the body's own tissues. The aetiology of the illness is unknown. In essence the fundamental rules of tolerance are violated and autorreactive B and T cell clones cooperate, proliferate and lead the production of pathogenic auto-antibodies. The development of lymphomas and autoimmunity involves an intrincate interplay among various pathogenic factors. Besides genetic abnormalities, a variety of environmental and microbial factors, as well as abnormal immune-regulatory processes and tolerance mechanisms can lead to autoimmunity and the generation of different lymphoma subtypes. Within germinal centers, naïve B cells undergo activation, proliferation, somatic hypermutation of rearranged V regions genes, isotype switching, and subsequent positive and/or negative selection by antigen. However, the germinal center exclusion of autorreaction is defective in SLE and the existence of a defective check point in the maintenance of peripheral B cell tolerance appears to be specific to patients with SLE. This is important because, some autorreactive B cells may initiate germinal center reactions and autorreactivity arises de novo in the germinal center through somatic mutations. Moreover, in patients with active SLE a marked B cell lymphopenia that affects naïve B cells leads to a relative predominance of memory B cells with multiple somatic mutations. Somatic mutations are introduced at a high rate in the germinal center and are implicated usually in single nucleotide exchanges. However, deletions and insertions may also occur. The involvement of the hypermutation machinery in deletions and insertions seem to be the main cause of generation of several lymphoproliferative disorders in these patients.
The aim of the present review is to summarize potential harmful steps in the development of lymphocytes, tolerance checkpoints (anergy, deletion, germinal centre exclusion, receptor editing and revision, memory check points, somatic hypermutation) and immune responses that induce the acquisition and proliferation of neoplastic lymphocytes in the contex of SLE. We also review the different subtypes of lymphoproliferative disorders associated with SLE and its management.

3. Development of B cell repertoire

B cells are derived from CD34+CD19-CD10+cells. The earliest lineage-committed B cell is the pro-B cell, which is characterized by a CD19+ phenotype (Wang et al., 1998). The pro-B

cell stage is defined by immunoglobulin (Ig) heavy chain rearrangement initiated via the recombinase activating genes RAG1 and RAG2 (Blom & Spits, 2006; LeBien & Tedder, 2008). In these cells, DH to JH gene rearrangements occur, often, but not always in both IgH alleles, which are located on chromosome 14 in humans (Cobett, et al., 1997; Ravetch, et al., 1981). In the next, step VH gene segment is rearranged to a DHJH (Cook & Tomlinson, 1995). If the first VH/DH/JH rearrangement is nonproductive, the B cell precursor has a second chance to generate a productive IgH gene rearrangement by using the second IgH allele. When heavy chain gene rearrangement is successful, then Ig class is expressed on the cell surface in association with μ heavy chain and the signal transducing molecules CD79a/b to form the pre-B cell receptor. This is accompanied by loss of CD34 and TdT expression and marks the transition to the pre-B-cell stage of development. Pre-B cells discontinue further IgH gene rearrangements, divide several times, and then initiate light chain gene rearrangements (Rajewsky, 1996). Internalization of the pre-B cell receptor and rearrangement of the light chains occur next, defaulting to the kappa gene. Lambda gene rearrangement and expression generally occur only if kappa gene rearrangement is unsuccessful. Successful light chain rearrangement induces the expression of sIgM composed by IgH and either κ or λ light chains. Failure to rearrange either the heavy or light chains induces apoptosis. If immature B cells react with self antigens, mechanisms of negative selection can induce apoptosis, receptor edition or anergy (LeBien, 2000).
Secondary B cell development is characterized by the migration of immature B cells to the spleen, where they differentiate into mature naïve B cells, now characterized by surface IgD in addition to IgM, CD21 and CD22, as well as a loss of CD10. Positive selection subsequently commences, with cells failing to react succumbing to cell death. Following this process, mature cells migrate to secondary lymphoid tissue whereupon they can further differentiate to plasma cells or establish a germinal center when they recognize an antigen (DiLillo, et al., 2008).

4. Germinal centre reaction

Within germinal centers, activated B cells undergo the process of somatic hypermutation. Centrally proliferating B cells are referred to as centroblasts, which divide to form smaller centrocytes that migrate to periphery of the germinal center. Centroblasts first remove the surface immunoglobulin, then undergo several rounds of division and then re-express mutated immunoglobulin receptors as centrocytes. Centrocytes expressing BCR with increased affinity will be able to appropriately interact with germinal centre T cells and follicular dendritic cells and be positively selected. Surviving centrocytes subsequently depend on CD40-based interactions with T cells to facilitate differentiation into long lived plasma cells and memory B cells (MacLennan, 1994).

5. Tolerance B cell check points

B cell precursors undergo immunoglobulin gene rearrangements to generate a population of mature B cells bearing surface immunoglobulin (sIg) with a range of specificities. Random V/D/J gene assembly generates many self-reactive B-cell receptors (BCR). To avoid autoimmunity, B cells displaying self-reactive immunoglobulin are deleted centrally in the bone marrow and at subsequent check points in the periphery (Yurasov et al., 2005a) **(Fig. 1).** Self reactivity arising during V/D/J recombination could be corrected by receptor editing, clonal deletion and anergy. In normal subjects the number of self reactive B cells decreases significantly as B cells progress though normal development. Nevertheless, central tolerance appears not enough to control self-reactive B cells in SLE patients. Significantly, the frequency of autoreactive antibodies declines from 75% in the bone marrow to 20% in the circulating naïve compartment (Yurasov et al., 2005b). However, several of these check points appear deficient in SLE patients (Yurasov S, et al., 2005b). In patients with SLE, mature naïve B cell compartment comprises 40% to 50% of autoreactive clones. This fact indicates that SLE patients have defects in censoring self reactive B cells early in development even in SLE patients in remission (Yurasov et al., 2006). Because signaling through the BCR is a primary mechanism for triggering deletion, anergy, or receptor edition abnormal BCR signaling is likely to play a role in breakdown tolerance (Kamradt & Mitchinson, 2001). Interestingly, circulating mature B cells from SLE patients demonstrate a heightened response to BCR crosslinking. Even more SLE patients have low levels of intracellular tyrosine kinase Lyn that can diminish BCR signaling through phosphorylation of inhibitory receptor such CD22 and FCRIIb (Flores-Borja, et al., 2005).

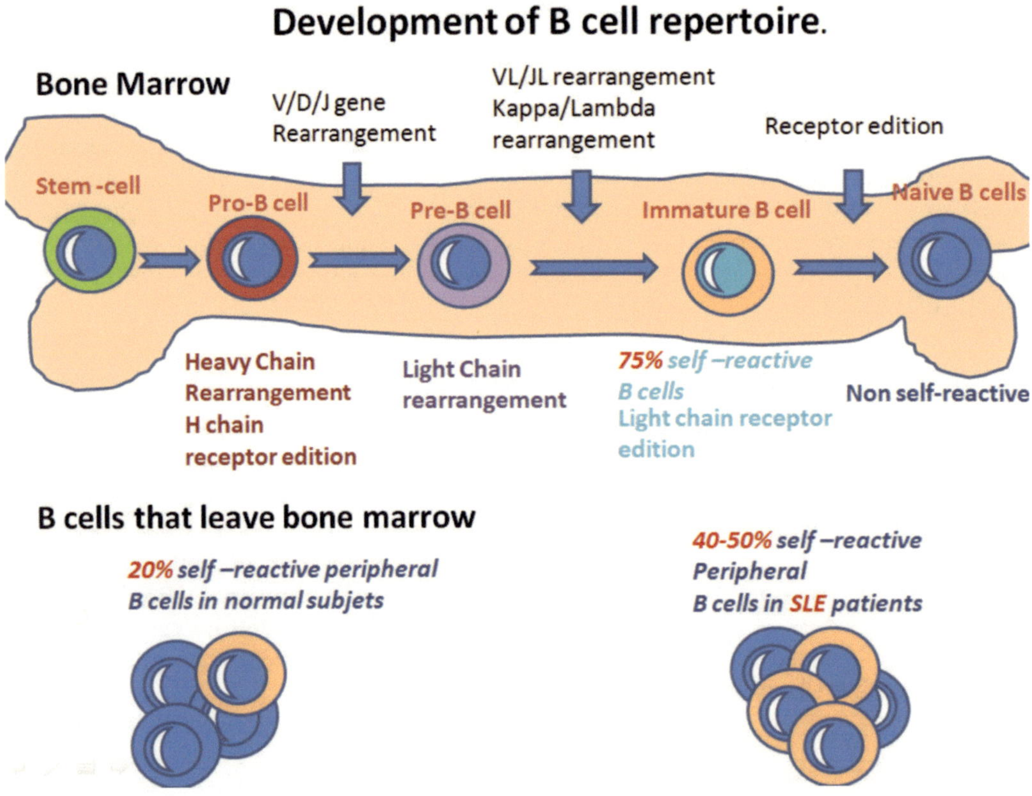

Fig. 1. Defective central tolerance in development of B cell repertoire in SLE.
Patients with SLE have increased numbers of self-reactive B cells. We speculate that defects in complement could contribute to this phenomena. We propose that although receptor edition works well in SLE patients if immature B cells cannot test their BCR with self-antigens it is possible that they mature to naive self-reactive B cells and leave bone marrow and migrate to secondary lymphoid organs.

During central tolerance in bone marrow, receptor editing appears to be the preferred mechanism to establish early B cell self-tolerance (Tiegs et al., 1993; Gay et al., 1993; Halverson et al., 2004). Self reactive BCR can apparently be purged by receptor editing, a mechanism through which antigen binding in bone marrow induces continued rearrangement of immunoglobulin gene segments; this process results in a change in the specificity of a previously autorreactive BCR (Melamed, et al., 1997). Interestingly, although receptor editing works well in patients with SLE, it is possible that it could be insufficient to avoid the development of self-reactive B cells (Dörner, et al., 1999) and subsequent emigration to lymph nodes or spleen. However, the basic question as to whether receptor editing is increased or decreased during lupus requires further study (Luning-Prak et al., 2011). Interestingly, receptor edition can contribute to generating lymphoproliferative disorders (Chiorazzi, et al., 2005; Wang, et al., 2008; García-Muñoz et al., 2009; Hatzidimitriou, et al., 2009).

There are also data showing that regulatory checkpoints exist for B cells in the periphery in germinal center and in the late stages of B cell differentiation to memory or long-lived plasma cells (Cappione A 3rd et al., 2005; William et al., 2006)

Germinal center exclusion of self reactive B cells (9G4 B cells) that express self-reactive antibodies encoded by the IGVH 4-34 gene is an important peripheral checkpoint to avoid interaction of autoreactive B cells with T cells and subsequent generation of autoantibodies. For this reason, 9G4 B cells are present only in 5-10% of the naïve B cell in healthy donors as well as in the IgM memory compartment and these cells participate in less than 1 % of germinal centers of tonsil biopsies. However, germinal center exclusion is defective in SLE patients and evaluation of lymphoid tissue from tonsillar biopsies and spleens reveals that the frequency of germinal center 9G4 B cells in this population is 15% to 20% (Cappione A 3rd et al., 2005). The expression of *IGHV4-34* heavy chains in antibodies is synonymous of autoreactivity against N-acatyllactosamine (NAL) determinants expressed by the iI blood group antigen and other self glycoproteins including CD45 (Silberstein et al., 1991; Pugh-Bernard et al., 2001. Cappione AJ, et al., 2004). Importantly, antibodies against anti-B cell CD45 and a significant fraction of anti-native double stranded DNA (anti-DNA) use *VH4-34* heavy chain and are detected in patients with SLE (Pugh-Bernard et al., 2001) and represent about 10-45% of total serum IgG in this patients. However, *IGHV4-34* antibodies are virtually undetectable in healthy sera because *IGHV4-34* cells are censored at multiple check points during B cell development to avoid autoimmunity (Pugh-Bernard et al., 2001).

Preventing the generation of self-reactive memory B cells or long lived plasma cells is another important peripheral checkpoint to stay away from autoimmunity. B cells expressing self reactive antibodies and broadly bacterially reactive antibodies are continuously removed from the repertoire in the transition from naïve to IgM memory B cells and selection against self reactive antibodies is implemented before the onset of somatic hypermutation (Tsuiji et al., 2006). This checkpoint is supported by data showing a decrease in frequency of autoreactive IgM+ memory B cells to 2% from 20% in the mature naive B cell population in healthy individuals (Tsuiji et al., 2006). Even when dysfunction of this checkpoint in SLE is not yet determined, the fact that memory B cells with IGHV4-34 have been detected in patients with SLE (Odendhal et al., 2000) provides indirect support for some deficiency in this checkpoint.

The presence of extensive somatic mutations seen in autoantibodies derived from SLE patients strongly supports the notion of germinal center maturation of pathogenic, self reactive B cells and support defects at several check points.

6. Lymphomagenesis in SLE

Chronic immune stimulation by self antigens and infectious agents together with genetic variations of TNF-α and IL-10 expression have been suggested to explain lymphomagenesis in SLE (Dias et al., 2011; Bertansky et al., 2009). However, the mechanism underlying the association between SLE and lymphoma remains unexplained. Lymphoproliferative neoplasm could arise from precursor B cells development and in pre-germinal center, germinal center or post germinal center differentiation. During development and maturation of B cells, they can acquire mutations, deletions or translocations that direct the generation of lymphomas. Rearrangements of V/D/J genes, receptor editing, somatic hypermutation, and class switching are responsible for DNA strand breaks that lead chromosomal aberrations that are in part responsible for lymphomagenesis (Küppers et al.,1999). A reasonable hypothesis is that the accumulation of clonally expanded self-reactive B cells that recognize self-antigens in the lymph nodes may predispose these B cells to DNA breaks, facilitating tumorigenesis (Xu et al., 2001). In support of this viewpoint, lymph nodes of patients with SLE have extensive necrosis with apoptotic debris (self antigens), with numerous plasma cells within germinal centers. On the one hand, these histopathologic features suggest that in lymph nodes it is possible that self reactive B cells can suffer somatic hypermutation, class switching and receptor edition/revision induced by apoptotic bodies increasing the risk of suffering DNA breaks and translocations. On the other hand, B cells with self-reactive specificity are likely to present self peptides to autoreactive T cells (Chan et al., 1999). In this context, T cells contribute to rescuing and supporting the maturation of self-reactive B cells to plasmatic B cells or memory B cells. Significantly, during this process it is possible that some cells acquire translocations and DNA alterations that contribute to development of lymphoma. In addition, in combination with recognition of self antigens in lymph nodes, self reactive B cells also recognize self antigens in bone marrow and acquire translocations or genetic alterations during B cell development. Autoreactive B cells may suffer receptor editing and V/D/J gene recombination in bone marrow. Recent evidence shows that L chain receptor editing occurs not only in bone marrow with a pre-B/immature B cell phenotype but also in immature/transitional splenic B cells. Nevertheless, editing at the H chain locus appears to occur exclusively in bone marrow cells with pro-B phenotype (Nakajima et al., 2009). Receptor editing appears to work well in patients with SLE. However, a feature of SLE is an increased production of self-reactive B cells that migrate from bone marrow to secondary lymphoid organs. This implies that other mechanisms or defects are necessary to maintain central tolerance in bone marrow. Significantly, defects in elimination of apoptotic cells and defects in complement components have been proposed to explain impaired central tolerance in bone marrow (Carrol, 2004). Interestingly, this model suggest that autoantigens from apoptotic cells are presented to immature B cells by immune complexes containing C1q, C4b and IgM in bone marrow. In support of this model Tripodo, et al., discovered C1q production by bone marrow stromal cells, an important part of complement that is involved in clearance of apoptotic cells (Tripodo et al., 2007).

We speculate that the impaired elimination of apoptotic cells in bone marrow and lymph nodes could contribute to persistent autoantigenic overstimulation leading to refractoriness of autoimmunity and increased risk of chromosomal alterations and lymphomas **(Fig. 2).**

7. Hypothetical immunologic mechanisms implicated in generation of lymphomas in patients with SLE (Fig 2)

Deficiency in self-antigen retention induced by defects in complement components or impaired clearance of apoptotic B cells will possibly lead to an increased release of self-reactive B cells from bone marrow to periphery. On the one hand, defects in the complement system might produce deficient presentation of antigens in bone marrow and diminish the protection of receptor edition mechanism. On the other hand, impaired clearance of apoptotic cells in bone marrow induces increased stimulation of immature self-reactive B cells that could suffer increased receptor edition in bone marrow or avoid tolerance. Importantly, receptor edition also can produce polyreactive B cells or a simple change in recognition from an auto-antigen for others that recognize the new edited BCR in an immature B cell. These two mechanisms could be implicated in generation of mantle cell lymphoma (García-Muñoz et al.,2009) or chronic lymphocytic leukemia with unmutated

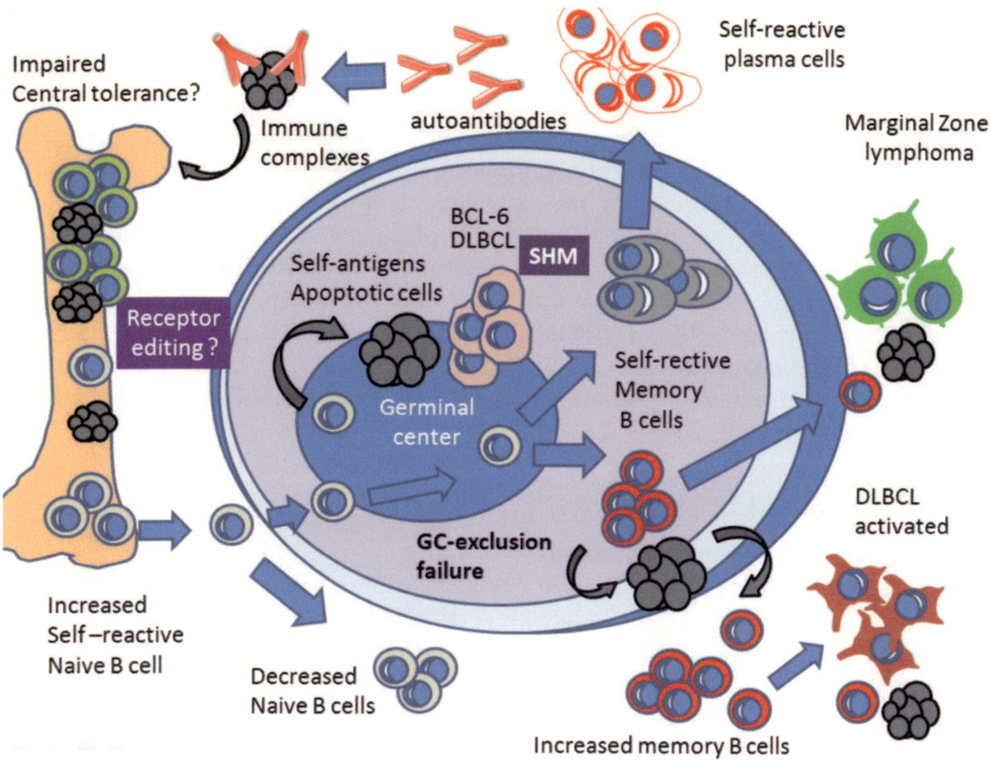

Fig. 2. Lymphoma development in patients with SLE.
Impaired clearance of apoptotic cells in concert with insufficiency in germinal centre exclusion of self-reactive B cells might induce constant stimulus of these B cells. Naive self-reactive B cells recognize auto-antigens and become memory B cells and plasma cells that produce auto antibodies. Continuous activation of memory B cells raises the risk of transformation into DLBC (activated subtype) and marginal zone B cell lymphomas. SLE activity and decrease in complement components could contribute to a defect in both central tolerance and clearance of apoptotic cells.

IGHV genes (Hadzidimitriou et al. 2009). Increased variable region gene recombination and heavy or light chain receptor edition in self-reactive B cells of patients with SLE in bone marrow could in theory contribute to lymphomagenesis. Self reactive B cells that leave bone marrow, enter germinal centres because germinal center exclusion is defective in patients with SLE. Within germinal centers, self-reactive B cells recognize self-antigens from apoptotic cells and suffer somatic hypermutation, receptor revision, and class switch-recombination. Some of this self-reactive B cells can be converted into memory B cells or plasmatic B cells that produce autoantibodies and return to the sites of antigen stimulation. During this process self-reactive B cells can acquire translocations, deletions or mutations that make a subtype of lymphoma. Germinal center derived lymphomas are derived by transformation from either variable region gene recombination (BCL-2-IgH) in follicular lymphoma, somatic hypermutation (BCL-6) in diffuse large B cell lymphoma, or class switching in c-myc sporadic Burkitt´s lymphoma (Küppers et al.,1999). **(Fig. 3)** Post-germinal center B cell lymphomas are marginal zone lymphoma, small lymphocytic lymphoma/chronic lymphocytic leukemia and plasmacytoma and are derived from memory B cells and plasma cells (Jaffe ES et al., 2008) **(Fig. 3)**. Interestingly, post-germinal center derived lymphomas are commonly associated with antigen stimulation by self-antigens or infectious agents (Suarez et al., 2006). In a study of 24 patients with malignant lymphoma and rheumatic diseases including SLE the majority of diffuse large B cell lymphomas exhibited activated phenotype and EBV associated lymphoma comprised only a small fraction (Kojima et al., 2006).

8. Lymphoma and SLE; Therapy

8.1 Lymphoma subtypes in SLE patients

Patients with SLE have an increased risk to develop lymphomas specially diffuse large B cell lymphoma (Löfstrom et al., 2007; Bernatsky et al., 2005; Bernatsky et al., 2006: King & Costenbader, 2007; Lin et al., 2003; Rossi et al., 2011; Biasiotta et al., 2010; Simon et al., 2007) and marginal zone lymphomas (Maeda et al., 2008; Gonzalez et al., 2009; Tektonidou, 2010) however, several subtypes have been reported.

8.2 Highly aggressive B cell lymphomas

Burkitt lymphoma is a highly aggressive B cell malignancy typically characterized by a rapid proliferation rate and the translocation of c-myc [t(8;14), t(8;22) or t(2;8)]. The typical immunophenotype of Burkitt lymphoma is sIg+, CD10+,CD19+, CD20+, TdT -, Ki-67+ (90-100% of cells), bcl-2 -, bcl-6 + (Ferry, 2006) Patients with Burkitt lymphoma often present with symptoms of a rapidly enlarging abdominal mass and B symptoms. Bone marrow involvement is found in up to 70% of patients, and leptomaningeal spread is common (Perkins et al., 2008). Data from patients with SLE and Burkitt lymphoma are scarce, however: some case reports or case series include patients with SLE that develop this rare malignancy (Posner et al., 1990; Bernatsky et al., 2005). The treatment of Burkitt lymphoma is based on intensive chemotherapy. Some highly effective regimens include CODOX-M (cyclophosmphamide, vincristine, doxorubicin, high dose methotrexate) alternating with IVAC (ifosfamide, etoposide and high-dose cytarabine)(Magrath et al., 1996.) or Hyper-CVAD (hyper fractioned cyclophosphamie, vincristine, doxorubicin, dexametasona) (Thomas et al., 2006) both plus Rituximab.

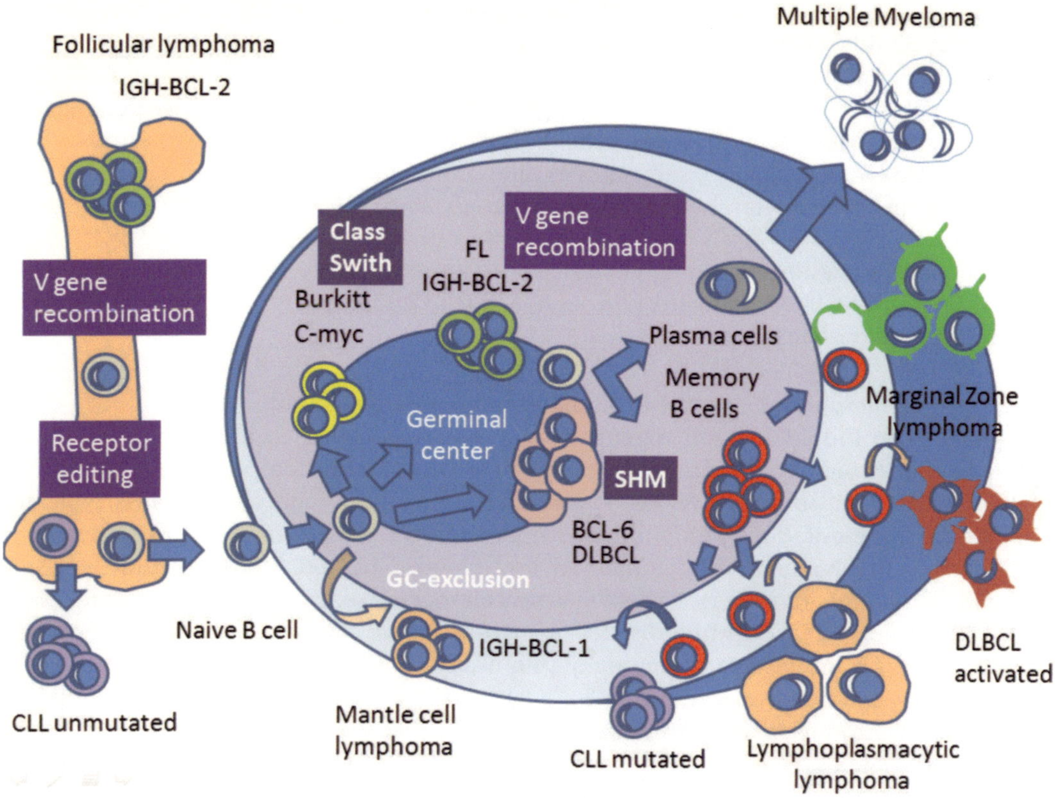

Fig. 3. Origin of Non Hodgkin B cell lymphomas and mechanisms related to their development
During development B cells can acquire translocations, deletions or mutations that make a subtype of lymphoma. Pre-germinal center derived lymphomas are CLL unmutated and mantle cell lymphoma and some follicular lymphomas. Germinal center derived lymphomas are derived by transformation from either variable region gene recombination (BCL-2-IgH) in follicular lymphoma, somatic hypermutation (BCL-6) in diffuse large B cell lymphoma, or class switching in c-myc sporadic Burkitt´s lymphoma. Post-germinal center B cell lymphomas are marginal zone lymphoma, small lymphocytic lymphoma/chronic lymphocytic leukemia and plasmacytoma and are derived from memory B cells and plasma cells.

8.3 CD5+ B cell lymphomas

CD5+ B cell lymphomas comprises Mantle Cell lymphoma (MCL) and Chronic lymphocytic leukemia/Small lymphocytic lymphoma (CLL/SLL). Sometimes patients with SLE develop this subtypes of lymphomas (Munzert et al., 1997; Lugassy et al., 1992).

8.3.1 Mantle cell lymphoma

MCL can have a varied initial presentation and clinical course. Most patients are diagnosed when they already present an advanced stage disease. Common sites of involvement include lymph nodes, spleen, bone marrow gastrointestinal tract and the lymphoid tissue of

Waldeyer´s ring. MCL is characterized by the translocation t(11;14)(q13;q32) which leads to the overexpression of cyclin D1. Mutation analysis of the rearranged immunoglobulin´s heavy chain variable region (IGHV) genes shows a major subset with unmutated IGHV and a smaller subset displaying mutated IGHV genes (Swerdlow et al., 2008). The treatment of MCL is by intensive chemotherapy with R-HyperCVAD (rituximab, cyclophosphamide, vincristine, doxorubicin and Dexametasone) alternating with R-MA (Rituximab plus high-dose methotrexate and cytarabine) (Romaguera et al., 2005) followed by consolidation with myeloablative chemotherapy with autologous stem cell transplant in selected patients in first complete remission (Dreyling et al., 2005). However, other less intensive treatment options include R-CHOP (Howard OM, et al., 2002), Bendamustine (Rummel et al., 2005) and Bortezomib (Fisher et al., 2006).

8.3.2 Chronic lymphocytic leukemia/small lymphocytic lymphoma

CLL/SLL is an indolent B cell malignancy, which is believed to originate in memory antigen-experienced B-cells. Tumors usually involve not only the peripheral blood and bone marrow but also lymph nodes, spleen and liver. The diagnosis of SLL is typically applied if the presentations predominantly nodal and the diagnosis of CLL is made when the principal involvement is bone marrow and blood. CLL remains an incurable tumor and clinical features have very variable presentation, course, and outcome. Risk markers and stratification in CLL can be divided in two different entities. High risk phenotype usually expresses unmutated immunoglobulin heavy variable genes (Hamblin et al.,1999) CD38 surface marker (Damle et al.,1999), zeta-associated protein 70 (ZAP-70)(Crespo et al., 2003) and chromosomal aberrations as 17p (the site of the tumor protein p53) or 11q23 deletions (the site of the ataxia telangiectasia mutated ATM)(Dörner et al., 2000). Low risk phenotype habitually expresses mutated IGVH, lack CD38 and ZAP-70 and has a normal karyotype or 13q14 deletion. Additional adverse predictive factors include advanced Rai (Rai et al., 1975) and Binet clinical staging (Binet et al., 1981), usage of VH3-21 independent of VH mutation status (Throsélius et al., 2006) and short lymphocyte doubling time (Montserrat et al., 1986). There is no evidence that early treatment of asymptomatic patients benefits them. The current advice is that patients who are asymptomatic should be managed by watchful waiting until they present symptoms or International Workshop on Chronic Lymphocytic Leukemia indications for treatment are met (Hallek et al., 1996). First line treatment includes chlorambucil, fludarabine, Bendamustine or fludarabine plus cyclophosphamide, either alone or in combination with Rituximab (Hallek, 2010) . The choice of therapy is influenced by co-morbidities and status performance of patients.

8.4 Follicular lymphoma

Coexistence of follicular lymphoma (FL) and SLE has previously been reported (Löftröm et al., 2007; Suvajdzic et al., 2011). FL is a neoplasm composed of follicle center (germinal center) B cells (typically both centrocytes and centroblast) which usually has at least a partial follicular pattern. FL is genetically characterized by the translocation t(14;18)(q32;q21) and BCL-2 rearrangements.

FL involves lymph nodes, spleen, peripheral blood and Waldeyer ring. FL may occasionally be primary in extranodal sites. Most patients have widespread disease at diagnosis, including peripheral and central (abdominal and thoracic) lymphadenopathy and splenomegaly. Despite widespread disease, patients are usually otherwise asymptomatic (Harris et al., 2008). Multiple treatment options exist for patients with newly diagnosed FL, ranging from observation only to a variety of combined chemoimmunterapy regimens (Bendandi, 2008; Cheson et al., 2011).

8.5 Diffuse large B-cell lymphomas

Studies specifically investigating lymphoma and SLE have noted that DLBCL are the most common histology when lymphoma occurs in these patients (Gayed et al., 2009). This aggressive subtype makes up 30% of lymphomas in the general population, but in SLE groups, it accounts for between 38% and 53% of lymphomas (Smedby et al., 2006; Bernatsky et al., 2005a). Although DLBCL can occur at any age, it is, in general, a disease of middle-aged and older adults. Unlike indolent Iymphomas that are almost always widely disseminated at diagnosis, DLBCL present as early-stage disease in approximately 30% of cases. Clinically, presentation with a rapidly enlarging symptomatic mass is very common, with B symptoms (fever, unexplained weight loss > 10% over 6 month interval, or night sweats) in one-third of the cases. Extranodal disease in DLBCL can be present in up to 40% of cases; common sites include the gastrointestinal tract, bone, and CNS.

With the application of microarray techniques, three subgroups of DLBCL with distinctive gene-expression profiles have been identified on the basis of hierarchical clustering: germinal-center B-cell-like, activated B-cell-like, and type 3 DLBCL (Rosenwald et al., 2002). A number of recent studies have attempted to define germinal-center and non-germinal center phenotypes in DLBCL, using immunohistochemistry markers such as bcl-6, CD10 for germinal center and MUM1, IRF4 and CD38 for post-germinal center. In general, a germinal center immunophenotype, particularly including Bcl-6 expression, has been associated with a better prognosis (Lossos et al., 2004).

8.5.1 Therapy

For nearly 20 years anthracycline-based chemotherapy has been the mainstay of treatment, because of its proven efficacy, the CHOP (cyclophosphamide/doxorubicin/vincristine/ prednisone) regimen being the gold standard of therapy for aggressive NHL. Application of this treatment resulted in curing 30% of patients with DLBCL. The standard chemotherapy regimen has changed little in the past three decades, but a variety of strategies have been tested to identify regimens that might increase the disease-free survival rate for aggressive lymphomas. Monoclonal-antibody therapy has been added to the armamentarium and represents an advance in therapeutic options. The anti-CD20 monoclonal antibody rituximab has been combined with the chemotherapy regimen of CHOP in an attempt to improve outcomes; increased remission and survival have been reported with no additional toxicity (Friedberg JW & Fisher RI., 2006).

8.5.2 Limited stages

Classically, external beam radiation therapy was employed as a single modality in the therapy for localized DLBCL, with prolonged disease-free survival of approximately 35%. However with the success of anthracycline based chemotherapy in treating advanced stage DLBCL, the combination of CHOP with radiotherapy emerged as the strategy of choice for treating localized DLBCL (Miller et al., 1998). Several cooperative groups have developed clinical assays in order to elucidate which is the best chemotherapy regimen to combine with radiotherapy in these patients. The SWOG group showed advantage for progression-free survival (PFS) and overall survival (OS) in patients receiving 3 cycles of CHOP followed by involved field radiation (40-50 Gy) versus those who received 8 cycles of CHOP alone (Miller et al., 2001). Results worsened with the acquisition risk factors. Similar results in advantage for disease-free survival but not for OS were published for the ECOG group of patients receiving 8 cycles of CHOP followed by radiotherapy consolidation (Horning et al., 2004). The GELA group has also addressed this issue in several clinical trials suggesting no advantage for patients receiving radiotherapy and a short course of chemotherapy compared to those receiving standard chemotherapy (Reyes et al., 2005). Recent reports about the addition of rituximab showed advantages in PFS and OS to the historical experience without rituximab therapy (Persky, 2008). Nowadays, R-CHOP rather than CHOP would be recommended for these patients. However, no data exist to support the use of three courses of R-CHOP chemotherapy with radiation consolidation for limited stage disease. In view of the activity of R-CHOP in more advanced disease and in spite of the lack of a randomized trial to demonstrate its superiority in the setting of three rather than six courses, most clinicians prefer to use R-CHOP rather than CHOP.

8.5.3 Advanced stages

After rituximab was found to have activity in B cell NHL, the GELA group conducted a randomized trial to compare CHOP alone vs. R-CHOP in elderly patients (60 to 80 years old) with DLBCL. Chemotherapy courses were given every 3 weeks. Patients were randomly assigned to receive either eight cycles of CHOP every 21 days or eight cycles of R-CHOP. They concluded that the addition of rituximab to the CHOP regimen increases the complete remission rate and prolongs event-free and OS in this group of patients, without a clinically significant increase in toxicity (Coiffier et al., 2002). Once the GELA group proved the superiority of R-CHOP-21, Pfreundschuh et al. decided to conduct the trial known as MabThera International Trial (MInT) to evaluate CHOP-21, R-CHOP-21, CHOEP-21 and R-CHOEP-21 in patients aged 18–60 years with favorable prognosis (0-1 adverse risk factors according to age-adjusted International Prognostic Index). They concluded that rituximab added to six cycles of CHOP is an effective treatment for young patients with good-prognosis DLBCL (Pfreundschuh et al., 2006). The addition of rituximab to CHOP seems to eliminate the advantage of CHOEP over CHOP. This study also proved for the first time that rituximab when added to CHOP or CHOEP is effective in patients younger than 60 with favorable IPI. Following these results, the RICOVER-60 trial was developed to asses whether six courses were as effective as eight cycles and whether the addition of rituximab to CHOP-14 could improve outcome of patients treated with the CHOP-14 regimen. Conclusions of this study were that six cycles of R-CHOP-14 significantly improved event-free, PFS and OS over six cycles of CHOP-14 treatment. The other major conclusion of this study was that six cycles of chemotherapy with or without rituximab was as effective as eight cycles (Pfreundschuh et al., 2008). The RICOVER trial has been criticized for not including an arm with R-CHOP-21. As CHOP-14 is superior to CHOP-21, and R-CHOP-14 is superior to CHOP-14, it is logical to think that R-CHOP-14 should also be superior to R-CHOP-21. However, many investigators refuse to accept that R-CHOP-14 is the gold standard for treatment of DLCL until a randomized study with a control arm of R-CHOP-21 is carried out (Cabanillas, 2010).

8.5.4 Special considerations in DBCL and SLE therapy

When treatment options for DLBCL in the context of SLE are considered, special caution should be taken in order to manage the prognostic factors related to the tumor (e.g. histology, genetics and stage) as well as patient-specific factors (e.g. age, comorbidity, and general health status), because many lymphoma treatments are gruelling, particularly for old or frail individuals (Sehn et al., 2007). Patients with SLE often have both the hematopoietic reserve reduced and the immune function altered due to immunossupressive drugs thus being therapy-related infections a major problem in these patients. In this particular subset of patients with SLE and DLBCL, aggressive surveillance, prophylaxis, and treatment of infections are essential to prevent morbidity and mortality. Granulocyte colony stimulating factors (G-CSF) are largely used in the treatment of hematologic disorders to improve the myelosuppression indirectly induced by the chemotherapy regimen. G-CSF reduces the depth and duration of neutropenia in lymphoma patients and thus allows the design of more dose intense chemotherapy regimens which were shown to improve outcome particularly in patients with DLBCL (Lionne-Huyghe et al., 2006).

Besides, many SLE patients have deteriorated the glomerular filtration rate and a delay in drug excretion, needing the adjust of cytotoxic drugs to creatinine clearance. For this reason, management of tumor lysis syndrome in these patients can also be problematic. In order to avoid these problems, patients with SLE and renal impairment should be handled following chemotherapy schedules with a prephase treatment, in the same way on which are treated very aggressive lymphomas and elderly patients (Pfreundschuh, 2004, 2010). Sufficient fluid intake must be ensured, and appropriate supportive measures must be provided, including frequent electrolyte controls and allopurinol or even rasburicase administration to prevent hyperuricemia and tumor lysis syndrome.

SLE is associated with high cardiovascular morbidity and mortality. Clinically silent pulmonary hypertension, right ventricular dysfunction and myocardial perfusion defects usually asymptomatic are common in SLE patients (Plazak et al., 2011). A careful evaluation by means of echocardiography preferably with tissue doppler study and lung function test should be part of the pre-treatment studies to prevent anthracycline toxicity (Buss et al., 2010). Recommendations for therapy should be similar to elderly DLBCL patients. R-CHOP should be administered with close functional monitoring or even excluded if they present with cardiac-failure New York Heart Association > 2 and/or an ejection fraction < 50% or have a forced expiratory volume in 1 second (FeV1) level < 50% or a diffusion capacity < 50%. If cardiomyopathy is the only limiting condition, doxorubicin should be replaced by liposomal doxorubicin under close monitoring of the cardiac function. (Pfreundschuh, 2010; Zaja et al., 2006)

8.6 Marginal zone lymphoma

The marginal zone of lymphoid tissues is a unique B-cell compartment that contains B cells with a high surface density of IgM and complement receptor 2, and which exhibits a rapid activation and immunoglobulin secretion in response to blood-borne T-independent (Weill et al., 2009). This micro-anatomic compartment is well developed in lymphoid organs such as spleen, mesenteric lymph nodes and mucosa-associated lymphoid tissue or MALT where circulation of antigens occurs. Marginal B-cell lymphomas (MZL) are a well categorized group of indolent B-cell NHL that arise from the marginal zone of lymphoid tissues. The WHO-classification of tumors of hematopoietic and lymphoid tissues distinguish three different MZL types: extranodal, splenic and nodal (Isaacson et al., 2008).

Despite its common cell origin these three subtypes display differences in their frequency and clinical presentation and features according to the organ where the lymphoma arises. Extranodal MZL, also known as low-grade B-cell lymphoma of mucosa-associated lymphoid tissue (or MALT lymphoma) is the most common MZL subtype accounting for approximately 70% of all MZLs (Isaacson et al., 2004, 2008). These subtypes can arise at virtually any extranodal site and are commonly associated with chronic antigenic stimulation, either as a result of infection (eg, Helicobacter pylori in the stomach) or autoimmune disease. Splenic MZL accounts for approximately 20% of all MZLs. (Matutes et al., 2008). Patients typically present with an enlarged spleen, involvement of abdominal lymph nodes, and bone marrow disease. Liver and leukemic involvement are not infrequent. Nodal MZL is the least common, representing approximately 10% of all MZLs. (Arcaini et al., 2009). Patients with nodal MZL, by definition, have lymph node-based disease without involvement of the spleen or extranodal sites.

8.6.1 Therapy

Therapy of patients with MZL and SLE should not differ from that administered to patients without the latter condition. While some patients obtain cure of MALT lymphoma with an antibiotic treatment of the infectious causing agent, as occurs in the case of the infections for *H. pylori*, other patients require treatment with radio chemotherapy and immunotherapy (Martinelli et al., 2005; Zucca E & Dreyling M., 2008). Approximately 75 % of patients with gastric MALT lymphoma achieve a remission following the elimination of H. pylori with antibiotics (Du & Isaccson, 2002; Wundisch et al., 2005). The interval of histological regression following this treatment is variable, ranging from 1 to 25 months. In the cases both of persistent infection or resistant lymphoma, a second attempt with the antibiotic therapy is usually recommended (Psyrri et al., 2008). Although antibiotics have demonstrated efficacy in early stages of disease, its use is also recommended in patients with advanced stages, in those without apparent infection for *H. pylori*, as in those with primary non-gastric disease. However, a therapeutic consensual guide for these patients has not yet established, much less for patients with the rare condition of MALT lymphoma and SLE.

In addition, the therapeutic role of treatments against infectious pathogens in non-gastric MALT lymphoma is less defined. The therapeutic application of antibiotics against B. Bugdorferi in cutaneous MALT lymphoma has been described, as well as the treatment against *C. psittaci* in MALT lymphoma of ocular adnexa (Bertoni & Zucca, 2005; Ferreri et al., 2005). However the association of these pathogens with MALT lymphoma seems to show a marked geographical variation and the antibiotic effectiveness of the treatments has not been confirmed yet (Husain et al., 2007).

Treatment with the anti-CD20 monoclonal antibody rituximab, chemotherapy and radiation therapy as single agents or in combination are alternative therapies for patients failing to treatment with antibiotics. Rituximab has demonstrated efficacy in gastric MALT lymphoma without *H. pylori* evidence, in cases of refractory disease, in relapses and in advanced disease as well as in localized disease in non-gastric MALT lymphoma (Martinelli et al., 2005; Thieblemont & Coiffier, 2006). The combined administration of rituximab with chemotherapy increases the efficacy of the monoclonal antibody.

The regimens of chemotherapy include alkylating agents, commonly used in low-grade lymphomas, analogues of purines, like the fludarabine, whose use combined with rituximab has proven to be efficacious in patients with gastric and non-gastric MALT lymphoma (Levy et al., 2002). Recently, the combination of bendamustine (a new agent combining the alkylating and the purine analogue properties) with rituximab has demonstrated a great efficacy in achieving remission in MALT lymphoma of any origin with a very successful toxicity profile (Kahl et al., 2010). Anthracycline based regimes are occasionally used for young patients with aggressive gastric disease and for refractory patients to conventional treatments.

Splenic MZL is a disease with a relatively indolent course, but the optimal treatment strategy and outcome of splenic MZL remains undefined. Patients without a marked lymphocytosis, anemia or thrombocytopenia may not require treatment. However there is a significant group of patients who die from the lymphoma in a short interval of time (Chacón et al., 2002). Before rituximab, the recommended treatment for splenic MZL with symptomatic splenomegaly or threatening cytopenia was splenectomy, since chemotherapy had limited efficacy. Responses to splenectomy occurred in approximately 90% of patients (Sagaert X & Tousseyn T, 2010). Chemotherapy with CHOP and purine analogues such as fludarabine or pentostatine demonstrated objective responses (Franco et al., 2003). Presently, treatment of such patients with rituximab administered as a single agent or in combination has shown remarkable responses with an overall survival comparable to that reported following splenectomy (Bennett M & Schechter GP., 2010). Rituximab in combination with purine nucleosides may provide further improvement in PFS; however, confirmatory prospective trials are necessary.

As shown, in MZL chronic infections and autoimmune diseases such as SLE induce a chronic antigenic stimulation in B lymphocytes, through BCR. This constant stimulation induces the molecular NF-κB way, which probably plays a role in the initiation of the development of subsequent lymphoma (Thome, 2004; Ngo et al., 2011) Regarding therapy we can speculate with the future utility of drugs interacting the NF-κB way such as proteosome inhibitors (O'Connor, 2005).

8.7 Other lymphomas

Interestingly, a wide variety of lymphomas types with low prevalence has been reported in SLE patients. These subtypes include lymphoplasmacytic lymphoma (Papadaki et al., 2003), intravascular lymphoma (Sanchez-Cano et al., 2007), Franklin´s disease (García-Muñoz et al., 2008.), subcutaneous panniculitis-like T cell lymphoma (Pincus et al., 2009.), ALK-negative T cell anaplastic large cell lymphoma (Suvajdizc et al.,2003), peripheral T cell lymphoma (Löfström et al., 2007) and T cell leukemia/lymphoma (Frisch Stork et al.,2009).

9. Conclusions

SLE has an excess of lymphoma unrelated to immunosuppressive therapy. The mechanisms underlying the association between SLE and lymphoma remain unknown, but it is possible that impaired clearance of apoptotic cells in bone marrow and lymph nodes induces amplified stimulation of self-reactive B cells, increasing the risk to DNA damage and lymphomagenesis. Patients with SLE have shown an increased risk of marginal zone lymphoma, predominantly of the MALT type, and of DLBCL. Treatment of lymphoproliferative disorders in SLE does not differ from that administered to patients without SLE. Because the outcome is dependent on treatment, patients with SLE and suspected lymphoma should be evaluated jointly by both a rheumatologist and a hematologist with experience in lymphoproliferative disorders.

10. References

Arcaini L, Lucioni M, Boveri E, Paulli M. (2009). Nodal marginal zone lymphoma: current knowledge and future directions of a heterogeneous disease. Eur J Haematol. 2009;83:165-173.

Bassiota A, Frati A, Salvati M, Raco A, Fazi M, D´Elia A, Cruccu G.(2010). Primary hypothalamic lymphoma in a patient with systemic lupus erythematosus: case report and review of the literature. Neurol Sci 2010 Oct;31(5):647-52.

Bendandi M. (2008). Aiming at a curative strategy for follicular lymphoma.CA Cancer J Clin 2008;58:305-317.

Bennett M & Schechter GP. (2010). Treatment of splenic marginal zone lymphoma: splenectomy versus rituximab. Semin Hematol. 2010 Apr;47(2):143-7.

Bernatsky S, Ramsey-Goldman R, Rajan R, Boivin JF, Joseph L, Lachance S, Cournoyer D, Zoma A, Manzi S, Ginzler E, Urowitz M, Gladman D, Fortin PR, Edworthy S, Barr S, Gordon C, Bae SC, Sibley J, Steinsson K, Nived O, Sturfelt G, St Pierre Y & Clarke A. (2005a) Non-Hodgkin's lymphoma in systemic lupus erythematosus. Ann Rheum Dis. 2005 Oct;64(10):1507-9.

Bernatsky S, Boivin JF, Joseph L, Rajan R, Zoma A, Manzi S, Ginzler E, Urowitz M, Gladman D, Fortin PR, Petri M, Edworthy S, Barr S, Gordon C, Bae SC, Sibley J, Isenberg D, Rahman A, Aranow C, Dooley MA, Steinsson K, Nived O, Sturfelt G, Alarcón G, Senécal JL, Zummer M, Hanly J, Ensworth S, Pope J, El-Gabalawy H, McCarthy T, St Pierre Y, Ramsey-Goldman R, Clarke A. (2005b). An international cohort study of cancer in systemic lupus erythematosus. Arthritis Rheum. 2005 May;52(5):1481-90.

Bernatsky S, Ramsay-Goldman R, Lachance S, Pineau CA, Clarke AE. (2006). Lymphoma in a patient with systemic lupus erythematosus. Nat Clin Prac Rheumatol 2006 Oct;2(10):570-574.

Bernatsky S, Ramsey-Goldman R, Clark AE. (2009). Malignancy in systemic lupus erythematosus: what have we lerned? *Best Pract Res Clin Rheumatol.* 2009 August ; 23(4): 539–547.

Bertoni F & Zucca E. (2005). State-of-the-art therapeutics: marginal-zone lymphoma. J Clin Oncol. 2005 Sep 10;23(26):6415-20

Binet JL, Auquier A, Dighiero G, et al. (1981). A new prognostic classification of CLL derived from a multivariate survival analysis. Cancer 1981;48:198-206

Blaes AH & Morrison VA. (2010). Post-transplant lymphoproliferative disorders following solid-organ transplantation. Expert Rev Hematol. 2010 Feb;3(1):35-44.

Bloom B, Spits H. Development of human lymphoid cells. (2006). Ann Rev Immunol 2006;24:287-320.

Buss SJ, Wolf D, Korosoglou G, Max R, Weiss CS, Fischer C, Schellberg D, Zugck C, Kuecherer HF, Lorenz HM, Katus HA, Hardt SE, Hansen A. (2010). Myocardial left ventricular dysfunction in patients with systemic lupus erythematosus: new insights from tissue Doppler and strain imaging. J Rheumatol. 2010 Jan;37(1):79-86.

Cabanillas F. Front-line management of diffuse large B cell lymphoma (2010). Curr Opin Oncol. 2010 Nov;22(6):642-5.

Cappione AJ, Pugh-Bernard AE, Anolik JH, Sanz I. (2004) Lupus IgG VH4-34 antibodies bind to a 220-kDa glycoform of CD45/B220 on the surface of human B lymphocytes. J Immunol. 2004;172:4298-4307.

Cappione A 3rd, Anolik JH, Pugh-Bernard A, Barnard J, Dutcher P, Silverman G, Sanz I. Germinal center exclusion of autoreactive B cells is defective in human systemic lupus erythematosus. (2005) J Clin Invest. 2005;115:3205-3216

Carroll MC. (2004) A protective role for innate immunity in systemic lupus erythematosus. Nat Rev Immunol 2004;4:825-831

Chacón JI, Mollejo M, Muñoz E, Algara P, Mateo M, Lopez L, Andrade J, Carbonero IG, Martínez B, Piris MA, Cruz MA. (2002). Splenic marginal zone lymphoma: clinical characteristics and prognostic factors in a series of 60 patients. Blood 2002 Sep 1;100(5):1648-54.

Chan OT, Hannum LG, Haberman AM, et al. (1999) A novel mouse with B cells but lacking serum antiboy reveals an antibody-independent role for B cells in murine lupus. J. Exp. Med. 1999;189(10):1639-1648.

Cheson BD. (2011) New Agents in Follicular Lymphoma. Best Pract Res Clin Haematol. 2011 Jun;24(2):305-12.

Chiorazzi N, Hatzi K, Albesiano E. (2005) B cell chronic lymphocytic leukemia, a clonal disease of B lymphocytes with receptors that vary in specificity for (auto)antigens. Ann N Y Acad Sci. 2005 Dec;1062:1-12

Cobett SJ, Tomlinson IM, Sonnhammer EL, et al. (1997) Sequence of the human immunoglobulin diversity (D) segment locus: a systematic analysis provides no evidence for the use of DIR segments, inverted D segments, "minor" D segents or D-D recombination. J Mol Biol 1997;270:587-597

Coiffier B, Lepage E, Briere J, Herbrecht R, Tilly H, Bouabdallah R, Morel P, Van Den Neste E, Salles G, Gaulard P, Reyes F, Lederlin P, Gisselbrecht C. (2002). CHOP chemotherapy plus rituximab compared with CHOP alone in elderly patients with diffuse large-B-cell lymphoma. N Engl J Med. 2002 Jan 24;346(4):235-42.

Cook GP, Tomlinson IM. (1995) The human immunoglobulin VH repertoire. Immunol Today 1995;16:237-242.

Crespo M, Bosch F, Villamor N, et al. (2003) Zap-70 expression as a surrogate for IgV-region mutations in CLL. N Engl J Med 2003;348:1764-1775.

Damle RN, Wasil T, Fais et al, (1999) IGVH gene mutation status and CD38 expression as novel prognostic indicators in CLL. Blood 1999:94:1840-1847.

Diaz C, Isenberg DA. (2011) Susceptibility of patients with rheumatic disease to B cell non Hodgkin lymphoma. Nat Rev Rheumatol. 20011;7:360-368

DiLillo DJ, Hamaguchi Y, Ueda Y et al. (2008) Maintenance of long lived plasma cells and serological memory despite mature and memory B cell depletion during CD20 immunotherapy in mice. J Immunol 2008;180:361-71.

Döner T, Farner NL, Lipsky PE. (1999) Ig lambda and heavy chain gene usage in early untrated systemic lupus erythematosus suggest intensive B cell stimulation. J Immunol. 1999 Jul 15;163(2):1027-36

Döhner H, Silgenbauer S, Benner A, et al. (2000) Genomic aberrations and survival in CLL. N Engl J Med. 2000:343:1910-1916.

Dreyling M, Lenz G, Hoster E, et al. (2005) Early consolidation by myeloablative radiochemotherapy followed by autologous stem cell transplant in fist remission significantly prolongs progression-free survival in mantle-cell lymphoma: results of a prospective randomized trial of the European MCL Network. Blood 2005;105;2677-2684.

Du MQ, Isaccson PG. (2002). Gastric MALT lymphoma: from aetiology to treatment. Lancet Oncol. 2002 Feb;3(2):97-104.

Ferreri AJ, Ponzoni M, Guidoboni M, De Conciliis C, Resti AG, Mazzi B, Lettini AA, Demeter J, Dell'Oro S, Doglioni C, Villa E, Boiocchi M, Dolcetti R. (2005) Regression of ocular adnexal lymphoma after Chlamydia psittaci-eradicating antibiotic therapy. J Clin Oncol. 2005 Aug 1;23(22):5067-73.

Ferry JA. (2006) Burkitt Lymphoma: Clinicopathologic features and differential diagnosis. Oncologist.2006;11(4):375-383.

Fisher RI, Bernstein SH, Kahl BS, et al. (2006) Multicenter phase II study of botezomib in patients with relapsed or refractory mantle cell lymphoma. J Clin Oncol 2006;24:4867-4874.

Flores-Borja F, Kabouridis PS, Jury EC, et al. (2005) Decreased Lyn expression and traslocation of lipid raft signalling domains in B lymphocytes from patients with systemic lupus erythematosus. Arthritis Rheum. 2005;52(12):3955-3965

Franco V, Florena AM, Iannitto E. (2003). Splenic marginal zone lymphoma. Blood. 2003 Apr 1;101(7):2464-72.

Friedberg JW & Fisher RI. (2006). Diffuse large B-cell NHL. In Hodgkin´s and non-Hodgkin´s Lymphoma. Leonard JP and Coleman M, 121-140. Springer.

Fritsch-Stork RD, Leguit RJ, Derksen RH. (2009) Rapidly fatal HTLV-1 associated T cell leukemia/lymphoma in a patient with SLE. Nat Rev Rheumatol. 2009 May;5(5):283-7.

García-Muñoz R, Panizo E, Rodriguez-Otero P, Mugueta-Uriaque MC, Rifon J, Llorente L, Panizo C. (2008) Systemic lupus erythematosus and Franklin´s disease: when the somatic mutation mechanism makes a mistake. Rheumatology (Oxford)2008 Jul;47(7):1105-6

García-Muñoz R, Panizo C, Bendandi M, Llorente L. (2009) Autoimmunity and lymphoma: is mantle cell lymphoma a mistake of the receptor editing mechanism? Leuk Res. 2009 Nov;33(11):1437-9

Gay D, Saunders T, Camper S, Weigert M.(1993) Receptor editing: an approach by autoreactive B cells to escape tolerance. J. Exp. Med. 1993;177:999-1008

Gayed M, Bernatsky S, Ramsey-Goldman R, Clarke A, Gordon C. (2009) Lupus and cancer. Lupus. 2009 May;18(6):479-85

Gonzalez N, Xicoy B, Olive A, Jove J, Ribera JM, Feliu E. (2009) Systemic lupus erythematosus in a patient with primary MALT lymphoma of the laryx. Ear Nose Throat J 2009 Aug;88(8):E4-5.

Hadzidimitriou A, Darzentas N, Murray F, et al. (2009) Evidence for the significant role of immunoglobulin light chains in antigen recognition and selection in chronic lymphocytic leukemia. Blood. 2009 Jan 8;113(2):403-11.

Hallek M, Cheson BD, Catovsky D, et al. (2008) Guidelines for the diagnosis and treatment of chronic lymphocytic leukemia: a report from the international Workshop on chronic lymphocytic leukemia updating the National Cancer Institute-Working Group 1996 guidelines. Blood 2008;111:5446-56.

Hallek M. (2010) Therapy of chronic lymphocytic leukemia. Best Pract Res Clin Haematol. 2010 Mar;23(1):85-96.

Hamblin TJ, Davis Z, Gardiner A et al. (1999) Unmutated IGVH genes are associated with a more aggressive form of CLL. Blood 1999;94:1848-1854.

Halverson R, Torres RM, Pelanda R.(2004) Receptor editing is the main mechanism of B cell tolerance toward membrane antigens. Nat. Immunol. 2004;645-650

Harris NH, Swerdlow SH, Jaffe ES, Ott G, Nathwani BN, de Joug D, Yoshino T, Spagnolo D. (2008). Follicular lymphoma In: WHO Classification of Tumours of Haematopoietic and Lymphoid Tissues. Swerdlow SH, Campo E, Harris NL. IARC Press. Lyon, France, 229-232

Horning SJ, Weller E, Kim K, Earle JD, O'Connell MJ, Habermann TM, Glick JH. (2004). Chemotherapy with or without radiotherapy in limited-stage diffuse aggressive non-Hodgkin's lymphoma: Eastern Cooperative Oncology Group study 1484. J Clin Oncol. 2004 Aug 1;22(15):3032-8.

Howard OM, Gribben JG, Neuberg DS, et al. (2002) Rituximab and CHOP induction therapy for newly diagnosed mantle-cell lymphoma: molecular complete responses are not predictive of progression-free survical. J Clin Oncol 2002;20:1288-1294.

Husain A, Roberts D, Pro B, McLaughlin P, Esmaeli. (2007). Meta-analyses of the association between Chlamydia psittaci and ocular adnexal lymphoma and the response of ocular adnexal lymphoma to antibiotics. B.Cancer. 2007 Aug 15;110(4):809-15.

Isaacson PG, Du MQ. (2004) MALT lymphoma: from morphology to molecules. Nat Rev Cancer. 2004;4:644-653.

Isaacson PG, Chott A, Nakamura S. (2008). Extranodal marginal zone lymphoma of mucosa-associated lymphoid tissue (MALT lymphoma). In: WHO Classification of Tumours of Haematopoietic and Lymphoid Tissues. Swerdlow SH, Campo E, Harris NL. IARC Press. Lyon, France, 214-217.

Jaffe ES, Harris NL, Stein H, et al. (2008) Introduction ans overview of the classification of the lymphoid neoplasm. In Swerdlow SH, Campo E, Harris NL, et al (eds.) Who Classification of Tumours of Haematopoietic and Lymphoid Tissues. 2008 (4th ed.) pp.158-66. Lyon: IARC

Kahl BS, Bartlett NL, Leonard JP, Chen L, Ganjoo K, Williams ME, Czuczman MS, Robinson KS, Joyce R, van der Jagt RH, Cheson BD. (2010). Bendamustine is effective therapy in patients with rituximab-refractory, indolent B-cell non-Hodgkin lymphoma: results from a Multicenter Study. Cancer. 2010 Jan 1;116(1):106-14.

Kamradt T, Mitchinson NA. (2001) Tolerance and autoimmunity. N Engl J Med 2001;344(9):655-664

Kojima M, Itoh H, Shimizu K, Saruki N, Murayama K, Higuchi K, et al. (2006) Malignant lymphoma in patients with systemic rheumatic diseases (Rheumatoid arthritis, Systemic lupus erythematosus, systemic sclerosis and dermatomyositis): a clinicopathologic study of 24 Japanese cases. Int J Surg Pathol. 2006 Jan;14(1):43-8.

King JK, Costenbader KH. (2007) Characteristics of patients with systemic lupus erythematosus (SLE) and non Hodgkin´s lymphoma (NHL). Clin Rheumatol 2007 Sep;26(9):1491-4

Küppers R, Klein U, Hansmann ML, Rajewsky K. (1999) Cellular origin of human B cell lymphomas. N Engl J Med. 1999 Nov 11;342(20):1520-9

LeBien TW. (2000) Fates of B cell precursors. Blood 2000;96:9-23

LeBien TW, Tedder TF. (2008) B lymphocytes: how they develop and function. Blood 2008;112:1570-80.

Levy M, Copie-Bergman C, Traulle C, Lavergne-Slove A, Brousse N, Flejou JF, de Mascarel A, Hemery F, Gaulard P, Delchier JC; Groupe d'Etude des Lymphomes de l'Adulte (GELA). (2002). Conservative treatment of primary gastric low-grade B-cell lymphoma of mucosa-associated lymphoid tissue: predictive factors of response and outcome. Am J Gastroenterol. 2002 Feb;97(2):292-7.

Lionne-Huyghe P, Kuhnowski F, Coiteux V, Bauters F, Morschhauser F. (2006). Indications of G-CSF administration in hematologic disorders. Bull Cancer. 2006 May;93(5):453-62.

Lin MH, Huang JJ, Chen TY, Chen FF, Chang KC, Liu MF, Huang WT, Su WC, Tsao CJ. (2003) EBER-1 positive diffuse large cell lymphoma presenting as lupus nephritis. Lupus 2003:12(6):486-9.

Löftröm B, Baclin C, Sundström C, Ekbom A, Lundberg IE. (2007) A closer look at non-Hodgkin´s lymphoma cases in a national Swedish systemic lupus erythematosus cohort: a nested case control study. Ann Rheum Dis 2007;66:1627-1632.

Lossos IS, Czerwinski DK, Alizadeh AA, Wechser MA, Tibshirani R, Botstein D, Levy R. (2004). Prediction of survival in diffuse large-B-cell lymphoma based on the expression of six genes. N Engl J Med. 2004 Apr 29;350(18):1828-37.

Lugassy G, Lishner M, Polliak A. (1992) Systemic lupus erythematosus and chronic lymphocytic leukemia; rare coexistence in three patients, with comments on pathogenesis. Leuk Lymphoma 1992 Oct;8(3):243-5.

Luning Prak ET, Monestier M, Eisenber RA. (2011) B cell receptor editing in tolerance and autoimmunity. Ann N Y Acad Sci. 2011 Jan 5;1217:96-121

MacLennan IC. (1994) Germinal centers. Ann Rev Immunol 1994;12:117-139.

Maeda A, Hayama M, Nakata M, Masaki H, Tanemoto K. (2008) Mucosa-associated lymphoid tissue lymphoma in the thymus of a patient with systemic lupus erytematosus. Gen Thorac Cardiovasc Surg 2008 Jun;56(6):288-91.

Magrath I, Adde M, Shad A, et al. (1996) Adults and children with small non-cleaved-cell lymphoma have a similar excellent outcome when treated with the same chemotherapy regimen. J Clin Oncol 1996;14:925-934.

Martinelli G, Laszlo D, Ferreri AJ, Pruneri G, Ponzoni M, Conconi A, Crosta C, Pedrinis E, Bertoni F, Calabrese L, Zucca E. (2005). Clinical activity of rituximab in gastric marginal zone non-Hodgkin's lymphoma resistant to or not eligible for anti-Helicobacter pylori therapy. J Clin Oncol. 2005 Mar 20;23(9):1979-83.

Matutes E, Oscier D, Montalban C, Berger F, Callet-Bauchu E, Dogan A, Felman P, Franco V, Iannitto E, Mollejo M, Papadaki T, Remstein ED, Salar A, Solé F, Stamatopoulos K, Thieblemont C, Traverse-Glehen A, Wotherspoon A, Coiffier B, Piris MA. (2008) Splenic marginal zone lymphoma proposal for a revision of diagnostic, staging and therapeutic criteria. Leukemia. 2008;22:487-495.

Melamed D, Nemazee D. (1997) Self-antigen does not accelerate immature B cell apoptosis but stimulates receptor editing as a consequences of developmental arrest. Proc Natl Acad Sci USA 1997 Aug 19;94(17):9267-9272.

Miller TP, Dahlberg S, Cassady JR, Adelstein DJ, Spier CM, Grogan TM, LeBlanc M, Carlin S, Chase E, Fisher RI. (1998) Chemotherapy alone compared with chemotherapy plus radiotherapy for localized interrnediate- and high-grade non-Hodgkin's lymphoma. N Engl J Med. 1998 Jul 2;339(1):21-6.

Miller TP, LeBlanc M, Spier C. (2001). CHOP alone compared to CHOP plus radiotherapy for early stage aggressive non-Hodgkin's Iymphomas: Update of the Southwest Oncology Group (SWOG) randomized trial. Blood 98:724-5a, 2001.

Montserrat E, Sánchez-Bisono J, Vinolas N, Rozman C. (1986) Lymphocyte doubling time in CLL: analysis of its prognostic significance. Br J Haematol 1986; 62:567-575.

Munzert G, Frickhofen N, Bauditz J, Schreiber S, Hermann F. (1997) Concomitant manifestation of systemic lypus erythematosus and low-grade non-Hodgkin´s lymphoma. Leukemia 1997 Aug;11(8):1324-8

Nakajima PB, Kieffer K, Price A et al. (2009) Two distinct populations of H chain edited B cells show differential surrogate L chain dependence J Immunol. 2009;182:3583-3596

Ngo VN, Young RM, Schmitz R, Jhavar S, Xiao W, Lim KH, Kohlhammer H, Xu W, Yang Y, Zhao H, Shaffer AL, Romesser P, Wright G, Powell J, Rosenwald A, Muller-Hermelink HK, Ott G, Gascoyne RD, Connors JM, Rimsza LM, Campo E, Jaffe ES, Delabie J, Smeland EB, Fisher RI, Braziel RM, Tubbs RR, Cook JR, Weisenburger DD, Chan WC, Staudt LM. (2011). Oncogenically active MYD88 mutations in human lymphoma. Nature 2011 Feb 3;470(7332):115-9.

O'Connor OA, Wright J, Moskowitz C, Muzzy J, MacGregor-Cortelli B, Stubblefield M, Straus D, Portlock C, Hamlin P, Choi E, Dumetrescu O, Esseltine D, Trehu E, Adams J, Schenkein D, Zelenetz AD. (2005). Phase II clinical experience with the novel proteasome inhibitor bortezomib in patients with indolent non-Hodgkin's lymphoma and mantle cell lymphoma. J Clin Oncol. 2005 Feb 1;23(4):676-84

Odendahl M, Jacobi A, Hansen A, et al. (2000) Disturbed peripheral B lymphocytes homeostasis in systemic lupus erythematosus. J Immunol 2000;165;5970-5979.

Papadaki HA, Xylouri I, Katrinakis G, Foudoulakis A, Kriticos HD, Stathopoulos EN, Boumpas DT, Eliopoulos GD. (2003) Non-Hodkin´s lymphoma in patients with systemic lupus erythematosus. Leuk Lymphoma 2003;Feb;44(2):275-9.

Perkins AS, Friedberg JW. (2008) Burkitt´s lymphoma in adults. Haematology 2008;341-8.

Persky DO, Unger JM, Spier CM, Stea B, LeBlanc M, McCarty MJ, Rimsza LM, Fisher RI, Miller TP; Southwest Oncology Group. (2008). Phase II study of rituximab plus three cycles of CHOP and involved-field radiotherapy for patients with limited-stage aggressive B-cell lymphoma: Southwest Oncology Group study 0014. J Clin Oncol. 2008 May 10;26(14):2258-63

Pfreundschuh M, Trümper L, Kloess M, Schmits R, Feller AC, Rübe C, Rudolph C, Reiser M, Hossfeld DK, Eimermacher H, Hasenclever D, Schmitz N, Loeffler M; German High-Grade Non-Hodgkin's Lymphoma Study Group. (2004). Two-weekly or 3-weekly CHOP chemotherapy with or without etoposide for the treatment of elderly patients with aggressive lymphomas: results of the NHL-B2 trial of the DSHNHL. Blood. 2004 Aug 1;104(3):634-41.

Pfreundschuh M, Trümper L, Osterborg A, Pettengell R, Trneny M, Imrie K, Ma D, Gill D, Walewski J, Zinzani PL, Stahel R, Kvaloy S, Shpilberg O, Jaeger U, Hansen M, Lehtinen T, López-Guillermo A, Corrado C, Scheliga A, Milpied N, Mendila M, Rashford M, Kuhnt E, Loeffler M; MabThera International Trial Group.(2006). CHOP-like chemotherapy plus rituximab versus CHOP-like chemotherapy alone in young patients with good-prognosis diffuse large-B-cell lymphoma: a randomised controlled trial by the MabThera International Trial (MInT) Group. Lancet Oncol. 2006 May;7(5):379-91.

Pfreundschuh M, Schubert J, Ziepert M, Schmits R, Mohren M, Lengfelder E, Reiser M, Nickenig C, Clemens M, Peter N, Bokemeyer C, Eimermacher H, Ho A, Hoffmann M, Mertelsmann R, Trümper L, Balleisen L, Liersch R, Metzner B, Hartmann F, Glass B, Poeschel V, Schmitz N, Ruebe C, Feller AC, Loeffler M; German High-Grade Non-Hodgkin Lymphoma Study Group (DSHNHL). (2008). Six versus eight cycles of bi-weekly CHOP-14 with or without rituximab in elderly patients with aggressive CD20+ B-cell lymphomas: a randomised controlled trial (RICOVER-60). Lancet Oncol. 2008 Feb;9(2):105-16.

Pfreundschuh M. (2010). How I treat elderly patients with diffuse large B-cell lymphoma. Blood. 2010 Dec 9;116(24):5103-10.

Pincus LB, LeBoit PE, McCalmont TH, Ricci R, Buzio C, Fox LP, Oliver F, Cerroni L. (2009) Subcutaneus panniculitis.like T cell lymphoma with overlapping clinicopathologic features of lupus erythematosus coexistence of 2 entities?. Am J Dermatopathol 2009 Aug;31(6):520-6.

Plazak W, Gryga K, Milewski M, Podolec M, Kostkiewicz M, Podolec P, Musial J. (2011). Association of heart structure and function abnormalities with laboratory findings in patients with systemic lupus erythematosus. Lupus. 2011 Jun 2

Posner MA, Gloseter ES, Bonagura VR, Valacer DJ, LLowite NT. (1990) J Rheumatol 1990 Mar;17(3):380-2.

Psyrri A, Papageorgiou S, Economopoulos T. (2008). Primary extranodal lymphomas of stomach: clinical presentation, diagnostic pitfalls and management. Ann Oncol. 2008 Dec;19(12):1992-9

Pugh-Bernard, A.E. et al . (2001) Regulation of inherently autoreactive VH4-34 B cells in the maintance of human B cell tolerance. J Clin Invest. 2001;108:1061-1070.

Rai KR, Sawitsky A, Cronkite EP, et al. (1975) Clinical staging of CLL. Blood 1975;46:219-234.

Rajewsky K. (1996) Clonal selection and learning in the antibody system. Nature 1996;381:751-758.

Ravethc JV, Siebenlist U, Korsmeyer S, et al. (1981) Structure of the human immunoglobulin mu locus: characterization of embryonic and rearranged J and D genes. Cell 1981;27:583-591.

Reyes F, Lepage E, Ganem G, Molina TJ, Brice P, Coiffier B, Morel P, Ferme C, Bosly A, Lederlin P, Laurent G, Tilly H; Groupe d'Etude des Lymphomes de l'Adulte (GELA). (2005) ACVBP versus CHOP plus radiotherapy for localized aggressive lymphoma. N Engl J Med. 2005 Mar 24;352(12):1197-205

Romaguera JE, Fayad L, Rodriguez MA, et al. (2005) High Rate of durable remissions after treatment of newly diagnosed aggressive mantle cell lymphoma with Rituximab plus HyperCVAD alternating with Rituximab plus High dose Methotrexate and Cytarabyne. J Clin Oncol 2005;23(28):7013-7023.

Rosenwald A, Wright G, Chan WC, Connors JM, Campo E, Fisher RI, Gascoyne RD, Muller-Hermelink HK, Smeland EB, Giltnane JM, Hurt EM, Zhao H, Averett L, Yang L, Wilson WH, Jaffe ES, Simon R, Klausner RD, Powell J, Duffey PL, Longo DL, Greiner TC, Weisenburger DD, Sanger WG, Dave BJ, Lynch JC, Vose J, Armitage JO, Montserrat E, López-Guillermo A, Grogan TM, Miller TP, LeBlanc M, Ott G, Kvaloy S, Delabie J, Holte H, Krajci P, Stokke T, Staudt LM; Lymphoma/Leukemia Molecular Profiling Project. (2002) The Use of Molecular Profiling to Predict Survival after Chemotherapy for Diffuse Large B-Cell Lymphoma. N Engl J Med. 2002 Jun 20;346(25):1937-47.

Rossi E, Catania G, Truini M, Ravetti GL, Grassia L, Marmont AM. (2011) Patients with systemic lupus erythematosus (SLE) having developed malignant lymphomas. Complete remission of lymphoma following high-dose chemotherapy, but not of SLE. Clin Exp Rheumatol 2011 May-Jun;29(3)555-9.

Rummel MJ, Al-Batran SE, Kim S-Z, et al. (2005) Bendamustine plus Rituximab is effective and has a favorable toxicity profile in the treatment of mantle cell and low grade non Hodgkin´s lymphoma. J Clin Oncol 2005;23(15):3383-3389

Sagaert X & Tousseyn T. (2010). Marginal zone B-cell lymphomas. Discov Med. 2010 Jul;10(50):79-86.

Sanchez-Cano D, Callejar-Rubio JL, Vilanova-Mateu A, Gómez-Morales M, Ortego-Centeno N. (2007) Intravascular lymphoma in a patient with systemic lupus erythematosus; a case report. Lupus 2007;16(7):525-8.

Sehn LH, Berry B, Chhanabhai M, Fitzgerald C, Gill K, Hoskins P, Klasa R, Savage KJ, Shenkier T, Sutherland J, Gascoyne RD, Connors JM. (2006). The revised International Prognostic Index (R-IPI) is a better predictor of outcome than the standard IPI for patients with diffuse large B-cell lymphoma treated with R-CHOP. Blood. 2007 Mar 1;109(5):1857-61.

Silberstein LE, et al. (1991) Variable region gene analysis of pathologic human autoantibodies to the related i and I red blood cell antigens. Blood. 1991;78:2372-2386.

Simon Z, Tarr T, Ress Z, Gergely L, Kiss E, Illes A. (2007) Successful rituximab-CHOP treatment of systemic lupus erythematosus associated with diffuse large B-cell non Hodgkin lymphoma. Rheumatol Int 2007 Dec;28(2)179-83.

Smedby KE, Hjalgrim H, Askling J, Chang ET, Gregersen H, Porwit-MacDonald A, Sundström C, Akerman M, Melbye M, Glimelius B, Adami HO. (2006). Autoimmune and chronic inflammatory disorders and risk of non-Hodgkin lymphoma by subtype. J Natl Cancer Inst 2006; 98: 51–60

Smedby KE, Vajdic CM, Falster M, Engels EA, Martínez-Maza O, Turner J, Hjalgrim H, Vineis P, Seniori Costantini A, Bracci PM, Holly EA, Willett E, Spinelli JJ, La Vecchia C, Zheng T, Becker N, De Sanjosé S, Chiu BC, Dal Maso L, Cocco P, Maynadié M, Foretova L, Staines A, Brennan P, Davis S, Severson R, Cerhan JR, Breen EC, Birmann B, Grulich AE & Cozen W. (2008a) Autoimmune disorders and risk of non-Hodgkin lymphoma subtypes: a pooled analysis within the InterLymph Consortium. Blood. 2008 Apr 15;111(8):4029-38.

Smedby KE, Askling J, Mariette X, Baecklund E. (2008b). Autoimmune and inflammatory disorders and risk of malignant lymphomas--an update. J Intern Med. 2008 Dec;264(6):514-27.

Suarez F, Lortholary O, Hermine O, Lecuit M. (2006) Infection-associated lymphomas derived from marginal zone B cells: a model of antigen-driven lymphoproliferation. Blood. 2006 Apr 15;107(8):3034-44

Suvajdzic N, Stojanovic-Milenkovic R, Tomasevic Z, Cemerikic-Martinovic V, Mihalijevic B, Atkinson HD. (2003) ALK-negative T cell anaplastic large cell lymphoma associated with systemic lupus erythematosus. Med Oncol. 2003;20(4):409-12.

Suvajdzic N, Djurdjevic P, Todorovic M, Perunicic M, Stojanovic R, Novkovic A, Mihaljevic B. (2011) Clinical characteristics of patients with lymphoproliferative neoplasms in the setting of systemic autoimmune diseases. Med Oncol 2011.

Swerdlow SH, Campo E, Harris NL, et al, (2008) WHO Classification of Tumours of Haematopoietic and Lymphoid Tissues. Lyon, France: IARC Press

Swerdlow SH, Campo E, Seto M, Müller-Hermelink HK. (2008). Mantle cell lymphoma In: WHO Classification of Tumours of Haematopoietic and Lymphoid Tissues. Swerdlow SH, Campo E, Harris NL. IARC Press. Lyon, France, 229-232

Tekonidou MG. (2010) MALT lymphoma of the lacrimal gland in the contexto f systemic lupus erythematosus: complete remission after treatment with rituximab. Lupus 2010 Sep;19(10):1243-5.

Thieblemont C & Coiffier B. (2006). Management of marginal zone lymphomas. Curr Treat Options Oncol. 2006 May;7(3):213-22

Thomas DA, Farderl S, O´Brien S, Bueso-Ramos C, et al. (2006) Chemoimmunotherapy with hyper-CVAD plus Rituximab for the treatment of adult Burkitt and Burkitt-type lymphoma or acute lymphoblastic leukemia. Cancer 2006;106(7):1569-1569-1580.

Thome M. (2004). CARMA1, BCL-10 and MALT1 in lymphocyte development and activation. Nat Rev Immunol. 2004 May;4(5):348-59

Throsélius M, Krober A, Murray F, et al.(2006) Striklingly homologous immunoglobulin gene rearrangements and poor outcome in VH3-21 using CLL patients independent of geographic origin and mutational status. Blood 2006;107:2889-94.

Tiegs SL, Russell DM, Nemazee D. (1993) Receptor editing in self-reactive bone marrow B cells. J. Exp. Med. 1993;177:1009-1020.

Tripodo C, Porcasi R, Guarnotta C, Ingrao S, Campisi V, Florena AM, et al. (2007) C1q production by bone marrow stromal cells. Scand J Immunol 2007;65:308-309.

Tsuiji M, Yurasov S, Velinzon K, Thomas S, Nussenzweig MC, Wardemann H. (2006) A check point for autorreactivity in human IgM memory B cell development. J Exp Med 2006;203(2):393-400

Wang YH, Nomura J, Faye-Petersen OM, Cooper MD. (1998) Surrogate light chain production during B cell differentiation: differential intracellular vs cell surface expression. J Immunol 1998; 161:1132-9

Wang JH, Alt FW, Gostissa M, et al. (2008) Oncogenic transformation in the absence of Xrcc4 targets peripheral B cells that have undergone editing and switching. J Exp Med. 2008 Dec 22;205(13):3079-90

Weill JC, Weller S, Reynaud CA.(2009). Human marginal zone B cells. Annu Rev Immunol. 2009;27:267-85.

William J, Euler C, Primarolo N et al. (2006) B cell tolerance checkpoints that restrict pathways of antigen-driven differentiation. J Immunol. 2006;176(4):2142-2151.

Wündisch T, Thiede C, Morgner A, Dempfle A, Günther A, Liu H, Ye H, Du MQ, Kim TD, Bayerdörffer E, Stolte M, Neubauer A. (2005). Long-term follow-up of gastric MALT lymphoma after Helicobacter pylori eradication. J Clin Oncol. 2005 Nov 1;23(31):8018-24.

Xu Y, Wiernik P. Systemic lupus erythematosus and B cell hematologic neoplasm. Lupus 2001;10(12):841-50.

Yurasov S, Wardemann H, Hammersen J, et al. (2005a) Defective B cell tolerance checkpoints in systemic lupus erythematosus. J Exp Med 2005. Feb 28;201(5):703-711

Yurasov S, Hammersen J, Tiller T et al. (2005b) B cell tolerance checkpoints in healthy humans and patients systemic lupus erythematosus. Ann N Y Acad Sci. 2005. Dec;1062:165-174

Yurasov S, Tiller T, Tsuiji M, Velinzon K, Pascual V, Wardemann H, Nussenzweig MC. (2005c) Persistent expression of autoantibodies in SLE patients in remission. J Exp Med 2006;203:2255–2261.

Zaja F, Tomadini V, Zaccaria A, Lenoci M, Battista M, Molinari AL, Fabbri A, Battista R, Cabras MG, Gallamini A, Fanin R. (2006). CHOP-rituximab with pegylated liposomal doxorubicin for the treatment of elderly patients with diffuse large B-cell lymphoma. Leuk Lymph 2006;47(10):2174-2180.

Zucca E & Dreyling M; ESMO Guidelines Working Group. (2008). Gastric marginal zone lymphoma of MALT type: ESMO clinical recommendations for diagnosis, treatment and follow-up. Ann Oncol. 2008 May;19 Suppl 2:ii70-1

19

Infections and Systemic Lupus Erythematosus

C. Alejandro Arce-Salinas and Pablo Villaseñor-Ovies
Hospital Central Sur de Alta Especialidad, PEMEX
Instituto Nacional de Rehabilitación, SSA
México City
México

1. Introduction

Notwithstanding that life expectancy in patients with systemic lupus erythematosus (SLE) has improved progressively in the last few decades, the mortality rates remain three times higher as compared with the general population (Uramoto et al, 1998). Reported causes of death vary according to the region of the world, yet there is agreement on the bimodal curve of mortality rate in these patients, with an initial peak occurring early after diagnosis, strongly related with disease activity and infections, and a later escalade associated with cardiovascular disease, accrued damage, and infections too (Rubin et al, 1985). It may be due to its complexity that infectious disease is often considered a grim topic in SLE, but it is undeniable that infections are important contributors of mortality in every stage of the disease.

The range of infections in lupus patients varies widely, from opportunistic infections - attributable in some level to immunological dysfunction- to common bacterial and viral infections with typical or atypical presentations. Moreover, patients with lupus exhibit increased proclivity to hospital acquired infections than hospitalized patients with other diagnosis. Some authors have stressed out the association that certain conditions have with the risk of infections in patients with lupus. Some of these include: high disease activity, specific immune dysregulation; drug-induced immune deficiency; and organ failure due to irreversible damage.

On the other hand, several clinical manifestations like fever, lymphadenopathy, unexplained confusion, pulmonary infiltrates, skin and mucosal injuries, coagulation disorders, and others, represent true diagnostic challenges for the clinician who may take them as clues of a lupus flare, or may be compelled to commence a trial of antimicrobial treatment because these may also be the clinical expression of a life-threatening infection, or perhaps, as it often occurs in the field treat both conditions simultaneously. Some evidence suggests that certain infections, particularly of viral nature, might participate in disease initiation, disease flare or worsening of an active lupus condition.

In this chapter we will review the current information regarding infections in patients with SLE, and recommendations to prevent and treat them.

2. Immune dysfunction and infection in SLE

Patients with SLE are known to have defects both in the humoral and the cellular branches of the immune system. Some of these defects participate in the inadequacy of immune defense against pathogens. The relationship between altered immune function and infections in SLE is exceedingly complex, as infectious agents can interact with the immune system in several ways, and the immune system itself works as an intricate, overlapping and sometimes redundant network of signals and checkpoints under different levels of control. Of course, the defective immune function is not universal and as in other aspects of the disease, its expression is not homogenous among lupus patients and hence susceptibility to different pathogens is reasonably variable. The potential role of macrophage and polymorphonuclear defects, reduced numbers and dysfunction of T-cells and B-cells, defects in the production of immunoglobulin and altered function of the reticuloendothelial system are all considered to take part in the altered immune response against pathogens that is present in a proportion of patients with SLE (Sebastiani & Galeazzi, 2009; Iliopoulos & Tsokos, 1996).

All this is further complicated by the almost obligated use of immunosuppressant drugs to control disease activity. Nevertheless, the young readers will be surprised to know that 60 years ago, lupus was not treated with steroids or immunossuppresants and despite that, infection was still one of the major causes of death in lupus patients. (Klemperer, et al 1941)

2.1 Defects in the complement system

The complement system plays a crucial role in host defense against pathogens and the increased infection rates observed in SLE patients have been attributed in part to defects of the complement system that are in turn, frequent in SLE. Genetic deficiencies of early components of the classical pathway are major risk factors for the development of lupus, particularly C1q deficiency. Since C1q plays an important role in complement activation through the recognition and clearance of apoptotic material, antibodies and structural proteins on bacteria and viruses, it is not surprising that a deficient state would increase susceptibility to infection. Also the consumption of complement components by immune complexes is also considered to limit the amount of complement available to be used against invading pathogens. Reduction of other components of the complement system comes with various risk degrees of specific infections, i.e. C3: encapsulated bacteria, C5-C9: Neisserial infections. (Pickering et al, 2000; Figueroa & Densen, 1991)

2.2 Mannose-Binding Lectin (MBL) and Infections in SLE

The lectin pathway of complement activation is also implicated in the pathogenesis of lupus and most likely in the increased propensity to infections in this disease, as well. MBL is a serum protein that serves as a recognition particle in the lectin pathway of complement activation. Additionally, MLB may directly opsonise pathogenic microorganisms and activate phagocytes. Several studies have demonstrated that variant alleles of MBL are associated with an increased risk for the development of SLE. Furthermore, among patients with SLE, those homozygous for MBL allelic variants had an increased risk of serious infections in comparison with patients heterozygous of homozygous for the normal allele (M.Y. Mok et al, 2007a). Other studies have failed to demonstrate a connection between functional MBL activity and the occurrence of infections (Bultink et al, 2006). This discrepancy between the genotypic and phenotypic data could be explained by the fact that functional activity of MBL is not only determined by mutations on its encoding gene. Also, the immune system has redundancies and in most cases, increased susceptibility to infection with MBL deficiency arises when other factors are inducing immune dysfunction (i.e.

immunosuppressive drugs). In fact, low levels of MBL are associated with poorer outcomes in severe infections, even in otherwise immunocompetent individuals. In synthesis, a proportion of patients with lupus appear to have increased frequency of infections related to allele variants of MBL; such infections are for the most part from encapsulated bacteria, and most likely owing to defective opsonization (Monticielo et al, 2008; Super et al. 1989).

2.3 Cellular immune defects

The diminished phagocytic activity observed in monocytes from patients with lupus, may be due to a decrease in the production of TNF-α, deficit in the generation of superoxide, or by the presence of specific autoantibodies against receptor Fcγ. These autoantibodies may have a wider effect over the immune system because these receptors also exist on the surface of B-cells, natural killer cells, and some T-cells (Boros et al, 1993; Yu et al, 1989). Defective phagocytosis has also long been noticed in polymorphonuclear leukocytes in patients with lupus. Although the presence of antibodies against neutrophil cytoplasmic components, some of which are directly involved in pathogen fighting (i.e. lactoferrin, elastase and lysozyme), has been reported in SLE, its clinical significance is still obscure. Their presence has no influence over total number of neutrophils and their precise contribution to the increased susceptibility to infections in SLE, remains to be determined (Lee et al, 1992; Schnabel et al, 1995).

T-cell lymphopenia is the most common quantitative disorder observed in the blood of patients with lupus. Lymphopenia correlates with disease flares and responds to immunosuppressive treatment. It is generally considered to be a major contributor in the increased propensity to infections. T-cells also exhibit important functional deficits. Impaired T-cell cytolytic activity is largely attributable to a decreased production of interleukin-2 and γ-interferon and is more prominent within the CD8+ T-cell population. On top of the reduced delayed hypersensitivity skin response that happens in patients with SLE. A group of studies pointed out that an important proportion of patients with SLE have altered *in vitro* immune responses to alloantigens and recall antigens, and that such dysfunction correlates with higher disease activity. (Yu et al, 1989; Gumma et al, 1994).

In general, B-cell functions seem unaltered in SLE. Antibody production and immunization are preserved in the majority of cases, but some B-cell and immunoglobulin alterations have been described. Scattered reports of transient or permanent hypogammaglobulinemia with an increased risk of infections were informed prior to the use of anti-CD20 therapies. Alternatively, many patients with SLE display a prominent polyclonal B-cell activation and hypergammaglobulinemia (Yong et al, 2008, Karim 2006; Battafarano et al 1998).

Transient or permanent spleen dysfunction is associated with diverse autoimmune diseases including SLE. In SLE, functional asplenia, defined as failure of splenic uptake of a radiolabeled colloid is present in approximately 5% and seems to correlate with disease activity. Asplenia increases vulnerability to pneumoccocal and Salmonella infections (Fishman & Isenbert, 1997). **Table 1** summarizes factors predisposing SLE patients to infections.

3. Epidemiology of infections in systemic lupus erythematosus

Although infections in SLE remain as an important clinical concern that should have a prominent place in the research agenda in lupus, there is a notorious absence of high-quality studies addressing this phenomenon. The majority of studies involve hospitalized patients, a population that certainly has a selection bias and limits their external validity; also, we

Cellular immunity	
T-cell lymphopenia	
Impaired T-cell cytotoxic activity	
Altered recall of antigens	
Diminution of NK-cell function and number	
Humoral immunity	
Antibodies against Fcγ receptor	
Antibodies against neutrophil cytoplasmic components	
Hypogammaglobulinemia	
Phagocytic deficiency	
Mononuclear cell defective phagocytosis	
Deficit in superoxide generation	
Cytokine defects and other immune anomalies	
Mannose-binding lectin allelic variants	
Hypocomplementemia	
Decrease in the production of TNF-α	
Decrease of IL-2 production	
Other cytokine imbalance (IL-10, γ-interferon, IL-1)	
Disease related	
Disease activity and/or glucocorticoid use	
Transient or permanent spleen dysfunction	
Accrued damage (irreversible damage, i.e. ESRD, lung fibrosis, etc.)	
Treatment related	
Immunosuppressive drugs	
Glucocorticoids	
Immune targeted biologic agents	

Table 1. Summary of factors related to infection propensity in SLE

found a great number of patient series and case reports of outstanding features but only a few prospective cohorts in most of which the outpatient setting had been neglected.

Morbidity of lupus patients varies with the chronological stage of the disease. In subjects with short disease duration, the most important causes of hospitalization and medical attention are related to disease activity and common bacterial or viral infections and few opportunistic infections. With the improved survival rates and longer disease duration, other morbid conditions are commonly identified in longstanding disease; the most regularly described are accelerated atherosclerosis and cardiovascular disease, osteoporosis, osteonecrosis, cognitive dysfunction, chronic fatigue, fibromyalgia, malignancies and the coexistence with other chronic illnesses such as diabetes mellitus and systemic hypertension. However, infectious disease is still one of the most important causes of hospitalizations and death in this group.

In a large cohort of patients with SLE followed in several European countries, the annual incidence of infection was 27% during the first 5 years. A follow-up report indicates that infections continued to be the cause of one fifth of all hospitalizations in the second half of the 10 year follow-up, with a notorious reduction in the diagnosis of sepsis in this later period (Cervera et al, 2003). Other authors have reported on the burden of infectious disease in SLE: close to 15% of patients with lupus are hospitalized for major infections every year; the risk of major infection is 60% higher in SLE as compared with other chronic diseases, and many of them are treated in the ICU. A bacterial etiology is detected in the majority of cases and lower respiratory tract is the most important site of infection. Mexican researchers performed a study to determine the incidence of infections in their group; among the ambulatory patients, 57% of hospitalizations were due to infection of any kind, and although diagnostic confirmation was achieved only in one third of their cohort, all patients with suspicion of infection, received complete antibiotic courses. They found 12.5% of nosocomial infections in non-infected subjects admitted for other reasons (Navarro-Zarza et al, 2010). Furthermore, Al-Arfaj in Arabia found, in patients followed by almost 30 years with a remarkable long-term survival, that 50% of deceases were related to severe bacterial sepsis, mainly in subjects with renal failure (Al-Arfaj & Khalil, 2009). Other groups in different regions of the world report similar rates of infections in SLE, emphasizing that these complications remain as a significant problem both in the outpatient care and in the hospital setting.

Infections are also a prominent cause of death among lupus patients. On the early 1980's, a multicenter evaluation in more than 1,000 lupus patients was reported, revealing that one third of registered deaths were caused by infections and another third because of disease activity. Other authors, in different regions of the world, have assessed the issue of mortality due to infections, and with different methodological approaches, mortality rate associated to this cause is reported from 14 to 50% of all deaths (Cervera et al, 2003; Zandman-Goddard & Shoenfeld, 2003; Gladman et al, 2002).**Table 2** depicts impact of infections in general mortality of SLE patients.

The nature of most infections in lupus patients either in the ambulatory or nosocomial settings is mainly of bacterial origin, being lower respiratory and urinary tract infections the most frequently registered, with less cases of sepsis of unknown cause, soft tissue & skin and other common bacterial infections (Gladman et al, 2002; Iliopoulos & Tsokos, 1996). Nevertheless, it should be underlined that non-complicated infections occurring on ambulatory settings are not usually recorded, and it is possible these may be underestimations of the true burden they give. In a prospective study of an outpatient clinic, an incidence of 32% of infections along 2 years of follow-up was observed. Urinary tract infections (UTI) due to *Escherichia coli*, skin infections produced by *Staphylococcus aureus*, and simultaneous infections of different sites were the most frequently registered; the majority were treated on ambulatory basis with good results (Zonana-Nacach et al, 2001).

Nosocomial infections are a noteworthy issue to address in this scenery. Some investigators reported that more than a half of infections diagnosed in SLE patients are of a nosocomial source, mostly upper and lower respiratory and bloodstream infections; patients with organ dysfunctions and with high-steroid dose are more susceptible to acquire nosocomial infections. The most important information in this regard comes from Navarro-Zarza's cohort, indicating an incidence rate of 12.5% among patients who had neither symptoms nor clinical suspicion of infection at admission, and afterward develop nosocomial infections; higher disease activity score measured by the Mex-SLEDAI (Guzmán et al, 1992), high damage scores (SLICC/ACR), immunosuppressive treatment and length of hospital stay were all risk factors for the development of nosocomial infection (Navarro-Zarza et al, 2010).

Consequently, lupus patients admitted for hospital care are at higher risk of infection and any action to lower their incidence, by every member of the healthcare team should be implemented with emphasis.

Author, year/Site	# of patients followed by time	# of deaths	Survival	% of deceases due to infections
C.C.Mok, 2000/China	186 by 7 y	9	93% - 5 y	75%
Kasitanon, 2002 /Thailand	349 by 14 y	52	84% - 5 y; 75% - 10 y	35%
Cervera, 2003/Europe	1,000 by 10 y	68	97% - 5 y; 92% - 10 y	25%
Pons-Estel 2004/Latin America	1,214 by 3 y	34	ND	58%
Bernatsky, 2006/North-America§	9,547 by 30 y	1,255	ND	5%
Wadee, 2007/South Africa	226 by 15 y	55	72% - 5 y; 58% - 10 y	44%
Nossent, 2007/Europe	2,500 by 5 y	91	ND	57%
Al-Arfaj, 2009/ Saudi Arabia	624 by 30 y	25	98% - 5 y; 97% - 10 y	48%
Goldblatt, 2009/UK	104 (of 407) by 29 y¶	67	ND	25%

¶ Only reports results of 104 patients hospitalized form a cohort of 470
§ Study in 23 Centers of US, Canada and UK, only 1 in Sweden and 1 in Iceland

Table 2. Percentage of deaths due to infections in some studies around the world.

Infectious diseases in SLE patients admitted to the ICU require an additional comment. Most admissions to the ICU in lupus patients are related to infection, and a considerable mortality is usually observed (45-86%); the most often reported predictive markers are: higher APACHE-II scores, length of stay in the ICU, and inadequate initial selection of antibiotics. It has been shown that not infected patients with SLE admitted to the ICU with lupus flares, exhibit high mortality rates (75-95%), and nosocomial acquired infections are a relevant complication in most cases. These reports, as well as others (Alzeer et al, 2004), highlight the importance of pneumonia and bacterial sepsis of unknown origin as the most frequent reason for admission to ICU, and their relationship with poor outcomes.

3.1 Usual bacterial infections

Common microorganisms underlie the majority of infections among lupus patients. Pneumonia and respiratory tract infections are the most recognized (Petri, 2008). Some immune defects increase susceptibility to certain bacteria, but no comparative studies have made clear the possible connection that such defects may have with specific infections. Continuing on the subject of common infections, *S. aureus* and *Streptococcus pyogenes* persist as the most frequent etiology of respiratory infections. However, as mentioned, information related to respiratory infection in the outpatient setting is scarce, and not surprisingly pathogens differ in the hospitalized subject; gram-negative bacteria appear as key pathogens in respiratory infections in these circumstances, being *Klebsiella sp, Pseudomonas aeruginosa,* and *E. coli* mainly involved. *Streptococcus pneumoniae* has been reported as a cause of septicemia; interestingly, lower rates of pneumococcal septicemia have been seen after the implementation of routine vaccination.

Bladder dysfunction seems to be more prevalent among women with SLE; in an outpatient cohort, near to 10% suffered of recurrent infection and depict abnormal voiding function tests, with small bladder capacity, reduced bladder sensation, residual urine and abnormal urinary flows. These data were alike to those reported by others, and also shows a possible association of these abnormalities and disease activity. Urinary tract infections are very common among women with SLE, and the functional derangements previously mentioned are found often, particularly in cases of recurrent infections. *E coli* and *Streptococcus agalactiae* were the most prevalent recovered microorganisms (Durán-Barragán et al, 2008).

Infections due to *Salmonella* species are important cause of bacteremia after ingestion of contaminated food; inasmuch as underdeveloped countries have more risk conditions to this infection, it has been reported more frequently in these regions of the world. Lupus patients' conditions are prone to develop primary bacteremia, extra-intestinal collections, osteomyelitis, septic arthritis, infective endocarditis, bloodstream and endovascular infections, even in absence of gastrointestinal symptoms. Infections of different *Salmonella* serogroups are also related to high mortality, as it has been shown after bacteremia episodes. Risk factors for mortality due to *Salmonella* infection are re-infection, older age and concomitant infection with other microorganisms; a high index of suspicion is vital, insofar as salmonellosis and SLE have similarities in clinical manifestations like fever, rash, pleurisy, abdominal complaints and synovitis. **Table 3** describes the main pathogens observed in prospective or relevant studies in different regions of the world.

3.2 Infections due to Mycobacteria

Infections as a consequence of *Mycobacterium* species are of two groups: infections due to *M tuberculosis,* that trend to occur early in the course of lupus, related to disease activity and treatment, and usually resulting mainly from reactivation of latent infection or to reinfection; and infections to non-tuberculous *Mycobacterium* (NTM), presenting later in the course of disease and predominantly as a new infection, including *M. avium* complex, *M. chelonae, M. haemophilum* or *M. fortitum* (Cuchacovich & Gedalia, 2009). Mok et al (M.Y. Mok et al, 2007b) describes 11 cases of NTM infections localized in skin and soft tissues, in patients with long disease duration and long cumulative prednisone dose. In transplant patients, SLE remains as a risk factor for tuberculosis with a substantial increase of mortality among patients with this infection.

Mycobacterium tuberculosis infections represent a great problem to many countries around the world. The HIV pandemic and use of biologic immune-regulator agents for other rheumatic conditions are related to rise of tuberculosis (TB) in regions where TB was believed near to ending (Mathers & Loncar, 2006). In point of fact, since the first use of high-steroid doses in rheumatic diseases, an increase of TB infections was noticed, as well as reactivation of previously treated TB once steroids were newly administered (Yun et al, 2002); besides, occurrence of TB is closely and directly interrelated to the mean daily doses or cumulative steroid-dose. In lupus patients, TB is a major contributor of morbidity and mortality. There seems to be a higher risk for this infection and clinical illness in these patients is often extra-pulmonary (miliary) where hematogenous dissemination is usually

Author, year/Site	# patients observed	# of infections	Main pathogens (Percentage of total)	Characteristics
Oh, 1993/Singapore	28	38	*S. aureus* (21%) *P. aeruginosa* (11%) *Klebsiella sp.* (11%) *E. coli* (7%) *M. tuberculosis* (7%)	Hospitalized patients followed by 8 months
Zonana-Nacach, 2001/Mexico	200	65	*E. coli* (25%) *S. aureus* (8%) *Candida sp.* (6%) *M. tuberculosis* (2%) *Salmonella sp.* (2%)	Outpatient only. Two years of observation
Leone, 2007/Brazil	71	48	*S aureus* (50%) *P. aeruginosa* (17%) *Candida sp.* (17%) *Aspergillus sp.* (17%)	Juvenile SLE, 18 deaths.
Ramírez-Gómez, 2007/Colombia	ND	123	*E. coli* (22%) *Staphylococcus sp.* (15%) *Klebsiella sp.* (9%) *Candida sp.* (9%) *P. aeruginosa* (4%)	All nosocomial acquired. High disease activity (SLEDAI > 11). Three years of observations
Ruiz-Irastorza, 2009/Spain	249	88	*E. coli* 16% *S. aureus* 14% *M. tuberculosis* 12% *S. pneumoniae* 9% *Candida sp.* 7%	Major infections (organ dysfunction, hospitalized)
Navarro-Zarza, 2010/Mexico	473	268 (confirmed 96)	*E. coli* (48%) *Candida sp.* (21%) *Staphylococcus sp.* (15%) *Streptococcus sp.* (12%) *M. tuberculosis* 4.5%	Community acquired infections seen along 5 years

Table 3. Pathogens frequency in some prospective studies around the world

the mechanism involved (Hou et al, 2008). Extra-pulmonary tuberculosis presents a wide range of symptoms, which may confound with other diseases, or with disease activity; symptoms like arthritis, lymphadenopathy, lung nodules, pulmonary infiltrates, pleural effusion, weight loss and renal abnormalities offer this challenge, so, workup to identify mycobacteria is imperative. Moreover, in a review of patients with central nervous system involvement, *M. tuberculosis* represents a frequent cause of meningitis that requires prompt recognition and treatment, since it is linked to high mortality and severe functional sequels (Yang et al, 2007). Burden of TB in SLE is higher in countries were TB is endemic; for instance, incidence may vary from less than 1% in industrialized countries to 11.6% in India (Falagas et al, 2007) with a 6-fold risk of TB among SLE patients in Spain to 15-fold in Hong

Kong and 60-fold in India. In a study of overall infections among lupus patients, TB was the most frequently diagnosed and extra-pulmonary localization was present in one quarter of patients. In addition, TB was found during the first year of lupus diagnosis in 60% and 80% in the first 24 months, mainly linked to a major organ dysfunction or aggressive treatment (Shyam & Malaviya, 1996).

Diagnosis of TB and NTM infections in lupus patient represents a challenge for clinicians due to the overlap of symptoms and laboratorial abnormalities produced by both conditions; however, search for mycobacteria in tissues and corporal fluids, cultures and serological test, even with genetic material amplification, as well as ADA assay, tuberculin test, and γ-interferon assays seem to be equally accurate than in non-SLE patients. It's fair to mention that some variations have been reported in the diagnostic yield of some of these tests that require further assessment. (Prabu et al, 2010). Treatment of TB and NTM infections should be provided accordingly to WHO guidelines taking into account the local antimicrobial resistance rates. The question of isoniazid prophylaxis in these patients will be discussed later.

3.3 Opportunistic infections

Immunological abnormalities in lupus patients related to dysregulation of both, humoral and cellular responses have been extensively documented. Besides, drugs used to treat SLE exert diverse degrees of immune system turndown that deepen the problem of immune fighting against pathogens (I. Kang et al, 2003). Opportunistic infections, considered as those caused by non-pathogenic microorganisms not often seen in individuals with normal immune conditions, which lead to clinically significant consequences in immunocompromised subjects, are frequently reported in SLE patients. Furthermore, its difficult to know the real load that this type of infections represent in SLE since frequency rates are yet to be determined for most of them. On the other hand, case-reports and small case series are abundant on this topic. Nonetheless, in all cohorts describing lupus patients with infectious diseases there are cases with opportunistic infections either of bacterial, fungal, protozoan or viral origin; lot of cases had overlapping manifestations between disease activity and infection leading to treatment delay and poor outcomes.

3.3.1 Opportunistic infections of viral origin

Viral infections in SLE have been suspected to play a pathogenic role on development, trigger and flare of disease. Some authors have demonstrated activation of immune system and antibodies production during acute viral infections, as we mentioned before. On the other hand, besides its suggested pathogenic role in autoimmune diseases, acute viral infections are frequently reported as partners of disease flares or at disease presentation, confusing and favoring misinterpretation of clinical signs and deferral of adequate treatment (Ramos-Casals et al, 2008).

Herpes zoster (HZ) is the symptomatic reactivation of the varicella-zoster virus (VZV), an infection frequently acquired at childhood; virus prevails in a latent stage in the dorsal root ganglia for long periods of time; more than 90% of adults have serologic evidence of a previous VZV infection. Control of latent virus at ganglia is exerted by humoral and cellular mechanisms; its reactivation requires a change of immune system balance. The incidence rate of HZ is 32.5/1,000 patients-year, from a group of prospectively followed lupus patients, which is at least 2-3 fold greater than the general population (T.Y. Kang et al, 2005).

In a national survey in an Asian country, SLE was the most important risk factor to develop HZ at population level. Major complications of HZ are visceral dissemination with CNS, lung and liver involvement. Use of immunosuppressant drugs is the most relevant risk factor for complicated HZ; presence of lupus nephritis and disease activity has been also mentioned. Particular genetic abnormalities have not been found in association with HZ infection. Lupus patients have more severe forms of infection, with disseminated disease in 11-20% of cases, higher number of cases with ocular involvement, and post-herpetic neuralgia (Borba et al, 2010). Treatment of this condition should be carried out accordingly to current guidelines. A live attenuated varicella virus vaccine has not been tested in SLE patients and is not recommended in patients using any type of immunosuppressant.

Cytomegalovirus (CMV) infection is a life-threatening that endangers organ function in immunocompromised host, either as primary infection or as a reactivation of latent CMV. Although in other conditions associated with immune dysfunction reports of visceral, eye, CNS involvement and graft rejection due to this viral disease are ubiquitous. CMV infection is also relevant in pregnant women since it is a frequent cause of newborn morbidity and mortality. Seroprevalence of CMV antibodies in healthy population have been found to range from 50 to 80% in US. In lupus patients, clinical infections often come from reactivation of latent virus when aggressive immunosuppressive therapy is installed. Clinical pictures are wide: pneumonia and alveolar hemorrhage, skin ulcers, proteinuria and renal failure, thrombocytopenia, pancytopenia, hepatitis, vasculitis, retinitis and encephalitis. It may be underseeked and hence underdiagnosed but only few cases with any of these complications are reported in SLE (Ramos-Casals et al, 2008). Diagnosis of CMV is made with serology, although a note of caution should be taken: false positive reactions are not infrequent, presumably because of secondary production by auto-reactive B-cells. Other tools for diagnosis are DNA amplification of viral material as well as the characteristic cellular changes seen in biopsies. Antiviral agents to treat this disease should be initiated once a reasonable suspicion is present because it is linked to a considerable mortality and irreversible organ dysfunction, and in the clinical arena it is often difficult to wait for an unquestionable diagnosis; ganciclovir and its pro-drug valganciclovir, foscarnet and cidofovir are currently used in this setting, with the necessity of a tight monitoring due to its potential serious adverse effects. Up till now, attempts to develop an effective vaccine to prevent CMV infection by several researches around the world, either in the general population or in some special groups, have not been successfully (Gandhi & Khanna, 2004).

Epstein-Barr virus (EBV) infection importance resides in its temporal relationship with lupus initiation; moreover, EBV infection is relevant because of the immunological abnormalities found during and after exposure to this virus (Barzilai et al, 2007), the defective control of latent infection seen in lupus patients (I. Kang, 2004) and the higher prevalence of serum antibodies against EBV observed in subjects with SLE as compared with other patient groups. In Ramos-Casals' review, only a few cases with EBV infection were obtained, and no patient had organ-specific involvement; such cases had lymphadenopathy, fever and rash often considered manifestation of disease activity may well represent mild infections with EBV. We found very interesting a report of lymphoma with EBV infection in a patient receiving azathioprine that regressed after withdrawal of immunosuppressive therapy (Evans et al, 2008). No specific treatment for this condition has been described.

Human papillomavirus infection has demonstrated to be cause of genital, rectal and laryngeal cancer. Uterine cancer is the most important malignancy of those linked to HPV infection, due to its high incidence in third world countries. In 2010 it remains a public health problem in poor countries, in spite of the many healthcare programs of prevention, early detection and treatment of pre-malignant lesions (Clifford et al, 2005). Lupus women have higher prevalence of HPV infection compared with a control group, as well as high-risk variants of the virus (Klumb et al, 2010). Furthermore, there might be more risk of squamous intraepithelial lesion because of a higher prevalence of identified factors of disease progression, such as persistence of high-risk HPV variants and the use of cyclophosphamide. Progression to neoplasia is probably more frequent among SLE patients also. Therefore, SLE women require close follow-ups, particularly in women with sexual activity and/or presence of the virus in the cervix. Treatment of those with high-risk variants and adherence to management guidelines of squamous epithelial lesions and cervical intraepithelial neoplasia should be warranted. No evidence of impact of recently applied programs of vaccination in these patients can be made due to current short length of follow-up.

Parvovirus infection has also been associated with pure red-cell aplasia, hydrops fetalis and acute and chronic arthropathy; other clinical manifestations such as rash, fever, lymphadenopathy, and blood cell abnormalities may also puzzle the clinician into a misdiagnosis of SLE. Careful assessment and follow-up will differentiate between both conditions (Severin et al, 2003). Diagnosis of infection is made by serology or viral DNA amplification, no treatment for this condition has been described as a great majority of cases have self-limited disease. No methods of prevention are available.

Hepatitis C-virus (HCV) infection has a worldwide distribution and is endemic in some regions. It is the most common cause of chronic liver disease and the global prevalence has been estimated in 2%, more than 120 million people around the world might be currently infected (Shepard et al, 2005). Coexistence of SLE and HCV infection is therefore not an unusual treat. HCV infection is the viral illness with the most described muscle skeletal and autoimmune manifestations resembling rheumatic conditions, mostly acute and chronic polyarthritis, vasculitis, glomerulonephritis, neuropathy, thrombocytopenia, cryoglobulinemia and other laboratory anomalies, including positive antinuclear antibodies, low complement levels and anti-DNA antibodies, which are indistinguishable of the idiopathic diseases. In a comparison of lupus patients with and without HCV infection, some authors found a large prevalence of infection among SLE patients belonging from the same population, with lower frequency of cutaneous features and anti-dsDNA antibodies, as well as a higher prevalence of cryoglobulinemia, hypocomplementemia and liver test abnormalities (Ramos-Casals et al, 2000). HCV infection may mimic not only SLE, but Sjögren syndrome, polyarteritis nodosa and rheumatoid arthritis also (Sharlala & Adebajo, 2008; Becker & Winthrop, 2010) and may play a pathogenic role in autoimmune thyroiditis and Behçet´s disease. On the other hand, α2-interferon therapy used for the treatment of chronic HCV may induce SLE which may or may not regress after withdrawal. Also, clinicians should bear in mind that SLE has been described as a remarkable cause of false positive serology for HCV.

Other viral infections in lupus patients such as mumps, measles, herpesvirus-6, or herpes simplex virus are seldom reported and seem not to have relevance interactions of these viral agents and SLE (Ramos-Casals et al, 2008).

3.4 Rare bacterial infections

Listeria monocytogenes is a ubiquitous pathogen that causes disease in animals and humans. Outbreaks of listeriosis in relation to contaminated food have been reported in immunocompetent hosts. In immune deficient patients it is frequently a fatal infection with sepsis and CNS involvement. In an analysis of 38 lupus patients with CNS infections, Yang et al (Yang et al, 2007) found tuberculosis in a half, *L. monocytogenes* in 3, other gram-positive and gram-negative bacteria in 3 cases, *Cryptococcus neoformans* in 12 and *Aspergillus fumigatus* in 1; high steroid dose and low albumin were related to unfavorable outcome. In other series, listeriosis mainly manifested as meningitis in SLE patients with remarkable high mortality (Kraus et al, 1994). Antibiotic regimen in acute bacterial meningitis in lupus patients should include an agent with anti-listerial activity.

The *Nocardia* genus includes a group of soil gram-positive saprophyte aerobic actinobacteria. *Nocardia* causes human infections that are difficult to diagnose because of unspecific clinical or histological manifestations. There are reports of several lupus cases complicated with *Nocardia* infections; lungs were the most common site of involvement (81%), followed by the central nervous system (C.C. Mok et al, 1997). A high degree of suspicion to identify this infection is required.

3.5 Opportunistic Infections of fungal origin

Fungal infectious disease is more often recognized in hospitalized patients owing to the more extensive use of broad-spectrum antibiotics. In lupus patients, the most common fungal infections are, as in other chronic immune deficient states, those produced by *Candida* species, which may affect pharynx, esophagus, and the urinary tract or may present themselves as a primary bloodstream infection. A relationship with high steroid doses and intense immunosuppression is suggested by many. *Pneumocystis jiroveci* (formerly *carinii*) has been acknowledged as a cause of severe pulmonary involvement in chronic disease with deficient immune function. There are several reports of *P. jiroveci* pneumonia in patients with rheumatic disorders after intense immunosuppression. It has been suggested that SLE patients have more dramatic disease behavior and higher mortality rates, but this remains speculative. Patients receiving high dose steroids (>40 mg of prednisone or equivalent, for more than three months) or a combination of immunosuppressants, and with lung involvement of SLE (i.e. autoimmune alveolitis) may be considered for a prophylactic trial of antimicrobials. (Vernovsky & Dellaripa, 2000).

C. neoformans is ubiquitous encapsulated yeast that causes severe neurological infections and other disseminated diseases in immunocompromised hosts. In several fatal cases of lupus patients with meningeal infection, *C. neoformans* has been seen as a causative agent. Moreover, in a group of lupus patients with invasive fungal infections, *C. neoformans* represented almost 70% of cases, with both meningeal and disseminated disease. Prompt initiation of active antifungal treatment is mandatory in accordance to the elevated mortality registered in these cases. Other fungal agents such as *Aspergillus fumigatus* and mucor species have been reported and recently reviewed (Arce-Salinas et al, 2010).

3.6 Parasitic infections in SLE

Parasitic diseases remain as a major cause of morbidity and mortality in the tropical areas and in the underdeveloped world. Malaria persists in at least 109 countries and affects 300 million people around the world. No relevant association with clinical manifestations of lupus or with its treatment has been reported. Also, no particular clinical picture of malaria in this population has been mentioned. Nevertheless, relationship of the parasite and lupus resides in the production of antibodies cross-reacting against *Plasmodium* parasites found in some patients (Zanini et al, 2009); and the fact that anti-ribosomal P protein antibodies produced by lupus patients cross-react with the ribosomal phosphoprotein P0 of *Plasmodium falciparum* and exert a potent inhibition of the parasite growth *in vitro* (Singh et al, 2001), the clinical significance of this interesting observation remains elusive. On the other hand, IgM anti-phospholipid antibodies have been recognized in patients with active malaria infection (Jakobsen et al, 1993), mainly against phosphatidylinositol, phsophatidylcholine and cardiolipin; high titers correlated with infection severity and poor outcome.

Exposure to *Toxoplasma gondii* accordingly to seroprevalence studies is widely distributed; its importance increases in pregnant women (increased risk of fetal neurological damage), and in immune deficient hosts, in whom encephalitis, retinal damage, pneumonitis and other severe manifestations may occur. In lupus patients there are a few case-reports of patient with neurological or ocular involvement, as well lymphadenopathy and fever, again mimicking disease activity (Seta et al, 2002).

Strongyloides stercoralis, a soil worm that infects humans in tropical areas should be in mind of every clinician caring for SLE patients. *S. stercolaris* clinical infection has a prevalence that ranges from 0.1 to 11% depending the way in which it is sought (serum antibodies, stool ova or other methods). Generally its infection produces a few intestinal symptoms and its relevance, besides its infectivity, is a consequence of the autoinfection cycle that permits blood larvae migration. Without effective cellular immune control disseminated disease develops. Some lupus cases complicated with overwhelming strongyloidosis have been described; some authors suggest that stool examination looking for parasite's ova and preventive treatment could be recommended for patients at risk who will receive intense treatment for SLE. Albendazol or ivermectin have been used in chronic and disseminated infection, and the few reports describing this condition are related with poor outcome (Caramaschi et al, 2010).

4. Approach to fever in SLE

Fever in lupus patients represents a challenge for the clinician, who must face up with finding ways to determine the most likely origin between a lupus flare and active infection, bearing in mind that often both require prompt treatment. In an old report Harvey, said fever was a manifestation of disease activity in at least 86% of their patients, later Daniel Wallace draw attention to the decline of fever as a symptom of disease activity in reports of the 1980's and early 1990's; he thought that such decrease was related with frequent and earlier use of NSAIDs and glucocorticoids. Moreover, febrile lupus patients are habitually seen in both the outpatient clinic and the hospital wards. The workup requires an intelligent and sequential approach to recognize the true nature of fever. Lupus patients with fever may show certain patterns of clinical behavior that correspond, more or less, to clinical scenarios that entail different actions. Firstly, a patient recently diagnosed, without treatment and with active lupus disease including fever among other manifestations; in these cases, treatment beginning, particularly with steroids, produces a rapid disappearance of fever; when fever persists, the search of an infectious source is mandatory with appropriate cultures. Secondly, patients with fever who have inactive disease or mild disease activity in their last follow-up visits, often in the outpatient situation, and may or may not be receiving low steroid dose, antimalarials or a mild immunosuppressive regimen; in this cases, a thorough clinical assessment and studies in hunt of common bacterial infections followed by currently recommended empirical antibiotic treatment is warranted and associated with resolution of fever.

In a lupus patient hospitalized because of persistent fever, a meticulous clinical evaluation is critical, followed by the workup study based on its findings and suspected diagnosis; an assessment of disease activity with a validated index is also suggested, activity biomarkers are not perfect discriminative elements and are not always available. Adjustment of lupus treatment or initiation of a trial of empiric antibiotics should be determined based on the initial findings and patient status. Often both are required initially and tailored when a clearer scenario is at hand. An extensive assessment of a lupus cohort tested two hypotheses, demonstrating that fever is rarely associated with lupus flares in patients taking low dose of prednisone (median 10 mg per day), with only one case presenting with fever among 73 flare episodes (Rovin et al, 2005). And also, in SLE patients with recent onset fever, moderate doses of prednisone (20 to 40 mg/day) were related with a rapid resolution of the symptom, except in cases when infection was the cause.

Differentiation between infection and disease activity is highly important but difficult. Acute infections, systemic response to infection and disease activity share many clinical and laboratorial abnormalities. Certain biomarkers have been proposed as discriminative elements in such scenarios. C-reactive protein could be a useful tool to differentiate both conditions (Roy & Tan, 2001), although others reports do not support this, it is our believe that the issue remains inconclusive. Procalcitonin, a precursor of calcitonin hormone is a novel marker of bacterial infection; nowadays, determination of serum level is routinely performed in hospitals as a bedside rapid measurement to provide evidence of bacterial infection, in circumstances when clinical or bacteriological diagnosis is not clear. It was suggested, that procalcitonin might be useful for distinction of infection or disease activity; however, a recent careful evaluation rejected this hypothesis; procalcitonin exerted a poor diagnostic accuracy for differentiation of both conditions, and is no longer being used with this purpose (Lanoix et al, 2011).

Systemic lupus is also reported as a cause of fever of unknown origin (FUO) in different settings, corresponding to a relevant proportion of cases with this entity being in some reports a repeated diagnosis among the inflammatory non-infectious conditions, which represent at least one third of all causes of FUO (Arce-Salinas et al, 2005).

5. Prevention strategies

Preventive strategies should begin with the identification and amendment of factors that predispose SLE patients to infections. This is, however easier said than done. Even though infection rates were as high as 40% prior to the widespread use of corticosteroids for the treatment of SLE, several studies have demonstrated that high dose steroids, the current angular stone of SLE treatment, increase the risk of infection. Weaker associations have been reported with the use of cyclophosphamide. Other commonly reported risk factors for infection in SLE are: high disease activity, damage accrual, nephritis and neurologic disease activity (Gladman et al, 2002; Fessler 2002). No published evidence has shown that the steroids effect over the risk of infection is independent of disease activity, and this will probably remain as it is, in view of the difficulty to dissect these two conditions. Considering this information it seems fair to admit that measures aimed at lowering disease activity should be considered the backbone of the preventive strategy against infection in SLE, even given their immunosuppressive nature.

Although inconclusive evidence suggests that certain measures of prophylaxis against infective pathogens may be in order for specific subgroups of patients based on their particular risks (**Table 4**), there are no guidelines as to which subgroups of patients may benefit the most, the agents that should be used, and the best timing to do so.

Respiratory Infections	• Influenza vaccination safe and effective (antibody response) in SLE. (Abu-Shakra et al, 2007) • Pneumococcal vaccine safe. Significant minority left unprotected (risk factors: high disease activity and immunosuppressive use). (Battafarano et al, 1998)
Tuberculosis	• Screening for latent TB is critical prior to high dose PDN and other lupus drugs (anergy is frequent). (ATS, 2005) • In endemic areas prophylaxis with isoniazid may reduce the risk of developing TB in patients taking > 15 mg/day of PDN (Hernández-Cruz B et al, 1999).
Herpes Zoster	• Frequency of herpes zoster is higher in patiens taking CFM than other lupus drugs. Lower doses of CFM reduce risk (Houssiau F et al, 2002). • No data on (live attenuated) vaccine use in patients with SLE.
B & C Hepatitis	• Minimal data on the course of HBV and HCV infections, antiviral treatment in SLE, and effect of lupus drugs in viral replication and hepatic necrosis. • Increase risk of autoimmune symptoms after HBV vaccine (Geier D.A. & Geier M.R., 2005). • Effect of SLE on response to HBV vaccination not clear.
Fungal infections	• No primary prevention is suggested for *Candida, Cryptotoccus* or *Aspergillus.* • Prophylaxis for pneumocystis in severe lupus mostly with lung involvement is suggested (Vernovsky & Dellaripa, 2000). No real data.
Other	• Meningococcal vaccination recommended in asplenia but not formally examined in SLE • *Haemophilus influenzae* type B recommended in asplenia. Safe and effective in SLE (antibody response). (Battafarano et al, 1998)

Table 4. Preventive Management of Selected Infection in SLE.

A common problem that physicians often face is whether immunization is a safe and effective strategy to prevent infections in patients with SLE or not. Concern has been raised from a group of reports that link vaccination to autoimmune manifestations. However, data from observational cohorts denotes that vaccinations are safe for the majority of SLE patients, when inactivated and component vaccines are used. For instance, a group of 70 patients with SLE received pneumococcal, tetanus and *H. influezae* type B vaccines, and none had a disease flare or any significant change in the activity status. (Battarfarano et al, 1998).
The efficacy of vaccination in SLE remains elusive for the majority of vaccines. While most patients with SLE show an antibody response to vaccination, this does not imply that the patients actually gain an advantage against the pathogen. No study so far, has looked into the true protective effect (i.e.: rates of pneumonia infection) that vaccines are supposed to offer, in patients with SLE.

The reader is encouraged to read the guidelines proposed by the British Society for Rheumatology (www.rheumatology.org.uk). Here it is recommended that live vaccines should not be used in patients taking immunosuppressive drugs or a few months after cessation of them. They also recommend that when non-live vaccines are given, an assessment of response should be sought, and to consider a booster when antibody titers are low. Finally, Barber et al proposed a set of strategies for prevention of opportunistic infections in SLE, briefly: yearly influenza vaccination, quinquenal pneumococcal vaccination, regular pap smears, TB skin test prior to starting immunosuppressive treatment and treatment with isoniazid for patients with latent TB infection. Hepatitis B, hepatitis C and HIV serology should be screened at baseline, as well as *S. stercoralis* in endemic areas (Barber et al, 2011).

6. Final remarks

It has been said that infections loom, like the Sword of Democles, over patients with SLE, and this is certainly not an understatement. About half of the patients with SLE will suffer a major infection in their lives and a great proportion of them will have an infection attributable death. In spite of this, only a few studies have addressed the issues that would provide clinicians with better management alternatives for infectious disease in SLE and its prevention. It is believed that SLE patients are at high risk for infections owing to intrinsic underlying immunological derangements and to the use of therapeutic regimens with immunosuppressive agents.

The use of high dose glucocorticoids, high disease activity, organ dysfunction and use other immunosuppressants, are the strongest risk factors for the development of an infection in SLE.

Fever, among other findings challenges the clinician into a discriminative endeavor to establish its relation with disease activity and/or infection. Workup in such scenarios depends on a thorough physical exam. Some biomarkers have been proposed to be discriminative in this situation.

Specific measures of prophylaxis may offer benefit in patients with lupus against infection, but for the most, no controlled studies support their use. Reports of autoimmune induction with vaccination are scarce and for the majority of patients, vaccination is a safe procedure. Pneumococcal and influenza vaccinations are recommended, but no probe of true efficacy exist for these or other vaccines in patients SLE.

Many questions remain unanswered in the field of infections and SLE, among others: 1) Determining true predictors of infection in SLE such as specific immune defects, genetic markers or other biomarkers that indicates proclivity to infection. 2) Studying which specific immune derangements underlie the increase susceptibility to specific infections. 3) Evaluating which measures is likely to prevent infectious disease in SLE patients, who should receive them and what is the best timing to do so; these include studies of long-term efficacy vaccines and cost-effectiveness of their routine application in SLE. 4) Testing of proposed biomarkers that may help clinician solve a frequent diagnostic dilemma between disease activity and active infections.

7. References

Al-Arfaj, A.S. & Khallil, N. (2009). Clinical and immunological manifestations in 624 SLE patients in Saudi Arabia. *Lupus*, Vol.18, No.5 (April), pp.465-473.

Alzeer, A.H.; Al-Arfaj, A.; Basha, S.J. et al. (2004) Outcome of patients with systemic lupus erythematosus in intensive care unit. *Lupus* Vol.13, No.7 (July), pp. 537-42.

American Thoracic Society; Centers for Disease Control and Prevention; Infectious Diseases Society of America. (2005). American Thoracic Society/Centers for Disease Control and Prevention/Infectious Diseases Society of America: controlling tuberculosis in the United States. *Am J Respir Crit Care Med,* Vol.172, No.9 (November 1st), pp.1169-1227.

Arce-Salinas, C.A. & Pérez-Silva, E. (2010). Mucormycosis complications in systemic lupus erythematosus. *Lupus,* Vol.19, No.1 (July), pp.985-988.

Arce-Salinas, C.A.; Morales-Velázquez, J.L.; Villaseñor-Ovies, P. & Muro-Cruz, D. (2005) Classical fever of unknown origin (FUO): current causes in Mexico. *Rev Invest Clin* Vol.57, No.6 (November-December), pp.762-9.

Barber, C.; Gold, W.L. & Fortin, P.R. (2011). Infections in the lupus patient: perspectives on prevention. *Current Op Rheumatol,* Vol.23, No.4 (July), pp.358-365.

Barzilai, O.; Ram, M. & Shoenfeld, Y. (2007). Viral infection can induce the production of autoantibodies. *Curr Opin Rheumatol* Vol.19, No.6 (November), pp.636-643.

Battafarano, D.; Battafarano, N.; Larson, L. et al. (1998). Antigen-specific antibody responses in lupus patients following immunizations. *Arthritis Rheum,* Vol.41, No.10 (October), pp.1828-1834.

Becker, J. & Winthrop K.L. (2010). Update on rheumatic manifestations of infectious diseases. *Curr Opin Rheumatol* Vol.22, No.1 (January), pp.72-77.

Bernatsky, S.; Boivin J.-F-; Joseph, L. et al. (2006). Mortality in systemic lupus eryhtematosus. *Artthritis Rheum,* Vol.58, No.8 (August), pp.2250-2257.

Borba, E.F.; Ribeiro, A.C.M.; Martin, P.; Costa, L.P.; Guedes, L.K.N. & Bonfá, E. (2010). Incidence, risk factors, and outcome of herpes zoster in systemic lupus erythematosus. *J Clin Rheumatol* Vol.16, No.3 (April), pp.119-122.

Boros, P.; Muryoi, T.; Spiera, H.; Bona, C. & Unkeless, J.C. (1993). Autoantibodies directed against different classes of FcγR are found in sera of autoimmune patients. *J Immunol,* Vol.150, No.5 (March), pp.2018-2024.

Bultink, I.E.; Hamann, D.; Seelen, M.A.; Hart, M.H.; Dijkmans, B.A.; Daha, M.R. & Voskuyl, A.E. (2006). Deficiency of functional mannose-binding lectin is not associated with infections in patients with systemic lupus erythematosus. *Arthritis Res Ther.* Vol.8, No.6 (June), pp.R183.

Caramaschi, P.; Marocco, S.; Gobbo, M. et al. (2010). Systemic lupus erythematosus and strongyloidiasis: a multifaceted connection. *Lupus* Vol.19, No.7 (July), pp.872-874.

Cervera, R.; Khamashta, M.A.; Font, J. et al. (2003) Morbidity and mortality in systemic lupus erythematosus during a 10-year period. A comparison of early and late manifestations in a cohort of 1,000 patients. *Medicine* Vol.82, No.5 (September), pp.299-308.

Clifford, G.M.; Gallus, S.; Herrero, R. et al. (2005). Worldwide distribution of human papillomavirus types in cytologically normal women in the International Agency for research on cancer HPV prevalence surveys; a pooled analysis. *Lancet* Vol.366, No. 9490 (September 17-23), pp.991-998.

Cuchacovich, R. & Gedalia, A. (2009). Pathophysiology and clinical spectrum of infections in systemic lupus erythematosus. *Rheum Dis Clin North Am,* Vol.35, No.1 (February), pp.75-93.

Durán-Barragán, S.; Ruvalcaba-Naranjo, H.; Gutiérrez-Rodríguez, L. et al. (2008). Recurrent urinary tract infections and bladder dysfunction in systemic lupus erythematosus. *Lupus*, Vol.17, No.12 (December), pp.1117-1121.

Evans, S.J.; Watson, D.K. & O'Sullivan, M. (2008). Reversible Hodgkin's lymphoma associated with Epstein-Barr virus occurring during azathioprine therapy for SLE. *Rheumatology* Vol.47, No.7 (July), pp.1103-1104.

Falagas, M.E.; Voidonikola, P.T. & Angelousi, A.G. (2007) Tuberculosis in patients with systemic rheumatic or pulmonary diseases treated with glucocorticosteroids and the preventive role of isoniazid: A review of the available evidence. *Int J Antimicrob Agents* Vol.30, No.6 (December), pp.477-486.

Fessler, B. (2002). Infectious diseases in systemic lupus erythematosus: risk factors, management and prophylaxis. *Best Pract Res Clin Rheumatol*, Vol. 16, No.2, (April), pp.281-291.

Figueroa, J.E. & Densen, P. (1991). Infectious diseases associated with complement deficiencies. *Clin Microbiol Rev*, Vol.4, No.3 (July), pp.359-95.

Fishman, D. & Isenberg, D.A. (1997). Splenic involvement in rheumatic diseases. *Semin Arthritis Rheum*, Vol.27, No.3 (December), pp.141-155.

Gandhi, M.K. & Khanna, R. (2004). Human cytomegalovirus: clinical aspects, immune regulation, and emerging treatments. *Lancet Infect Dis* Vol.4, No.12 (December), pp.725-738.

Geier, D.A. & Geier, M.R. (2005). A case-control study of serious autoimmune adverse events following hepatitis B immunization. *Autoimmunity*. Vol.38, No.4 (June), pp.295-301.

Gladman, D.; Hussain, F.; Ibañez, D. & Urowitz, B.M. (2002). The nature and outcome of infection in systemic lupus erythematosus. *Lupus* Vol.11, No.4 (April), pp.234–239.

Goldblatt, F.; Chambers, A.; Rahman, A. & Isenberg, D.A. (2009). Infections in British patients with systemic lupus erythematosus: hospitalisations and mortality. *Lupus*, Vol.18, No.8 (July), pp.682-689.

Guzmán, J.; Cardiel, M.H.; Arce-Salinas, C.A.; Sánchez-Guerrero, J. & Alarcón-Segovia, D. (1992). Measurement of disease activity in systemic lupus erythematosus. Prospective validation of 3 clinical indices. *J Rheumatol* Vol.19, No.10 (October), pp.1551–1558.

Hernández-Cruz, B.; Ponce-de-León-Rosales, S.; Sifuentes-Osornio, J.; Ponce-de-León-Garduño, A. & Díaz-Jouanen, E. (1999). Tuberculosis prophylaxis in patients with steroid treatment and systemic rheumatic diseases. A case-control study. *Clin Exp Rheumatol*, Vol.17, No.1 (January-February), pp.81-87.

Houssiau, F.; Vasconcelos, C.; D'Cruz, D. et al. (2002). Immunospuressive therapy in lupus nephritis: the Euro-Lupus Nehritis Trial, a randomized trial of low-dose versus high-dose intravenous cyclophosphamide. *Arthritis Rheum*, Vol.46, No.8 (August), pp.2121-2131.

Iliopoulos, A.G. & Tsokos, G.C. (1996). Immunopathogenesis and spectrum of infections in systemic lupus erythematosus. *Semin Arthritis Rheum* Vol.25, No.5 (April), pp.318-336.

Jakobsen, P.H.; Morris-Jones, S.D.; Hviid, L. et al. (1993). Anti-phospholipid antibodies in patients with *Plasmodium falciparum* malaria. *Immunology* Vol.79, No.4 (August), pp.653-657.

Kang, I. & Park, S.H. (2003). Infectious complications in SLE after immunosuppressive therapies. *Curr Opin Rheumatol*, Vol.15, No.5 (September), pp.528-534.

Kang, I.; Quan, T.; Nolasco, H. et al. (2004) Defective control of latent Epstein-Barr virus infection in systemic lupus erythematosus. *J Immunol* Vol.172, No.2 (January), pp.1287-1294.

Kang, T.Y.; Lee, H.S.; Kim, T.H.; Jun, J.B. & Yoo, D.H. (2005). Clinical and genetic risk factors of herpes zoster in patients with systemic lupus erythematosus. *Rheumatol Int*, Vol.25, No.2 (March), pp.97-102.

Karim MY. (2006). Immunodeficiency in the lupus clinic. *Lupus*, Vol.15, No.3 (March), pp.127-131.

Kasitanon, N.; Louthrenoo, W.; Sukitawut, W. & Vichainun, R. (2002). Causes of death and prognostic factors in Thai patients with systemic lupus erythematosus. *Asian Pac J Allergy Immunol*, Vol.20, No.2 (June), pp.85-91.

Klemperer, P.; Pollack, A. & Baehr, G. (1941). Pathology of disseminated lupus erythematosus. *Arch Pathol*, Vol.32 (July), pp.569-631.

Klumb, E.M.; Pinto, A.C.; Jesus, G.R. et al. (2010). Are women with lupus at higher risk of HPV infection? *Lupus* Vol.19, No.13 (November), pp.1485-1491.

Kraus, A.; Cabral, A.R.; Sifuentes-Osornio, J. & Alarcón-Segovia, D. (1994). Listeriosis in patients with connective tissue diseases. *J Rheumatol*, Vol.21: No.4, (April), pp.635-638.

Lanoix, J.P.; Bourgeois, A.M.; Schmidt, J. et al. (2011). Serum procalcitonin does not differentiate between infection and disease flare in patients with systemic lupus erythematosus. *Lupus*, Vol.20, No.2 (February), pp.125-130.

Lee, S.S.; Lawton, J.W.; Chan, C.E.; Li, C.S.; Kwan, T.H. & Chau, K.F. (1992). Antilactoferrin antibody in systemic lupus erythematosus. *Br J Rheumatol*, Vol.31, No.10 (October), pp.669-673.

Leone, F.C.; Campos, L.M.A.; Febrônio, M.V.; Marques, H.H.S. & Silva, C.A. (2007). Risk factors associated with the death of patients hospitalized for juvenile systemic lupus erythematosus. *Br J Med Biol Res*, Vol.40, No.7 (July), pp.903-1002.

Mathers ,C.D. & Loncar, D. (2006). Projections of global mortality and burden of disease from 2002 to 2030. *PLoS Med*, Vol.3, No.11 (November), pp.e442.

Mok, C.C.; Yuen, K.Y. & Lau, C.S. (1997). Nocardiosis in systemic lupus erythematosus. *Semin Arthritis Rheum*, Vol.26, No.4 (February), pp.675-863.

Mok, C.C.; Lee, K.W.; Ho, C.T.K.; lau, C.S. & Wong, R.W.S. (2000). A prospective study of survival and prognostic indicators in systemic lupus erythematosus i a southern Chinese population. *Rheumatology*, Vol.39. No.4 (April), pp.399-406.

Mok, M.Y.; Ip, W.K.; Lau, C.S.; Lo, Y; Wong, W.H., & Lau, Y.L. (2007). Mannose-binding lectin and susceptibility to infection in Chinese patients with systemic lupus erythematosus. *J Rheumatol*, Vol.34, No.6 (June) pp.1270-1276.

Mok, M.Y.; Wong, S.S.; Chan, T.M.; Fong, D.Y.; Wong, W.S. & Lau, C.S. (2007). Non-tuberculous mycobacterial infection in patients with systemic lupus erythematosus. *Rheumatology* Vol.46, No.2 (February), pp.280-284.

Monticielo, O.A.; Mucenic, T.; Xavier, R.M.; Brenol, J.C. & Chies, J.A. (2008). The role of mannose-binding lectin in systemic lupus erythematosus. *Clin Rheumatol*, Vol.27, No.4 (April), pp.413-419.

Navarro-Zarza, J.E.; Álvarez-Hernández, E.; Casasola-Vargas, J.C. et al. (2010). Prevalence of community-acquired and nosocomial infections in hospitalized patients with systemic lupus erythematosus. *Lupus*, Vol.19, No.1 (January), pp.43-48.

Nossent, J.; Cikes, N.; Kiss, E. et al. (2007). Current causes of death in systemic lupus erythematosus in Europe, 2000-2004: relation to disease activity and damage accrual. *Lupus*, Vol.16, No.5 (May), pp.309-317.

Oh., H.M.; Chng, H.H.; Boey, M.L. & Feng, P.H. (1993). Infections in systemic lupus erythematosus. *Singapore Med J*, Vol. 34, No.5 (October), pp.406-408.

Petri, M. Infection in systemic lupus erythematosus. (2008). *Rheum Dis Clin North Am*, Vol.24, No.2 (May), pp.423-456.

Pickering, M.C.; Botto, M.; Taylor, P.R.; Lachmann, P.J. & Walport, M.J. (2000). Systemic lupus erythematosus, complement deficiency, and apoptosis. *Adv Immunol*. Vol.76, pp.227-324.

Pons-Estel. B.; Catoggio, L.J.; Cardiel, M.H. et al. (2004). The GLADEL multinational Latin American prospective inception cohort of 1,214 patients with systemic lupus erythematosus. Ethnic and disease heterogeneity among "hispanics". *Medicine*. Vol. 83, No.1 (January), pp.1-17.

Prabu, V. & Agrawal, S. (2010). Systemic lupus eryhtematosus and tuberculosis: A review of complex interactions of complicated diseases. *J Postgrad Med*. Vol.56, No.3 (July-September), pp.244-250.

Ramírez-Gómez, L.A.; Velásquez, J.F.; Granda, P.; Alfonzo-Builes, C. & Jaimes, F. (2007). Association between disease activity and risk of nosocomial infection in patients from a University Hospital at Medellín: prospective study 2001-2004. *Rev Col Reumatol*, Vol.24, No.3 (September), pp.177-186.

Ramos-Casals, M.; Font, J.; García-Carrasco, M.; Cervera, R. et al. (2000) Hepatitis C virus infection mimicking systemic lupus erythematosus: study of hepatitis C virus infection in a series of 134 Spanish patients with systemic lupus erythematosus. *Arthritis Rheum*, Vol.43, No.12 (Decemeber), pp.2801-2806.

Ramos-Casals, M.; Cuadrado, M.J.; Alba, P. et al. (2008). Acute viral infections in patients with systemic lupus erythematosus: description of 23 cases and review of the literature. *Medicine*. Vol.87, No.6 (Novemeber), pp.311-318.

Rovin, B.H.; Tang, Y.; Sun, J. et al. (2005). Clinical significance of fever in the systemic lupus erythematosus patient receiving steroid therapy. *Kidney Int*, Vol.68, No.2 (August), pp.747-759.

Roy, S. & Tan K.T. (2001). Pyrexia and normal C-reactive protein (CRP) in patients with systemic lupus erythematosus: always consider the possibility of infection in febrile patients with systemic lupus erythematosus regardless of CRP levels. *Rheumatology*, Vol.40, No.3 (March), pp.349-350.

Rubin, L.A.; Urowitz, M.B. & Gladman, D.D. (1985). Mortality in systemic lupus erythematosus: the bimodal pattern revisited. *Q J Med*, Vol.55, No.216 (April), pp.87-98.

Ruiz-Irastorza, G.; Olivares, N.; Ruiz-Arruza, I.; Martínez-Berriotxoa, A.; Egurbide, M.V. & Aguirre, C. (2009) Predictors of major infections in systemic lupus eryhtematosus. *Arthritis Res Ther*, Vol.4, No.11, pp.R109.

Schnabel, A.; Csernok, E.; Isenberg, D.A.; Mrowka, C. & Gross, W.L. (1995). Antineutrophil cytoplasmic antibodies in systemic lupus erythematosus. Prevalence, specificities, and clinical significance. *Arthritis Rheum*, Vol.38, No.5 (May), pp.633-637.

Sebastiani, G.D. & Galeazzi, M. (2009). Infection-genetics relationship in systemic lupus erythematosus. *Lupus*, Vol.18, No.13 (November), pp.1169-1175.

Seta, N.; Shimizu, T.; Nawata, M. et al. (2002) A possible novel mechanism of opportunistic infection in systemic lupus erythematosus, based on a case of toxoplasmic encephalopathy. *Rheumatology*, Vol.41, No.9 (September), pp.1072-1073.

Severin, M.C.; Levy, Y. & Shoenfeld, Y. (2003). Systemic lupus erythematosus and parvovirus B19. Casual coincidence or causative culprit? *Clin Rev Allergy Immunol*, Vol.25, No.1 (August), pp.41-8.

Sharlala, H. & Adebajo, A. (2008). Virus-induced vasculitis. *Curr Rheumatol Rep*, Vol.10, No.6 (December), pp.449-452.

Shepard, C.W.; Finelli, L. & Alter, M.J. (2005), Global epidemiology of hepatitis C virus infection. *Lancet Infect Dis*, Vol.5, No.9 (September), pp.558-567.

Shyam, C. & Malaviya, A.N. (1996) Infection-related morbidity in systemic lupus erythematosus: a clinical-epidemiological study from northern India. *Rheumatol Int*, Vol.16, No.1, pp.1-3.

Singh, S.; Chatterjee, S.; Sohoni, R.; Badakere, S. & Sharma, S. (2001). Sera from lupus patients inhibit growth of *P. falciparum* in culture. *Autoimmunity*, Vol.33, No.4, pp.253-263.

Super, M.; Thiel, S.; Lu, J.; Levinsky, R.J. & Turner, M.W. (1989). Association of low levels of mannan-binding protein with a common defect of opsonisation. *Lancet*, Vol.2, No.8674 (Novemeber 25th), pp.1236-1239.

Uramoto, K.M.; Michet, C.J.; Thumboo, J. et al. (1999). Trends in the incidence and mortality of systemic lupus erythematosus, 1950-1992. *Arthritis Rheum*, Vol.42, No.1 (January), pp.46-50.

Vernovsky, I. & Dellaripa, P.F. (2000). Pneumocystis carinii pneumonia prophylaxis in patients with rheumatic diseases undergoing immunosuppressive therapy: prealence and associated features. *J Clin Rheumatol*, Vol.6, No.2, (April), pp.94-101.

Wadee, S.; Tikly, M. & Hopley, M. (2007). Causes and predictors of death in South Africans with systemic lupus erythematosus. *Rheumatology*, Vol.46, No.9 (September), pp.1487-1491.

Yang, C.D.; Wang, X.D.; Ye, S. et al. (2007). Clinical features, prognostic and risk factors of central nervous system infections in patients with systemic lupus erythematosus. *Clin Rheumatol*, Vol.26, No.6 (June), pp.895-901.

Yong, P.F.; Aslam, L.; Karim, M.Y. & Khamashta, M.A. (2008). Management of hypogammaglobulinaemia occurring in patients with systemic lupus erythematosus. *Rheumatology*, Vol.47, No.9 (September), pp.1400-14005.

Yu, C.L.; Chang, K.L.; Chiu, C.C. et al. (1989). Defective phagocytosis, decreased tumour necrosis factor-alpha production, and lymphocyte hyporesponsiveness predispose patients with systemic lupus erythematosus to infections. *Scand J Rheumatol*, Vol.18, No.2 (February), pp.97-105.

Yun, J.E.; Lee, S.W.; Kim, T.H. et al. (2002). The incidence and clinical characteristics of *Mycobacterium tuberculosis* infection among systemic lupus erythematosus and rheumatoid arthritis patients. *Clin Exp Rheumatol,* Vol.20, No.2 (March-April), pp.127-132.

Zandman-Goddard, G. & Shoenfeld, Y. (2003). SLE and infections. *Clin Rev Allergy Immunol,* Vol.25, No.1 (August), pp.29-39.

Zanini, G.M.; De Moura Carvalho, L.J.; Brahimi, K. et al. (2009). Sera of patients with systemic lupus erythematosus react with plasmodial antigens and can inhibit the in vitro growth of *Plasmodium falciparum. Autoimmunity,* Vol.42, No.6 (September), pp.545-552.

Zonana-Nacach, A.; Camargo-Coronel, A.; Yañez, P.; Sánchez. L.; Jiménez-Balderas, F.J. & Fraga, A. (2001). Infections in outpatients with systemic lupus erythematosus: a prospective study. *Lupus,* Vol.10, No.7 (July), pp.505-510.

20

Anti-Tumour Necrosis Factor-α Induced Systemic Lupus Erythematosus

Hani Almoallim[1,2] and Hadeel Khadawardi[1]
[1]*Umm Alqura University, Makkah*
[2]*King Faisal Specialist Hpspital, Jeddah*
Saudi Arabia

1. Introduction

There are new drugs in medicine represent a revolution in therapeutics in the current era. These drugs are produced by different molecular biological techniques. Anti-tumor necrosis factor- α (anti-TNF-α) agents are important new class of the biological therapy of disease modifying antirheumatic drugs (DMARD). They target specific proteins of tumor necrosis factor- α (TNF-α) in the immune systems known to increase the inflammatory processes. Anti-TNF–α agents are increasingly used for a rapidly expanding number of rheumatic autoimmune diseases including rheumatoid arthritis (RA), ankylosing spondylitis (AS), crohn's disease (CD), ulcerative colitis (UC), psoriasis, and psoriatic arthritis (PsA). They can increase odds of remission in both randomized controlled trials and clinical practice in early and established rheumatoid arthritis. They can withhold the radiological progression of certain diseases like RA. They can produce a dramatic normalization of acute phase reactants. Due to prolonged follow up periods, side effects profile for these agents is growing. This is in addition to their ability to neutralize specific immune pathways resulting in many adverse events. Autoimmune syndromes with cutaneous and systemic manifestations including systemic lupus erythematosus may occur in patients receiving anti-TNF-α therapies (Ramos-Casals, Brito-Zeron et al. 2007). These agents represent a challenge for the practicing clinician with a range of judgments for optimal use and management of adverse events. In this chapter an overview of TNF-α will be demonstrated including its wide use in clinical practice. A more focus on anti-TNF-α agents side effects profile will be presented particularly anti-TNF-α induced lupus erythematosus (ATIL). The chapter will address the various aspects related to ATIL including clinical manifestations, autoantibodies profile, management, prognosis and preventive strategies.

2. Tumor necrosis factor-α (TNF-α)

TNF and TNF receptors are members of a family of molecules (including Fas-ligand/fas, CD40 ligand/CD40) possessing crucial regulatory functions that include activation and apoptosis. TNF-α is an attractive therapeutic target owing to its abundant expression in the rheumatoid joint and plethora of proinflammatory effects that include regulation of other proinflammatory mediators. TNF-α is a cytokine produced primarily by monocytes and macrophages but may also be produced by other cell types (e.g., B cells, T cells, mast cells, fibroblasts). TNF-α may further contribute to the pathogenesis of RA by induction of proinflammatory cytokines such as interleukin (IL)-1 and IL-6, enhancement of leukocyte migration by increasing endothelial layer permeability and expression of adhesion molecules by endothelial cells and leukocytes, activation of neutrophils and eosinophils, induction of the synthesis of acute-phase reactants, and the induction of tissue-degrading enzymes (matrix metalloproteinase enzymes) produced by synoviocytes and/or chondrocytes (Cush, Kavanaugh et al. 2011). It is expected then to have numerous biological effects in vivo with agents that inhibit the production or function of this cytokine.

3. Anti-tumor necrosis factor-α (TNF-α) agents

There are two strategies for inhibition of TNF-α which can be achieved either with monoclonal antibody such as infliximab (Remicade), adalimumab (Humira), certolizumab pegol (Cimzia), and golimumab (Simponi), or with a circulating receptor fusion protein such as etanercept (Enbrel) (Fig 1).

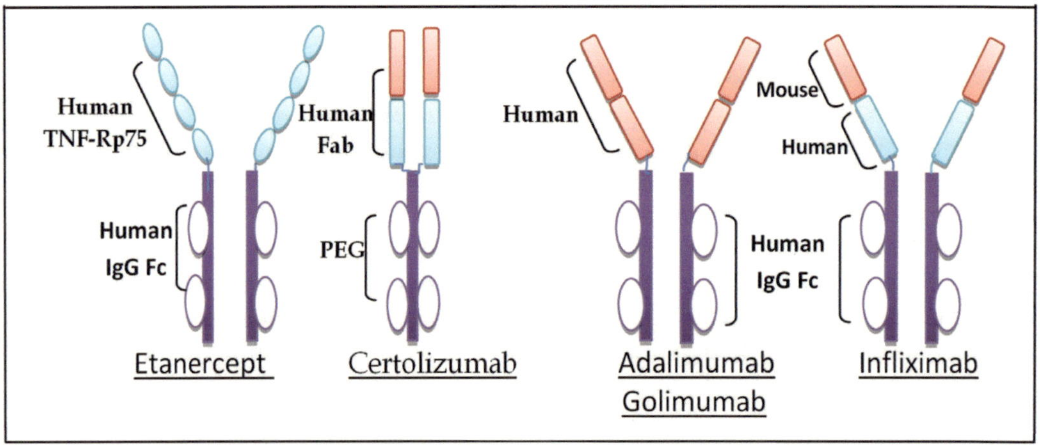

Fig. 1. Structure of anti- TNF-α agents.

3.1 Infliximab (Remicade)

Infliximab (Remicade) is a human/mouse chimeric monoclonal antibody against TNF-α and it was the first anti-TNF-α agent used to treat inflammatory disease. It was initially approved by the U.S. Food and Drug Administration (FDA) for the treatment of Crohn's disease in August 1998. Later on, it was approved by the FDA for the treatment of ulcerative colitis. Infliximab works by blocking the action of TNF-α by preventing it from binding to its receptor in the cell and neutralizing its action. However, the powerful action of infliximab that it causes programmed cell death of TNF-α expressing activated T lymphocytes, a cell type mediating inflammation, which explains its efficacy in Crohn's disease.(Van den Brande, Braat et al. 2003). This is in contrast to another TNF-α neutralizing medication, etanercept, which is worse than a placebo in Crohn's disease.(Van Den Brande,

Peppelenbosch et al. 2002) Infliximab is administered as an intravenous infusion, on a 2-4 weekly initially and then on a 6-8 weekly basis.

3.2 Etanercept (Enbrel)

Etanercept (Enbrel) is a p75 TNF--α receptor fusion protein produced through expression of recombinant DNA and conjugated to the Fc region of human immunoglobulin G (IgG1) which inhibits the binding of TNF to its cell surface receptor. Etanercept was developed by researchers at Immunex, and was released for commercial use in late 1998, soon after the release of infliximab. There are two types of TNF receptors: those found embedded in white blood cells that respond to TNF by releasing other cytokines, and soluble TNF receptors which are used to deactivate TNF and blunt the immune response. Etanercept mimics the inhibitory effects of naturally occurring soluble TNF receptors, the difference being that etanercept, because it is a fusion protein rather than a simple TNF receptor, has a greatly extended half-life in the bloodstream, and therefore a more profound and long-lasting biologic effect than a naturally occurring soluble TNF receptor. (Madhusudan, Muthuramalingam et al. 2005) The FDA has licensed etanercept for moderate to severe rheumatoid arthritis, moderate to severe polyarticular juvenile idiopathic arthritis, psoriatic arthritis, ankylosing spondylitis, and moderate to severe plaque psoriasis. Etanercept is administered as a subcutaneous injection with a dose of 25 mg twice weekly or 50 mg once weekly.

3.3 Adalimumab (Humira)

Adalimumab (Humira), the third approved TNF-α inhibitor after infliximab and etanercept, is a human anti-TNF-α monoclonal antibody. It binds to TNF-α preventing the activation of TNF receptors; adalimumab was constructed from a fully human monoclonal antibody, while infliximab is a mouse/human chimeric antibody. In 2008, adalimumab has been approved by the FDA for the treatment of rheumatoid arthritis, ankylosing spondylitis, psoriatic arthritis, and crohn's disease. It is administered subcutaneously bi-weekly as preloaded 0.8 mL syringes or preloaded pen devices.

3.4 Other anti- TNF-α agents

Other two monoclonal antibodies targeting TNF-α are golimumab (Simponi), and certolizumab pegol (Cimzia); which is a Fab fragment of human anti-TNF-α antibody attached to a polyethylene glycol (PEG) moiety. In 2008, the FDA approved Cimzia for use in the treatment of crohn's disease in people who did not respond sufficiently or adequately to standard therapy. Large, randomized, double-blind trials in patients with rheumatoid arthritis have shown that golimumab in combination with methotrexate was more effective than methotrexate alone.(Oldfield and Plosker 2009).

4. Indications

The introduction of the TNF- α blocking therapies (anti-TNF) in 1998 marked the beginning of a new era in the treatment of chronic inflammatory human diseases, including RA, AS, psoriasis and PsA, and inflammatory bowel diseases. Infliximab, Etanercept, and adalimumab are the most common anti- TNF-α agents to be used with great response and disease control in the treated patients. The U.S FDA has approved the indications of anti TNF-α therapy (table 1).

Indication	Etanercept	Infliximab	Adalimumab
Rheumatoid arthritis (RA)	Yes [1]	Yes [1R]	Yes [1]
Early RA	Yes	Yes	Yes
Polyarticular juvenile arthritis	Yes [2]	--	--
Psoriatic arthritis	Yes [3E]	Yes [3]	Yes [3]
Ankylosing spondylitis	Yes [4]	Yes [4]	Yes [4]
Psoriasis	Yes [5]	Yes	--
Crohn disease	--	Yes [6]	Yes 6
Ulcerative colitis	--	Yes [7]	--

1- Indicated for reducing signs and symptoms, inhibiting the progression of structural damage, and improving physical function for patients with moderately to severely active rheumatoid arthritis. It can be initiated alone or in combination with methotrexate.

1R- Infliximab is approved for use in combination with methotrexate only.

2- Indicated for reducing signs and symptoms of moderately to severely active polyarticular course juvenile rheumatoid arthritis patients who have had an inadequate response to one or more DMARDs.

3- Indicated for reducing signs and symptoms of active arthritis in patients with psoriatic arthritis.

3E- Only etanercept is indicated to inhibit the progression of structural damage and improve physical function for patients with moderately to severely active psoriatic arthritis. It can be used in combination with methotrexate in patients who do not respond adequately to methotrexate alone.

4- Indicated for reducing signs and symptoms in patients with active ankylosing spondylitis.

5- Indicated for the treatment of adult patients (>18 years) with chronic moderate to severe plaque psoriasis who are candidates for systemic therapy or phototherapy.

6- Indicated for reducing signs and symptoms and inducing or maintaining clinical remission in patients with moderately to severely active Crohn's disease who have had an inadequate response to conventional therapy. Infliximab is also indicated for reducing the number of enterocutaneous and rectovaginal fistulas and maintaining fistula closure in fistulizing Crohn disease.

7- Only infliximab is indicated for reducing signs and symptoms, achieving clinical remission and mucosal healing, and eliminating corticosteroid use in patients with moderately to severely active ulcerative colitis who have had an inadequate response to conventional therapy.

Table 1. U.S. Food and Drug administration-approved indications for anti-TNF-α therapy (Cush, Kavanaugh et al. 2011).

4.1 Rheumatoid Arthritis (RA)

RA is a chronic inflammatory autoimmune disease associated with debilitating and destructive polyarthritis and other systemic manifestations. DMARDs are used for treatment of patient with well-established RA and ongoing inflammation like methotrexate, sulfasalazine or hydroxychloroquine. If a patient had an inadequate response or intolerance to the usual treatment, biological therapy of anti-TNF-α can be used as monotherapy or in combination with other DMARDs. These recommendations have recently been modified because large controlled trials in early RA patients now allow their use as the initial DMARDs in RA.

4.2 Ankylosing Spondylitis (AS)

AS is a chronic inflammatory disease, that affect young males. It is characterized by its association with HLA B27 antigen and spinal inflammation mainly in form of sacroilitis. Patients with active AS who did not respond to conventional therapies can be managed with anti -TNF-α therapy.

4.3 Psoriasis and psoriatic arthritis

Psoriatic arthritis is a potentially debilitating disease that may affect small and large peripheral joints, and the axial skeleton, seen in more than 10% of patients with plaque psoriasis. Arthritis may precede onset of skin disease. The conventional therapy of psoriatic arthritis includes non-steroidal anti-inflammatory drugs (NSAID), systemic and intra-articular corticosteroids, and disease-modifying anti rheumatic drugs (DMARD) such as sulfasalazine or methotrexate. Recent trials in Psoriatic arthritis have shown excellent results with anti TNF-α therapy which have positive effects not only on joints, but also on the skin lesions.

4.4 Inflammatory Bowel Diseases (IBD)

Crohn's disease (CD) and ulcerative colitis (UC) are chronic inflammatory disorders of the gastrointestinal tract. Although the primary etiological defect still remains unknown, genetic, environmental and microbial factors have been reported in activation of the mucosal immune response. TNF-α is one of the central cytokines in the underlying pathogenesis of mucosal inflammation which is responsible for the effectiveness of anti - TNF-α therapy. Infliximab, adalimumab and certolizumab all seems to be effective in CD. Infliximab is the only anti-TNF agent currently approved for UC. Although etanercept is a TNF-α blocker, it is not approved and marketed for IBD. A randomized, controlled trial showed that etanercept was no better than placebo in IBD (Sandborn, Hanauer et al. 2001). Both etanercept and infliximab neutralized TNF-α, but only infliximab bounds to T lymphocytes and induces apoptosis of these cells (Van den Brande, Braat et al. 2003).

4.5 Relative contraindications

Due to the accumulative experience developing from the worldwide use of these drugs, certain conditions considered relative contraindications for the use of anti-TNF-α agents. Most of these conditions were obtained mainly from observations in randomized controlled trials and post-marketing phase IV trials. These conditions include systemic lupus erythematosus, lupus overlap syndrome, a history of demyelinating disorder (multiple sclerosis, optic neuritis), untreated active or latent tuberculosis, congestive heart failure, and pregnancy. The use of a TNF-α inhibitor in these conditions is currently experimental in terms of risks and benefits.

5. Side effects

Short- and long-term therapy with anti-TNF-α agents is well tolerated; however, the increased risk of infrequent but serious complications warrant sustained vigilance on the part of physicians and patients alike.

5.1 Injection site reaction

Administration of anti -TNF-α either by intravenous infusion or subcutaneous injection may result in site reactions including development of redness, swelling, itching or even skin rash. Some patients report an allergic response to infliximab, possible reason may be due to its chimeric monoclonal antibody that has human part and mouse part.

5.2 Infections

TNF-α is a cytokine that plays a crucial role in the body's immune defense against bacterial infections. Infections are mainly consisting of upper respiratory tract infections, bronchitis and urinary tract infections. A systematic review of adverse effects of anti- TNF-α therapies as they were used in rheumatoid arthritis concluded that patients taking these agents are at 2.0 time higher risk for serious infections. Serious infections that were observed, included pneumonia, sepsis and pyelonephritis (Leombruno, Einarson et al. 2009).

It has been documented well in the literature that treatment with anti-TNF-α agents is associated with increased rate of tuberculosis, in form of miliary, lymphatic, peritoneal, as well as pulmonary tuberculosis. Most of the cases of tuberculosis occurred within the first eight months after initiation of anti -TNF-α therapy.(Gomez-Reino, Carmona et al. 2003) As a result, it is recommended that patients should be screened with a TB skin test prior to starting these medications. If there is evidence of prior exposure with positive skin test, treatment for TB can be given in combination with the anti-TNF-α agents.

Other reported infections in patients on TNF-α inhibitors are fungal infections, such as pulmonary and disseminated histoplasmosis, coccidioidomycosis, and blastomycosis. It is recommended that patients with active infections should not be started on anti -TNF-α agents until their infection resolve. Furthermore, these agents should be temporarily discontinued in those patients who develop an infection while on therapy.

5.3 Malignancy

The use of anti-TNF-α agents is accompanied by some worries about their long-term safety. Thus, it seems important to investigate whether blocking the action of this TNF-α cytokine might lead to an increased risk of malignancy. The particular worry concerns of lymphoproliferative malignancies, because these malignancies occur at an increased rate in immunosuppressed patients. There are concomitant risk factors that may predispose to lymphoma in patients with RA who are using anti-TNF-α therapy. Patients with RA per se have an increased risk for developing lymphoma(Van den Brande, Braat et al. 2003). Patients specifically treated with anti -TNF-α agents are likely to have more severe disease regarding both disease duration and disease severity, which may increase the risk of malignant transformation. The accompanying use of medication, especially cyclophosphamide and azathioprine may increase the risk of developing malignancy (Van den Brande, Braat et al. 2003). In one study, it has been observed that there is an increased risk of lymphoproliferative malignancies in patients with RA who were treated with high-dose azathioprine compared with non– azathioprine-treated RA controls (Silman, Petrie et al. 1988). In another study, an increased risk of bladder and skin cancer was observed in patients with RA who were treated with cyclophosphamide (Radis, Kahl et al. 1995). Most of the reported cases of lymphoma in patients with RA who were treated with methotrexate are related to Epstein-Barr virus (EBV) (Georgescu and Paget 1999). Methotrexate exposure is almost a universal practice in anti -TNF-α treated patients and could be an important confounder of the subsequent risk for lymphoproliferative malignancies. In response to this risk of lymphoma, the US Food and Drug Administration (FDA) convened a meeting in March 2003 to review the safety data on TNF-α antagonists, focusing on the risk of malignancy in general and lymphoproliferative malignancies in particular(Kovacs, Vassilopoulos et al. 1996; Cush JJ 2003). Six lymphomas were found among 6303 RA patients treated with TNF-α inhibitors in controlled clinical trials, but none were observed in placebo-treated patients. A total of 23 lymphomas were observed (9 etanercept, 4 infliximab, 10 adalimumab) during drug treatment, with an increased standardized incidence ratio (SIR, relative risk) of 3.47, 6.35, and 5.42, respectively (Cush JJ 2003). However, the 95% confidence intervals for these SIRs were particularly wide and overlapping, thus not permitting any separation of lymphoma risk due to drug or active RA alone. Rates of solid tumors were not increased when anti-TNF-α agents associated malignancies were compared with population expectations at an FDA meeting in 2003. Similarly, in registry studies, no overall increase in risk has been reported in RA patients whether or not exposed to TNF inhibitors (Cush JJ 2003). For all this evidence, there is no clear answer regarding the risk of developing lymphoma in patients with RA and on anti -TNF-α therapy, either if it is related to anti-TNF-α therapy or to RA itself and other confounding factors.

5.4 Autoimmune diseases

Anti-TNF-α agents are widely being used for a large number of patients with different rheumatic and systemic autoimmune diseases. As a result of this use, these agents have been associated with an increasing incidence of autoimmune diseases as adverse effects, principally vasculitis, lupus like syndrome, antiphospholipid-like features, and interstitial lung disease. Other autoimmune diseases have been described, such as sarcoidosis, autoimmune hepatitis, uveitis, and thyroiditis (Ramos-Casals, Brito-Zeron et al. 2008). The clinical characteristics, outcome and pattern of autoimmune diseases following TNF-α targeted therapies have been analyzed through a baseline Medline search of articles published between January 1990 and May 2008. A total of 379 cases have been reported with drug induced autoimmune diseases (table 2) (Ramos-Casals, Brito-Zeron et al. 2008).
The reported cases of vasculitis have been classified into cutaneous vasculitis and visceral vasculitis (table 3) (Ramos-Casals, Brito-Zeron et al. 2008). Most of these cases of vasculitis overwhelmingly presented as cutaneous lesions, in form of purpura, ulcerative lesions, nodules or digital vasculitis. Regarding the biopsy, 75% of specimens were leukocytoclastic vasculitis, 15% necrotizing vasculitis, 5% lymphocytic vasculitis, and 2% urticarial vasculitis(Ramos-Casals, Brito-Zeron et al. 2008). Other patients may develop visceral vasculitis including peripheral nerve, renal, lung, and CNS involvements. Peripheral neuropathy may present in a form of axonal peripheral neuropathy, mononeuropathy multiplex, multifocal motor neuropathy with conduction block, or chronic inflammatory demyelinating polyradiculoneuropathy (Ramos-Casals, Brito-Zeron et al. 2008). Patients on anti -TNF-α agents may develop glomerulonephritis (GN) with a biopsy of pauci-immune GN, crescenting necrotizing GN or IgA GN (Ramos-Casals, Brito-Zeron et al. 2008). Pulmonary involvement has been described in association with patients who are having perinuclear anti-neutrophil cytoplasmic antibodies (pANCA) focal segmental necrotizing GN and crescentic GN. Rare cases have been reported with CNS involvement presented as central retinal artery occlusion, confusion of unclear origin and seizure(Ramos-Casals, Brito-Zeron et al. 2008). Systemic vaculitis has been reported in a form of temporal arteritis, Henoch-Schonlein purpura, and polyarteritis nodosa (Ramos-Casals, Brito-Zeron et al. 2008).

Interstitial lung disease (ILD) has been developed after starting anti -TNF-α therapy in a form of interstitial pneumonitis, pulmonary hemorrhage and bronchiolitis obliterans organizing pneumonia. The specific feature of the ILD associated with anti-TNF-α therapy is the poor prognosis in spite of cessation of these agents. Therefore initiation of corticosteroids and immunosuppressive agents is mandatory (Ramos-Casals, Brito-Zeron et al. 2008).

	Reported cases (*n*)	Mean age ± SEM (years)	Female (%)	Underlying disease: RA, Sp, IBD (%)	Biological agent: INF, ETA, ADA, other (%)
a) Systemic autoimmune diseases					
• DIL	**140**	**49.51 ± 1.68**	77	72, 7, 11	**37, 33, 25, 6**
• Vasculitis	**139**	**51.55 ± 2.68**	79	92, 7, 8	**43, 42, 7, 7**
• APS/ APS-like disease	**42**	**50.00 ± 3.79**	70	26, 11, 26	**45, 41, 5, 9**
• Sarcoidosis	**38**	**49.41 ± 2.05**	65	60, 37, 0	**26, 61, 10, 3**
b) Organ-specific autoimmune diseases					
• Optical neuritis[a]	**123**	**43.47 ± 3.29**	63	37, 17, 25	**43, 49, 7, 1**
• Interstitial lung disease	**118**	**62.79 ± 1.98**	77	77, 6, 4	**43, 47, 3, 7**
• Inflammatory ocular disease	**87**	**45.96 ± 2.16**	81	41, 48, 0	**18, 79, 2, 0**
• MS/MS-like[a]	**55**	**42.83 ± 1.99**	70	59, 17, 12	**20, 51, 27, 2**
• Peripheral neuropathies[b]	**44**	**52.47 ± 2.16**	66	61, 16, 16	**74, 12, 14, 0**
• Autoimmune hepatitis	**19**	**45.24 ± 2.83**	76	32, 47, 21	**79, 10, 10, 0**

DIL: drug-induced lupus; APS: antiphospholipid syndrome; MS: multiple sclerosis; RA: rheumatoid arthritis; Sp: spondyloarthropathies; IBD: inflammatory bowel disease; INF: infliximab; ETA: etanercept; ADA: adalimumab; SEM: standard error of the mean.
a Eight patients had the two processes.
b Excluding those appearing in patients with vasculitis.

Table 2. Characteristic of main autoimmune diseases associated with biological agents (BIOGEAS Registry, last update July 15, 2009)(Ramos-Casals, Roberto Perez et al.).

Clinical characteristics of Vasculitis	Number of cases
Cutaneous vasculitis	96
Leukocytoclastic	44
Necrotic	8
Lymphocytic	5
Urticaria	2
Not biopsied	37
Peripheral neuropathy	18
Glomerulonephritis	17
Central nervous system	6
Pulmonary involvement	3
Systemic vasculitis	5

Table 3. Clinical characteristics of 145 patients with vasculitis related to TNF-α targeted therapy.

6. Anti-TNF-α Induced Lupus Erythematosus (ATIL)

Drug induced lupus is a syndrome with symptoms, signs, and laboratory findings similar to idiopathic SLE. The diagnosis requires a temporal relationship between symptoms and therapy for at least four American Congress of Rheumatology criteria for SLE (Ramos-Casals, Brito-Zeron et al. 2007). More than 80 drugs have been implicated in drug-induced lupus, with sulfadiazine being the first reported in 1945 (Vasoo 2006). The relationship between drugs and induced lupus was confirmed by the disappearance of symptoms with drugs withdrawal.

Treatment with anti-TNF-α agents have been reported to be associated with drug-induced lupus erythematosus, most commonly with infliximab and etanercept, and rarely related to adalimumab (Haraoui and Keystone 2006; van Rijthoven, Bijlsma et al. 2006), as infliximab and etanercept have been used wider and for longer period than adalimumab. Lupus-like syndrome and ATIL were the most common in a registry of autoimmune diseases associated with anti-TNF-α agents (Ramos-Casals, Brito-Zeron et al. 2007). In this study, analysis of 92 cases with ATIL revealed that all had clinical and immunological features suggestive of SLE, 94% had positive autoantibodies, 89% had cutaneous features, 39% had musculoskeletal manifestations and general symptoms were presented in 29% (Ramos-Casals, Brito-Zeron et al. 2007).

Majority of patients with ATIL were diagnosed with RA as it will be shown below. It can be argued that the development of ATIL was actually due to a change induced by anti-TNF-α agents from RA to SLE? It is well recognized clinically that patients may evolve from one disease to another. It can be argued as well that those RA patients who developed ATIL were actually carrying the diagnosis of SLE but with a predominant presentation of polyarthritis and the use of anti-TNF-α agents had just triggered other lupus manifestations? This notion is supported, as it will be shown below by the fact that some patients with ATIL had positive ANA prior to initiation of Anti-TNF-α agents. All these arguments remain areas for ongoing research to help clinicians learn more about Anti-TNF-α agents and the actual pathogenesis of ATIL. It has to be noted that ATIL developed not only in RA patients but in patients with PsA, CD, and AS as well. The abundance of case reports and case series support the notion that anti-TNF-α therapy can induce a lupus-like syndrome as a separate and well recognized clinical entity. Rigorous exclusion of SLE prior to initiation of Anti-TNF-α agents is extremely important as a preventive action (see below).

6.1 Role of TNF-α in the pathogenesis of SLE

TNF-α is pleiotropism cytokine that has both immunoregulatory and proinflammatory effects, and its blockage has been proposed to be beneficial for the majority of patients with rheumatoid arthritis or inflammatory bowel disease. However, anti-TNF-α therapy has led in some cases to a significant incidence of drug-induced autoantibodies production and ATIL. TNF-*a* blocking could relieve the inflammation induced by TNF-*a*, at the same time the immunoregulatory and antiapoptotic effects of TNF-*a* could also be blocked which may lead to autoimmunity (Ramos-Casals, Brito-Zeron et al. 2007).

6.1.1 Immunoregulatory effects and apoptosis of TNF-α in SLE

In an experimental study, a heterozygous mice was generated which has reduced TNF-*a* production, by crossing NZB mice with TNF-*a* deficient mice. These mice developed enhanced autoimmunity and severe renal disease similar to the classic mice model of SLE. Autoimmune responses were associated with an early spontaneous increase in serum levels of antinuclear antibodies (ANA) and hyperproliferating B cells which readily express anti-double stranded DNA antibodies (anti-ds DNA) antibodies specificities in response to polyclonal and T helper stimuli. These findings demonstrate a physiological role for TNF-*α* in suppressing the emergence of autoreactive lymphocytes in the NZB model and indicate that defective TNF-*α* function may be causative of the autoimmune and pathological phenomena in lupus. Loss of physiological TNF-*α* production in an autoimmunity prone background suffices to exacerbate antinuclear autoimmunity and the development of disease (Kontoyiannis and Kollias 2000).

Apoptosis (programmed cell death (PCD)) plays an important role in the homeostasis of the immune response. Peripheral blood lymphocytes (PBLs) from SLE patients exhibit increased spontaneous and diminished activation induced apoptosis. Increased spontaneous apoptosis of PBLs has been linked to chronic lymphopenia and release of nuclear autoantigens in patients with SLE (Gergely, Grossman et al. 2002). The appearance of high numbers of autoreactive lymphocytes in the peripheral blood of patients with SLE might be a consequence of defective activation-induced cell death (Emlen, Niebur et al. 1994). It has been showed that permeabilitized lupus T cells displayed significantly lower amounts of TNF-*α*, a functional Fas/Fas-ligand path and adequate amounts of intracellular TNF-*α* were needed for the CD3-mediated T cell death. Prolonged survival of autoreactive T cells can lead to increased autoantibody production. Defective activation-induced apoptosis in lupus would worsen under TNF blockage (Kovacs, Vassilopoulos et al. 1996).

The clinical reports about the levels of TNF-*α* in SLE patients' were controversial. In most studies, TNF-*α* is found to be increased and appeared to be bioactive in the sera of patients with active SLE, and levels of TNF-*α* have been shown to correlate with SLE disease activity (Aringer, Feierl et al. 2002; Aringer and Smolen 2003). In another study, it has been found that SLE patients had elevated plasma levels of TNF-*α* with no correlation of disease activity (Zhu, Landolt-Marticorena et al. 2010). Furthermore, in a third study, it has been demonstrated that TNF-*α* levels were higher in patients with inactive disease compared with patients with very active disease, suggesting that TNF-*α* could be a protective factor in SLE patients (Gomez, Correa et al. 2004).

HLA-DR2 and DQwl positive subjects frequently exhibit low production of TNF-*α* whereas DR3 and DR4 positive subjects show high levels of TNF-*α* production. DR2 and DQwl positive SLE patients show low levels of TNF-*α* inducibility; this genotype is also associated with an increased incidence of lupus nephritis (LN). DR3 positive SLE patients, on the other hand, are not predisposed to nephritis, and these patients have high TNF-*α* production. DR4 haplotype is associated with high TNF-*α* inducibility and is negatively correlated with LN. These data suggested that low TNF-*α* production may be involved in the genetic predisposition to LN, and may help explain the association between HLADR2/DQwl and susceptibility to LN (Jacob, Fronek et al. 1990).

As TNF receptor1 (TNFR1)—TNFR associated death domain (TRADD)--Fas-associated death domain (FADD) system leading to apoptotic signaling, the down regulation of TRADD, FADD in patients with SLE may promote an anti-apoptotic effect. Defects in expression of these genes may increase the likelihood that lymphocytes avoid the normal processes used by the immune system to eliminate unwanted lymphocytes or to down-regulate an immune response. If patients carry this autoimmune gene expression signature, signaling pathways essential for the maintenance of tolerance may not function properly.

This may permit lymphocytes to escape tolerance and adopt a pro survival agenda that increases the likelihood of autoimmune diseases (Rosen and Casciola-Rosen 2001), (Balomenos and Martinez 2000).
The dysregulation of programmed cell death is suggested to be involved in the generation of autoantibodies. The low expression of TRADD, receptor-interacting protein 1 (RIP-1), and TNF receptor associated factor 2 (TRAF-2) might be one of the etiopathogeneses leading to redundant apoptotic death in SLE patients. It has been indicated that decreased expression of TRADD, RIP-1, and TRAF-2 and restrained pathogenesis for the loss of immune tolerance and redundant apoptotic cell death, leading to massive production of autoantibodies in SLE patients (Zhu, Yang et al. 2007).

6.1.2 Inflammatory effects of TNF-α in the pathogenesis of SLE

TNF-α is the most important proinflammatory cytokine and a harbinger of tissue destruction, and it is at the top of a pro-inflammatory "cascade" leading to tissue damage. In contrast to the complex role of TNF-α in apoptosis and in immune regulation, its powerful proinflammatory effects are unequivocal. It has been found that TNF-α is clearly expressed in glomeruli of LN patients, mainly by infiltrating macrophages but also by endothelial cells, glomerular visceral epithelium, and mesangial cells, with WHO class III and IV LN, while no TNF-α is detected in healthy kidney tissues. Most of the conducted studies have demonstrated that TNF-α is expressed in LN of all WHO classes and high TNF-α expression is associated with high histological disease activity. Also, it has been found that upregulation of renal expression of TNF-α in class III and class IV LN by immunohistochemical studies, and the upregulation of TNF-α was correlated with increased number of proliferating cell nuclear antigen (PCNA-)positive cells, CD68-positive cells and the activity index of renal pathologic changes (Aringer and Smolen 2004).

6.2 Clinical trials of anti- TNF-α therapy in SLE

SLE is a multifactorial autoimmune disease characterized by breakdown of self-tolerance, B cell hyperactivity, autoantibody production, aberrant formation of immune complexes, and inflammation of multiple organs. As TNF-α is a proinflammatory cytokine, participate in inflammatory tissue damage and in SLE pathogenesis, few clinical trials have been conducted regarding the use of anti TNF-α agents in patients with active SLE.
In 2008, an open-label study was reported about the safety and efficacy of TNF-blockade in SLE. Seven patients with SLE were treated with infliximab at weeks 0, 2, 6, and 10 in combination with azathioprine or methotrexate. Autoantibodies to ds-DNA increased in 5 of 7 patients. Histone levels were increased in 4 of 7 patients, and IgM anti-cardiolipin antibodies were also increased in 4 of 7 patients, peaking 4–10 weeks after the last infliximab infusion. This trial suggested that while anti-TNF-*a* agent was clinically effective, the majority of SLE patients treated with infliximab showed an increase in autoantibodies to nuclear antigens and phospholipids. These increases were transient and were not associated with disease flares (Aringer and Smolen 2008). A long-term follow up study was conducted of 13 patients about the adverse events and efficacy of TNF-*a* blockade with infliximab in SLE patients. It indicated that short-term therapy with four infusions of infliximab in combination with azathioprine was relatively safe and had remarkable long-term efficacy for LN and, potentially, also interstitial lung disease. Long-term therapy with infliximab, however, was associated with severe adverse events in two out of three SLE patients, which

may have been provoked by infliximab and/or by their long-standing refractory SLE and previous therapies(Aringer, Houssiau et al. 2009).

6.3 Development of autoantibodies

The induction of autoantibodies and anti-TNF-α therapy has been widely documented (De Bandt, Sibilia et al. 2005). Most of patients who were treated with anti-TNF-α agents developed antibodies that normally found almost exclusively in patients with SLE, however, these patients do not have any clinical features suggestive of SLE (Charles, Smeenk et al. 2000). Therefore, discontinuation of these agents is not indicated but this evident do not exclude potential induction of clinical lupus signs or symptoms and patients need further close follow up and observation (Charles, Smeenk et al. 2000). TNF-α antagonists lead into an elevated titers of ANA with a homogeneous pattern in patients who already started treatment with positive serology of ANA. In addition, new onset of positive ANA may develop in previously negative ANA patients treated with TNF-α inhibitors (FDA 2008; Lin, Ziring et al. 2008). Development of new onset of anti-ds DNA antibodies, more specific antibodies of SLE, was reported during anti- TNF-α therapy which represents a strong evidence for diagnosis of induction of lupus-like syndrome following treatment with these agents. However, anti-ds DNA antibodies are found in 50-70% of patients with idiopathic SLE while their prevalence is from 9% to 33% in patients treated with anti- TNF-α (FDA 2008; Lin, Ziring et al. 2008). It has been reported that patients on anti-TNF-α agents had serum antibodies to ds DNA of IgG, IgM, and IgA subtypes. In all reported patients, most common induced antibodies were solely of the IgM subtype. This finding is in marked contrast to the patients with idiopathic SLE, in whom although IgM antibodies to ds DNA are fairly common, it is extremely rare to find this response without accompanying IgG anti-ds DNA antibodies (Charles, Smeenk et al. 2000). Anti-histone antibodies are detected in 57% among patients with ATIL in one study (Costa, Said et al. 2008) and only in 17% in another study (De Bandt, Sibilia et al. 2005). It should be noted that anti-histone antibodies are not pathognomonic for drug-induced SLE and occur in more than 95% of cases, they are also found in 75% of cases with idiopathic SLE (Katz and Zandman-Goddard 2010). Hypocomplementemia is found in up to 59% of patients with ATIL while this finding is extremely rare in other drug-induced lupus (Costa, Said et al. 2008). The occurrence of anticardiolipin (ACL) antibodies were detected in anti-TNF-α treated patient. Up to 25% of patients on anti- TNF-α agents for RA developed IgG or IgM ACL, but thrombosis is observed in much fewer patients (about 4%) (Cambien, Bergmeier et al. 2003). It is also known that TNF-α has potent antithrombotic properties. It is therefore conceivable that the association of ACL antibodies and inhibition of TNF-α could lead to an increase risk of thrombosis. The presence of anti-Smith antibodies is almost exclusive of idiopathic SLE and rarely found in drug-induced SLE. Anti-nucleosome antibodies of the IgG subtype are considered to be a more sensitive marker for SLE than anti-dsDNA and anti-histone antibodies (Amoura, Koutouzov et al. 2000). Although there are number of patients who develop anti-nucleosome antibodies during treatment with anti- TNF-α agents, this number is not statistically significant. Positive ENAs also may develop in patients on these agents (Costa, Said et al. 2008). A comparison of different autoantibodies produced in ATIL reported in three different studies is presented in (table 4) (Williams, Gadola et al. 2009).

It has been confirmed that the induction of ANA and anti-dsDNA antibodies occur in patients who started treatment with anti-TNF-α agents, and the presence of this serological finding is unrelated to the genetic background or the underlying disease process. The development of only anti-dsDNA antibodies with absence of other lupus specific antibodies in the consequence of anti- TNF-α therapy is reassuring in terms of the safety of this treatment; however, long term observation is mandatory.

Among laboratory findings, the hematological results that have been reported secondary to anti-TNF-α agents that are typical of idiopathic SLE which include leukopenia, thrombocytopenia, and lymphopenia (Costa, Said et al. 2008).

Autoantibody	Costa et al., 2008, (Britain), (n=33)	Ramos et al., 2007, (Spain), (n=72)	De Bandt et al., 2005, (French), (n=12)
ANA, n (%)	**32/32 (100)**	**57 (79)**	**12 (100)**
dsDNA, n (%)	**29/32**	**52 (72)**	**11 (92)**
Histone, n (%)	**16/28 (57)**	**Not reported**	**2 (17)**
aPL, n (%)	**Not reported**	**8 (11)**	**6 (50)**
ENAs, n (%)	**10/19 (53)**	**Anti-Sm 7 (10)** **Anti-Ro/La 9 (12)** **Anti-RNP 5 (7)**	**5 (42)**

Table 4. Comparison of the developed antibodies in ATIL reported in three different studies (Williams, Gadola et al. 2009). ANA: antinuclear antibodies, dsDNA: double stranded DNA, aPL: antiphospholipid antibodies, ENAs: extractable nuclear antigens.

6.4 Clinical manifestations of anti-TNF-induced SLE (ATIL)

The true incidence of ATIL is difficult to establish due to the paucity of data and lack of double blind placebo-controlled prospective studies, difficulty to establish causality and lack of universal recognition of this relatively new entity (Katz and Zandman-Goddard). Post marketing studies on the three licensed anti-TNF-α agents have suggested an estimated incidence of ATIL of 0.19%-0.22% for infliximab, 0.18% for etanercept and 0.10% for adalimumab (De Bandt, Sibilia et al. 2005; Schiff, Burmester et al. 2006). However, the prevalence of ATIL in the main randomized controlled trials (RCTs) using anti-TNF agents is higher, with 14 (0.76%) cases in the 1842 patients included in 17 studies (Ramos-Casals, Roberto Perez et al.). It has to be realized that this is an accumulative figure and it does not represent the exact prevalence. The mean duration of disease before initiation of anti-TNF-α therapy was 13.5 years in one cohort (range, 1-35 years)(Wetter and Davis 2009). Onset of symptoms ranges from less than one month to more than 4 years (Williams and Cohen). In another larger report, the mean latency time until the manifestations of ATIL was 41 weeks (Ramos-Casals, Brito-Zeron et al. 2007). There was, in this series, a 5:1 female : male ratio. The most common disease for which anti-TNF-α was used for was RA (Ramos-Casals, Brito-Zeron et al. 2007; Costa, Said et al. 2008). Other diseases include but not limited to juvenile idiopathic arthritis, PsA, AS, CD. In one cohort, most patients who developed ATIL were having CD (Wetter and Davis 2009). The most common anti-TNF-α agent in use currently is infliximab as it is the first to be approved and introduced to clinical practice. Obviously, most of the cases of ATIL were due to infliximab use followed by etanercept and adalimumab respectively (Ramos-Casals, Brito-Zeron et al. 2007; Costa, Said et al. 2008). (Table 5) demonstrates the clinical characteristics of 92 patients with ATIL reported in the literature up to December 2006 (Ramos-Casals, Brito-Zeron et al. 2007). (Table 6) demonstrates comparison of different features of ATIL reported in some studies (Williams, Gadola et al. 2009).

Main Characteristic	No. (%)
Underlying rheumatic disease (n=92)	
Rheumatoid arthritis	**77 (84%)**
Crohn disease	**8 (9%)**
Ankylosing spondylitis	**2 (2%)**
Psoriatic arthritis	**2 (2%)**
Other	**3 (3%)**
Anti-TNF agent (n=62)	
Infliximab	**40 (44%)**
Etanercept	**37 (40%)**
Adalimumab	**15 (16%)**
Demographic characteristics (n=62)	
Female/male	**52/10**
Mean age at diagnosis of vasculitis (yr±SEM)	**50.9 ± 2.3**
Length of anti-TNF treatment ± SEM (wk)	**41.2 ± 5.7**
SLE criteria (n=72)	
ANA	**57 (79%)**
Anti-dsDNA	**52 (72%)**
Cutaneous features	**48 (67%)**
Arthritis	**22 (31%)**
Cytopenia	**16 (22%)**
Serositis	**9 (12%)**
aPL	**8 (11%)**
Anti-Sm antibodies	**7 (10%)**
Nephropathy	**5 (7%)**
Oral ulcers	**3 (4%)**
CNS involvement	**2 (3%)**
Number of SLE criteria fulfilled (n=72)	
≥ 4 (defined SLE)	**37 (51%)**
3 (lupus-like syndrome)	**17 (24%)**
1-2 (isolated lupus features)	**18 (25%)**
Outcome (n=72)	
Improvement	**71**
Time of improvement (mo ± SEM)	**9.9 ± 1.4**
Rechallenge phenomenon	**2/8 (33%)**

Table 5. Clinical characteristics of 92 patients with lupus related to TNF-targeted therapy (Ramos-Casals, Brito-Zeron et al. 2007).

ACR diagnostic criteria for lupus	BSRBR data, (Britain), (n=41)	Coasta et al., 2008, (USA), (n=33)	Ramos-Casal et al., (Spain), (n=72)	De Bandt et al., 2005, (France), (n=12)
Malar rash. N (%)	**Not reported**	**Not reported**	**Not reported**	**5 (42)**
Discoid rash, n (%)	**25 (61)**	**24 (73)**	**48 (67)**	**0**
Photosensitivity, n (%)	**4 (10)**	**Not reported**	**Not reported**	**5 (42)**
Oral ulcer, n (%)	**5 (12)**	**1 (3)**	**3 (4)**	**0**
Arthritis, n (%)	**3 (7)**	**17 (52)**	**22 (31)**	**6 (50)**
Serositis, n (%)	**0**	**3 (18)**	**9 (12)**	**3 (25)**
Renal Disorder, n (%)	**0**	**3 (9)**	**5 (7)**	**0**
Neurological disorder, n (%)	**0**	**0**	**2 (3)**	**0**
Hematological disorder, n (%)	**1(2)**	**20 (61)**	**Cytopenia-16 (22)**	**6 (50)**
Immunological disorder, n (%)	**4 (10)**	**29 (88)**	**dsDNA-52 (72), anti-Sm-7 (10)**	**11 (92)**
Anti-nuclear antibodies, n (%)	**13 (32)**	**32 (97)**	**57 (79)**	**12 (100)**

Table 6. Features of patients with ATIL based on case reports and case series in some studies (Williams, Gadola et al. 2009).

6.4.1 Development of cutaneous manifestations

ATIL may present in variable forms of clinical features, either in form of isolated cutaneous manifestations or systemic manifestations. Most of the reported clinical features of anti-TNF-α-induced SLE are in form of cutaneous lesions (tables 5 and 6). Most of these symptoms are similar to that symptoms present with idiopathic SLE. The cutaneous features of ATIL are most commonly malar rash, pruritic rash, photosensitive rash or purpura (Ramos-Casals, Brito-Zeron et al. 2008). Other cutaneous features are discoid rash, mucosal ulcers, and alopecia (Ramos-Casals, Brito-Zeron et al. 2008). The diagnosis of these cutaneous symptoms is based upon the clinical features in combination with concurrent use of an implicated drug. Therefore, many of the reported cases did not have skin lesions biopsied for diagnosis (Wetter and Davis 2009). When described, the pathological changes of this adverse effect are similar to those observed in patients with non-drug-associated idiopathic SLE (De Bandt, Sibilia et al. 2005; Costa, Said et al. 2008).

6.4.2 Development of systemic manifestations

Patients on anti- TNF-α therapy may develop systemic features of SLE that usually resolve after discontinuation of the offending drug. The associated general features include constitutional symptoms of fever, malaise, and weight loss which are considered as common symptoms of SLE after anti- TNF-α therapy and they often present in association with positive serology of autoantibodies. Other systemic symptom that reported is induction of new onset of polyarthritis or progression to worsening symptoms of presented arthritis in form of joint tenderness, swelling, and effusion, some other patients develop arthralgia without evidence of arthritis (De Bandt, Sibilia et al. 2005). Arthritis was the first sign to develop in 71% in a cohort of patients in one center (Wetter and Davis 2009). It was also the most debilitating sign. Other rare and serious clinical characteristics may develop as side effects in patients on anti-TNF-α agents include serositis with pleurisy or pericarditis, pleural or pericardial effusions, deep venous thrombosis, life-threating pneumonitis, and neuritis (Costa, Said et al. 2008) (Table 7). Two cases of biopsy-confirmed proliferative lupus nephritis were described in patients treated with etanercept for juvenile RA (Mor, Bingham et al. 2005; Stokes, Foster et al. 2005). Renal biopsies revealed severe hypercellularity, endocapillary proliferation, wire loops and intraluminal deposits. Immunofluoresence shared positive staining for all immunoglobulin isotypes as well as C3 and Clq. Extensive electron-dense deposits were visualized by electron microscopy. Of note, focal proliferative lupus nephritis (Class III) was described with adalimumab (Stokes, Foster et al. 2005).

Clinical manifestation	Number of reported cases	% of reported cases
Rash	24/33	73 %
Polysynovitis	17/33	52 %
Fever	17/33	52 %
Myalgias	8/33	24 %
Pericardial/pleural effusion	3/33	9 %
Nephritis	3/33	9 %
Valvulitis	1/33	3 %
Pneumonitis	1/33	3 %
Deep venous thrombosis	1/33	3 %
Oral ulcer	1/33	3 %

Table 7. Clinical features of 33 reported cases with ATIL (Costa, Said et al. 2008).

ATIL may present with unusual manifestation that is even uncommon feature of idiopathic SLE. This requires clinical suspension for ATIL in any patient presenting with unusual clinical findings. Invasive methods may be required to confirm the diagnosis. In a case that we reported (Almoallim 2011), adalimumab was initiated in a patient to control her symptoms of RA. She presented with prolonged morning stiffness and severe polyarthritis evident by swelling and tenderness in her metacarpophalangeal joints (MCPs), elbows, shoulders, knees and ankles. Serology for RF, anti-citrullinated protein antibodies (ACPA), and ANA (1:160) were all positive. While the patient was on adalimumab therapy, she showed significant improvement with complete remission of her disease. Within one year of this treatment, she developed diffuse muscle weakness mainly proximal rather than distal which made her unable to get up from the bed, climb stairs or even stand from sitting position. She had signs of active arthritis in two MCP joints in the right and bilateral wrist joints. She had mild hyperpigmented area around the mouth with no skin rashes elsewhere. She had a very high titer of ANA (1:1280) with emerging of a new onset of strongly positive anti-ds DNA antibodies, her creatinine kinase was entirely normal. Electromyograghy (EMG) was suggestive of inflammatory myopathy. MRI deltoid and thigh showed mild edema involving the right triceps muscle with minimal enhancement in the post contrast sequence (Figure.2). Deltoid biopsy showed focal mild perivascular and endomysial lymphohistiocytic which revealed inflammatory myositis (Figure.3). Based on the clinical findings, the positive serology of ANA and anti-ds DNA, and the biopsy findings, the diagnosis of adalimumab induced lupus myositis was made. Given the profound muscle weakness that she had, she received 1 gm of pulse methylprednisolone intravenously daily for three days then she was maintained on 60 mg/day, in addition she received rituximab 1000 mg intravenously, two doses in two weeks. This regimen was well tolerated and she recovered fully. Ten months later, she was asymptomatic with normal power, negative serology for anti-dsDNA antibodies and off treatment. In another case report, the patient developed severe myositis as a part of complex overlap syndrome following treatment with adalimumab, with positive serology for ANA and anti-dsDNA antibodies (Liozon, Ouattara et al. 2007).

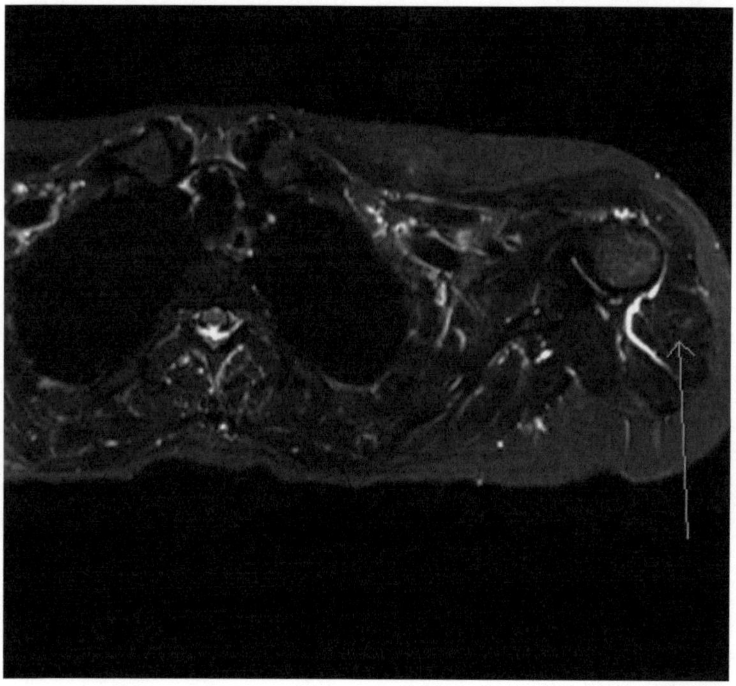

Fig. 2. MRI right arm showed mild edema involving the right triceps muscle with minimal enhancement in the post contrast sequence in comparison to other muscles which appeared mildly atrophied.

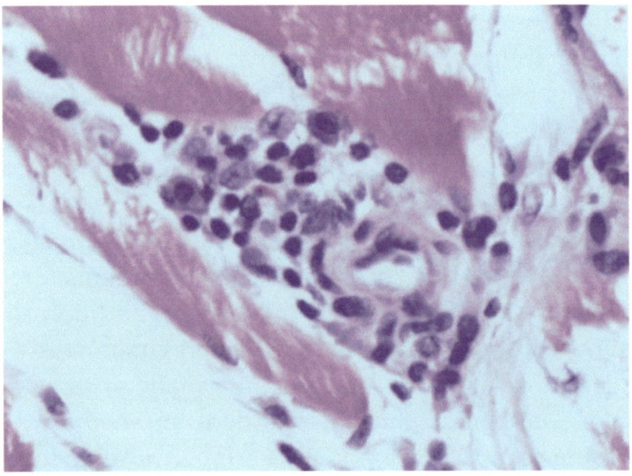

Fig. 3. Biopsy from right arm (triceps muscle) using Hematoxylin and Eosin stain, original magnification 400, which revealed inflammatory myositis (focal mild perivascular and endomysial lymphohistiocytic inflammation).

6.5 Differences between ATIL and classic Drug Induced Lupus Erythematosus (DILE)

These comparisons are observations based on the abundance of case reports in the literature. Skin rashes for example are thought to be more common in ATIL in comparison to DILE (Costa, Said et al. 2008). It is noticed that the classical cutaneous features of SLE is rare in DILE (Katz and Zandman-Goddard). While myalgias is more common in DILE (Yung and Richardson 1994) in comparison to ATIL. The incidence of fever is similar in both diseases in one series (Costa, Said et al. 2008). (Table 8) represents the prevalence of clinical manifestations and laboratory features in ATIL, DILE and SLE as reported in three different studies (Ramos-Casals, Brito-Zeron et al. 2007).

Feature	Anti-TNF-related lupus (%)	Procainamide-realted lupus (%)	Idiopathic SLE (%)
ANA	**79**	**>95**	**99**
Anti-dsDNA	**72**	**<5**	**90**
Rash/cutaneous involvement	**67**	**<5**	**54-70**
Arthritis	**31**	**20**	**83**
Fever/general symptoms	**23**	**45**	**42**
Hypocomplementemia	**17**	**<5**	**48**
Leukopenia	**14**	**15**	**66**
Serositis	**12**	**50**	**28**
Anticardiolipin antibodies	**11**	**5-20**	**15**
Glomerulonephritis	**7**	**<5**	**34**
Thrombocytopenia	**6**	**<5**	**31**
Neuropsychiatric	**3**	**<5**	**12**
Anti-histone antibodies	**Not reported**	**>95**	**50-60**

Table 8. Prevalence of clinical manifestations and laboratory features in lupus related to anti-TNF agents compared with idiopathic SLE (Ramos-Casals, Brito-Zeron et al. 2007).

6.5 Diagnosis of Anti-TNF-α-induced lupus erythematosus

Development of SLE in patients who is being treated with anti-TNF-α agents is well documented throughout the literature and the diagnosis of this side effect is crucial. The clinical presentation of ATIL can vary, and specific diagnostic criteria have not been established. However, in the most reported cases, the diagnosis was made on the basis of the development of one or more symptoms compatible with SLE, ongoing exposure to an anti-- TNF-α agent, no prior history of SLE, and resolution of symptoms when the offending drug is discontinued. The strict application of the American College of Rheumatology criteria for idiopathic SLE (ACR criteria) would probably exclude the diagnosis of ATIL in many patients receiving anti-TNF-α therapy. Therefore, for the purpose of early diagnosis; the following criteria can be considered (De Bandt, Sibilia et al. 2005): (1) a temporal relationship between symptoms and anti-TNF-α-therapy; (2) at least 1 serologic finding that compatible with ACR criteria eg, ANA, anti-dsDNA antibodies, and (3) at least 1 non serologic finding that compatible with ACR criteria eg, arthritis, serositis, hematologic disorder, malar rash. The musculoskeletal symptoms were taken into account only if they reappeared with other lupus symptoms in a patient in whom they had previously disappeared while receiving anti- TNF-α therapy as in the case reported above in section 6.4.2. Isolated positive results for ANAs or anti-dsDNA antibodies were not considered for diagnosis, given their high frequency in patients receiving this therapy (De Bandt, Sibilia et al. 2005).

6.6 Treatment of Anti-TNF-α-induced Lupus Erythematosus (ATIL)

The main approach regarding the treatment of ATIL is the withdrawal of offending drug. The time until symptoms resolution ranges from three weeks to six months (De Bandt, Sibilia et al. 2005; Wetter and Davis 2009). The level of autoantibodies have been either normalized or decreased in response to drug withdrawal (De Bandt, Sibilia et al. 2005; Wetter and Davis 2009). However, some investigators have suggested that TNF-α antagonists do not need to be discontinued if the patient has isolated induction of autoantibodies without any clinical manifestations of lupus (Ramos-Casals, Brito-Zeron et al. 2007; Kerbleski and Gottlieb 2009). It has to be realized that autoimmune diseases may coexist and there is always the possibility of latent idiopathic SLE triggered by anti-TNF-α agents. Strongly positive autoantibodies should raise the suspicion for ATIL. In addition to discontinuing of anti- TNF-α therapy, many patients required to be treated by the traditional therapy for idiopathic SLE to achieve full resolution of their lupus symptoms. The Spanish Study Group of Biological Agents in Autoimmune Diseases (BIOGEAS) classified all patients with autoimmune diseases secondary to the use of biologic agents into two groups, i.e. mild (with cutaneous, articular or general features) and severe (with pulmonary, renal or neurological involvement) disease (Ramos-Casals, Brito-Zeron et al. 2007). For mild disease, it has been suggested to withdraw TNF-α antagonists and for severe disease, immediate cessation of the offending drug and addition of corticosteroids and other immunosuppressive agents. The British Society for Rheumatology's (BSR) guidance for suspected ATIL recommends withdrawal of anti-TNF- α therapy, but does not specify additional treatment measures (Ledingham, Wilkinson et al. 2005). It has been reported that lupus-like symptoms in patients receiving anti-TNF-α therapy disappeared in most of the cases after withdrawal of the anti- TNF-α therapy (Ramos-Casals, Brito-Zeron et al. 2007). Forty per cent of the patients also received corticosteroids, while 12% required additional immunosuppression with azathioprine, cyclophosphamide, leflunomide, methotrexate, mycophenolate or cyclophosphamide in one of the largest series of ATIL (Ramos-Casals,

Brito-Zeron et al. 2007). In a reported case of a patient who developed ATIL in a form of a pruritic photo-distributed skin rash after initiation of etanercept therapy, patient has been treated with hydroxychloroquine beside drug discontinuation and systemic corticosteroids(Williams and Cohen 2011). We reported case of a patient who developed lupus myositis after treatment with adalimumab for rheumatoid arthritis. She received pulse steroid therapy and two doses of rituximab. The treatment was well tolerated with complete recovery. The patient was then maintained on hydroxychloroquine and azothioprine. She remained asymptomatic for 10 months of follow up (Almoallim 2011). An important question is whether patients with ATIL can safely receive an alternative anti-TNF-α agent? There are limited evidences that support the safety of re-challenging with alternative anti-TNF-α agents. Reports regarding this issue are scarce, but one author described 4 patients who were re-challenged with the same or different agents and had no recurrence of lupus symptoms (3 received etanercept and 1 received adalimumab)(Cush 2004). In another study, 4 of 5 patients tolerated an alternative TNF inhibitor (adalimumab for 3 patients, etanercept for 1) without recurrence of ATIL after discontinuation of infliximab (Wetter and Davis 2009). Nevertheless, these findings should be interpreted cautiously, given the small number of patients who were re-challenged. In addition, some of these reports were conducted on patients with ATIL with mild disease and few clinical findings. The successful continued therapy with an alternative anti-TNF-α agent reported for one patient (Williams and Cohen), was actually manifested with only cutaneous findings. The clinical decision to continue an alternative anti-TNF-α agent in ATIL patients with severe and systemic involvement is really hard to make. Exposing patients to the risk of developing another serious complication from an offending drug, even if it were another drug in the same class is against the basic principles of safe practice.

6.7 Prognosis of Anti-TNF-α -induced Lupus Erythematosus (ATIL)

Most patients who developed ATIL had a good prognosis upon discontinuation of these agents. Normalization of the emerged autoantibodies and resolution of lupus symptoms occur when the offending drugs is stopped without recurrence. Some patients might need to be started on corticosteroids and immunosuppressive agents for full recovery as described above. However, patients who developed serious side effects in form of renal or neurological involvements may have residual effects (Ramos-Casals, Brito-Zeron et al. 2007).

6.8 Prevention of Anti-TNF-α-induced Lupus Erythematosus (ATIL)

ATIL is a well documented entity. Physicians need to use these biological agents in caution with close follow up. It is not known whether ATIL and other autoimmune phenomena are a contributing factor for the high rate of long-term drug failure/discontinuation of anti-TNF-α therapy(Papagoras, Voulgari et al.) Rigorous follow up and early recognition of any complication developing while patients receiving anti-TNF-α agents, are essential to assure patients safety on the long term. This should help clinicians to learn more about these agents and identify appropriate approaches in different clinical settings encountered. As the use of anti-TNF-α agents has become more widely spread, the incidence of ATIL will likely also increase. There are currently no recommendations for prevention of ATIL. It has been suggested that concurrent use of immunosuppressive agents may reduce the incidence of autoantibody formation and thereby reduce the incidence of ATIL (Eriksson, Engstrand et al. 2005). Indeed, methotrexate can exert a suppressive effect on the production of autoantibodies in patients with isolated cutaneous lupus (Boehm, Boehm et al. 1998).

Although direct comparison between studies is difficult, as the majority of patients on anti-TNF will also be taking MTX, data from clinical trials of infliximab in patients with RA suggest that concurrent therapy with DMARDs is not protective (Charles, Smeenk et al. 2000; Eriksson, Engstrand et al. 2005). It has to be noted also that some RA patients had lupus features before the initiation of anti-TNF-α agents (Ramos-Casals, Brito-Zeron et al. 2007). Use of anti-TNF-α agents may have triggered or unmasked the symptoms of SLE in some patients. For this reason, assuring the diagnosis of RA prior to initiation of anti-TNF-α therapy is an extremely important aspect in the prevention process. Presence of SLE is considered a contraindication to the use of anti-TNF-α therapy. Therefore, it is recommended to perform a thorough baseline immunological screening for any patient with definite polyarthritis to assure accurate diagnosis. It is recommended to perform a detailed immunological screening for any patient whom you are considering anti-TNF-α therapy for. Some recommendations have been suggested for each patient upon starting anti-TNF-α therapy which will help in the therapeutic approach for autoimmune diseases induced by these biological agents (Ramos-Casals, Brito-Zeron et al. 2007). First, perform baseline immunological analysis and chest X-ray before treatment. Second, maintain specific follow up centered on the possible development of cutaneous, articular, or pulmonary manifestations. Third, evaluate adverse effects related to anti-TNF-α accurately, discarding the existence of undiagnosed autoimmune diseases (mainly systemic vasculitis). Fourth, preexisting SLE, especially in the presence of sever organ involvement (renal, pulmonary, or neurogical), should be considered as a precautionary scenario for the use of anti-TNF-α therapy. Finally, anti-TNF-α agents should not be used in patients with preexisting interstitial lung disease (table 9).

1.	Perform baseline immunological analysis and chest X-ray before treatment.
2.	Maintain specific follow up centered on the possible development of cutaneous, articular, or pulmonary manifestations.
3.	Evaluate adverse effects related to anti-TNF-α accurately, discarding the existence of undiagnosed autoimmune diseases (mainly systemic vasculitis).
4.	Preexisting SLE, especially in the presence of sever organ involvement (renal, pulmonary, or neurogical), should be considered as a precautionary scenario for the use of anti-TNF-α therapy.
5.	Anti-TNF-α agents should not be used in patients with preexisting interstitial lung disease.

Table 9. Some recommendations for each patient upon starting anti-TNF-α therapy. Adopted with modifications from (Ramos-Casals, Brito-Zeron et al. 2007).

7. Acknowledgments

The work to produce this chapter was supported by Alzaidi's Chair of research in rheumatic diseases- Umm Alqura University.

8. References

Almoallim, H. A., A. Khadawardi, H (2011). Lupus myositis with normal creatinine kinase levels following adalimumab use in a rheumatoid arthritis patient. *Turkish Journal of Rheumatology*, Volume 26, Number 4, Page(s): 328-332

Amoura, Z., S. Koutouzov, et al. (2000). "The role of nucleosomes in lupus." *Current opinion in rheumatology* 12(5): 369-73.

Aringer, M., E. Feierl, et al. (2002). "Increased bioactive TNF in human systemic lupus erythematosus: associations with cell death." *Lupus* 11(2): 102-8.

Aringer, M., F. Houssiau, et al. (2009). "Adverse events and efficacy of TNF-alpha blockade with infliximab in patients with systemic lupus erythematosus: long-term follow-up of 13 patients." *Rheumatology* 48(11): 1451-4.

Aringer, M. and J. S. Smolen (2003). "SLE - Complex cytokine effects in a complex autoimmune disease: tumor necrosis factor in systemic lupus erythematosus." *Arthritis research & therapy* 5(4): 172-7.

Aringer, M. and J. S. Smolen (2004). "Tumour necrosis factor and other proinflammatory cytokines in systemic lupus erythematosus: a rationale for therapeutic intervention." *Lupus* 13(5): 344-7.

Aringer, M. and J. S. Smolen (2008). "Efficacy and safety of TNF-blocker therapy in systemic lupus erythematosus." *Expert opinion on drug safety* 7(4): 411-9.

Balomenos, D. and A. C. Martinez (2000). "Cell-cycle regulation in immunity, tolerance and autoimmunity." *Immunology today* 21(11): 551-5.

Boehm, I. B., G. A. Boehm, et al. (1998). "Management of cutaneous lupus erythematosus with low-dose methotrexate: indication for modulation of inflammatory mechanisms." *Rheumatol Int* 18(2): 59-62.

Cambien, B., W. Bergmeier, et al. (2003). "Antithrombotic activity of TNF-alpha." *The Journal of clinical investigation* 112(10): 1589-96.

Charles, P. J., R. J. Smeenk, et al. (2000). "Assessment of antibodies to double-stranded DNA induced in rheumatoid arthritis patients following treatment with infliximab, a monoclonal antibody to tumor necrosis factor alpha: findings in open-label and randomized placebo-controlled trials." *Arthritis Rheum* 43(11): 2383-90.

Costa, M. F., N. R. Said, et al. (2008). "Drug-induced lupus due to anti-tumor necrosis factor alpha agents." *Semin Arthritis Rheum* 37(6): 381-7.

Costa, M. F., N. R. Said, et al. (2008). "Drug-induced lupus due to anti-tumor necrosis factor alpha agents." *Seminars in arthritis and rheumatism* 37(6): 381-7.

Cush, J., A. Kavanaugh, et al. (2011). Tumor necrosis factor blocking therapies. *Rheumatology*. M. Hochberg, A. Silman, J. Smolen, M. Weinblatt and M. Weisman. Philadelphia, mosby
elsevier. 1: 577.

Cush, J. J. (2004). "Unusual toxicities with TNF inhibition: heart failure and drug-induced lupus." *Clinical and experimental rheumatology* 22(5 Suppl 35): S141-7.

Cush JJ, K. A. (2003) "FDA Meeting March 2003: Update on the safety of new drugs for rheumatoid arthritis. Part I: The risk of lymphoma with rheumatoid arthritis (RA) and TNF " *www.rheumatology.org/research/hotline/0303TNF-L.htm* Volume, DOI:

De Bandt, M., J. Sibilia, et al. (2005). "Systemic lupus erythematosus induced by anti-tumour necrosis factor alpha therapy: a French national survey." *Arthritis research & therapy* 7(3): R545-51.

De Bandt, M., J. Sibilia, et al. (2005). "Systemic lupus erythematosus induced by anti-tumour necrosis factor alpha therapy: a French national survey." *Arthritis Res Ther* 7(3): R545-51.

Emlen, W., J. Niebur, et al. (1994). "Accelerated in vitro apoptosis of lymphocytes from patients with systemic lupus erythematosus." *Journal of immunology* 152(7): 3685-92.

Eriksson, C., S. Engstrand, et al. (2005). "Autoantibody formation in patients with rheumatoid arthritis treated with anti-TNF alpha." *Ann Rheum Dis* 64(3): 403-7.

Eriksson, C., S. Engstrand, et al. (2005). "Autoantibody formation in patients with rheumatoid arthritis treated with anti-TNF alpha." *Annals of the rheumatic diseases* 64(3): 403-7.

FDA (2008) "FDA labels for TNF inhibitors." *FDA Drug Safety Newsletter >> www.fda.gov/cder/dsn/default.htm* Volume, DOI:

Georgescu, L. and S. A. Paget (1999). "Lymphoma in patients with rheumatoid arthritis: what is the evidence of a link with methotrexate?" *Drug safety : an international journal of medical toxicology and drug experience* 20(6): 475-87.

Gergely, P., Jr., C. Grossman, et al. (2002). "Mitochondrial hyperpolarization and ATP depletion in patients with systemic lupus erythematosus." *Arthritis and rheumatism* 46(1): 175-90.

Gomez-Reino, J. J., L. Carmona, et al. (2003). "Treatment of rheumatoid arthritis with tumor necrosis factor inhibitors may predispose to significant increase in tuberculosis risk: a multicenter active-surveillance report." *Arthritis Rheum* 48(8): 2122-7.

Gomez, D., P. A. Correa, et al. (2004). "Th1/Th2 cytokines in patients with systemic lupus erythematosus: is tumor necrosis factor alpha protective?" *Seminars in arthritis and rheumatism* 33(6): 404-13.

Haraoui, B. and E. Keystone (2006). "Musculoskeletal manifestations and autoimmune diseases related to new biologic agents." *Current opinion in rheumatology* 18(1): 96-100.

Jacob, C. O., Z. Fronek, et al. (1990). "Heritable major histocompatibility complex class II-associated differences in production of tumor necrosis factor alpha: relevance to genetic predisposition to systemic lupus erythematosus." *Proceedings of the National Academy of Sciences of the United States of America* 87(3): 1233-7.

Katz, U. and G. Zandman-Goddard "Drug-induced lupus: an update." *Autoimmun Rev* 10(1): 46-50.

Katz, U. and G. Zandman-Goddard (2010). "Drug-induced lupus: an update." *Autoimmunity reviews* 10(1): 46-50.

Kerbleski, J. F. and A. B. Gottlieb (2009). "Dermatological complications and safety of anti-TNF treatments." *Gut* 58(8): 1033-9.

Kontoyiannis, D. and G. Kollias (2000). "Accelerated autoimmunity and lupus nephritis in NZB mice with an engineered heterozygous deficiency in tumor necrosis factor." *European journal of immunology* 30(7): 2038-47.

Kovacs, B., D. Vassilopoulos, et al. (1996). "Defective CD3-mediated cell death in activated T cells from patients with systemic lupus erythematosus: role of decreased intracellular TNF-alpha." *Clinical immunology and immunopathology* 81(3): 293-302.

Ledingham, J., C. Wilkinson, et al. (2005). "British Thoracic Society (BTS) recommendations for assessing risk and managing tuberculosis in patients due to start anti-TNF-{alpha} treatments." *Rheumatology (Oxford)* 44(10): 1205-6.

Leombruno, J. P., T. R. Einarson, et al. (2009). "The safety of anti-tumour necrosis factor treatments in rheumatoid arthritis: meta and exposure-adjusted pooled analyses of serious adverse events." *Ann Rheum Dis* 68(7): 1136-45.

Lin, J., D. Ziring, et al. (2008). "TNFalpha blockade in human diseases: an overview of efficacy and safety." *Clinical immunology* 126(1): 13-30.

Liozon, E., B. Ouattara, et al. (2007). "Severe polymyositis and flare in autoimmunity following treatment with adalimumab in a patient with overlapping features of polyarthritis and scleroderma." *Scandinavian journal of rheumatology* 36(6): 484-6.

Madhusudan, S., S. R. Muthuramalingam, et al. (2005). "Study of etanercept, a tumor necrosis factor-alpha inhibitor, in recurrent ovarian cancer." *J Clin Oncol* 23(25): 5950-9.

Mor, A., C. Bingham, 3rd, et al. (2005). "Proliferative lupus nephritis and leukocytoclastic vasculitis during treatment with etanercept." *The Journal of rheumatology* 32(4): 740-3.

Oldfield, V. and G. L. Plosker (2009). "Golimumab: in the treatment of rheumatoid arthritis, psoriatic arthritis, and ankylosing spondylitis." *BioDrugs* 23(2): 125-35.

Papagoras, C., P. V. Voulgari, et al. "Strategies after the failure of the first anti-tumor necrosis factor alpha agent in rheumatoid arthritis." *Autoimmun Rev* 9(8): 574-82.

Radis, C. D., L. E. Kahl, et al. (1995). "Effects of cyclophosphamide on the development of malignancy and on long-term survival of patients with rheumatoid arthritis. A 20-year followup study." *Arthritis and rheumatism* 38(8): 1120-7.

Ramos-Casals, M., P. Brito-Zeron, et al. (2008). "Vasculitis induced by tumor necrosis factor-targeted therapies." *Current rheumatology reports* 10(6): 442-8.

Ramos-Casals, M., P. Brito-Zeron, et al. (2007). "Autoimmune diseases induced by TNF-targeted therapies: analysis of 233 cases." *Medicine (Baltimore)* 86(4): 242-51.

Ramos-Casals, M., P. Brito-Zeron, et al. (2007). "Autoimmune diseases induced by TNF-targeted therapies: analysis of 233 cases." *Medicine* 86(4): 242-51.

Ramos-Casals, M., P. Brito-Zeron, et al. (2008). "Autoimmune diseases induced by TNF-targeted therapies." *Best practice & research. Clinical rheumatology* 22(5): 847-61.

Ramos-Casals, M., A. Roberto Perez, et al. "Autoimmune diseases induced by biological agents: a double-edged sword?" *Autoimmun Rev* 9(3): 188-93.

Rosen, A. and L. Casciola-Rosen (2001). "Clearing the way to mechanisms of autoimmunity." *Nature medicine* 7(6): 664-5.

Sandborn, W. J., S. B. Hanauer, et al. (2001). "Etanercept for active Crohn's disease: a randomized, double-blind, placebo-controlled trial." *Gastroenterology* 121(5): 1088-94.

Schiff, M. H., G. R. Burmester, et al. (2006). "Safety analyses of adalimumab (HUMIRA) in global clinical trials and US postmarketing surveillance of patients with rheumatoid arthritis." *Ann Rheum Dis* 65(7): 889-94.

Silman, A. J., J. Petrie, et al. (1988). "Lymphoproliferative cancer and other malignancy in patients with rheumatoid arthritis treated with azathioprine: a 20 year follow up study." *Ann Rheum Dis* 47(12): 988-92.

Stokes, M. B., K. Foster, et al. (2005). "Development of glomerulonephritis during anti-TNF-alpha therapy for rheumatoid arthritis." *Nephrology, dialysis, transplantation : official publication of the European Dialysis and Transplant Association - European Renal Association* 20(7): 1400-6.

Stokes, M. B., K. Foster, et al. (2005). "Development of glomerulonephritis during anti-TNF-alpha therapy for rheumatoid arthritis." *Nephrol Dial Transplant* 20(7): 1400-6.

Van den Brande, J. M., H. Braat, et al. (2003). "Infliximab but not etanercept induces apoptosis in lamina propria T-lymphocytes from patients with Crohn's disease." *Gastroenterology* 124(7): 1774-85.

Van Den Brande, J. M., M. P. Peppelenbosch, et al. (2002). "Treating Crohn's disease by inducing T lymphocyte apoptosis." *Ann N Y Acad Sci* 973: 166-80.

van Rijthoven, A. W., J. W. Bijlsma, et al. (2006). "Onset of systemic lupus erythematosus after conversion of infliximab to adalimumab treatment in rheumatoid arthritis with a pre-existing anti-dsDNA antibody level." *Rheumatology* 45(10): 1317-9.

Vasoo, S. (2006). "Drug-induced lupus: an update." *Lupus* 15(11): 757-61.

Wetter, D. A. and M. D. Davis (2009). "Lupus-like syndrome attributable to anti-tumor necrosis factor alpha therapy in 14 patients during an 8-year period at Mayo Clinic." *Mayo Clin Proc* 84(11): 979-84.

Wetter, D. A. and M. D. Davis (2009). "Lupus-like syndrome attributable to anti-tumor necrosis factor alpha therapy in 14 patients during an 8-year period at Mayo Clinic." *Mayo Clinic proceedings. Mayo Clinic* 84(11): 979-84.

Williams, E. L., S. Gadola, et al. (2009). "Anti-TNF-induced lupus." *Rheumatology (Oxford)* 48(7): 716-20.

Williams, E. L., S. Gadola, et al. (2009). "Anti-TNF-induced lupus." *Rheumatology* 48(7): 716-20.

Williams, V. L. and P. R. Cohen "TNF alpha antagonist-induced lupus-like syndrome: report and review of the literature with implications for treatment with alternative TNF alpha antagonists." *Int J Dermatol* 50(5): 619-25.

Williams, V. L. and P. R. Cohen (2011). "TNF alpha antagonist-induced lupus-like syndrome: report and review of the literature with implications for treatment with alternative TNF alpha antagonists." *International journal of dermatology* 50(5): 619-25.

Yung, R. L. and B. C. Richardson (1994). "Drug-induced lupus." *Rheum Dis Clin North Am* 20(1): 61-86.

Zhu, L., X. Yang, et al. (2007). "Decreased expressions of the TNF-alpha signaling adapters in peripheral blood mononuclear cells (PBMCs) are correlated with disease activity in patients with systemic lupus erythematosus." *Clinical rheumatology* 26(9): 1481-9.

Zhu, L. J., C. Landolt-Marticorena, et al. (2010). "Altered expression of TNF-alpha signaling pathway proteins in systemic lupus erythematosus." *The Journal of rheumatology* 37(8): 1658-66.

Part 3

Pregnancy and SLE

21

SLE and Pregnancy

Hanan Al-Osaimi and Suvarnaraju Yelamanchili
King Fahad Armed Forces Hospital, Jeddah
Saudi Arabia

1. Introduction

Systemic lupus erythematosus (SLE) is an autoimmune disease that affects multiple organs. Disease flares can occur at any time during pregnancy and postpartum without any clear pattern.

The hormonal and physiological changes that occur in pregnancy can induce lupus activity. Likewise the increased inflammatory response during a lupus flare can cause significant complications in pregnancy. Distinguishing between signs of lupus activity and pregnancy either physiological or pathological can be difficult [Clowse, 2007].

Pregnancy is a crucial issue that needs to be clearly discussed in details in all female patients with SLE who are in the reproductive age group. There are two essential concerns. The first one is the Lupus activity on pregnancy and the second one is the influence of pregnancy on Lupus. That is the reason why pregnancy should be planned at least six months of remission with close follow-up for SLE flares.

Women with SLE usually have complicated pregnancies out of which one third will result in cesarean section, one third will have preterm delivery and more than 20% will be complicated by preeclampsia [Clowse, 2006; Clark, 2003]. Rarely an SLE patient with a controlled disease activity may deteriorate as pregnancy advances, but still the pregnancy outcome can be better if pregnancy is well timed and managed.

2. Physiology of pregnancy

There are increased demands by the mother, fetus and the placenta during pregnancy which is to be met by the mother's organ systems. Therefore there are some cardiovascular, hematological, immunological, endocrinal and metabolic changes in the mother in normal pregnancy.

2.1 Cardiovascular system

The most important physiological changes that occur in pregnancy are the increase in cardiac output, retention of sodium and water leading to increase in the blood volume, reduction in systemic vascular resistance and blood pressure. These changes begin as early as fourth week of pregnancy [Chapman, 1998], reaching their peak during the second trimester, and then remain relatively constant until delivery. As the increase in the red cell volume is proportionately less than the increase in plasma volume there is hemodilution (physiological anemia) by the end of second trimester [Table 1]. The plasma volume gain is between 1000ml to 1500ml while the blood volume at term is about 100ml/kg which could commonly present as mild pedal edema [Jansen, 2005]

The increased levels of plasma erythropoietin is responsible for steady increase in the red cell mass by 20-30% who take iron supplements and by 15-20% in those who do not take iron supplements. The physiological anemia that occurs in pregnancy reduces the cardiac work load and helps for better placental perfusion by decreasing the blood viscosity.

It also decreases the risk of thrombosis in utero-placental circulation. The increased blood volume also protects against the usual blood loss in the peripartum period [Stephansson, 2000]. The hemoglobin begins to increase from the third postpartum day and the blood volume returns to non-pregnant level by two months postpartum.

Cardiac output- It increases by 30-50% during normal pregnancy [Robson, 1989]. This is as a result of increase in the preload due to rise in blood volume, decrease in afterload due to decrease in systemic vascular resistance and increase in the maternal heart rate by 15-20 beats/min without any change in the ejection fraction. Twin pregnancy increase the cardiac output by another 20%. However, maternal heart rate, stroke volume, and cardiac output during pregnancy may vary when mother changes from lateral to supine position [Lang,1991, Kametas,2003].

Hemodynamic changes related to labor and delivery – Normal labor and delivery is associated with significant hemodynamic changes due to anxiety, exertion, labor pains, uterine contractions, uterine involution, and bleeding. Cardiovascular effects also occur in some women due to infection, hemorrhage, or the administration of anesthesia or analgesia. The cardiac output and systemic vascular resistance gradually return to non-pregnant levels over a period of three months [Capeless, 1991].

2.2 Hematological changes

The total white cell count is increased up to 40% due to the increase in neutrophils as a result of demargination seen in pregnancy. Therefore the WBC count increases gradually in pregnancy as follows:

1st trimester- 3000-15,000 (Mean increase 9500/mm3)

2nd and 3rd trimesters- 6000-16,000 (mean 10,500)

During labor-may increase up to 30,000/ mm3

The platelet count gradually decreases till the term although they do not fall below 100,000/cu mm, most of the time they are in the lower range of normal values. This is as a result of dilutional effect, increased destruction and turn over.

The RBC increased by 20% due to increased production of erythropoietin but as the plasma volume is increased more than the red cell volume there is a drop in the hemoglobin causing physiological anemia [McColl, 1997].

2.3 Changes in systemic coagulation

Pregnancy is associated with changes in several coagulation factors that result in a 20 percent reduction of prothrombin and the partial thromboplastin times. The main changes are:

- Increased Resistance to activated protein C in the second and third trimesters
- Decreased levels of Protein S
- Increased levels of Factors I, VII, VIII, IX, and X
- Increased Activity of the fibrinolytic inhibitors PAI-1 and PAI-2, although total fibrinolytic activity may not be impaired

PARAMETER IN PREGNANCY	CHANGE (+/-)
Stroke volume	+30%
Heart rate	+15%
Cardiac output	+40%
Oxygen consumption	+20%
SVR (systemic vascular resistance)	-5%
Systolic BP	-10mmHg
Diastolic BP	-15mmHg
Mean BP	-15mmHg
Blood volume	+30%
Plasma volume	+40%
Red blood cell volume	+20%
Renal plasma flow	+35%
Glomerular filtration rate (GFR)	+50%
Polymorphonuclear leukocytes	+40%
Hemoglobin (11 g%)	-1-2G%
Leucocytosis (15,000/cmm)	+40%
Platelet (may drop upto 100,000)	Decreased
ESR (may go up to 40mm/Hr	Increased
Fibrinogen (up to 4.5G %)	+50%
Factor II,III,V,XII	No change
Factors I,VII,VIII,IX,X	Increased
Factors XI,XIII	Decreased
PT & APTT	Reduced
Bleeding time & clotting time	Unchanged
Fibrinolytic activity	Decreased
Complement C3, C4 levels	+10-50%

Table 1. Changes in maternal physiology in pregnancy
(Christopher Ficiliberto & Gertic F.Marx.(1998). Physiological changes associated with pregnancy. Physiology, 9(2):1-3)

The net effect of these pregnancy-induced changes is to produce a hypercoagulable state, which is a double-edged sword, both for protection (e.g., hemostasis contributing to reduced blood loss at delivery) and increased risk (e.g., thromboembolic phenomenon). Venous thrombosis in pregnancy occurs in approximately 0.7 per 1000 women, and is three to four folds higher in the puerpurium than during pregnancy. The risk is increased in women with underlying inherited thrombophilia (e.g. factor V Leiden or the prothrombin gene mutation) [Talbert, 1964; Hellgren, 1981].

2.4 Changes in the maternal immune system

The local adaptation of the maternal immune system is responsible for the successful coexistence between the mother and the fetus/placenta expressing both maternal (self) and paternal (non-self) genes [Mor, 2009; Robertson, 2010]. The cell- mediated adaptive immune responses are diminished, bypassed or even eliminated but the anti-body mediated immunity is altered while the natural immunity (innate immunity) remains intact which continues to provide the host defense against infection [Nagamatsu, 2010].

During insemination, transforming growth factor β1 (TGF- β1), found in the seminal fluid stimulates the production of granulocyte-macrophage colony- stimulation factor (GM-CSF) and recruitment of inflammatory cell infiltrates in the uterus. During implantation of the fertilized ovum, the majority of the lymphocytes infiltrating the decidua are distinctive uterine natural killer (NK) cells which are CD56++, CD16- & CD3- and express various receptors. Uterine decidua and the feto-placental unit produces large number of cytokines which contribute to shift of the immune response from T helper -1 (Th1) to T helper-2 (Th2) response where cytokines IL-10, IL-4, IL-5,IL-6 and IL-13 predominate while pregnancy rejection is mediated by Th1 response where IFN-α, TNF-β, IL-2, and IL-12 predominate [Lim,2000].

There are many specific mechanisms for immunological protection against the fetus. The most important one is altered HLA expression.

2.4.1 HLA class I

Very specific expression of the HLA class I molecules in trophoblasts is the main factor for protection against paternal HLA class I antigen. The extra-villous trophoblasts (EVT) will not express the HLA class Ia antigens-A, B, C or HLA II antigens but instead they express weak antigens of HLA class Ib – G, E & F which dampen the immune response by interacting with leukocyte inhibitory receptor (LIRs) on uterine natural killer (NK) cells and macrophages and with the T-cell receptors on CD8+ cells [Tilburgs, 2010; Le, 1997; Hunt, 2006).

2.4.2 Natural killer cells

There is a change in the relative population of lymphocytes in the uterus. The T & B cells become scarce and the uterine natural killer (NK) cell population shifts from endometrial NK cells to decidual NK cells.

2.4.3 Progesterone

The role of progesterone, the hormone of pregnancy, seems to be crucial in the maintenance of pregnancy. Progesterone leads to release of progesterone-induced blocking factor (PIBF), which controls cytokine production (IL-10 & others) and NK cell behavior. Increased embryo loss is associated with decreased levels of PIBF & IL-10 and increased levels of IL-12 and IFN-α [Ito, 1995; Nilsson, 1994].

2.5 Hormonal changes in pregnancy

Maternal changes in pregnancy involve hypothalamus, pituitary, parathyroid, adrenal glands, and ovaries to accommodate the needs of the fetal-placental-maternal unit. The hypothalamus still regulates much of the endocrine system through hypothalamic-pituitary axis, directly affecting the function of the above mentioned endocrine organs. Hence an intact hypothalamus is very much essential for normal pregnancy [Chrousos, 1995].

2.5.1 Hypothalamus

Secretes stimulatory hormones like gonadotropin-releasing hormone (GnRH), corticotrophin-releasing hormone (CRH), growth hormone-releasing hormone (GHRH), thyrotropin-releasing hormone (TRH) and inhibitory hormones like somatostatin and prolactin-inhibiting factors. These hormones are present in high concentrations in portal circulation where they are biologically active and the circulating concentrations of many of these hormones are also elevated in pregnancy due to placental production of identical or variant hormones. The most important changes are seen in the following hormones [Stojilkovic, 1994].

GnRH levels increases during pregnancy whose main source is placenta and plays a main role in placental growth and function. It also produces kisspeptin (KISS-1) which controls the gonadotropic axis and placental kisspeptin gradually increases with pregnancy which has a role in placentation [Bilban, 2004].

CRH from hypothalamus is involved in stress response in pregnancy and delivery. It is also secreted by placenta, chorionic trophoblasts, amnion and decidual cells. The placental CRH do not stimulate ACTH secretion but helps in initiation of labor. Besides CRH the gestational tissues also secretes urocortin which shares the same function of placental CRH, and urocortin-2 (stresscopin- related peptide) and urocortin-3 (stresscopin) which controls the tone of vascular endothelium also play a major role in parturition [Imperatore,2006; Florio, 2007].

2.5.2 Pituitary gland

Changes occur both in the anterior as well as the posterior lobe of pituitary gland.

Anterior lobe of pituitary gland enlarges to 3-fold during gestation due to hypertrophy and hyperplasia of lactotrophs and it takes at least six months after delivery to return to normal volume. FSH, LH & TSH levels are decreased while GH, ACTH & PRL levels are increased (mainly due to placental synthesis) [Lonberg, 2003].

The serum **prolactin** concentration (PRL) increases throughout pregnancy, reaching a peak at delivery to prepare the breast for lactation (figure 1) [Tyson, 1972], though the magnitude of the increase is quite variable.

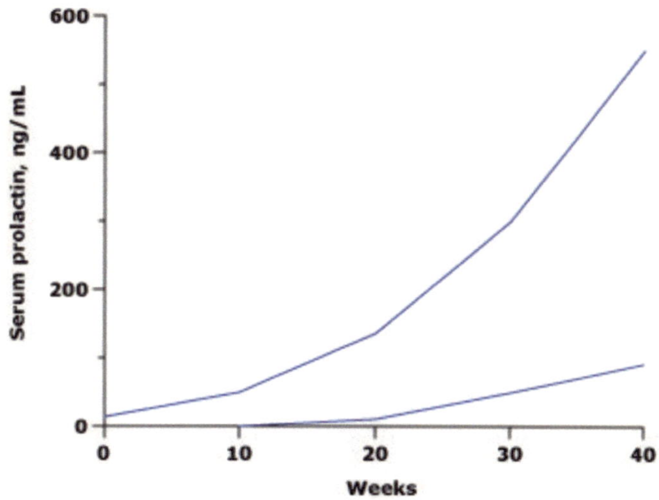

Fig. 1. Serum prolactin concentrations, as a function of time of gestation, showing the increase in prolactin as pregnancy progresses. The zone lines represent the range of values that can be seen. (Tyson, 1972)

The probable cause of hyperprolactinemia is the increasing serum estradiol concentration during pregnancy. By six weeks after delivery, estradiol secretion decreases and the basal serum prolactin concentration returns to normal range as in non-breast feeding mother. In women who are nursing, the decline in serum prolactin level is slower and marked by intermittent hyperprolactinemia related to suckling. Pregnancy appears to permanently reduce pituitary prolactin secretion. The serum prolactin concentration was lower in parous women at up to 12 years postpartum [Musey, 1987].

Posterior lobe of pituitary gland is a storage terminal for antidiuretic hormone (ADH) and oxytocin produced by supraoptic and paraventricular hypothalamic nuclei.

ADH- Its concentration remains in the non-pregnant range throughout pregnancy. Its metabolic clearance is increased due to vasopressinase released by placenta. The plasma sodium concentration falls by 5 meq/ L due to resetting of osmoreceptors as a result of increased levels of HCG.

Oxytocin- Its levels increases gradually throughout gestation and is involved in parturition and lactation [Lindheimer, 1991].

2.5.3 Thyroid gland

The size of the thyroid gland remains the same throughout the pregnancy but there is increase in the thyroxin-binding globulin (TBG). This leads to increased levels of both serum total thyroxin (T4) and triiodothyroxin (T3) but not the physiologically important serum free T4 & free T3 levels [Glinoer, 1990].

2.5.4 Adrenal gland

This gland does not undergo morphological changes during pregnancy. The renin-angiotensin-aldesterone system is stimulated during pregnancy due to decrease in peripheral vascular resistance and blood pressure and progressive decline in vascular responsiveness to angiotensin II. The aldesterone levels increased by 4-6 folds and the blood pressure usually reduced by 10mmHg. Relaxin, which is produced by the placenta, is a vasodilator factor, and aldesterone are critical in maintaining sodium balance in the setting of peripheral vasodilatation. During pregnancy there is increase in the levels of maternal & placental ACTH, cortisol-binding protein, atrial natriuretic peptide (ANP), plasma rennin activity (PRA), sex hormone-binding protein and testosterone levels [Homsen, 1993; Clerico, 1980].

2.6 Changes in the renal system in pregnancy

Both kidneys increase in size by 1 to 1.5 cm during pregnancy. Kidney volume increases by 30 percent, primarily due to an increase in renal vascular and interstitial volume. The renal pelvises and caliceal systems may be dilated as a result of progesterone effects and mechanical compression of the ureters at the pelvic brim. Dilatation of the ureters and renal pelvis (hydroureter and hydronephrosis) is more prominent on the right than the left and is seen in up to 80 percent of pregnant women [Beydoun, 1985]. All the above changes may not resolve until 6 to 12 weeks postpartum. Urinary frequency, nocturia, dysuria, urgency, and stress incontinence are the common symptoms during pregnancy [Nel, 2001].

Renal hemodynamics – Normal pregnancy is characterized by widespread vasodilatation with increased arterial compliance and decreased systemic vascular resistance. These global hemodynamic changes are accompanied by increases in renal perfusion and glomerular filtration rate. In late gestation, assumption of the left lateral position is associated with increases in glomerular filtration rate and sodium excretion [Almeida, 2009]. The increase in GFR which is approximately 40-50% is mainly due to increased glomerular plasma flow than increased intraglomerular capillary pressure. The renal blood flow increases by 80% above non-pregnant levels. As a result, the serum creatinine and BUN falls below the non-pregnant levels.

The mechanisms for decreased vascular resistance and increased renal plasma flow during pregnancy are not fully understood. Reduced vascular responsiveness to vasopressors such as angiotensin II, norepinephrine, and vasopressin is well-documented. Nitric oxide synthesis increases during normal pregnancy and may contribute to the systemic and renal vasodilatation and the fall in blood pressure [Danielson', 1995].

The ovarian vasodilator hormone, relaxin, appears to be a key upstream mediator of enhanced nitric oxide signaling in pregnancy. Relaxin increases endothelin and nitric oxide production in the renal circulation, leading to generalized renal vasodilatation, decreased renal afferent and efferent arteriolar resistance, and a subsequent increase in renal blood flow and GFR. There is increased urinary protein excretion up to 200 mg/day in the third trimester [Novak, 2001].

3. Distinguishing lupus activity from signs and symptoms of pregnancy

Systemic lupus erythematosus (SLE) primarily affects women in their reproductive years of life, making the issue of pregnancy important to many of these patients. Pregnancy changes affecting disease severity can be attributed to placental or maternal hormones, increased circulation, increased fluid volume, increased metabolic rate, hemodilution, circulating fetal cells, or other factors. Lupus flares are common in pregnancy at rate of 0.06-0.136 per patient-month [Table 2].

Likewise, the increased inflammatory response during a lupus flare can cause significant pregnancy complications. Distinguishing lupus activity from signs of both healthy and pathologic pregnancy is not straight forward and can be very difficult at times [Table 4]. Therefore, activity scales specific for pregnancy which takes into account these issues, have been established. One of them, the Lupus Activity Index in Pregnancy is actually validated, showing high sensitivity, specificity and predictive values for detecting flares during pregnancy [Clowse, 2006].

There is an increase in disease activity during pregnancy, according to many studies. In some patients, this will mean a dramatic worsening of symptoms that can be life threatening. Most patients, however, will have a modest increase in symptoms making pregnancy uncomfortable but not affecting their long-term survival. The increasing levels of estrogens that are seen in normal pregnancy to promote physiologic and immunologic changes required may also increase the lupus activity [Cohen-Solal, 2006; Grimaldi, 2006]. Even though it is highly debated, at least some studies have found a two- to threefold increase in SLE activity during pregnancy [Petri, 1997; Lim, 1995; Il Dong, 2011].

40-50% of the patients will have increased SLE activity, majority of which are mild but in 1/3 of cases it may be moderate to severe [Cortes-Hernandez., 2002]. Fortunately, the majority of SLE activity in pregnancy is not severe and in most studies, it is the skin, joint, and constitutional symptoms that are commonly seen. The physiological changes that occur

in pregnancy interfere with assessment of disease activity in SLE. So the signs and symptoms of pregnancy can easily be mistaken for increased lupus activity.
Fatigue can be a distressing complaint throughout normal pregnancy. The fatigue of fibromyalgias increases during pregnancy. As there is no inflammation in this condition the excess sex hormones as well as steroids do not relieve pain.
Palmar erythema and **facial blush** are also seen in pregnancy due to increased secretion of estrogens.

Impact of pregnancy on SLE activity

- Pregnancy probably increases lupus activity:
- About 50% of women will have measurable SLE activity during pregnancy
- Most of the disease activity will be mild to moderate
- 15% to 30% of women will have highly active SLE in pregnancy
- Most common types of SLE activity in pregnancy:
    1. Cutaneous disease (25-90%)
    2. Arthritis (20%)
    3. Hematologic disease (10-40%)
- Risk factors for increased lupus activity:
    1. Active lupus within the 6 months before conception
    2. Multiple flares in the years before conception
    3. Discontinuation of hydroxychloroquin

Table 2. Impact of pregnancy on lupus activity (adopted from Megan, 2007)

Arthralgias, joint effusions, headaches and low back pain are also common in pregnancy due to the effects of relaxin, increased levels of estrogens and fluid retention. The increased **shortness of breath** is due to elevation of diaphragm as a result of upward growth of gravid uterus. The **hair loss** particularly during puerpurium and post-partum is a common finding in normal pregnancy.
The HAQ (Health assessment questionnaire) score increases for normal pregnant women from 0.02 in the first trimester to 0.16 in the second and 0.48 in the third trimester.
As the blood volume increases in pregnancy by 50% there is an effect of hemodilution in the body which **decreases hemoglobin and platelets**, however the hemolytic anemia and platelets less than 100,000/c mm do not occur in normal pregnancy, if present suspect either lupus activity, severe preeclampsia or HELLP (Hemolysis, Elevated Liver enzymes, Low Platelets) [Buyon, 1999].
The risk for skin disease during pregnancy is higher (25-90%) than arthritis (20%), thrombocytopenia (10-40%) or nephritis (4-30%). Women with previous history of lupus nephritis have a higher chance for relapse of nephritits (20-30%).
Due to **increased blood volume and glomerular filtration rate** the **serum creatinine falls** gradually and **proteinuria** increases during normal pregnancy. Therefore a stable serum creatinine that is maintained during pregnancy without a fall suggests renal insufficiency. Only proteinuria which is more than double the baseline is to be taken as abnormal, as proteinuria up to 300mg/24 hours can occur in normal pregnancy. A serum creatinine level

>140 μmol/L is associated with a 50% pregnancy loss and this increases to 80% if the level is >400 μ mol/L [Megan, 2007].

Symptoms of pregnancy that can mimic lupus activity	
Constitutional	Fatigue that can be debilitating in entire pregnancy.
Skin	Palmar erythema and a facial blush due to increased estrogen.
Face	Melasma: "mask of pregnancy." A macular, photosensitive Hyperpigmented area over cheeks and forehead.
Hair	Increased hair growth and thickness during pregnancy. Hair loss in the weeks to months postpartum.
Pulmonary	Increased respiratory rate from progesterone. Dyspnea from enlarging uterus late in pregnancy.
Musculoskeletal	Back pain in second and third trimesters. -Relaxin loosens sacroiliac joint and symphysis pubis -Gravid uterus increases lumbar lordosis. Joint effusions: non-inflammatory in lower extremities.
Central nervous system	Headache can be part of normal pregnancy or associated with hypertension. Seizures occur in eclampsia. Cerebral vascular accidents can be caused by preeclampsia or antiphospholipid syndrome.

Table 3. Symptoms in pregnancy that mimics lupus activity
(Adopted from Tsokos GC et al. Systemic lupus erythematosus, A companion to rheumatology. St. Louis: Mosby; 2007)

Complement C3, C4, anti-dsDNA titer, autoimmune target testing (AITT) and lupus activity

The activity of the lupus cannot accurately be assessed by the C3/C4 level and anti-dsDNA titers as in non-pregnant lupus patients. C3 and C4 may be decreased with increased lupus activity because these proteins are consumed in the inflammatory process [Ho A, 2001]. In pregnancy, however, the complement levels may increase 10-50% in response to increased hepatic protein synthesis [Buyon, 1992].
During pregnancy, C3 and C4 may rise to supranormal levels, and thus a flare with complement activation may occur despite apparently normal levels of C3 and C4. Conversely C3and C4 may be low in the absence of a flare, probably due to synthetic defects. However, if C3 or C4 levels drop by >25%, this may be reasonably ascribed to disease activity [Buyon, 1999]. Therefore, the utility of complement measurement in pregnancy is unclear. However, the combination of low complement levels and high-activity lupus leads to a 3-5-fold increase in pregnancy loss and preterm birth [Clowse, 2004].

AITT uses the macrophage cell line (IT-1) as a substrate that is wider than the ANA test in clinical applications

The anti- dsDNA titer is very sensitive for the diagnosis of lupus and can be indicative of increased lupus activity, especially if the kidney is involved [Ho A, 2001]. Increased dsDNA which is considered for diagnosis and increased activity of the disease can be seen in 43% of pregnant lupus women without disease activity, but rising titers of dsDNA is suggestive of increased lupus activity [Table 4]. However, this antibody does not predict pregnancy outcomes. Instead, the combination of a positive anti-dsDNA titer and highly active SLE contribute toward a 4-6-fold increase in perinatal mortality and a 2-3-folds decrease in full-term birth [Clowse, 2004].

Criteria	**For Lupus Flare**	
SYSTEM	*"VALID"*	"INVALID"
Cutaneous	Inflammatory rash	Cloasma or Palmar erythema , Post partum alopecia
Musculoskeletal	Inflammatory arthritis	Arthralgias Bland effusion
Hematological	New leucopenia New Thrombocytopenia (PLT <80,000)	Mild anemia ESR up to 40 mm
Serological	Rising titer anti-dsDNA	
Constitutional	Fever not due to infection	Fatigue
Pulmonary	Pain on inspiration	Mild SOB, Hyperventilation 2° to Progesterone
Source: JP Buyon MD	**Rheumatologia**	**2(4) 199 (2004)**

Table 4. Criteria for lupus flare

LE cell phenomenon is seen in lupus patient's blood. LE cell test was the first autoimmune disease test of using this phenomenon that showed lower sensitivity and specificity. So HEp-2 cell using the conventional antinuclear antibody (ANA) test is currently being used as a standard test. However AITT uses the macrophage cell line (IT-1) as a substrate that is wider than the ANA test in clinical applications.

The ESR is unreliable in pregnancy because it increases significantly in normal pregnancy but if it is very high (>40mm/hr) it can be taken for increased lupus activity. In non-pregnant SLE patients, CRP may increase with a lupus flare. The use of CRP has not been systematically tested in SLE pregnancies [Ho A, 2001]. As CRP is not elevated in pregnancy, it is to be considered for increased activity of the disease. Therefore elevated CRP is a better indicator for increased lupus activity than elevated ESR [Ruiz, 2004; Megan, 2007].

In a study (Table 5), complement C3 levels were statistically significant in hematuria, leucopenia, hypertension, high serum CRP levels, and preterm premature rupture of membranes. Complement C4 levels were statistically significant in kidney disease status, hematologic diseases and admissions to NICU. Anti-dsDNA was statistically significant in oligohydramnios, elevated CRP and neonatal anti-SSB (La) antibody detection. It is helpful to predict neonatal diseases. AITT is statistically significant in high ESR values and Apgar score. This helps to predict state of the newborn immediately after birth [II Dong Kim, 2011].

Complement C3	Complement C4	Anti-dsDNA	AITT
Leucopenia	Hematological disease	Anti-SSB/La antibodies (in neonates)	
Elevated CRP		Elevated CRP	Elevated ESR
Hypertension	Proteinuria		
Hematuria	Hematuria		
Premature rupture of Membranes (PRM)	Admission to NICU	Oligohydramnios	1 & 5 minute Apgar score
AITT= Auto-immune	Target Testing		

Table 5. Correlation of pregnancy complications with C3, C4, Anti-dsDNA and AITT
Source: II Dong Kim et al. Korean J Obstet Gynecol 2011; 54:17-25

In conclusion, although it is difficult to differentiate lupus activity from changes that occur in pregnancy, one needs to consider carefully all the above factors in a lupus pregnancy with high clinical suspicion of active disease for the diagnosis of increased lupus activity.

4. Influence of pregnancy on SLE

SLE patients suffer from different kinds of pregnancy related complications more than non-SLE women. The following are the common pregnancy related complications.

4.1 Hypertension

Blood pressure levels tend to drop during pregnancy starting from the first trimester and increases at term. Hypertension complicates 5% to 7% of all pregnancies. About 25% of lupus patients will develop hypertension and proteinuria in the second-half of pregnancy. In case of prior nephropathy of any type, hypertension develops in 41% of patients during pregnancy [How, 1985]. Pre-existing hypertension is the most common predisposing factor for preeclampsia.

The risk of preterm birth, IUGR, and fetal loss, all increase in hypertensive pregnant lupus patients. Yasmeen, et al identified 555 deliveries in women with SLE and compared those pregnancy outcomes with outcomes in control group of 600,000 deliveries in women without SLE. The results showed that women with SLE had higher rates of adverse outcomes of pregnancy, including hypertensive complications, preterm delivery, cesarean delivery, IUGR, and fetal deaths, than did women without SLE. The rate of hypertensive disorders of pregnancy were found to be 2.9% as compared to the controlled population which is only 0.4% [Yasmeen, 2001]. Hypertension can present in pregnancy as

- Pregnancy-induced hypertension or gestational hypertension (blood pressure ≥ 140/90mmHg seen first time during pregnancy, returns to normal levels 12 weeks post partum)
- Chronic hypertension (blood pressure ≥ 140/90mmHg before pregnancy or diagnosed before 20 weeks of gestation or hypertension first diagnosed after 20 weeks of gestation and persistent after 12 weeks post partum)
- Preeclampsia (blood pressure ≥ 140/90mmHg after 20 weeks of gestation with proteinuria of ≥ 300mg/24hrs)
- Eclampsia (preeclampsia with seizures)

4.2 Lupus flares

There is conflicting data on whether SLE activity increases during pregnancy. The risk of lupus flare is increased if the woman has had active lupus in the last 6 months of pregnancy. Therefore, inactive disease at the onset of pregnancy provides optimum protection against the occurrence of flare during pregnancy [Urowitz, 1993].

Lupus may flare during any trimester of pregnancy or post partum period. The flares are usually mild mainly involving the joints, skin and blood. Some of the physiological changes of pregnancy can mimic the symptoms of the active disease such as palmar erythema, arthralgia, myalgia and lower limb edema [Table 4].

High prolactin levels, presence of lupus anticoagulant and increased SLE activity, have poor outcome in pregnancy [Jara, 2007a]. Oral Bromocriptine may play a role in the prevention of maternal-fetal complication such as premature rupture of membrane, preterm birth and active disease as reported in one of the clinical trials but this needs to be confirmed by further trials [Jara, 2007b].

The most important laboratory data to differentiate lupus flare in pregnancy from pregnancy changes include rising titer of anti-double strand DNA antibodies, presence of red blood cell casts in the urine, positive direct Coomb's test and presence of antiplatelet antibody with thrombocytopenia. Complement levels can be in normal range as complement levels increases during pregnancy due to estrogen-induced hepatic synthesis of complements.

In normal pregnancy the increased glomular filtration rate observed in the second trimester leads to increase in proteinuria. Thrombocytopenia is seen in pregnancy, although it is generally mild and occurs only in 8% of women [Burrow, 1988]. The lupus activity index in pregnancy (LAI-P) scale which is a modified activity scale specific for pregnancy, studied by Ruiz-Irastorza G, et al showed (LAI-P) high sensitivity to changes in lupus activity, and has a significant correlation with modified physician global assessment (M-PGA). This index has high sensitivity, specificity, predictive values, and likelihood ratios for diagnosing SLE flares during pregnancy and puerpurium [Riuz, 2004].

4.3 Preeclampsia

SLE in general and hypertension and/or renal disease in particular were agreed upon by most studies to increase the risk for preeclampsia [Clowse, 2007]. Patients with class III and IV SLE nephritis have a significantly higher prevalence of preeclampsia (28% to 38%) as compared to class II or I (11.1%) or to lupus controls without nephritis (4.6%).

It is important to differentiate isolated preeclampsia from lupus nephritis during pregnancy, as the corner stone in preeclampsia management is delivery of the fetus. Preeclampsia as we mentioned previously is blood pressure levels of over 140/90 along with proteinuria of > 300mg per 24 hour after 20 weeks gestation [Table 6]. Sometimes it can be associated with features of HELLP syndrome. If preeclampsia presents very early (< 20 weeks) one should look for the presence of APS (Antiphospholipid antibody syndrome). Very severe cases of PET may evolve into eclampsia.

In patients with no previous history of renal involvement and with normal baseline urinary parameters, preeclampsia is strongly supported by the onset of proteinuria in the third trimester, new onset hypertension, inactive urinary sediment, absence of anti-DNA antibodies and normal complements levels.

PARAMETER	ACTIVE LUPUS NEPHRITIS	PREECLAMPSIA
High BP	Present or Absent	Diastolic BP > 90 mm Hg
Proteinuria	• >500 mg/24 hr if normal at baseline • Doubling if >500 mg/24 hr at baseline • Occur before 3rd trimester	• >300 mg/24 hr if normal at baseline • Occur during 3rd trimester
Edema	Present / Absent	Present / Absent
Active Sediment	Present / Absent	Absent
Uric Acid	Normal or Elevated	Elevated
C3, C4	Low	Normal
Anti-ds DNA Abs	Rising	Absent

Table 6. Broad Guidelines to differentiate Lupus Nephrites from Preeclampsia (Buyon, 2004)

Antiplatelet agents during pregnancy, particularly the use of low dose Aspirin as primary prevention in PET are associated with moderate but consistent reduction in the relative risk of premature birth before 34 weeks gestation, and of having a pregnancy without serious adverse outcome [Askie, 2007]. A systemic review showed that Aspirin reduces the risk of perinatal death and preeclampsia in women with a history of risk factors such as preeclampsia, chronic hypertension, diabetes, and renal disease. Given the importance of these outcomes and the safety along with low cost of aspirin, low dose aspirin should be considered in all women with the above risk factors [Coomarasamy, 2003]. Previous studies have suggested that several factors, including pre-existing hypertension, renal insufficiency, presence of APS, and active SLE, may increase the risk of preeclampsia in pregnancies complicated by SLE [Mascola, 1997]. The features which differentiate preeclampsia from lupus nephritis are given in Table 6.

4.4 Lupus Nephritis (LN)

Pregnant women with long-standing LN are at risk of spontaneous abortions and increased perinatal mortality. However, the outlook of pregnancy in patients with stable LN at conception is relatively favourable. Remission in lupus nephritis has been defined as stable renal function, a serum creatinine within the normal range, urinary red cells below 5/high power field, proteinuria below 0.5g/day and normal serum C_3 levels for the last 12-18 months (Table 6) [Gayed, 2007].

The incidence of obstetric complications and maternal mortality is high in patients with active lupus nephropathy associated with pre-existing hypertension. Pregnant women with LN require intense fetal and maternal surveillance for a better outcome of pregnancy [Rahman, 2005]. The increase in proteinuria can be secondary to the usual increase in glomerular filtration rate observed in the second trimester of pregnancy. Moderate renal impairment at the onset of pregnancy, as reflected by serum creatinine level of 120μmoles/L or greater, has a greater decline in renal function than would be expected in a non-pregnant patient for a similar time period [Hou, 1985].

The fetal loss in patients with active LN in pregnancy occurs in 36% to 52% of the pregnancies, as compared to fetal loss in pregnant patients with history of LN but with stable creatinine and minimal proteinuria during pregnancy, which is only 11% to 13% [Huong, 2001; Moroni, 2002]. A study of 24 pregnancies in 22 women with LN noticed flares in 50% with proteinuria, 42% with hypertension, and 25% with preeclampsia [Soubassi, 2004]. Lupus nephritis flare can be associated with other evidence of active lupus such as serositis, arthritis, and high titers of anti-DNA antibodies. The proteinuria of preeclampsia decreases after delivery but not that of active lupus patient.

4.5 Thrombocytopenia

It is not unusual to see this in pregnancy. It is encountered in at least 8% of all pregnancies. In gestational thrombocytopenia, the degree of thrombocytopenia is usually mild, with no history of bleeding or preconception history of thrombocytopenia. The platelet count usually returns to normal within 2-12 weeks post partum [Jeffrey, 2002]. Also, thrombocytopenia may occur for a variety of reasons in pregnancy such as SLE, APS, HELLP or medication particularly Heparin or expanding of circulatory volume.

4.6 Other complications

Pregnant lupus patients can face other problems like HELLP syndrome (**H**emolysis **E**levated **L**iver enzymes and **L**ow **P**latelets) and Gestational diabetes [Joya, 2010, Josephine, 2006].

5. Influence of SLE on pregnancy

5.1 Effect on fertility

Systemic lupus erythematosus (SLE) is not known to affect the fertility directly and therefore SLE patients are as fertile as any other female in general population [Kamashta, 1996]. Lowered fertility rate is seen in patients with active disease on high dose steroids, patients with established renal disease and moderate to severe renal failure [Hou, 1975]. End-stage renal disease secondary to lupus nephritis can result in amenorrhea, although amenorrhea in renal patients may also be due to ovarian failure secondary to cyclophosphamide or of auto-immune origin [Kong, 2006].

5.2 Effect of flare on conception

SLE patients can experience disease flare at anytime during pregnancy with potential negative effects on the conception. Lupus flares occur more during pregnancy and post partum period in SLE patients than non-SLE pregnant patients [Petri, 1991]. Increased lupus activity is seen after pregnancy in 1/3 of cases [Seng, 2008]. Therefore, for better outcome of lupus pregnancy it is essential to control disease activity and achieve clinical remission at least 6 months before pregnancy [Georgion, 2000].

Exacerbations or relapses occur during the course of pregnancy and immediate post partum period in 25% to 60% of cases. However, the likelihood of increased clinical activity of SLE during pregnancy is influenced by signs of activity present at onset of pregnancy. In the absence of signs of clinical activity for at least 6 months before conception, relapses occur only in one-third of cases, whereas in patients with clinical activity at onset of pregnancy, persistent activity or exacerbations occur in approximately two-thirds.

Fetal survival in these patients parallels with the incidence of SLE activity: Hence fetal survival is seen in 85% to 95% in the group with inactive disease at conception and 50% to 80% in subjects with active disease at the onset of pregnancy [Weyslett, 1991]. More recent studies have shown a 2-3 fold increase in SLE activity during pregnancy [Rehman, 2005]. Adverse live-birth outcome was significantly associated with low pre-gestational serum albumin level, elevated gestational anti-ds DNA antibody, and diabetes mellitus. Spontaneous abortion was directly associated with low levels of pre-gestational serum albumin, positive anticardiolipin IgA, anti-B_2-glycoprotein IgM, and anti-La antibodies.

Complication	Moderate to severely active SLE (n=57)	Inactive or mildly active SLE (n=210)	P-value
Miscarriage	7%	7%	0.9
Stillbirth:	16%	5%	<0.01
Extreme Preterm (<28 weeks gestation)	17%	6%	0.09
Late Preterm (28 to 37 weeks gestation)	49%	26%	<0.001
Small for gestational age baby (<10th percentile weight for gestational age)	30%	21%	0.23

Table 7. Increased Lupus Activity in Pregnancy Increases Pregnancy Complications (*Data from* Clowse MEB et al. The impact of increased lupus activity on obstetric outcomes. Arthritis Rheum, 2005. 52(2): p. 514–21)

5.3 Effect of lupus nephritis

The obstetric complications and maternal mortality is high in patients with active lupus nephropathy associated with pre-existing hypertension [Rahman, 2005]. Pregnant women with long-standing lupus nephritis are at high risk of spontaneous abortions and increased perinatal mortality. However, the outlook of pregnancy in patients with stable lupus nephritis at conception is relatively favorable [Table 7]. Patients with the combination of either high clinical activity of SLE and low complement or positive anti-ds DNA had the highest rate of pregnancy loss and preterm birth [Clowse, 2011].

Female recipients transplanted for renal failure secondary to lupus nephritis can maintain pregnancy successfully. Outcomes are comparable to renal recipients with other diagnoses. Newborns in both groups were often premature and had low birth weight [McGrory, 2003].

The second trimester Doppler ultrasound examination is the best predictor of late pregnancy outcome in systemic lupus erythematosus and/or the anti-phospholipids syndrome [Lethi, 2006].

Management of pregnant women with renal disease involves awareness of physiological changes such as decreased serum creatinine and increased proteinuria. Worsening proteinuria may be due to lupus flare but differential diagnosis also includes preeclampsia. In fact, women with severe renal impairment (serum creatinine over 300µmols/L) have a chance lower than 30% of having successful pregnancy [Germin, 2006].

5.4 Effect of Antiphospholipid Syndrome (APS)

Anti-phospholipids antibodies (APL), which include lupus anti-coagulant (LAC), anti-cardiolipin antibodies (ACL), and B_2glycoprotein are frequently found in patients with SLE, and their presence has been associated with increased fetal loss. If APL are present, the fetuses are susceptible to placental insufficiency. APL but not anti-Ro and anti-La

Term	Definition
Spontaneous abortions or miscarriages	Pregnancy loss <20 weeks of gestation
Recurrent abortion or recurrent miscarriages	≥3 spontaneous abortions
Fetal loss	Pregnancy loss from 10 weeks of gestation and onwards
Intrauterine fetal demise (IUFD) or stillbirth	Fetal death occurring at ≥20 weeks of gestation
Fetal wastage	Sum of spontaneous abortions and stillbirths
Neonatal death	Infant born live but died up to 28 days after birth
Small for gestational age	Birth weight <10th percentile
Low birth weight	Birth weight <2500 g
Very low birth weight	Birth weight <1500 g
Preterm birth or prematurity	Gestational age <37 weeks

Table 8. Adverse pregnancy outcomes
(Data from Josephine P et al-Lupus and pregnancy: complex yet manageable
Clin Med Res 2006 Dec; 4(4):310-321)

antibodies might have a role in direct placental damage. The levels of β-hCG are reduced in women with history of recurrent pregnancy loss or thromboembolic events. High titers of APL were found to cause the largest reduction in β-hCG. Anti-Ro and anti-La did not induce placental damage [Schwartz, 2007]. APL also have direct effect on trophoblast possibly through exposed anionic phospholipids and/ or adherent B_2glycoprotein "B_2GP1", resulting in altered trophoblast intercellular fusion, gonadotropin secretion and trophoblast invasiveness [Di Simone, 2005].

Typical fetal loss secondary to APS is characterized by progressive intrauterine growth restriction (IUGR) ultimately leading to fetal death [Birdsall, 1996]. Both early and late fetal deaths are associated with APS [Rai, 1995]. The live birth of an APS pregnancy rate increased from 19% in untreated patients to 70% in treated patients [Lima, 1996]. The risk of pregnancy loss in women with anti-phospholipids antibodies (APL) and with a previous pregnancy loss has been estimated at over 60%. APS pregnancy is not without complications in the mother [Table 9].

Beside those already mentioned, pregnancy confers a higher risk of thrombosis in women who are already at increased risk or with a past history of thrombotic events [Branch, 1992]. The incidence of extensive infarction, decidual vasculopathy, decidual thrombosis and perivillous fibrinoid change, which have been thought to be characteristic lesions of APS placenta, was significantly higher in LAC, or ACL or both LAC & ACL positive patients than in the patients without APL. LAC and ACL double-positivity is an important risk factor for fetal death in the SLE patient [Petri, 2004; Ogishima, 2000].

As the placenta positive for IgG-APL showed pathogenic findings such as infarction, degeneration, thrombus formation and fibrinoid deposits, it is suggested that IgG-APL bound to the placental tissue might cause direct pathologic damage to the placenta which results in IUFD, or IUGR by uteroplacental insufficiency [Katoro, 1995].

Fetal Risks	Maternal Risks
• Recurrent miscarriage (first and second trimester)	• Thrombosis
• Intrauterine growth restriction	• Severe early onset preeclampsia
• Fetal death	• Preterm labour, rupture of membranes
• Premature delivery	• Worsening of pre-existing thrombocytopenia
• Congenital malformations/ intracerebral haemorrhage (If Warfarin is administered)	• Placental abruption • Other bleeding complications

Table 9. Obstetric risks associated with anti-phospholipid syndrome (Adapted from S Stone, MA Khamashta, and L Poston [Stone, 2001])

Fetal risk had been reduced progressively in the past 40 years. Although it still continues to be higher than that occurring in pregnancies of healthy women. The presence of APL considerably worsens the fetal outcome [Moroni, 2005]. It is suggested that patients with early-onset severe preeclampsia be screened for APL, if antibodies are detected, then these women should be considered for prophylactic anticoagulation therapy [Branch, 1989].

A retrospective case-control study of 242 pregnancies in 112 patients concluded that the risk of fetal loss in SLE is 2.5 times higher than that in the normal population. The presence of LAC indicated a high risk of fetal loss, while the absence of APL is an indication of a favorable pregnancy outcome. No individual APL test seems to be clearly superior to the others to detect patients at high risk for fetal loss. However, by combining ACL with LAC, a reasonably good sensitivity and specificity can be achieved. Regardless of APL, infants of women with SLE are born more prematurely and are more retarded in growth than the infants in the normal population. Thus, factors other than APL also contribute to the adverse fetal outcome in lupus pregnancy [Heikki, 1993].

5.5 Effect of anti-ro/and or anti-la antibodies

SLE is the most recognized Rheumatic disease in which auto antibodies, anti-Ro and/or anti-La can pass from the mother to the fetus across the placenta during pregnancy. Anti-Ro/SSA antibodies are associated with neonatal lupus but do not negatively affect other gestational outcomes, and the general outcome of these pregnancies is now good. A large multi-centers cohort prospective controlled study of 100 anti-Ro/SSA positive women concluded that anti-Ro/SSA antibodies are responsible for congenital heart block but do not affect other outcomes of pregnancy, both in SLE and non-SLE women.

The general outcome for these pregnancies is now very good, if prospectively followed by multidisciplinary teams [Antonio, 2011; Brucato, 2002], although various studies considered the anti-Ro/SSA antibody as a possible causative factor for unexplained pregnancy loss. A significant greater fetal wastage is seen in black anti-Ro (SSA) positive women as compared to black anti-RNP positive women. No significant difference in fetal wastage was noted between the white SLE and the non-SLE women in either antibody group. These data suggest that black SLE patients with anti-Ro (SSA) antibody may be at increased risk of fetal wastage [Watson, 1986]. Hull et al reported three SLE patients with anti-Ro/SSA and a history of spontaneous abortions [Hull, 1983].

Ro52, Ro60 and La IgG antibodies all are transferred from the mothers to their fetus in utero and were present in the infant at birth as detected by enzyme-linked immunosorbent assay using recombinant antigens and a synthetic peptide. A significant decrease in Ro52, Ro60 and LA IgG auto antibody levels the infants was observed from birth to 4-5 weeks of the age. Ro- and La-specific IgA and IgM antibodies were detected in the serum from a subset of mothers. However, Ro- and La-specific IgA and IgM antibody levels were low or non-detectable in children raised both with and without breastfeeding. These findings support a role for placental materno-fetal transfer of the IgG auto antibodies in the pathogenesis of neonatal lupus erythematosus (NLE) and indicate that refraining from breast-feeding does not protect from NLE skin involvement [Klauinger, 2009].

Studies focusing on the neuropsychological development of SLE offspring show an increased number of learning disabilities in children with normal intelligence levels. The presence of anti-Ro/La antibodies and disease activity (flare) in mothers during pregnancy were significantly related to higher prevalence of learning disabilities in offspring. Mainly sons of women with SLE were significantly more likely to have learning disabilities than daughters of women with SLE or children of either sex in the control group as these maternal antibodies likely affect the fetal brain of male offspring and result in later learning problems. These findings should promote greater awareness and early educational intervention in those children [Ross, 2003].

5.6 Other risks

Prospective studies indicate that the majority of lupus mothers can sustain pregnancy without detrimental effects, provided that the pregnancy is planned during the inactive phase of the disease. Nevertheless the fetal risk, although progressively reduced during the last 40 years, continues to be higher, particularly in patients with anti-phospholipids antibodies (APL), than in pregnancies in healthy women [Moroni, 2003].

Premature rupture of membranes (PROM) is more common in pregnancies occurring in women with SLE which is the major etiology for preterm births [Johnson, 1995]. SLE is associated with increased risk of spontaneous abortion (pregnancy loss prior to 20 weeks gestation), preeclampsia, stillbirth (pregnancy loss after 20 weeks gestation), premature rupture of membrane (PROM), intrauterine growth restriction and fetal death.

The risk of thrombosis, infection, thrombocytopenia and requirement for transfusions is higher in women with SLE. Lupus patients also have a higher risk for cesarean sections, preeclampsia, and are also more likely to have other medical conditions like diabetes, hypertension, and thrombophilia which are also associated with adverse pregnancy [Clowse, 2008].

SLE women belong to category of high-risk pregnancy. Highly active lupus during pregnancy leads to increased premature birth and a decrease in live births, with almost one-quarter of these pregnancies resulting in fetal loss. The Hopkins Lupus Center Database has identified a combination of two factors: high clinical activity and serologic activity. These two are very important factors which predict preterm birth. Pregnancies in lupus patients must be closely watched and treated during all the three trimesters to improve pregnancy outcomes [Urowitz,1993; Chandran, 2005].

6. Conclusion

SLE is a chronic multisystem disease occurring in young women in their childbearing age. And therefore, the collaboration of rheumatologist and obstetrician who are experienced in high risk pregnancies management, are essential for managing these women with lupus who becomes pregnant to have a successful outcome as these women already have high risk in terms of fetal loss and spontaneous abortions [Georgion, 2000]. The manifestations of normal pregnancy can be mistaken as signs of lupus activity making the diagnosis and treatment challenging. Therefore, understanding of pregnancy and lupus interaction has resulted in better methods of monitoring and treating this particular clinical situation.

7. Acknowledgment

The work to produce this chapter was supported by Alzaidi's Chair of research in rheumatic diseases- Umm Alqura University.

8. References

Almeida FA, et al. (2009). The haemodynamic, renal excretory and hormonal Changes induced by resting in the left lateral position in normal pregnant women during late gestation. *BJOG*, 116:1749.

Antonio Brucato, Rolando Eimaz, et al. (2011). Pregnancy outcomes in patients with autoimmune diseases and anti-Ro/SSA antibodies. *Clinical Review in Allergy and Immunology* 40(1); 27-41.

Ashorson, et al. (1986). Systemic lupus erythematosus, antiphospholipid antibodies, chorea, and oral contraceptives. *Arthritis Rheum*, 29(12): 1535-1536.

Askie LM, et al. (2007). Antiplatelet agents for prevention of preeclampsia: a meta-analysis of individual patient data. *Lancet*, 369(9575): 1791-1798.

Beliver J, Pellicer A. (2009). Ovarian stimulation for ovulation induction and in vitro fertilization in patients with systemic lupus erythematosus and antiphospholipid syndrome. *Fertil Steril*, 92(6): 1803-10.

Beydoun SN. (1985). Morphologic changes in the renal tract in pregnancy. *Clin Obstet Gynecol*, 28:249.

Bilban M, et al. (2004) Kisspeptin-10, a KiSS-1/metastin-derived decapeptide, is a physiological invasion inhibitor of primary human trophoblasts. *J Cell Sci*, 117: 1319.

Birdsall MA, Lockwood. (1996). Anti-phospholipid antibodies in women having in-vitro fertilization. *Hum* reprod, 11(6): 1185-1189.

Blombäck M. S(1981). Studies on blood coagulation and fibrinolysis in pregnancy, during delivery and in the puerpurium. I. Normal condition. *Gynecol Obstet Invest*, 12: 141.

Bowes WA Jr. (1980). The effect of medication on lactating mother and her infant. Clinical Obstetrics & Gynecology, Dec. 23(4):1073-80

Branch DW, Andres R, Digne KB et al. (1989). The association of anti-phospholipid antibodies with severe Preeclampsia *Obstetric Gynecology*, 73(4): 541-5. (1992).

Antiphospholipid antibodies and fetal loss. *New English Journal of Medicine*, 326(4):951-2.

Briggs GG, Freeman RK, Yaffe SJ. (2002). *Drugs in pregnancy and lactation*. 6th ed. Philadelphia (PA): Lippincott Williams & Wilkins.

Brucato A, Doria A et al. (2002). Pregnancy outcome in 100 women with auto-immune diseases and anti-Ro/SSA antibodies: a prospective controlled study. *Lupus*, 11(11): 716-21.

Burrow RF, Kellen JG. (1988). Incidentally detected thrombocytopenia in healthy mothers and their infants. *N Engl J Med*, 319(3): 142-5.

Buyon et al. (1992). Activation of the alternative complement pathway accompanies disease flares in systemic lupus erythematosus during pregnancy. *Arthritis Rheum*, 35:55-61.

(1999). Assessing disease activity in SLE patients during pregnancy. *Lupus*, 8:677-84.

(2000). Neonatal Lupus: Bench to bedside and back. *Presented at the 66th annual meeting of the American College of Rheumatology*, October 2000.

(2004). Management of SLE during pregnancy: A decision tree. *Reumatologia*, 20 (4), 197-99

Capeless EL, Clapp JF. (1991). When do cardiovascular parameters return to Their reconception values? *Am J Obstet Gynecol*, 165:883.

Chandran V, Aggarwal A, Misra R. (2005). Active disease during pregnancy is associated with poor foetal outcome in Indian patients with systemic lupus erythematosus. *Rheumatol Int*, 26(2):152-6

Chapman AB, Abraham WT, Zamudio S, et al. (1998). Temporal relationships Between hormonal and hemodynamic changes in early human pregnancy. *Kidney Int*, 54:2056.

Christopher Ficiliberto & Gertic F.Marx.(1998). Physiological changes associated with pregnancy. Physiology, 9(2):1-3

Chrousos GP. (1995). The hypothalamic-pituitary-adrenal axis and immune-mediated inflammation. *N Engl J Med*, 332:1351.

Clark Ca et al. (2003).Preterm deliveries in women with systemic lupus erythematosus. *J Rheumatol*, 30:2127-32.

(2005).Decrease in pregnancy loss rates in patients with systemic lupus erythematosus over a 40-year period. *J Rheumatol*, 32:1709-12.

Clerico A, De et al. (1980). Elevated levels of biologically active (free) cortisol during pregnancy by a direct assay of diffusible cortisol in an equilibrium dialysis system. *J Endocrinol Invest*, 3:185.

(2006). National study of medical complications in SLE pregnancies. *Arthritis Rheum*, 54(9 Suppl):S263–4.

(2007). Lupus activity in pregnancy. *Rheum Dis Clin North Am*, 33:237-52.

(2008). A national study of the complications of lupus in pregnancy. *Am J Obstet Gynecol*, 199:127.e1-6.

(2010). The use of anti-TnFα medications for rheumatologic disease in pregnancy. *International Journal for Women's Health*, 9(2): 199-209.

(2010). Managing contraception and pregnancy in the rheumatologic diseases. *Best Pract Research in Clinical Rheumatology*, 24(3): 373-85.

(2011). The clinical utility of measuring complement and anti-ds DNA antibodies during Pregnancy in patients with systemic lupus erythematosus. *J Rheumatol*, 24(3): 373-85

Clowse ME. (2004). Complement and doublestranded DNA antibodies predict pregnancy outcomes in lupus patients. *Arthritis Rheum*, 50:S408.

(2005). The impact of increased lupus activity on obstetric outcomes. *Arthritis Rheum*, 52(2); 514-521 (2006). National study of medical complications in SLE pregnancies. *Arthritis Rheum*, 54(9 Suppl):S263–4.

(2006). National study of medical complications in SLE pregnancies. Arthritis Rheum, 54(9 supplement)5:263-264

(2007). Lupus activity in pregnancy. *Rheum Dis Clin North Am*, 33:237-52.

(2008). A national study of the complications of lupus in pregnancy. *Am J Obstet Gynecol*, 199:127.e1-6.

(2010). The use of anti-TnFα medications for rheumatologic disease in pregnancy. *International Journal for Women's Health*, 9(2): 199-209.

(2010). Managing contraception and pregnancy in the rheumatologic diseases. *Best Pract Research in Clinical Rheumatology*, 24(3): 373-85.

(2011). The clinical utility of measuring complement and anti-ds DNA antibodies during Pregnancy in patients with systemic lupus erythematosus. *J Rheumatol*, 24(3): 373-85

Cohen-Solal JF, Jeganathan V, Grimaldi CM, et al. (2006). Sex hormones and SLE: influencing the fate of autoreactive B cells. *Curr Top Microbiol Immunol*, 305:67–88.

Coomarasamy A, et al. (2003). Aspirin for prevention of preeclampsia in women with historical risk factors: a systemic review. *Obstet Gynecol* 2003, 101(6): 1319-32

Cortes- Cooper WO, Hernandez-Diaz, *et al.* (2006). Major Congenital malformations after first trimester exposure to ACE inhibitors. *New English Journal of Medicine*, 354(23): 2443-51.

Curran-Everett D, Morris KG Jr, Moore LG. (1991) Regional circulatory contributions to increased systemic vascular conductance of pregnancy. *Am J Physiol*, 261: H1842.

Danielson LA, Conrad KP. (1995). Acute blockade of nitric oxide synthase inhibits renal vasodilatation and hyperfiltration during pregnancy in chronically instrumented conscious rats. *J Clin Invest*, 96:482.

Di Simone N, Raschi E, Testoni C, et al. (2005). Pathogenic role of anti-B_2glycoprotein antibodies in antiphospholipid associated fetal loss: Characterization of B_2glycoprotein, binding to trophoblast cells and functional effects of anti-B_2glycoprotein, antibodies in vitero. *Annals of Rheumatic Disease*, 64: 462-7.

Dong kim et al. (2011). Complement C3,C4, DsDNA and AITT and Lupus activity. J Obstet Gynaecol, 54:17-25.

Duvekot JJ, et al. (1993). Early pregnancy changes in hemodynamics and volume homeostasis are adjustments by a primary fall in systemic vascular tone. *Am J Obstet Gynecol*, 169:1382

Florio P, Linton EA, Torricelli M, et al. (2007). Prediction of preterm delivery based on maternal plasma urocortin. *J Clin Endocrinol Metab*, 92:4734.

Fraga A, Mintz G, Orozco H. (1974). Fertility rate, fetal wastage and maternal morbidity in SLE. *J Rheumatology*1974; 1: 293-8.

(1974). The nature of pressor responsiveness to angiotensin II in human pregnancy. Obstet Gynecol, 43:854.

(1980). Control of vascular responsiveness during human pregnancy. *Kidney Int,* 18:253.

Gant NF et al. (1974). The nature of pressor responsiveness to angiotensin II in human pregnancy. Obstet Gynecol, 43:854.

(1980). Control of vascular responsiveness during human pregnancy. *Kidney Int,* 18:253.

Gayed and C. Gordon. (2007). Pregnancy in rheumatic diseases. *Rheumatology,* 46:1634-1640.

Georgion PE, Politi EN, Katsimbri P, Sakka V, Drosos AA. (2000). Outcome of Lupus pregnancy: a controlled study. *Rheumatology (Oxford),* 39(9): 1014.

Georgiou PG et al (2000). Outcome of lupus pregnancy. A controlled study. Rheumatology, 39(9):14-1019

Germin S, Nelsen-Piercy C. (2006). Lupus nephritis and renal disease in pregnancy. *Lupus,* 15(3): 148-155.

Glinoer D, de Nayer P, Bourdoux P, et al. (1990). Regulation of maternal thyroid during pregnancy. *J Clin Endocrinol Metab,* 71:276.

Grimaldi CM. (2006). Sex and systemic lupus erythematosus: the role of the sex hormones estrogen and prolactin on the regulation of autoreactive B cells. *Curr Opin Rheumatol,* 18(5):456–61

Handa R, U. Kumar, JP Wali. (2006, June). SLE and Pregnancy. *JAPI Suppl,* 54:19-21

Heikki Julkven, Tareli Jouhikainen. (1993). Fetal outcome in lupus Pregnancy: a retrospective case-control study of 242 pregnancies in 112 patients. *Lupus,* 2(2): 125-131.Hellgren M,

Hernandez J, Ordi-Ros J, Paredes F, et al. (2002). Clinical predictors of fetal and maternal outcome in systemic lupus erythematosus: a prospective study of 103 pregnancies. *Rheumatology* (Oxford) 41(6):643–50

Ho A, Barr SG, Magder LS, Petri M. (2001). A decrease in complement is associated with increased renal and hematologic activity in patients with systemic lupus erythematosus. *Arthritis Rheum,* 44:2350-7.

Homsen JK, et al (1993). Atrial natriuretic peptide (ANP) decrease during normal pregnancy as related to hemodynamic changes and volume regulation. *Acta Obstet Gynecol Scand,* 72:103.

How SH. (1985). Pregnancy in women with chronic renal disease. *N Engl J Med* 1985; 312(13):863-839.

Hou SH et al. (1985). Pregnancy in women with renal disease and moderate renal insufficiency. *American Journal of Medicine,* 78: 185-194.

(1985). Pregnancy in women with renal disease and moderate renal insufficiency. *Am J Med,* 1985; 78: 105-194.

Hull RG, Harris EN, Morgan SH, et al. (1983). Anti-Ro antibodies and abortions in women with SLE. *Lancet,* 11: 1138.

Hunt JS, Langat DK, McIntire RH, Morales PJ. (2006). The role of HLA-G in human pregnancy. *Reprod Biol Endocrinol,* 4 Suppl 1:S10.

Huong DL, et al. (2001). Pregnancy in the past or present lupus nephritis: a study of 32 pregnancies from a single center. *Ann Rheum Dis,* 60(6): 599-604.

(2002). Importance of planning ovulation induction therapy in systemic lupus erythematosus and antiphospholipid syndrome: a single center retrospective study of 21 cases and 114 cycles. *Semin Arthritis Rheum*, 32(3): 174-88

Imperatore A, Florio P, Torres PB, et al. (2006). Urocortin 2 and urocortin 3 are expressed by the human placenta, deciduas, and fetal membranes. *Am J Obstet Gynecol*, 195: 288.

Isenberg DA et al. (2004). Pregnancy in Rheumatic diseases: An overview. Oxford text book of Rheumatology 2004 3rd edition p 117-125

Ito I, Hayashi T, Yamada K et al. (1995). Physiological concentration of estradiol inhibits PMN chemotaxis via a receptor mediated system. *Life Sci*, 56:2247-2253.

Izmirly, Peter M, Kim et al. (2010). Evaluation of the risk of anti-SSA/Ro-SSB/La antibody-associated cardiac manifestations of neonatal lupus in fetuses of mothers with systemic lupus erythematosus exposed to hydroxychloroquine. *Annals of the Rheumatic Diseases*, 69(10):1827-1830, 1468-2060.

Izmirly, Peter M. et al. (2010, April). Cutaneous manifestations of neonatal lupus and risk of subsequent congenital heart block. *Arthritis & Rheumatism*, 62(4):1153-1157, 1529-0131.

Jansen AJ, van Rhenen DJ, Steegers EA, Duvekot JJ. (2005). Postpartum hemorrhage and transfusion of blood and blood components. *Obstet Gynecol Surv*, 60:663.

Jara LJ, et al. (2007). Prolactin levels are associated with lupus activity, lupus anticoagulant, and poor outcome in pregnancy. *Ann NY Acad Sci*, 1108; 218-26.

(2007). Bromocriptine during pregnancy in systemic lupus erythematosus: a pilot clinical trial. *Ann NY Acad Sci*, 1110; 297-304.

Jeffrey A. Levy, et al. (2007). Thrombocytopenia in pregnancy. *JABFP*, 15(4); 290-297.

Johnson MJ, Petri M, Witter FR, Repke JT. (1995). Evaluation of preterm delivery in a systemic lupus erythematosus pregnancy clinic. *Obstetric Gynecology*, 86(3): 396-399.

Josephine Patricia Dhar, et al. (2006). Lupus and pregnancy: complex yet manageable. *Clin Med Res*, 006 Dec; 4(4); 310-321.

Joya, Snee. (2010). Roy, et al. SLE in pregnancy. *BSMMUJ*, 3(1): 54-59.

Khamashta MA, Hughes GRV. (1996). Pregnancy in SLE. *Curropin Rheumatol*, 8: 424-429.

Kametas NA, McAuliffe F, Krampl E, et al. (2003). Maternal cardiac function in twin pregnancy. *Obstet Gynecol*, 102:806.

Katoro, K. Aoki. (1995). Specific anti-phospholipid antibodies (apL) eluted from placenta of pregnant women wit h apL-positive sera. *Lupus*, 4(4): 304-308.

Klauninger R, Skog A, Horvath et al. (2009). Serologic follow-up of children born to mothers with Ro/SSA auto-antibodies. *Lupus*, 18(9): 792-798.

Kong NC. (2006). Pregnancy of a lupus patient- a challenge to the nephrologist. *Nephrol Dial, Transplant*, 21(2): 268-272.

Kozer E, et al. (2003). Effects of aspirin consumption during pregnancy on pregnancy outcomes: meta-analysis. Birth Defects Res B Dev. *Reprod Toxicol*, 68(1): 70-84.

Lang, RM, Borow, KM. (1991). Heart disease. In: Medical Disorders During Pregnancy, Barron, WM, Lindheimer, MD, (Eds), *Mosby Year Book*, St. Louis. p. 184.

Le Bouteiller P, Mallet V. (1997). HLA-G and pregnancy. *Rev Reprod*, 2:7.

Lethi Hung D, Wechsler et al. (2006). The second trimester Dopplear ultrasound examination is the best predictor of late pregnancy outcome in systemic lupus erythematosus and/or the antiphospholipid syndrome. *Rheumatology (Oxford)*, 45(3): 332-338.

Lim KJH, Odukoya OA, Ajjan RA, et al. (2000). The role of T-Helper cytokines in human reproduction. *Fertil Steril*, 73:136-142.

Lima et al. (1995). Obstetric outcome in systemic lupus erythematosus. *Semin Arthritis Rheum*, 95;25(3):184–92.

(1996). A study of sixty pregnancies in patients with antiphospholipid syndrome. *Clinical Exp Rheumatology*, 14(2): 131-6.

Lindheimer MD, Barron WM, Davison JM. (1991). Osmotic and volume control of vasopressin release in pregnancy. *Am J Kidney Dis*, 17:105.

Lønberg U, et al. (2003). Increase in maternal placental growth hormone during pregnancy and disappearance during parturition. *Am J Obstet Gynecol*, 188:247.

Mascola MA, et al. (1997). Obstetric management of the high-risk lupus pregnancy. *Rheum Dis Clin North Am*, 23: 119-32.

McColl MD, Ramsay JE, Tait RC, et al. (1997). Risk factors for pregnancy associated venous thromboembolism. *Thromb Haemost*, 78:1183.

McGrory CH, McCloskey LJ, De Horatius et al. (2003). Pregnancy outcomes in female renal recipients: a comparison of systemic lupus erythematosus with other diagnoses. *American Journal of Transplant*, 3(1): 35-42.

Megan E.B. Clowse. Lupus Activity in Pregnancy. (2007). *Rheum Dis Clin N Am* 33:237–252

Molad Y, Borkowski T, Monselise et al. (2005). Maternal and fetal outcome of lupus pregnancy: a prospective study of 29 pregnancies. *Lupus*, 14(2); 145-151.

Mor, G, Abrahams, VM. (2009). The immunology of pregnancy. In: Creasy and Resnik's maternal-fetal *medicine: Principles and practice*, 6th ed, Creasy, et al, p.87.

Moroni G., et al. (2002). Pregnancy in lupus nephritis. *AMJ Kidney Dis*, 40(4): 713-20.

(2003). The risk of pregnancy in patients with lupus nephritis. *Journal of Nephrology*, 16 (2):161-167.

Moroni G, Ponticelli C. (2005). Pregnancy after lupus nephritis. *Lupus*, 14(1): 89-94.

Musey VC, Collins DC, Musey PI, et al. (1987). Long-term effect of a first pregnancy on the secretion of prolactin. *N Engl J Med*, 316:229.

Nagamatsu T, Schust DJ. (2010). The contribution of macrophages to normal and pathological pregnancies. *Am J Reprod Immunol*, 63:460.

Nel JT, Diedericks et al. (2001). A prospective clinical and urodynamic study of bladder function during and after pregnancy. *Int Urogynecol J Pelvic Floor Dysfunct*, 12:21.

Nilsson N Carlsten H. (1994). Estrogen induced suppression of natural killer cell cytotoxicity and augmentation of polyclonal B-cell activation. *Cell Immunol*, 158:131-139.

Novak J, Danielson LA, Kerchner LJ, et al. (2001). Relaxin is essential for renal vasodilatation during pregnancy in conscious rats. *J Clin Invest*, 107:1469.

Ogishima D, Matsumoto T, Nakamura et al. (2000). Placental pathology in systemic lupus erythematosus with antiphospholipid antibodies. *Pathol Int*, 50(3); 224-9.

Petri M et al. (1991). Frequency of lupus flare in pregnancy: the Hopki lupus pregnancy center experience. *Arthritis Rheum*, 34: 1538-45.

(1997). Hopkins Lupus Pregnancy Center: 1987 to 1996. *Rheum Dis Clin North Am*, 23(1):1–13.

(2004). Prospective study of systemic lupus erythematosus pregnancies. *Lupus*, 13:688-9.

Rahman EZ, et al. (2005). Pregnancy outcomes in lupus nephropathy. *Arch Gynecol Obstet,* 271(3): 222-6.

RA Levy, VS Vilela, MJ Cataldo, RC Ramos. (2001). Hydroxychloroquine (HCQ) in lupus pregnancy: double-blind and placebo-controlled study. *Lupus,* 10(6): 401-404.

Rai RS, Regan L, Clifford K, et al. (1995). Antiphospholipid antibodies and B_2glycoprotein-I in 500 women with recurrent miscarriage: result of a comprehensive screening approach. *Human Reprod,* 10(8): 2001-2005.

Robertson SA. (2010). Immune regulation of conception and embryo implantation-all about quality control? *J Reprod Immunol,* 85:51.

Robson SC, Hunter S, Boys RJ, Dunlop W. (1989). Serial study of factors influencing changes in cardiac output during human pregnancy. *Am J Physiol,* 256:H1060

Ross G, Sammaritano L, Nass R, Lockshin M. (2003). Effects of mother's autoimmune disease during pregnancy on learning disabilities and hand preference in their children. *Arch Pediatric Adolesc Med,* 157(4): 397-402.

Ruiz et al., (2004). Evaluation of systemic lupus erythematosus activity during pregnancy. *Lupus,* 13:679-82.

(2004). Measuring systemic lupus erythematosus activity during pregnancy: validation of the lupus activity index in pregnancy scale. *Arhthritis Rheum,* 51(1): 78-82.

(2004). MA Gordon Measuring SLE activity during pregnancy- *Arthritis Rheum,* 51:78-82

(2008). Lupus in Pregnancy: ten questions and some answers. *Lupus,* 17, 416–420

(2011, June). Integrating clues from the bench and bedside-*Eurj clin rest,* 41 (6):672-8

Schwartz N, Shoenfeld Y, Barzilai O. (2007). Reduced placental growth and hcG secretion in vitro induced by antiphospholipid antibodies but not by anti-Ro or anti-La: studies on sera from women with SLE/PAPs. *Lupus,* 16: 110-120.

Seng Yj, Liud Z et al. (2008). Predictors of maternal and fetal outcome in systemic lupus erythematosus: a restrospective study of 94 cases. *Zhonghua Neikezazhi,* 47(12): 1008-11.

Shnider, SM, Levinson, G. (1989). *Anesthesia for Obstetrics,* 3rd ed, Williams & Wilkins, Baltimore, 1989, p. 8.

Soubassi L, et al. (2004). Pregnancy outcome in women with pre-existing lupus nephritis. *J Obstet Gynaecol,* 24(6): 630-4.

Stephansson O, Dickman PW, Johansson A, Cnattingius S. (2000). Maternal hemoglobin concentration during pregnancy and risk of stillbirth. *JAMA,* 284:2611.

Stojilkovic SS, Reinhart J, Catt KJ. (1994). Gonadotropin-releasing hormone receptors: structure and signal transduction pathways. *Endocr Rev,* 15:462.

Stone S, Khamashta MA. (2001). Placenta, antiphospholipid syndrome and pregnancy outcome. *Lupus,* 10(2): 67-74

Talbert LM, Langdell RD. (1964). Normal values of certain factors in the blood clotting mechanism in pregnancy. *Am J Obstet Gynacol,* 90:44

Tilburgs T, Scherjon SA, Claas FH. (2010). Major histocompatibility complex (MHC)-mediated immune regulation of decidual leukocytes at the fetal-maternal interface. *J Reprod Immunol,* 85:58.

Tincanni A, Danieli E, Nuzzo M, et al. (2006). Impact of in utero environment on the offspring of lupus patients. *Lupus,* 15(11): 801-7

Tyson JE, Hwang P, Guyda H, Friesen HG. (1972). Studies of prolactin secretion in human pregnancy. *Am J Obstet Gynecol,* 113:14.

Urowitz MB, Glabman DD, Farewell VT, Stewart J, McDonald J. (1993). Lupus and pregnancy studies. *Arthritis Rheum*, 36(10); 1392-1397

Watson RM, Braunstein BL, Waston AJ, et al. (1986). Fetal wastage in women with anti-Ro antibody. *Journal of Rheumatology,* 13(1): 90-4.

Wayslett JP. (1991). Maternal and fetal complications in pregnant women with systemic lupus erythematosus. *American Journal of Kidney Diseases,* 17(2): 123-126.

Yasmeen S, et al. (2001). Pregnancy outcomes in women with systemic lupus erythematosus. *J Matern Fetal Med,* 10: 91-6.

22

Management of Pregnant Lupus

Hanan Al-Osaimi and Suvarnaraju Yelamanchili
King Fahad Armed Forces Hospital, Jeddah
Saudi Arabia

1. Introduction

The initiating point to manage pregnancy in lupus patient is ideally before the onset of pregnancy. Therefore, at preconception counseling, the physician not only estimates the risk profile of the patients but also reviews their drugs. This is to avoid known teratogenic drugs, to discontinue certain medications and to initiate other drugs as a golden goal to protect the mother and fetus from adverse effects of these medications. Hence, it is essential to observe the mother at least six months before attempting conception for a better outcome in lupus pregnancy.

The management of SLE pregnancy should be a multidisciplinary approach and needs good coordination and follow-ups with experts in the field like rheumatologist, obstetrician who is experienced in dealing with high risk pregnancies and nephrologist if the renal impairment is also present. Therefore, all lupus pregnancies should be closely monitored.

This chapter covers general guidelines for the management of SLE during Pregnancy and post partum period in addition to safety of contraceptive methods in lupus women.

2. Management issues

Once the pregnancy test results are positive we should have a baseline evaluation of the disease activity, its severity and major organ involvement [Table1].

- Prenatal care visits: Every 4 weeks up to 20 weeks, then every 2 weeks until 28 weeks, then weekly until delivery.

SLE presents several challenges in managing a pregnant woman and her fetus, as SLE affects almost every organ system in the body and shows a broad spectrum of disease manifestations ranging from mild to life-threatening conditions [Boumpas, 1995].

Due to the improvement of treatment modalities more and more women with this disease are able to become pregnant. Pregnancy outcomes have improved dramatically over the last 40 years, with a decrease in pregnancy loss rate from a mean of 43% in 1960-1965 to 17% in 2000 - 2003 [Clark, 2005].

Pregnant patients with SLE on immunosuppressive therapy need prophylaxis for infection, (including antibiotics for invasive procedures), and immunization with influenza & pneumococcal vaccine.

FIRST TRIMESTER	• Baseline CBC, electrolytes, serum creatinine, liver enzymes, uric acid.
	• Fasting blood glucose, fasting lipid profile if at high risk, for example if patient is nephritic or on steroids
	• Normal antenatal check up
	• ANA, Anti-DsDNA, anti-Ro and anti-La, antibody titers
	• Complements levels (C_3,C_4,CH_{50})
	• Anticardiolipin antibodies, lupus anticoagulant and β_2 glycoprotein
	• Urinalysis, 24-hour urine collection for measurement of protein and creatinine clearance
SECOND TRIMESTER	• Baseline laboratory studies
	• Anti-DsDNA
	• Complements levels (C_3,C_4,CH_{50}) , urinalysis
	• Obstetric ultrasound: Every 4 weeks from 20 weeks of gestation until delivery "to monitor fetal growth"
	• Mother with positive Anti-Ro and/or Anti-La antibodies, serial fetal echocardiography between 16-36 weeks of gestation
THIRD TRIMESTER	• Repeat laboratory studies
	• Urinalysis, 24-hour urine protein collection if proteinuria is present
	• Weekly fetal non-stress test (NST) and/or biophysical profile (BPP) scoring from 28 weeks gestation
	• Fetal Doppler ultrasonography to be done in presence of intrauterine growth restriction
EACH VISIT	• Careful blood pressure measurement
	• Urine dipstick for proteinuria

Table 1. Guidelines for assessment of pregnant patients with lupus

2.1 Safety of medications

SLE is common in women of childbearing age. Physicians should be aware of which medications to be used safely at preconception & conception, and effects on infants exposed to certain drugs.

The Food and Drug Administration (FDA) has a classification system for pregnancy risk (Table 2). The pharmacological management of SLE is challenging as it has an unpredictable clinical course, with the variable organ system involvement and the lack of clear understanding of disease pathogenesis [Francis L, 2009].

2.1.1 Antihypertensive drugs

Hypertensive disorders of pregnancy are the leading cause of maternal mortality and morbidity. Blood pressure tends to decrease in the first and second trimesters of pregnancy. The most appropriate blood pressure threshold and goal of antihypertensive treatment are controversial. For women with severe hypertension (defined as a sustained systolic BP of ≥160mmHg and/or a diastolic BP of ≥ 110mmHg), there is consensus that antihypertensive therapy should be given to lower the maternal risk of central nervous system complications. The target BP of safety in Pregnancy is less than 140/90 mm of Hg.

United States FDA Pharmaceutical Pregnancy Categories	
Pregnancy Category A	Adequate and well-controlled human studies have failed to demonstrate a risk to the fetus in the first trimester of pregnancy (and there is no evidence of risk in later trimesters).
Pregnancy Category B	Animal reproduction studies have failed to demonstrate a risk to the fetus and there are no adequate and well-controlled studies in pregnant women OR Animal studies have shown an adverse effect, but adequate and well-controlled studies in pregnant women have failed to demonstrate a risk to the fetus in any trimester.
Pregnancy Category C	Animal reproduction studies have shown an adverse effect on the fetus and there are no adequate and well-controlled studies in humans, but potential benefits may warrant use of the drug in pregnant women despite potential risks.
Pregnancy Category D	There is positive evidence of human fetal risk based on adverse reaction data from investigational or marketing experience or studies in humans, but potential benefits may warrant use of the drug in pregnant women despite potential risks.
Pregnancy Category X	Studies in animals or humans have demonstrated fetal abnormalities and/or there is positive evidence of human fetal risk based on adverse reaction data from investigational or marketing experience, and the risks involved in use of the drug in pregnant women clearly outweigh potential benefits.

Table 2. United States FDA pharmaceutical pregnancy categories

The bulk of evidence relates to use of parenteral hydralazine or labetalol, and oral nifedipine, labetalol or methyldopa [Magee, 2011]. It is essential to keep the blood pressure in the normal range. Patients with new onset hypertension in pregnancy should be evaluated for PET. The medications that are best studied are methyldopa and labetalol. Methyldopa is the only antihypertensive agent for which there has been long-term follow-up of children exposed in utero [Antonio, 2011].

Angiotensin converting enzyme inhibitors and angiotensin receptor blockers should be avoided prior to conception as they are contraindicated and cannot be considered safe. And these drugs are also associated with higher incidence of fetopathy [Cooper, 2006].

2.1.2 Aspirin

Treatment with low doses of Aspirin during pregnancy would be indicated in women with SLE, APS, hypertension, history of preeclampsia, and renal disease. Aspirin can cross the placenta and can cause congenital anomalies in animals but these are rare in human beings. Several large prospective studies failed to confirm a significant increase in cleft palate or congenital anomalies [Jick, 1981]. Low dose of Aspirin is safe throughout pregnancy. Women who took Aspirin had a significantly lower risk of preterm delivery than those treated with placebo but there is no significant difference in perinatal mortality [Kozer, 2003].

A meta-analysis showed reduction in the risk of preeclampsia, preterm delivery before 34 weeks of gestation and serious adverse outcomes among women taking low-dose Aspirin or dipyridamole [Aski, 2007].

Aspirin has anti-prostaglandin effects and therefore it is better discontinued 8 weeks prior the expected delivery to avoid prolonged gestation and labour. This also reduces bleeding during delivery and bleeding complications in the fetus.

2.1.3 Non-steroidal anti-inflammatory drugs (NSAIDs)

The effect of NSAIDs use on the fetus depends upon the term of pregnancy. A number of cohort studies looking at the teratogenic risk of NSAIDs use during the first trimester have not found an increased risk of congenital malformation [Janssen, 2000]. However, due to the shared property of inhibition of prostaglandin synthesis, adverse effects such as constriction of the ductus arteriosus in utero, persistent pulmonary hypertension, renal dysfunction in the neonate, increased maternal blood loss, and prolongation of pregnancy & labour are possible when administered to pregnant patients. NSAID should be given in the lowest effective dose, and should be withdrawn before 8 weeks of expected date of delivery [Ostensen, 1994].

Prostaglandins (PGs) increase uterine contractions, enhance platelet aggregation and increase the fetal renal blood flow. Therefore, NSAIDs by inhibiting the PG synthesis, may decrease the fetal urinary output. NSAIDs, by inhibiting cyclooxygenase, decrease the PG synthesis.

If NSAID is clinically indicated in the first or second trimester, Ibuprofen would be the preferred one.

NSAIDs can potentially inhibit contractions and thereby prolong gestation. Because of the later effect, indomethacin, a potent NSAID, has been used in the treatment of premature labour. NSAID inhibition of fetal urinary output may cause oligohydramnios and this is reversible once the NSAID is stopped. Inhibition of prostaglandin synthesis by NSAID may also result in constriction of the ductus arteriosus which can cause fetal pulmonary hypertension. In the studies with indomethacin, these effects were first noticed in the 27th week of gestation but most marked in the 32nd week of gestation [Janssen, 2000; En Hams, 2002].

2.1.4 Anti-malarial drugs

Hydroxychloroquine: "HCQ" is the commonest anti-malarial drug used in SLE. It has been used in pregnancy for malarial prophylaxis with no teratogenic effects [Lewis, 1973].

HCQ main mechanism of action is through inhibition of antigen processing and inflammatory cytokine release [Fox, 1996]. These drugs are highly effective for discoid lupus erythematosus (DLE) cutaneous lesions. HCQ improves photosensitive skin lesions and prevents lupus flares [Gladman, 1998]. Studies have shown that HCQ can prevent renal and central nervous system lupus. It also exhibits the role of a prophylactic agent against some of the major morbidities of SLE and its treatment, namely hyperlipidemia, diabetes mellitus and thrombosis [Mpetvi, 1996].

As it has a long half life of eight weeks and accumulates in the body, discontinuation of drug immediately after conception does not prevent the exposure of fetus to the drug. A systemic review of hydroxychloroquin use in pregnant patients with auto-immune diseases from 1980 to 2007 showed that HCQ is not associated with any increased risk of congenital defects, spontaneous abortions, fetal death, prematurity or decreased number of live births in patients with auto-immune disease [Sperber, 2009].

RA Levy et al observation in prospective randomized placebo controlled study revealed that HCQ can be used safely in pregnancy with additional benefits on the disease activity.

The neonatal results (Apgar score, weight and gestation age) were significantly better in the HCQ group with absence of teratogenic effects after 3 years of follow-up in children [Levy, 2001].
HCQ is often needed to manage hyperactivity of the disease, as it appears to be safe and decreases lupus activity during pregnancy.

2.1.5 Corticosteroids

It is relatively safe to use during pregnancy but we should pay attention to maternal hypertension, gestational diabetes, infection, weight gain, acne and proximal muscle weakness. Therefore close monitoring with the use of the lowest possible dose of corticosteroid needed to control disease flare along with vitamin D and calcium supplements. Although animal studies have suggested an increased risk of oral clefts associated with glucocorticoid, several human studies have failed to demonstrate either teratogenic or toxic effects [Raybum, 1992].
Corticosteroids (Prednisalone, Prednisone, and Methylprednisolone) are metabolized by placenta II-beta-hydroxy steroid dehydrogenase (II-beta-HSD) which converts active cortisone to inactive cortisone. Therefore, fetal blood levels are approximately 10% of the mother's level [69], while fluorinated corticosteroids (dexamethasone and betamethasone) do cross the placenta in an un-metabolized form. Therefore, neonates should be monitored for evidence of adrenal insufficiency.
If our concern is to treat the mother, the most suitable corticosteroid is prednisalone, prednisone or methylprednisolone. But if our concern is to treat the fetus, then it is either dexamethasone or betamethasone, which is not inactivated by placental 11-beta hydroxysteroid dehydrogenase and are best suited for fetal treatment as they clearly reduce the risk of death and respiratory distress syndrome in the preterm infants [NICHHD, 1994].
It is currently recommended that obstetricians give only a single course of antenatal corticosteroids to pregnant women to enhance lung maturity instead of giving repeated doses as weekly courses of antenatal corticosteroid which did not reduce composite neonatal morbidity compared with a single course of treatment. Weekly courses of antenatal corticosteroids should not be routinely prescribed for women at risk of preterm delivery [Guinn, 2001].
Separate meta-analysis of the data in the Cochrane review showed that betamethasone and not dexamethasone reduces neonatal morbidity [Crowley, 2000] as betamethasone may offer better long-term neuro developmental outcome for the fetus [Lee BH, 2008].
In patients with chronic corticosteroid treatment during pregnancy, "stress doses" of hydrocortisone are recommended for prolonged labor, delivery, caesarian section, or any emergency surgery.

2.1.6 Immunosuppressive agents

Cyclophosphamide

Fetal survival is strongly in doubt when cyclophosphamide is required to treat lupus during pregnancy. The high risk for loss of the fetus should be discussed with the patient prior to administration of cyclophosphamide [Clowse MEB, 2005]. Patients undergoing therapy with cyclophosphamide must avoid pregnancy during therapy, especially in the first trimester. Attempts of conception should be delayed until three months after cessation of therapy.

It is a teratogenic drug and should only be used after the first trimester unless the mother's life is threatened [Briggs, 2005]. To avoid fetal loss and malformations from inadvertent first trimester exposure during cyclophosphamide therapy, strict adherence to birth control measures, as well as a pregnancy test prior to pulse therapy should be the routine practice [Clowse MEB, 2005].

In patients with life-threatening disease, the use of cyclophosphamide may be considered after the first trimester.

Azathioprine (AZA)

It is a purine analogue which interferes with the synthesis of nucleic acid. Although azathioprine crosses the placenta, only minimal amount reaches the fetal blood. Azathioprine metabolites 6-thioguanine nucleotide (6-TGN) was slightly lower in the RBC of the infant than the mother, while other azathioprine metabolite 6-methylmercaptopurine (6-MMP) could not be detected in the infant which means the placenta forms a (relative) barrier to AZA and its metabolites [Da Boer, 2006].

Methotrexate (MTX)

It is contraindicated in pregnancy (FDA risk category x) because of severe adverse effects on both the fetus and the course of the pregnancy [Janssen, 2000]. Plan for conception should be taken after three months of methotrexate withdrawal as the active metabolites remain in the body for approximately two months after its discontinuation. MXT acts as a folate antagonist and therefore leads to folate depletion during MTX treatment. Hence folate supplementation should be continued throughout pregnancy.

Mycophenolate mofetil (MMF)

It is mainly used in renal lupus, and there are very few data concerning its use. It is advisable to switch to azathioprine before conception.MMF currently used as a maintenance therapy for lupus nephritis, and also used for resistant skin lupus, lupus disease activity and hematological manifestations [Karim, 2002].

Based on toxicity shown in animal studies, patients should not become pregnant while taking MMF. Women taking MMF who wish to become pregnant should discontinue the drug at least 6 weeks prior to conception.

Cyclosporine (CSA)

Cyclosporine is an immunosuppressant that was first used for pregnant transplant rejection. CSA does not appear to be a major human teratogen. It may be associated with increased rate of prematurity [Bar, 2001].

2.1.7 Biologic agents

Anti-tumor necrosis factor alpha (Anti-TNFα)

Maternal immunoglobulin (IgG) concentrations in fetal blood increase from early second trimester through term as maternal antibodies transported across the placenta to protect the new born. Most antibodies are acquired during the third trimester. The three commercially available TNF-α inhibitors (infliximab, etanercept, adalimumab) constructed based on IgG, so that these can cross the placenta to the fetus in the first trimester and more efficiently during the second and third trimesters.

Anti-TNFα medications have led to improvements in the treatment of inflammatory conditions. The safety of these drugs during pregnancy is an important issue. Prospectively collected data appear to be reassuring. However, an analysis of the FDA-reported anomalies has raised some questions. It appears that significant levels of these drugs cross the placenta as the pregnancy nears term, but very little passes into the breast milk. Prior to usage of these medications during pregnancy, their risks and benefits, other treatment options, and the ongoing inflammatory conditions, all must be carefully weighed by both doctor and patient [Clowse, 2010].

The FDA classified these biological agents as pregnancy risk category B, which means that no adverse pregnancy effect have been observed in animals studies but there have been insufficient controlled human studies. The published experience with anti-TNF during pregnancy consists of a limited number of case reports, series, and ongoing registry data.

Many patients have experienced successful pregnancies following TNF exposure. Patients with unplanned pregnancies exposed to TNF inhibitors either before or after conception does not require termination of pregnancy unless additional maternal-fetal assessments suggest untoward or dangerous effects. While most of the existing data on TNF inhibitors use in pregnancy have been generated during conception and the first trimester of pregnancy, there is limited and inadequate information regarding their use throughout pregnancy or during breast feeding [Ali, 2010]. At present the use of biological agents cannot be recommended throughout pregnancy [Sorensen, 2011]. Therefore, it is better to stop anti-TNF once the pregnancy test is positive.

Rituximab

It is a chimeric anti-CD_{20} monoclonal β-cell depleting antibody. One should continue to counsel the women to avoid pregnancy for up to 12 months after rituximab exposure [Chakra Varty, 2011]. Therefore, it must be withdrawn before a planned pregnancy. Experience with rituximab during pregnancy is too limited to allow any statement on safety in pregnancy. When administered in the second and third trimester, β-cell depletion occurs in the fetus. Long-term studies on β-cell and immune function of children exposed in utero are lacking [Ostensen, 2008]. Rituximab is potentially unsafe because of reversible fetal cytopenias including β-cell depletion have occurred in infants of mothers who are given this drug during pregnancy [Doria, 2008].

2.1.8 Other therapeutic measures

Intravenous Immunoglobulin (IVIG)

During pregnancy, intravenous Immunoglobulin (IVIG) may be used if needed to control severe maternal lupus activity. It does not appear to cause any fetal abnormalities. This drug has been used for many years without any adverse effects [Bonnie, 1995]. In a study comparing twelve SLE-suffered pregnant patients from recurrent spontaneous abortion (RSA) treated with a high dose of IVIG as against twelve SLE-RSA pregnant patients treated with prednisalone and NSAIDs showed a beneficial clinical response following IVIG treatment in all patients, and the antibodies and complement levels also tended to normalize in most of the patients. So IVIG is considered safe and effective [Perricone, 2008].

Plasmapheresis (PP)

It is safe, expensive, labor-intensive procedure. Its absolute indications include hyper viscosity, cryoglobulinemia, pulmonary hemorrhage and TTP. PP may be useful in cyclophosphamide resistant and serious organ–threatening disease [Erickson, 1994;

Wallance, 2001]. It is safe in children and pregnant females [Wallance, 2001]. Removal of anticardiolipin antibodies or Lupus anticoagulant by plasmapheresis during pregnancy or its use in those with recurrent thromboembolic episodes has been the subject of numerous case reports but no prospective studies have been done. However, it is believed that plasmapheresis during pregnancy definitely removes anticardiolipin antibodies. [Koblayash, 1992].

Aphaeresis is well tolerated among pregnant patients, and has been used to remove antiphspholipid antibodies and Anti-Ro (SSA). It has been suggested that weekly Plasmapheresis can decrease anti-52 kD reactivity and might prevent heart block if it is initiated in the first trimester [Vonderleij, 1994].

2.2 Delivery

Systemic lupus erythematosus is not an indication for delivery by cesarean section; although high rates of preeclampsia and cesarean section in connective tissue disease pregnancies were documented in a population based study they mainly emphasized on the importance of monitoring and obstetrical interventions [John Fredrick, 2000].

A team approach guarantees to the pregnant women with SLE, a safe vaginal delivery and allows performing a cesarean section for obstetric indications only.

In a study of 555 lupus pregnancies, cesarean sections were needed in 38.2% of these patients versus 19.7% of controls [Yasmeen, 2001] .The major indications for cesarean section are fetal distress and maternal preeclampsia. One should remember that, general anaesthesia in a pregnant women has a mortality rates of 16.7% which is much greater than that of epidural or subarachnoid anesthesia [Hawkins, 1997]. It is ideal that the obstetrician, the anesthesiologist and the rheumatologist should evaluate the condition of the mother and the fetus and plan the type of delivery accordingly.

Generally , in the case of vaginal delivery the anesthesiologist can guarantee an epidural analgesia with no greater risks than those of a healthy parturient. In the event of cesarean section we can usually administer a neuro-axial anesthesia as the preferred type of anesthesia reserving the general anesthesia only to obstetrical emergencies [Rawetz, 2004]. The indications for cesarean section include maternal causes such as avascular necrosis of the hips with inadequate hip abduction, placental abruption or fetal causes such as fetal distress, prolapsed umbilical cord, abnormal non- stress test, cephalo-pelvic disproportion and transverse presentation. Delivery should be in a hospital which has neonatal intensive care unit. Pregnant women with lupus treated with systemic steroid within two years of the anticipated delivery should receive steroid stress coverage during delivery.

2.3 Puerpurium

The optimum management is not over with the birth of a healthy baby. In fact, postpartum period should be considered as a high risk for pregnant lupus patients with several possible complications ahead. First, the mother can suffer a lupus flare, since several studies have confirmed the postpartum period is particularly high risk for increased lupus activity. A close surveillance in the first four weeks after delivery is thus warranted, especially in women with recent activity or with a previous history of severe disease. However no specific prophylactic therapy, such as increasing the dose of steroid, is recommended.

The puerpurium has also high risk for thromboembolic complications. This is especially true in women with APS, in whom adequate thrombo-prophylaxis with low molecular weight heparin (LMWH) should be extended 4-6 weeks after delivery. Those with previous history of thrombosis can be back on their usual full anticoagulant therapy within first 2-3 days postpartum. It should be remembered that both warfarin and heparin are safe during lactation [Guillermo Ruiz-Irastorza et al, 2009].

2.4 Lactation

The increasing prevalence of breast feeding along with the increased frequency of pregnancies in females with chronic medical conditions have increased the number of patients who face possible harmful effects on the newborn of medication excreted in breast milk. Generally, drugs known to be extensively protein bound are excreted in breast milk to a lesser extent than drugs that are poorly bound to plasma proteins.

Factors related to breast milk
Milk composition (lipid and protein concentrations)
Factors related to the mother
Renal and hepatic excretion Dose and duration of treatment Route of administration
Factors related to the infant
Age Drug Absorption Renal and hepatic excretion Volume of milk intake Safety of the drug for the infant
Factors related to the drug
Solubility in water and lipid Molecular size Oral bioavailability Toxicity Suppressive effect on milk production Long-acting drug x short-acting drug

Table 3. Factors that determine the safety of the drugs used during breastfeeding. (Adapted from Howard & Lawrence, 1999.)

There are multiple factors that determine the concentration of the drug in breast milk which include maternal, infant, and drug-related factors [Bowes, 1980] as shown in the table (Table 3). It is recommended to take the medication immediately after breastfeeding the baby, to ensure least possible concentration of the drug in breast milk. Safety of medication is very important during lactation.

2.4.1 Aspirin

Nursing mothers should avoid large doses of Aspirin. The American Academy of Pediatrics recommends that Aspirin be used cautiously by the mother of the nursing infant and large doses of it should be avoided [Pediatrics, 1994].

2.4.2 Non-Steroidal Anti-Inflammatory Drugs (NSAIDs)

The American Academy of Pediatrics considers Ibuprofen, Indomethacin, and Naproxen to be compatible with breastfeeding [Pediatrics, 1994], although most NSAIDs do not achieve high concentrations in breast milk [Ostensen, 1996]. Ibuprofen presents extremely low level in breast milk and has very short half-life; therefore it is considered to be a reasonable choice as an analgesic in the lactating women.

2.4.3 Hydroxychloroquin (HCQ)

The amount of HCQ received by children through lactation seems to be very low. HCQ should probably be maintained throughout pregnancy in patients with SLE as it is also safe in breastfeeding [Cosedoat, 2005]. The American Academy of Pediatrics classifies the drug as compatible with breastfeeding. Excretion into breast milk was very low (0.2mg/kg/day) and this level is not thought to be toxic [Costedoat, 2002]. Drug levels in milk reached a peak 2 hours after ingestion of hydroxychloroquine and declined after 9 hours. It was estimated that a nursing child would ingest between 0.06-0.2mg/kg/day or approximately 2% of the mother's weight-adjusted dose [Notionn, 1984; Ostensen, 1985]. Routine eye exams of breastfed children are not indicated as the follow-up studies of exposed children are re-assuring [Costedoat, 2002].

2.4.4 Corticosteroids

Corticosteroids do not enter breast milk in large quantities. The American Academy of Pediatrics has declared prednisone and prednisalone as safe and compatible with breastfeeding. Infant exposure to prednisalone through breast milk can be minimized by dosing prednisalone at infrequent intervals and avoiding nursing for at least 4 hours following a dose [Alan Kamada, 1994] as peak milk steroid levels occurred approximately 2 hours after a dose of prednisalone. No data are available on the use of dexamethasone or betamethasone in lactating women.

2.4.5 Cyclophosphamide

Lactation is contraindicated during cyclophosphamide use as it is found in substantial concentrations in human breast milk [Wiernik, 1971]. Patient with life-threatening condition, who received cyclophosphamide during second or third trimester, their offspring should be monitored for immunosuppression and the development of secondary malignancies.

2.4.6 Azathioprine (AZA)

Nursing is not recommended in patients on AZA, because of the long-term potential of immunosuppression and carcinogenesis [Pediatrics, 1994], although, there were no reports to confirm this. A report on a series of 4 patients treated with azathioprine while lactating, the breast milk samples were analyzed for 6-mercaptopurine (6-MP) in 2 of the mothers. Levels of 6-MP were undetectable. Therefore, relative infant dose would have been less than 0.09% of the maternal weight-adjusted dose. No adverse effects were encountered in any of the 4 infants. So, maternal azathioprine use during lactation does not appear to pose a significant immediate clinical risk to the suckling infant. Continued monitoring and long-term assessment of these infants are warranted [Moretti, 2006].

2.4.7 Methotrexate

The American Academy of Pediatrics considers methotrexate to be contraindicated during breastfeeding because of several patient problems, which include immunosuppression, neutropenia, adverse effects on growth, and carcinogenesis [Pediatrics, 1994]. So, breastfeeding during methotrexate treatment is not recommended.

2.4.8 Cyclosporine

The American Academy of Pediatrics considers cyclosporine to be contraindicated during lactation because of the potential long-term effects of immune-suppression, neutropenia, and a potential association with carcinogenesis [Pediatrics, 1994]. Breastfeeding should be discouraged in women using cyclosporine [Flecher, 1995].

2.4.9 Mycophenolate Mofetil (MMF)

There is no enough data regarding the excretion of MMF into breast milk. Lactation is not recommended while using MMF [EGRT, 2002].

2.4.10 Sulfasalazine

This is compatible with nursing. In eight mothers who were breastfeeding and taking sulfasalazine, analyses were done from mothers' serum, breast milk and serum from their children. The results showed that the amount of sulfasalazine and sulfa pyridine transferred to the child in the breast milk is negligible with regards to the risk of kernicterus [Eshjorner, 1987].

2.4.11 Tumor necrosis Factor α inhibitors (Anti-TNFα)

At present it is not known whether TNFα inhibitors are secreted into breast milk and can be ingested by mothers with breastfed child. Mothers who wish to breastfeed their children should be informed that there is insufficient knowledge to provide them with adequate information [Ostensen, 2008].

2.4.12 Rituximab

There is insufficient data to support breastfeeding in patients who are on Rituximab. So it is better to avoid Rituximab during lactation.

2.4.13 Intravenous Immunoglobulin (IVIG)

No data regarding IVIG excretion in breast milk. Therefore, we suggest avoiding breastfeeding while the patient is on IVIG.

2.5 Safety of contraception in SLE women

Premenopausal women with SLE should have access to safe and effective birth control measures. Women who have diminished fertility may seek hormonal manipulation to stimulate ovulation, and women receiving cyclophosphamide may need methods for preserving fertility. Furthermore, exogenous estrogen may be used not only to prevent glucocorticoid-induced osteoporosis but also to treat ovarian cysts, endometriosis, irregular menses, and menorrhagia.

The high rate of elective abortion among women with SLE may reflect the failure of the birth-control method used or the absence of an adequate birth-control program [Petri, 2005; Leona, 1981]. As the disease activity during pregnancy is generally high in women who conceive, pregnancy can be particularly risky in women with active disease or on teratogenic medications. So, pregnancy should be planned to begin during period of disease quiescence making contraception an important issue for these women. All women with rheumatologic disease have contraceptive options, including barrier methods, the intrauterine device (IUDs) and oral contraceptive pills (OCPs) [Wayslett, 1991; Clowse, 2010].

Progestin-only contraceptives are not widely used because of their effects on the endometrial bleeding pattern [Mintz, 1984]. Oral contraceptives (OCPs) remain one of the most effective forms of birth control [Lauterbach, 2000]. The Safety of Estrogens in Lupus Erythematosus National Assessment (SELENA) trial of oral contraceptives versus placebo was a prospective, randomized, double blind trial that examined the effects of oral contraceptives (containing 35mg ethinyl estradiol) i.e. low estrogen dose on disease activity in 183 premenopausal women with SLE. This concluded with only 7 severe flares occurring in 91 patients receiving oral contraceptives, the same number which was recorded for the 92 women receiving placebo. To the surprise of most physicians, OCP was equivalent to placebo in terms of severe flares. So, the available data support the use of OCPs containing estrogen as birth control choice for patients with inactive or stable SLE who are at low risk of thrombosis [Petri, 2005].

The SELENA trial does not pertain to women with very active SLE, such as active lupus nephritis, or those with the lupus anticoagulant or with high titer anticardiolipin, which were excluded. OCPs cannot be prescribed to all SLE women, but when appropriate, may demonstrably improve the quality of life [Petri, 2008]. Given the high prevalence of antiphospholipid antibodies in SLE, it seems prudent not to prescribe OCPs to women with lupus anticoagulant or medium-to-high titer anticardiolipin or anti-β_2 glycoprotein [Petri, 2001]. Despite a lack of randomized studies, evidence strongly suggests that the elevated risk of thrombosis makes estrogen-containing contraceptives unsuitable for patients with APS, prior thromboembolic episodes, and severe migraine. Decisions should be individualized according to the patients' medical status, personal preference and stage of reproductive life [Sammaritano, 2007; Ashorson, 1986].

Another study evaluating the safety of OCP was conducted as a randomized, single-blinded 12-month clinical trial in women with SLE to evaluate the effects on disease activity of combined oral contraceptives, as compared to progestin-only pill and IUD. Disease activity remained mild and stable in all groups throughout the study. There were no significant differences among the groups during the trial in disease activity, incidence or probability of flares on medication use. Thromboses occurred in four patients (two in each of the two groups receiving hormones) [Sanchez, 2005].

The risk of infection associated with IUD insertion is too small to warrant routine use of prophylactic antibiotics. Recently, FDA removed immunosuppression from list of contraindications to IUD use. The use of combined oral contraceptives is possible in stable premenopausal SLE, and who do not have any evidence of APS. Lupus patients who are APL positive or have APS should be treated with progestogens only pills (oral or Parenteral) or IUD.

2.6 Assisted reproductive therapy (ART)

Young lupus patient exposed to I.V. cyclophosphamide face the risk of premature ovarian failure. In vitro fertilization (IVF) and its associated technologies are used for infertility in patients with a wide range of etiologies, including those with SLE, and/or APS.

The first phase of ART is ovulation induction followed by in vitro fertilization (IVF) and embryo transfer (ET) in the uterus. The most threatening conditions in affected women undergoing ovarian stimulation are lupus flares and thrombosis, with the latter being especially associated with the occurrence of an overt ovarian hyper-stimulation syndrome (OHSS).

SLE manifestations in acute flares, badly controlled arterial hypertension, pulmonary hypertension, advanced renal disease, severe valvulopathy or heart disease, and major previous thrombotic events are situations in which to ARTs are to be discouraged. It is especially due to the high risk of complications in both mother and fetus during pregnancy and puerpurium. Therefore, ovarian stimulation for ovulation induction and IVF seems to be safe and successful in well-selected women with SLE and APS [Beliver, 2009].

The ovulation induction therapy (OIT) may precipitate SLE activity or APS. A careful review of the patient's history and appropriate laboratory tests should be undertaken before OIT. Clomiphene adverse effects are rare. When gonadotropins are prescribed, preventive anti-inflammatory therapy should be considered in women with SLE, in addition to heparin and/ or anti-aggregate therapy in patients with asymptomatic antiphospholipid antibodies or prior thrombotic events [Huong, 2002].

3. Pre-pregnancy counseling

Couples with SLE with or without recurrent pregnancy loss require empathy and understanding as early pregnancy loss is an emotionally traumatic experience, similar to that associated with still birth. As many patients with SLE are young women in reproductive age and some being young men, wanted to have healthy children they need to be reassured that if they follow the expert doctor's advice with careful follow-up during pregnancy, they could still have normal children. Therefore, one needs to stress the importance of preconception counseling (Table 4).

3.1 Fertility

The vast majority of patients have no problems with fertility. However occasionally some female patients may develop antibodies to ovarian tissue that interfere with development of ovum, others may have disrupted ovarian cycles which need further investigations. Infertility could be a problem in patients on long-term cyclophosphamide (more than 6 months) and its use can also cause congenital abnormalities. Therefore while the patients are on cyclophosphamide they need to be told to use reliable methods of contraception for the total duration on this drug and three months thereafter [Handa, 2006].

Preconception counseling
Assess for risk factors Stratify high/low risk Give realistic, evidence-based estimates for likely success and chance of problems Discuss prematurity and handicap Advise against pregnancy if appropriate Make and agree prospective plan of care

Table 4. Preconception Counseling (Ruiz, 2008)

For pregnancies with lupus, the risk of abortion, hypertension, and embryo deformity by a therapeutic agent is higher compared to healthy pregnancies. Lupus flares can occur at any time during pregnancy, as well as several months after delivery [Clowse, 2007]. Fortunately, the majority of gravidae do not have severe SLE activity but only mild flares mainly involving skin, joints, or constitutional symptoms [Izmirly, 2010].

Not all women with SLE have the same risk of complications during pregnancy. Thus, pre-pregnancy counseling is essential to estimate the chance of both fetal and maternal mortality and morbidity (Table 4).

To reduce the risk of pregnancy it is better to have a planned pregnancy. Therefore Pregnancy is usually undertaken when

- The disease has been in remission for at least 6 months
- Who require less than equivalent of 7.5 mg of prednisone per day
- No previous renal disease, hypertension, thrombocytopenia or anti-phospholipid antibodies

High-risk patients are shown in Table 5.

An obstetrician experienced in management of high risk pregnancies is particularly desirable for women with one of these features for a better outcome of pregnancy. A previous complicated pregnancy is, by itself, an important adverse prognostic variable. Likewise, the presence of APS is closely associated with maternal thrombosis and embryo-fetal demise. Maternal anti-Ro and anti-La antibodies may cause congenital heart block in 2% of babies.

This is fortunately a rare, but very serious condition, with a high mortality rate with or without cardiomyopathy and a high chance of permanent pacemaker for majority of children with CHB [Clowse, 2007). Defining a high risk pregnancy is not absolute as it differs from patient to patient due to the presence of other confounding factors.

The testing for Anti-SSA/SSB/ U1RNP antibodies are done only in high risk population like Women with SLE, Sjogren's syndrome, Undifferentiated connective tissue disease or other connective tissue diseases, since they comprise 50-60% of NLE mothers. It is also done in mothers with previous child having neonatal lupus as the risk of neonatal lupus in next pregnancy reaches up to 25%.

Management of a case of APS is shown in the flow chart (figure 1).

Chronic renal failure is also associated with other obstetric complications, such as hypertensive disorders and miscarriage, which are more likely to occur if renal impairment is more severe. Restrictive pulmonary disease may also worsen during pregnancy due to the thoracic compression by the growing uterus. Secondary APS is the main predictor of pregnancy complication in the form of miscarriage, fetal death, prematurity and preeclampsia. The disease activity has shown a clear association with fetal loss and prematurity and the lupus anticoagulant confers the highest risk of miscarriages among the antibodies of APS [Handa, 2006].

High Risk Lupus Pregnancy
Previous poor obstetric history
Renal involvement
Cardiac involvement
Pulmonary hypertension
Interstitial lung disease
Active disease
High-dose steroid therapy
Other immune-suppressive therapy (cyclophosphamide, Methotrexate, etc)
Antiphospholipid antibodies/syndrome
Extractable nuclear antigens (Ro, La)
Multiple pregnancy

Table 5. High Risk Lupus Pregnancy (Ruiz, 2008)

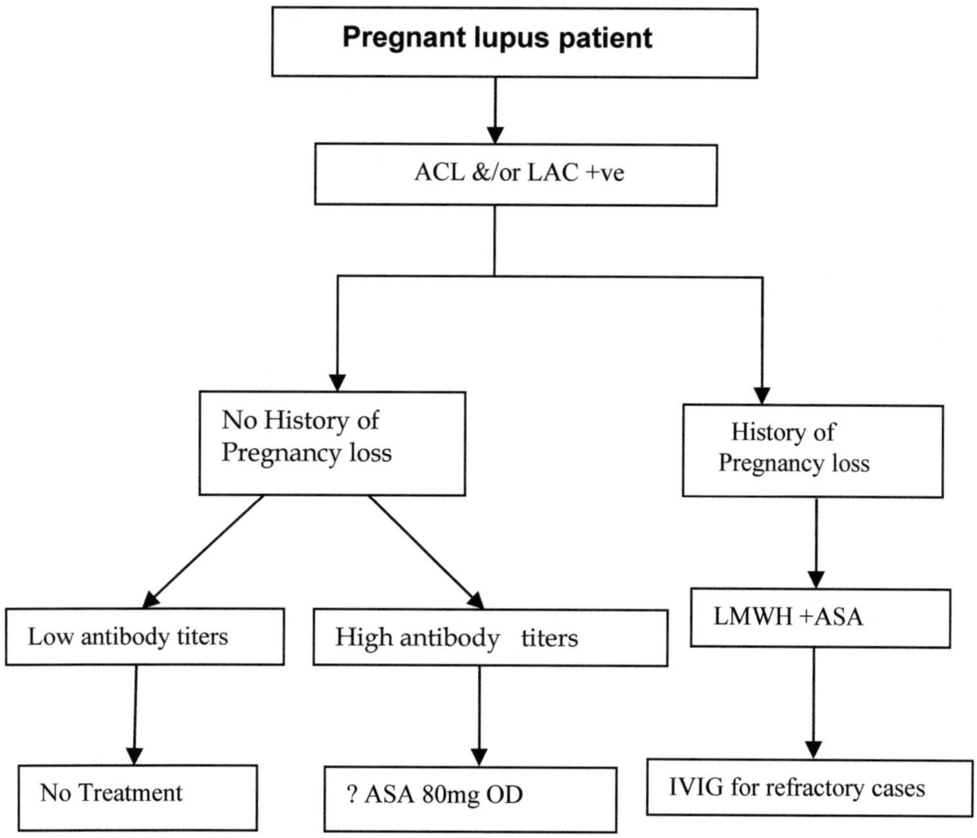

ACL=anti-cardiolipin antibody; LAC=lupus anticoagulant

Fig. 1. Flow Chart For Management Of APS Pregnant Patient (R. Handa, 2006)

Contraindications to Pregnancy in SLE (high maternal & fetal risk)
Severe pulmonary hypertension (PAP >50 mm Hg or symptomatic)
Restrictive lung disease (FVC <1 L)
Heart failure
Chronic renal impairment with Cr >250 μmols/L
H/O severe PET or HELLP (despite ASA/LMWH)
Stroke in <6 months
Severe lupus flare in<6 months
H/O arterial thrombosis or PE

Table 6. Contraindications to pregnancy in SLE (Ruiz, 2008)

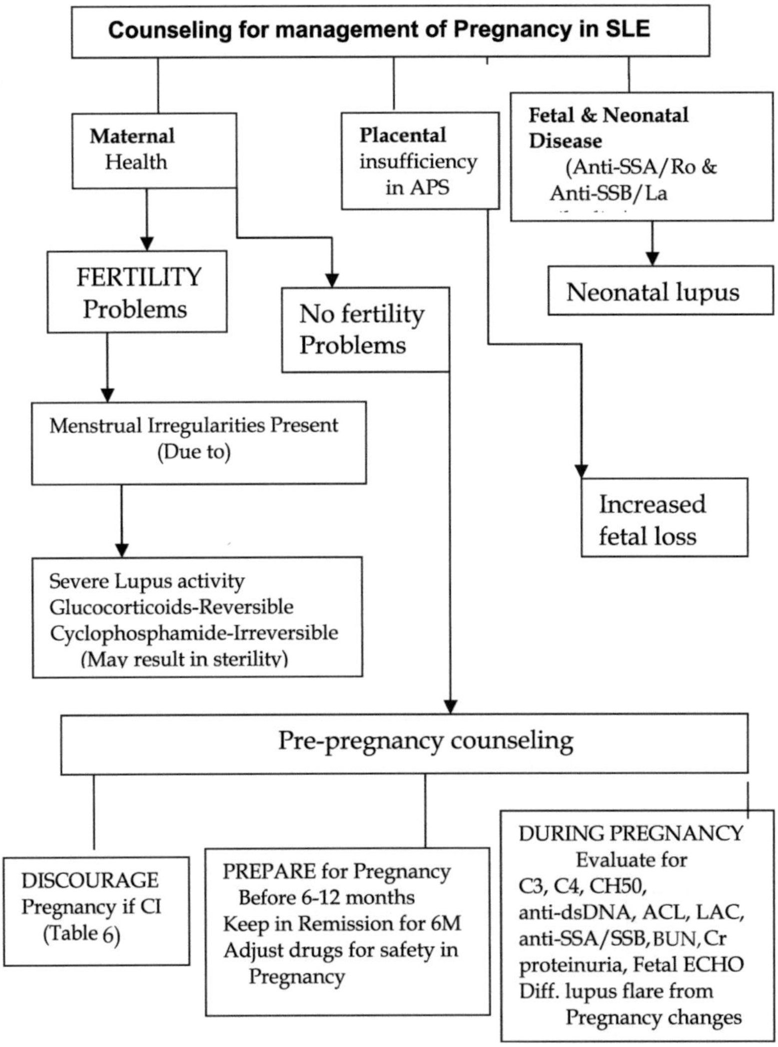

Fig. 2. Flow chart for counseling and management of pregnancy in SLE

In some extreme situations, the physicians should advise against pregnancy (Table 6). Women with current or recent lupus activity, particularly if affecting internal organs, should avoid pregnancy. The same recommendation applies to women with APS and recent thrombosis, particularly in the arterial bed. Women with severe kidney, lung or heart disease should also be discouraged from getting pregnant due to the high risk of maternal complications. Likewise, pregnancy should be considered an absolute contraindication in women with symptomatic severe pulmonary hypertension, which carries a higher than 30% maternal mortality during late pregnancy and the puerpurium.

In patients having a serum creatinine over 250 μmols/L the chance of having a successful pregnancy is <30%. Despite aggressive treatment of secondary anti-phospholipid antibody syndrome the risk of thrombo-embolism and fetal death is still high.

A major reason for discrepant results is in the definition of a lupus flare during pregnancy.

In applying the Systemic Lupus Activity Measure (SLAM) to the pregnant lupus patient, fatigue, alopecia, decreased hematocrit, and increase ESR may not represent lupus activity.

Suggestions for "valid" criteria attributable to a flare are characteristic dermatologic involvement, arthritis, hematuria, fever not secondary to infection, lymphadenopathy, leukopenia, alternative-pathway hypocomplementemia, and rising titers of antibodies to DNA. The patients with least risk in pregnancy are the patients who are in remission on < 7.5 mg of prednesalone per day, normal renal functions, no proteinuria, normal blood counts, normal BP, normal levels of complement levels and no detectable dsDNA.

The patients with moderate risk but still can be allowed to continue pregnancy with caution are-

- Patients with mild flare with arthritis, mild pleuro-pericarditis, recalcitrant skin lesions, requiring 10-15 mg of prednisalone daily for continued symptoms.
- Asymptomatic patients who have persistently elevated dsDNA and low levels of complement.

Because SLE is a progressive disease and is not curable we should not stop the couples from going for children as delaying may cause them not to have children at all. Hence, to have children earlier is better than later. Therefore one should weigh the risks and benefits and involve the patients fully in decision making.

Even platelets of 30,000-60,000, mild renal insufficiency (Cr=<200 μmols/L), proteinuria 1-2gm/day may have greater risk of flare and fetal demise but still may have successful pregnancy. Therefore such woman needs to be counseled about high likelihood of premature delivery, preeclampsia and potential need for early hospitalization for delivery [Buyon, 2004].

The minimum diagnostic work up of the couples with SLE before preconception counseling includes, detail history taking including medical, surgical, genetic, obstetrical and family history as well as thorough physical examination. Complete antibody profile needs to be done [Anti-SSA/Ro, anti-SSB/La, anti-U1 RNP antibodies, ANA, dsDNA, etc]. Anti-cardiolipin (ACL, both IgG & IgM), lupus anticoagulant (LA) are to be checked twice 6-8 weeks apart to exclude false positive results. Anti-dsDNA and complement levels to be checked every trimester, to assess the activity of the disease, along with it test for 24 hr urinary protein and serum albumin [Clowse, 2007].

Patients who are positive to anti-SSA/SSB/U1RNP needs to follow the flow chart [figure 3] for diagnosis and management of CHB which is the common presentation and has the highest mortality and morbidity in neonatal lupus [Buyon, 2004].

Screen for hypothyroidism as there is increased risk of miscarriage in subclinical hypothyroidism and incidence of hypothyroidism is found to be higher in SLE from recent studies. Test for diabetes mellitus and hyperprolactinemia and treat if present. If disease activity is present before pregnancy, the treatment needs to be started and patient should be free from disease activity at least for 6 months prior to pregnancy.

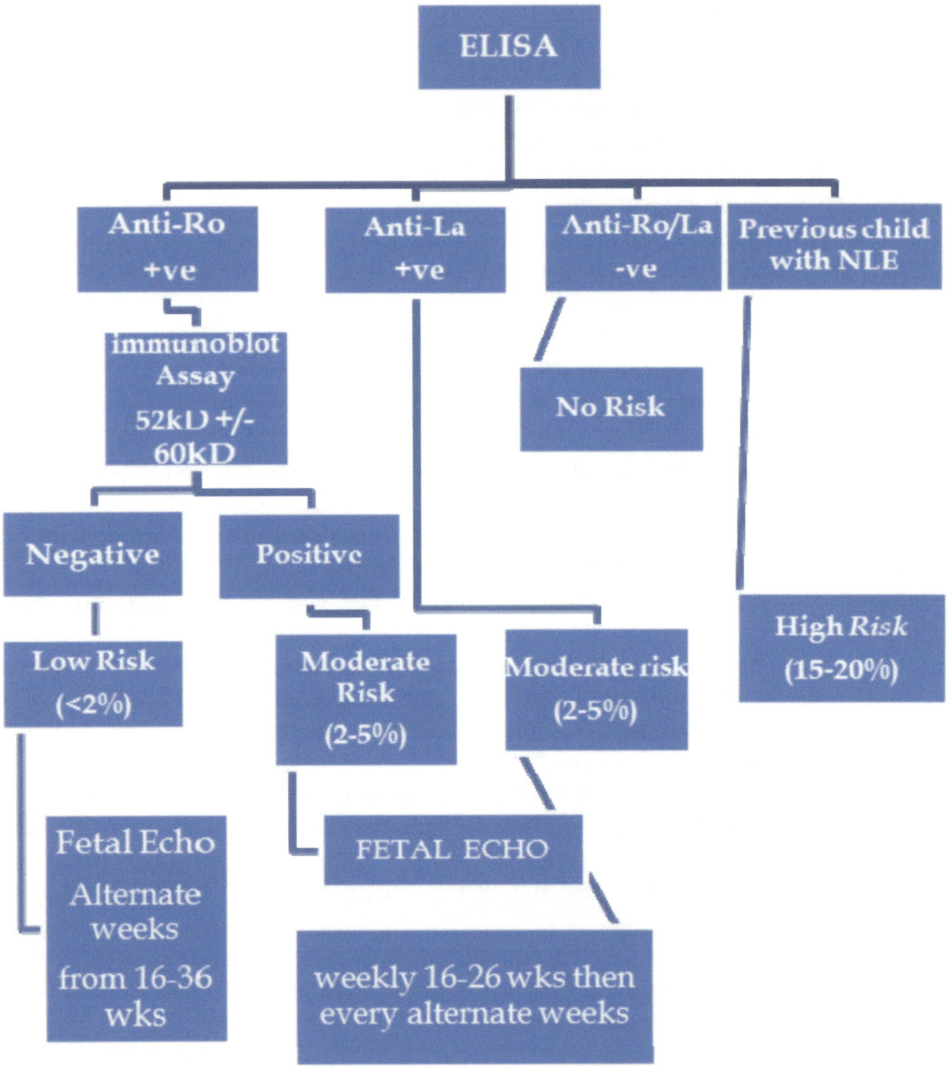

Fig. 3. Decision tree for diagnosis & management of CHB

High risk pregnancy needs a multi-disciplinary approach involving expert rheumatologist, experienced obstetrician skilled in managing high risk pregnancies, nephrologist, and neonatologist. Treatment of APS with aspirin or heparin as indicated before, during and after pregnancy.

The independent Risk Factors for pregnancy loss are Lupus activity in any trimester (but more in the first trimester), proteinuria, thrombocytopenia, hypertension in first trimester, APS and renal impairment, while the independent risk factors for pre-term delivery are increased lupus activity (before & during delivery), dose of prednisalone >7.5mg/day and hypertension [Ruiz, 2008).

Finally patients with severe active disease, high degree of end organ damage such as severe PAH, CHF, severe restrictive pulmonary disease, severe chronic renal failure are advised against becoming pregnant as they are absolute contraindications.

A significant rise in proteinuria and active sediment with or without falling complement values and rising DNA antibodies is justified to initiation the equivalent of 1 mg/kg per day of prednisalone. Moreover, the presence of proteinuria itself, even in the absence of active sediment, may warrant a trial of steroids. Persistent proteinuria > 3 grams/24 hr does not generally predict a good outcome for the mother or fetus.

In the absence of any response within two weeks, a reassessment of the situation is warranted with consideration given to the addition of cytotoxic agents and early termination, especially in the setting of deteriorating renal function and an active urinary sediment.

All patients have to practice hygienic way of living: No smoking, no alcohol, no recreational drugs, less caffeine consumption (<250mg/day) and to take folic acid supplements (at least 400 mcg/ day). All the medications prescribed needs to be checked by her attending physician and approved [Ruiz, 2011; Izmirly, 2010)].

4. Conclusion

Better outcome occurs by careful planning, patient education, close monitoring and aggressive management. All the above is important for a successful pregnancy outcome. Appropriate preconception counseling on management plans and shared care with special obstetrical & peri-natal attention will reduce the maternal and fetal morbidity and mortality.

In pregnant lupus patients the medication has to be adjusted to the patient needs depending on the disease activity, prior obstetric history, presence or absence of APS, presence of anti-SSA/Ro, SSB/La antibodies and the course of present pregnancy. So the disease manifestations, the course of pregnancy and the medications together will decide the morbidity of the mother and the child [Isenberg, 2004].

5. Acknowledgment

The work to produce this chapter was supported by Alzaidi's Chair of research in rheumatic diseases- Umm Alqura University.

6. References

Alan Kamada. (1994). Therapeutic controversies in treatment. *Pediatrics*,94(2): 270.

Ali, et al. (2010). Can tumor necrosis factor inhibitors be safely used in pregnancy? *Journal of Rheumatology*, 37(1): 9-17.

Ashorson et al. (1986). Systemic erythematosus, antiphospholipid antibodies, chorea, and oral contraceptives. *Arthritis Rheum*, 29(12):1535-1536

Aski LM et al. (2007). On behalf of PARIS collaborative group-antiplatelet agents for prevention of preeclampsia: a meta-analysis of individual patient data. *Lancet,* 369:1971-1980

Bar OZ, Benjamin Z, Hackman. (2001). Pregnancy outcome after Cyclosporine therapy during pregnancy: a meta-analysis 1. *Transplantation,* 71(8):1051-1055.

Baxter JD. (2000). Advances in glucocorticoid therapy. *Adv. Intern Med,* 45: 317-49.

Beliver J, Pellicer A. (2009). Ovarian stimulation for ovulation induction and in vitro fertilization in patients with systemic lupus erythematosus and antiphospholipid syndrome. *Fertil Steril,* 92(6):1803-10

Benediktsen R, Calder et al. (1997). Placenta II-β-hydroxysteroid dehydrogenase: a key regulation of fetal glucocorticoid exposure. *Clinical Endocrinology,* 46(2): 161-166.

Bonnie L, Bermas MD. (1995, Dec). Effects of immunosuppressive drugs during pregnancy. Dec; 38(12): 1722-1732

Boumpas DT, Austin HA, Fessler et al. (1995). Systemic lupus erythematosus: emerging concept, part 2: dermatologic and joint disease, the antiphospholipid antibody syndrome, pregnancy and hormone, morbidity and mortality, and pathogenesis. *Ann Intern Med,* 123(1): 42-53.

Briggs GG, Freeman RK, Yaffe SJ. (2005). *Drugs in pregnancy and lactation.* 7th ed. Philadelphia (PA): Lippincott Williams & Wilkins. 136-139.

Buyon et al. (2004). Management of SLE during pregnancy: A decision tree. *Rheumatologia,* 20 (4), 197-99

Carmona F, Font J, Cervera R et al. (1999). Obstetrical outcome of pregnancy in patients with systemic Lupus erythematosus: a study of 60 cases. *Eur J Obstet Gynecol Reprod Biol,* 83:137-42..

Chakra Varty. (2011). Pregnancy outcomes after maternal exposure to rituximab. *Blood,* 17(5):1499-506Clowse ME et al. (2005). Cyclophosphamide for lupus during pregnancy. *Lupus,* 14(8): 593-7.

Clark Ca et al. (2003).Preterm deliveries in women with systemic lupus erythematosus. *J Rheumatol,* 30:2127-32.

(2005).Decrease in pregnancy loss rates in patients with systemic lupus erythematosus over a 40-year period. *J Rheumatol,* 32:1709-12.

Clowse ME et al. (2004). Complement and doublestranded DNA antibodies predict pregnancy outcomes in lupus patients. *Arthritis Rheum,* 50:S408.

(2005). The impact of increased lupus activity on obstetric outcomes. *Arthritis Rheum,* 52(2); 514-521.

(2007) Lupus activity in pregnancy. *Rheum Dis Clin North Am,* 33:237-52.

(2008). A national study of the complications of lupus in pregnancy. *Am J Obstet Gynecol,* 199:127.e1-6.

Costedoat-Chalumeau N, et al. (2005). Safety of hydroxychloroquine use in pregnant patients with connective tissue diseases. *Autoimmune Rev,* 4(2):111-5.

Committee on Drugs, American Academy of Pediatrics. (1994). The transfer of drugs and other chemicals into human milk. *Pediatrics,* 93: 137-150.

Cooper WO et al. (2006). Major congenital malformations after first trimester exposure to ACE inhibitors. *New English Journal of Medicine*, 354(23):2443-5

Crowley P. (2000). Prophylactic corticosteroids for pre-term delivery. *Cochrane Database Syst. Rev*, 2: CD 000065.

Da Boer NK, Jarbandhan SV, de Gra FP. (2006). Azathioprine use during pregnancy: unexpected intrauterine exposure to metabolites. *Amj Gastroenerology*, 101(6): 1390-2.

Doria A, Tincani and M.Lockshin. (2008). Challenges of lupus pregnancy. *Rheumatology (Oxford)*, March 47 Suppl.3.iii 9-12.

En Hams. (2002). Antirheumatic drugs in pregnancy. *Lupus*, 10(11): 683-689.

Erickson RW, et al. (1994). Treatment of hemorrhagic lupus pneumonitis with plasmaphresis. *Semin Arthritis Rheum*, 24: 114-123.

Eshjorner E, Jarnerot et al. (1987). Sulphasalazine and sulphapyridine serum levels in children to mothers treated with sulphasalazine during pregnancy and lactation. *Acta Paediatric Scand*, 76(1): 137

European best practice guidelines for review transplantation. (2002)

Section IV: long-term management of the transplant recipient. IV-IOS Pregnancy in renal transplant recipients. *Nephrol Dial Transplant*, 17 (Suppl. 4): 50-55.

Flecher SM, Katz AR, Rogers AJ. (1985). The presence of cyclosporine in body tissues and fluids during pregnancy. *American Kidney*, 5(1): 60-3.

Francis L. Pharmacotherapy of systemic lupus erythematosus. (2009). *Expert Opin Pharmacother*, 10(9): 148-94.

Fox R. (1996). Antimalarial drugs: possible mechanisms of action in autoimmune disease and prospects for drug development. *Lupus*, 5(supp.): S4-S10.

Gladman DD, Urowitz MB, Senecal JL, *et al.* (1998). Aspects of use of antimalarials in systemic lupus erythematosus. *Journal of Rheumatology*, 25(5): 983-985.

Guillermo Riuz-Irastorza et al. (2009). Managing lupus patients during pregnancy. Best practice & research, clinical rheumatology, 23:575-582

Guinn DA, Atkinson MW, Sullivan et al. Weekly courses of antenatal corticosteroids for women at risk of preterm delivery: a randomized controlled trial. *JAMA*, 286(13): 1581-7.

Hawkins, et al. (1997). Anesthesia-related death during obstetric delivery in the United States,1979-1990. *Anesthesiology*, 86: 277-284.

Horlocker TT, Bajwa ZH, Ashraf et al. (2002). Risk assessment of hemorrhagic complications associated with non-steroidal anti-inflammatory medications in ambulatory pain clinic patients undergoing epidural steroid injection. *Anesth Analg*, 95(6): 1691-7.

Howard CR, Lawrence RA. (1994). Drugs and breastfeeding. *Clinical Perinatology*, 26: 447-78.

Huong DL, et al. (2001). Pregnancy in the past or present lupus nephritis: a study of 32 pregnancies from a single center. *Ann Rheum Dis*, 60(6): 599-604.

(2002). Importance of planning ovulation induction therapy in systemic lupus erythematosus and antiphospholipid syndrome: a single center retrospective study of 21 cases and 114 cycles. *Semin Arthritis Rheum*, 32(3): 174-88

Isenberg DA et al. (2004). Pregnacy in rheumatic disease- an overview. *Oxford text book of Rheumatology*, 2004, 3rd edition, p 117-125

Janssen NM, Genta M. (2000). The effects of immunosuppressive and anti-inflammatory medications on fertility, pregnancy and lactation. *Arch Intern*, 160: 610-619.

Jick H, et al. (1981). First trimester drug use and congenital disorders. *JAMA*, 246: 343-346.

John Fredrick. (2000). Pregnancy complications and delivery practice in women with connective tissue disease and inflammatory rheumatic disease in Norway. *AOGS* 79(6):490-495.

Karim MY, Alba P *et al.* (2002). Mycophenolate mofetil for systemic lupus Erythematosus refractory to alter immunosuppressive agents. *Rheumatology (Oxford)*, 41: 876-882.

Kiss E, Bhattoa et al. (2002). Pregnancy in women with systemic lupus erythematosus. *European Journal of Obstetric Gynecology Reproductive Biology* 2002; 101(2): 129-34.

Koblayash et al. Immunosorbent plasmapheresis for a patient with antiphospholipid antibody syndrome during pregnancy. *Ann Rheum dis*, 51:399-401.

Kozer E et al. (2003). Effects of aspirin consumption during pregnancy on pregnancy outcomes: meta-analysis. *Birth defects Res B Dev Reprod Toxicol*, 68(1):70-84

Lee BH, Stoll BJ, McDonald SA, Higgins RD. (2008). Neurodevelopmental outcomes of extremely low birth weight infants exposed prenatally to dexamethasone versus betamethasone. *Pediatrics*, 121(2): 1503-1510.

Lauterbach GL, et al. (2000). Women's health. *Rheum Dis Clinics NAM*, 25: 539-566.

Leona, et al. (1981). Systemic lupus erythematosus in pregnancy. *Ann Intern Med*, 94(5): 667-77.

Levy RA et al, (2001). Hydrozychloroquin in lupus pregnancy: Double blind and placebo controlled study. *Lupus*, 10(6):401-404

Lewis R, Laversen NH, Birnbaum S. (1972). Malaria associated with pregnancy. *Obstetric Gynecology*, 42: 696-700

Magee LA, Sibai B. (2011). How to manage hypertension in pregnancy effectively *British Clinical Pharmacology*, 10,111/j: 1365-2125.

Mintz, et al. (1984). Contraception with progestogens in systemic lupus erythematosus. *Contraception*, 30: 29-38.

Mpetvi. (1996). Hydroxychloroquine use in the Baltimore lupus cohort: effects on lipids, glucose and thrombosis. *Lupus*, (5): supp.1.

National Institutes of Health Report of the Consensus Development Conference. *(1994). On the effect of corticosteroids for fetal maturation on perinatal outcome. NIH publication no. 95-3784.*

Notion RL, Hackett LP, Dusci LJ, Ilett KF. (1984). Excretion of hydroxychloroquine in human milk. *British Journal of Clinical Pharmacology*, 17(3): 368-9.

Ostensen, ME etal. (1985). Hydroxychloroquine in human breast milk. *European Journal on Clinical Pharmacology*, 28(3): 357.

(1994). Optimisation of antirheumatic drug treatment in pregnancy. *Clinical Pharmacokinetics*, 27(6): 486-503.

(1996). Safety of non-steroidal anti-inflammatory drugs during pregnancy and lactation. *Inflammopharmacology*, 24(3), 4(1): 31-41.

(2006). Anti-inflammatory and immunosuppressive drugs and reproduction. *Arthritis Res Ther,* 8: 209-218

(2008). Update on safety during pregnancy of biological agents and some immunosuppressive anti-rheumatic drugs. *Rheumatology (Oxford),* 47 suppl.3: iii 28-31.

(2011). Treatment with biologics of pregnant patients with rheumatic diseases. *Curr Op in Rheumatology,* 23(3): 293-8.

Perricone R, C. De Carolis. (2008). Intravenous immunoglobin therapy in pregnant patients affected with systemic lupus erythematosus and recurrent spontaneous abortion.*Rheumatology (Oxford)*, 47(5): 646-651.

Petri M et al. (2001). Exogenous estrogen in systemic lupus erythematosus: oral contraceptives and hormone replacement therapy. *Lupus,* 10: 222- 226.

(2005). Combined oral contraceptives in women with systemic lupus erythematosus. *N Engl J Med.* 353: 2550-2558.

(2008). Editorial: oral contraceptives in systemic lupus erythematosus: the case for (and against). *Lupus,* 17: 708-710.

Rawetz. (2004). Anesthesiological aspects of pregnancy in patients with rheumatic disease. *Lupus,* 13: 699-702.

Raybum WF. (1992). Glucocorticoid therapy for rheumatic disease: maternal, fetal and breastfeeding considerations. *American Journal of Reproductive Immunology,* 28(3-4): 138-40.

Rahman P, Gladman DD, Urowitz MB. (1998). Clinical predictors of fetal outcome in systemic lupus erythematosus. J Rheumatol, 25:1526-30.

Ruiz et al. (2004). Evaluation of systemic lupus erythematosus activity during pregnancy. *Lupus,* 13:679-82.

Sammaritano LR. (2007). Therapy insight: guidelines for selection of contraception in women with rheumatic diseases. *N Clin Pract Rheumatol,* 3(5): 273-81.

Sanchez-Guerrero J, et al. (2005). A trial of contraceptive methods in women with systemic lupus erythematosus. *N Engl J Med,* 353: 2539-2549.

Simister NE. (2003). Placental transplant of immunoglobulin G. *Vaccine,* 21(24): 3365-9.

Sperber K, Hom C, Chao et al. (2009). Systemic review of Hydroxychloroquine use in pregnant Patients with autoimmune diseases. *Pediatric Rheumatology Online J,* 7: 9.

The American Academy of Pediatrics and the American College of Obstetricians and Gynecologist. (2002). *Antepartum Care. In: Guidelines for perinatal care, 5th edition*: Washington DC:73-127.

Vonderleij S, et al. (1994). Successful outcome of pregnancy after treatment of maternal anti-Ro (SSA) antibodies with immunosuppressive therapy and plasmapheresis. *Prenat Diagr* 14: 1003-1007

Wallance DJ, et al. (2001). Apheresis for lupus erythematosus: state of the art. *Lupus,* 10:193-196.

Wiernik PH, Duncan JH. (1971). Cyclophosphamide in human milk. *Lancet,* 1(7705): 912-914.

Yasmeen S, et al. (2001). Pregnancy outcomes in women with systemic lupus erythematosus. *J Matern Fetal Med*, 10: 91-6.

23

Neonatal Lupus Erythematosus (NLE)

Hanan Al-Osaimi and Suvarnaraju Yelamanchili
King Fahd Armed Forces Hospital, Jeddah
Saudi Arabia

1. Introduction

Neonatal lupus erythematosus (NLE) or neonatal lupus syndrome (NLS) is a rare syndrome seen in 1-2% of neonates with auto-antibodies to SSA/Ro, SSB/La and or U1 RNP, passively transferred transplacentally from the mother who is either asymptomatic or having manifestations of Sjogren's syndrome, SLE or other systemic rheumatic disease, characterized by cutaneous, cardiac or rarely both clinical manifestations.

The skin manifestations are seen at least in 30% of these patients, in the form of periorbital annular erythematous plaques later spreading to other areas of face, scalp, trunk and extremities which is non-scarring and non-atrophic. This is usually transient lasting for days to months. But, the cardiac manifestations are seen in up to 60% of the patients is mainly in the form of complete congenital heart block (CHB) which is irreversible and is associate with cardiomyopathy in at least 10% of the cases. Cardiomyopathy is associated with increased morbidity and mortality. Almost all the patients having cardiac lupus require permanent pacemaker. The recurrence rate of neonatal lupus is as much as 25% in the subsequent pregnancies. There has been better understanding of aetiopathogenesis of the disease which is due to the rapid advances in field of medicine [Buyon, 2001, 2007].

2. Historical aspects

The first case reported by Aylward in 1928, who described two siblings with CHB born to a mother who had Sjogren's syndrome. Plant & Stevens described CHB as a manifestation of NLE in 1945 [Plant, 1945). But the first report linking autoimmune disease in mother with cutaneous lupus was McCuistion and Schoch in 1954. In 1957 Hogg noted the possible relation between autoimmune disease of the mother and congenital heart block in her child. Finally in 1980 Weston reported the association of neonatal lupus (NLE) with maternal anti-Ro auto- antibodies [Lee LA, 1997].

The term, neonatal lupus erythematosus (NLE) has been challenged, because although cutaneous lupus resembles subacute cutaneous adult lupus, the cardiac manifestation of CHB is not seen in the adult lupus. So a better term could have been "Neonatal anti-Ro antibody associated disease", but the disease has become so popular with the name of neonatal lupus erythematosus (NLE). It is also called as Neonatal lupus syndrome (NLS) due to protean clinical manifestations of the disease.

3. Epidemiology

The prevalence of Anti-SSA antibodies in women is 1:200 while the incidence of neonatal lupus is only 1 in 20,000 live births [Neiman, 2000]. And less than 1:50 of women with anti-SSA antibodies will have child with CHB. Only 1-2% of the infants of mothers with anti-SSA/Ro with or without anti-SSB/La antibodies develop neonatal lupus, although it ranges from 0.6% to 25% with an average of 7.2% by various studies. The incidence increases to 3% if the mother has anti- La antibodies in addition to anti- Ra antibodies.

If the mother has also SLE along with anti-SSA antibodies the incidence of NLE may be up to 6-13%. This is much higher and reaches up to 25% if the mother already had a child with NLE. 15-20% present as CHB and 6% present as cutaneous lupus. A recent study reported that the overall recurrence rate for any manifestation of NLE was 49% out of which 18.2% were complicated by cardiac NLE, 29.9% by cutaneous NLE, and 1.3% by hematologic/hepatic NLE. On follow up studies it was found that there were no significant differences in the maternal risk factors for having a subsequent child with either cardiac or cutaneous NLE [Izmirly, 2010].

The incidence of CHB is seen in 50-60% while the cutaneous lupus is seen in 25-30% and the combination of cutaneous and cardiac manifestations seen only in 4-10% of the patients with NLE [Eronen, 2000]. The incidence of cutaneous lupus may be higher but under reported as the rash is transient and may not be noticed at times and these neonates are usually asymptomatic. The antibody titers are three fold higher for cardiac lupus as compared to cutaneous lupus.

Race: No racial predilection has been observed. However, NLE appears to be more common in African Americans, Latin Americans, and Asian children. So it is more common in non-white than white population (3:1).

Sex: Girls are affected more often than boys (2:1) and the cutaneous lupus is much more common in girls (3:1), whereas cardiac lupus is seen in equal ratio in males and females while anti-RNP neonatal cutaneous lupus is seen mainly in males [Jaeggie, 2010].

During a 20 year follow-up study of asymptomatic mothers with NLE, 50-60% of them have developed rheumatologic disease in the form of SLE, Sjogren's or undifferentiated connective tissue disease approximately in the ratio of 1:2:2. The incidence of rheumatologic disease is more in cutaneous lupus (up to 70%) and the incidence of Sjogren's disease is more common in mothers having infants with CHB than cutaneous lupus [Waltuck, 1994]. The overall risk of a woman with SLE having a child with CHB is 1:60 and it increases to 1:20 in presence of anti-SSA/Ra antibodies [Watson, 1986].

The prevalence of anti-SSA/Ro antibodies in general population (pregnant & non-pregnant) ranges from 1-10% and its average prevalence in SLE patients is up to 50%. The prevalence of anti-SSB/La antibodies in SLE is less than anti-SSA/Ro (15-20%) and usually associated with anti-SSA/Ro in 90% of cases. Rarely anti-SSB/La or anti-U1 RNP can be present without anti-SSA/Ro which may rarely cause cutaneous lupus [Singsen, 1986; Goldsmith, 1989].

4. Pathophysiology

NLE is presumed to result from trans-placental passage of maternal anti-SSA/Ro and/or anti-SSB/La auto-antibodies. The precise mechanism of injury to specific tissues, such as the skin and heart, is not known. The pathogenesis of disease probably involves more than simple trans-placental passage of antibodies because:

- The disease itself is very rare.
- The mothers who have these auto antibodies, half of them are asymptomatic.
- There is discordance of disease even in monozygotic twins.
- And finally the anti-Ro/SSA and anti-La/SSB are associated with a variety of clinical syndromes in adults.

4.1 Pathogenesis of CHB in NLE

The trans-placental passive transfer of IgG auto antibodies is the initiating factor. The auto antibodies are usually anti-SSA/Ro against usually 52kD or 60kD protein or anti-SSB/La against 48kD protein or rarely anti-U1RNP antibodies and the incidence for these antibodies in the mother for CHB and CNL (cutaneous neonatal lupus) is 100 and 91% for anti-SSA and 91 and 73% for anti-SSB and the incidence in the mother without NLE is only 47 and 15% respectively, strengthening the role of these antibodies in the pathogenesis. Anti-52 kD component of anti-SSA/Ro for a particular peptide fragment p200-239 has greatest risk for CHB than to p177-196, the later seen in unaffected children [Clansy, 2005].

Other autoantibody specificities reported to be associated with neonatal lupus include antibodies to calreticulin, a 57 kD protein, a 75-kD phosphoprotein, a-fodrin, the neonatal heart M1 muscarinic acetylcholine receptor, and the serotoninergic 5-HT4 receptor [Sontheimer,1996; Maddison 1995; Wang,1999; Miyagawa,1998; Borda, 2001; Eftekhari,2001]. Ro- and La-specific IgA and IgM antibodies were detected in the serum from a subset of mothers. However, Ro- and La-specific IgA and IgM antibody levels were low or non-detectable in children raised with or without breastfeeding [Klauinger, 2009]. This supports the role of transplacental passively transferred maternal antibodies than fetal antibodies in pathogenesis.

These auto antibodies later enter the myocardial cell causing exaggerated apoptosis which leads to expression of the antibodies on the surface of the cardiocyte. These results suggest that resident cardiocyte participate in physiologic clearance of apoptotic cardiocyte, but that clearance is inhibited by opsonization via maternal auto- antibodies, resulting in accumulation of apoptotic cells promoting inflammation , stimulating macrophages which secretes cytokines mainly, transforming growth factor-beta (TGF- β), that stimulates fibroblast proliferation later on leading to fibrosis of the conduction system (causing CHB) or myocardium (leading to cardiomyopathy or Endocardial fibroelastosis) or both as shown in Fig.1.

Histopathology of the affected heart shows fibrosis and calcification of the atrioventricular nodal region and replacement of that region with fibrous tissue explaining the irreversibility of the heart block in most patients [Lee LA, 1997). Infants exposed to low titers of anti-SSB/La or anti-U1 RNP were more likely to have non-cardiac manifestations of neonatal lupus or only cutaneous lupus while the antibody titers are at least three-fold higher in cardiac than cutaneous lupus [Jaeggie, 2010].

In addition to inducing tissue damage, anti-SSA/Ro and/or anti-SSB/La antibodies inhibit calcium channel activation or the cardiac L- and T-type calcium channels themselves. L-type channels are crucial to action potential propagation and conduction in the AV node [Xiao GQ, 2001; Silverman, 1995].

Very few neonates who have maternal antibodies develop neonatal lupus. Therefore factors other than attachment of the antibodies to the target antigens to be considered like fetal, uterine, viral and genetic factors.

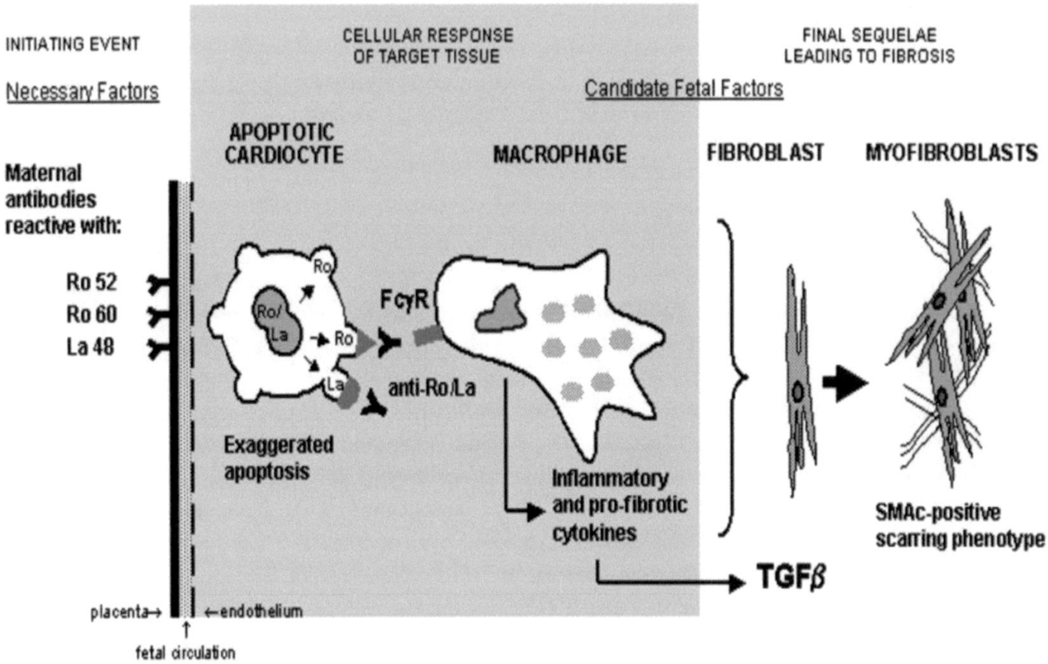

Fig. 1. Proposed pathologic cascade (Buyon, 2004)
(This leads from inflammation to fibrosis whereby maternal antibodies initiate events that lead to a persistent myofibroblasts, a phenotype associated with scarring. Apoptosis of cardiocyte results in the surface expression of SSA/Ro and SSB/La components, subsequent opsonization by cognate antibodies, and the secretion by macrophages of cytokines (e.g., TGF-β) which modulate fibroblasts into scar promoting myofibroblasts)

Genetic factors in particular the HLA alleles DR3, B8, DQw2 and DRw52 and a polymorphism in the promoter region of the gene for tumor necrosis factor alpha (-308A, associated with higher TNF-α production) may play a role at least in cutaneous lupus.
There are many questions that still remain. Why only few develop the disease while many do not develop? Why do some babies develop skin disease, others develop heart disease, and very few develop both? Studies from the laboratory failed to show differences between auto-antibodies from mothers who had babies with skin disease and auto-antibodies from mothers who had babies with cardiac disease. The sera were not different with regard to IgG antibody subclass, immunoblotting patterns against skin and heart extracts, and immuno-precipitation of Ro-associated hY RNAs. The only significant difference noted was, the lower titers of maternal anti-Ro60 in the skin disease subset, but the reason for that difference is also not clear [Lee LA, 1994, 1996; Bennion, 1990].
Again the discordance in the homozygotic twins goes against the genetic factors playing a major role in NLE. Post mortem studies in the neonates revealed deposition of IgG1 & IgG3 along with complement (including C1q, C4, C3d, C6, and C9), and fibrin [6. Silverman, 1995; Salomonsson 2002] leading initially to pancarditis and later on to fibroelastosis of the heart. Thus it can involve almost all the structures of the heart. So fibrosis starts near the AV nodal region and extends to the other regions of the heart. As the process of inflammation starts

mainly in the second trimester, when the organogenesis is complete, structural defects in the heart are rare.

It was also noticed that there is reduction of the protective molecules like the complement regulatory proteins (decay accelerating factor (DAF, CD55), protectin (CD59), and membrane cofactor protein (MCP, CD46) which predispose complement -mediated damage to the heart [Clancy, 2006; Miranda, 2000].

Some observational studies in monozygotic twins and triplets need clarification. Some neonates are affected while others are not affected. Even in the affected neonates each one will have different type of manifestations, regardless of them sharing a common placenta or not [Botard, 2000; Shimosegawa, 1997; Yazici, 2000]. Many studies revealed that type 1 interferon pathway is not involved in NLE pathogenesis [Niewold, 2002, 2008].

All the above indicate that the maternal antibodies to SSA/Ro and SSB/La recognize their respective antigens in the immature cardiac conduction system and the fetal myocardium, gain access perhaps through apoptosis, causing in utero an inflammatory reaction of the conduction system and endo-myo-pericardium, resulting in fibrosis of the conduction system with heart block and myocarditis.

4.2 Pathogenesis of cutaneous lupus

The same maternal antibodies recognize the antigens present in the neonatal skin exposed to UV light and high estradiol concentrations and cause the cutaneous manifestations of NLE. And the cutaneous lupus is due to deposition of anti-Ro IgG auto- antibodies throughout the epidermis and not the epidermo-dermal junction or dermis, which is seen even in the unaffected areas of skin. Probably deposition of antibodies in the affected organ is not leaving enough antibodies to be deposited in other organs to cause disease manifestations. And it is not known whether this could be the reason why usually only one organ is involved in one patient and other in another patient in neonatal lupus.

At this time, although there is compelling evidence that maternal auto- antibodies are a major factor in the genesis of disease, the factors that determine which child will be affected and which organs will be affected are largely unknown. These factors should be predictable so that one day it may be possible to identify the fetus at high risk, particularly for heart blocks, and target that particular fetus for prevention or effective treatment [Izmirly, 2007].

5. Patient history

The mother usually discovers her affected child either has skin rash shortly after birth or that her infant is highly sensitive to sunlight (intense photosensitivity). Mothers may be asymptomatic or have symptoms of lupus erythematosus, Sjogren's syndrome or undifferentiated CTD. When carefully questioned, they may report dry eyes, arthralgias, myalgias, or arthritis. A recent report linked the presence of hypothyroidism in mothers with anti-SSA/Ro with an increased risk of CHB. Cardiac involvement can be revealed in ultrasound exam of fetus from routine antenatal check-up from 20-24 weeks gestation in the form of bradycardia which may suggest cardiac lupus (CHB) or by physical exam at birth.

6. Clinical manifestations

A fetus/newborn can have either cutaneous or cardiac or both as the major manifestations of NLE. Cardiac manifestations usually occur at 18 to 24 weeks gestation. The rash is often present at birth, but can appear up to four months of age.

The commonest manifestation, CHB, is seen in 61%, cutaneous manifestations in 26.9% both cardiac & cutaneous manifestations in 8.7% and hepatic or hematological involvement in 3.2% but the recent literature shows that cutaneous, cardiac, hepatobiliary, and hematological involvement was found in 70.6%, 64.7%, 52.9%, and 35.3% of infants respectively with a mortality of 11.8% in 64.7% of asymptomatic mothers in recent literature [Wisuthsarewong, 2011]. NLE can also involve liver (6.2%), blood (5.2%), CNS (0.8%), lung (0.8%) and kidney (0.4%). It is usually common to see NLE with affection of one organ, although involvement of multiple organs can occur [Buyon, 2001].

6.1 Neonatal cutaneous lupus

This is seen in 15-30% of neonatal lupus and the incidence may be higher than this as it may be under reported because the skin rash is transient and majority of their mothers are usually asymptomatic. It is more common in female (3:1) than male neonates.

Cutaneous findings in neonatal lupus erythematosus [Wisuthsarewong, 2011]

- Annular erythematous plaques with a small scales characterize neonatal lupus erythematosus. Atrophic lesions may develop; however, over time, even these lesions leave little residual change. These lesions are usually not present at birth but may become evident shortly afterward, particularly in infants exposed to light therapy [Figure 2].

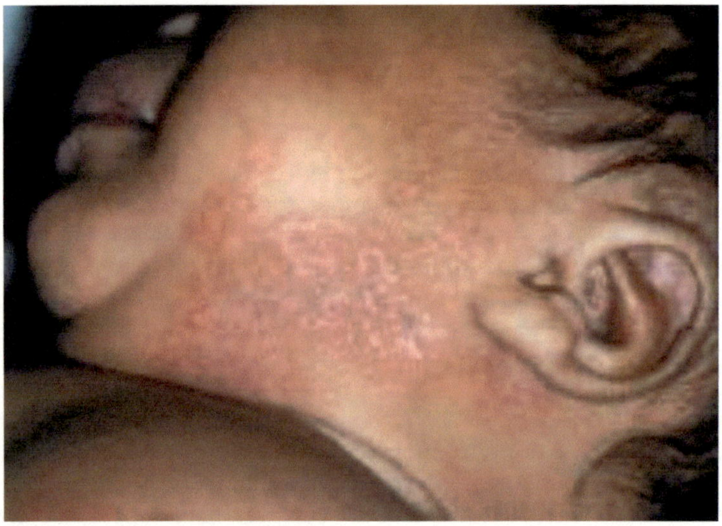

Fig. 2. Neonatal cutaneous lupus erythematosus

- These skin lesions are usually non-scarring and non-atrophic.
- The lesions are mainly seen on the face, scalp, trunk and extremities. The lesions are very dense in the periorbital area which gives an "eye-mask" or "owl-eye appearance (with ice-pick lesions located to the superior aspect of face, lateral edges of eyes, spreading into the temple regions bilaterally). Mild erythema on the face was observed at birth.
- An erythematosus raccoon-like patch began to develop on the face following sun exposure.

- It becomes plaque like and develop scaling and desquamation
- Intense photosensitivity is another striking feature in neonatal cutaneous lupus.
- Telangiectasia is often prominent and is the sole cutaneous manifestation reported in some patients, sometimes to the extent of forming muco-cutaneous and visceral hemangiomas [Spalding, 2007].
- Dyspigmentation is frequent, but, with time, this change spontaneously resolves. It may last as long as one year.
- Although histology is typical but it is not needed in most cases due to characteristic appearance of rash in the presence of auto-antibodies [Lee LA, 1993].

The lesional histology supports the clinical descriptions of sub acute cutaneous lupus with basal cell damage in the epidermis and a superficial mononuclear cell infiltrate in the upper dermis. As observed in sub acute cutaneous lupus, immunofluorescence is positive with the finding of a particulate pattern of IgG in the epidermis. The histopathology of the erythematous-desquamative lesions more closely resembles that of sub acute cutaneous lupus erythematosus (SCLE) than discoid lupus. Typical findings are vacuolar alterations at the dermo-epidermal interface and adnexal structures.

Some patients present with urticaria-like lesions that have superficial and deep perivascular and periadnexal lymphocytic infiltrates [Silverman, 2010, Penate, 2009]. The identification of cutaneous NL in an anti-SSA/Ro antibody-exposed infant is particularly important, since it predicts a 6-10-fold risk of a subsequent child developing cardiac NL [Izmirly, 2010].

6.2 Neonatal cardiac lupus

The commonest cardiac manifestation of neonatal lupus is congenital complete heart block and the next one is cardiomyopathy with or without heart failure. There are other rare cardiac manifestations that may be seen [Table 1).

6.2.1 Congenital complete heart block (CHB)

The most dangerous and life threatening cardiac manifestation of NLE is complete heart block (CHB) which is more common in female neonates (3:1) and usually appear in fetus from 20-24 weeks of gestation by fetal ultrasound exam and in 90% of cases it is seen by birth. It is mainly due to the anti-SSA/Ro with or without anti-SSB/La antibodies. Anti-SSB/La and anti-U1 RNP alone are not associated with cardiac lupus. It is seen in 62% cases of NLE as against 31% of cases with cutaneous lupus and together with cutaneous lupus it is seen only in 4% of cases. CHB is usually detected by fetal US exam as fetal bradycardia (40-80 beats/min) [Brucato, 1995, 2007; Agarwala, 1996]. NLE is responsible for 90-95% of CHB presenting in utero and only 5% of cases of CHB after birth. The incidence of CHB in the general population varies between 1 in 15,000 to 1 in 22,000 live-born infants [Michaëlsson, 1972].

Presentation in the neonate:

- Bradycardia
- Intermittent cannon waves in the neck,
- First heart sound that varies in intensity,
- Intermittent gallops and murmurs.
- The newborn at greatest risk has a rapid atrial rate, often 150 beats/min or faster, and a ventricular rate less than 50 beats/min. With junctional or atrioventricular (AV) nodal escape or ectopic rhythm

- First or second degree heart block found in infants at birth can progress to complete heart block [Jaggie, 2002].

It may take just one week for a neonate to develop CHB from a normal PR interval, so weekly fetal echo is very important between 16-24wks.

Presentation in the childhood:

Only 60% present before six years as the ventricular rate is adequate from the junctional release rhythm so they become symptomatic later in their life and the CHB is usually intermittent initially before becoming persistent. They are usually picked up for slow pulse which is not symptomatic. Some patients present with bradycardia-related symptoms like

- Reduced exercise tolerance and
- Pre-syncope or syncope (Stokes-Adams attacks) -26%
- Sudden death has also been described -6%

The sinoatrial (SA) node also may be involved and sinus bradycardia has been described in 3.8 percent of fetuses but is usually not permanent.
Other types of electrical disturbances can be there as reported in the table 1. There are host of other cardiac manifestations which are not that common.

Electrical	Mechanical	Structural
CHB II° Heart block I° Heart block RBBB Sinus bradycardia Stokes-Adams attacks Prolonged QT interval (sudden death)	Cardiomyopathy CHF Hydrops fetalis CHB with structural heart disease Libman-Sack's verrucous endocarditis Myopericarditis. Endocardial fibroelastosis (EFE) Valvular lesions (rare) Intramyocardial Vasculopathy 2° to APS	ASD PDA VSD Patent foramen ovale Pulmonary stenosis Pulmonary regurgitation Coarctation of Aorta Tetrology of Fallot Hypoplastic RV Anomalous Pulmonary Venous Drainage PV dysplasia, Fusion of chordae tendineae of the valves, causing MR & TR

Table 1. Cardiac disorders reported in neonatal cardiac lupus
(Data adopted from Buyon et al, 1998, 2007, Hornberger, 2010].

6.2.2 Cardiomyopathy/ CHF/ hydrops fetalis

This is the second most common cardiac abnormality commonly in the presence of CHB but can occur rarely in the absence of CHB. It may be due to various reasons. It may be due to the extension of fibrotic process into the myocardium causing myocardial fibrosis and CHF or it may be due to compensatory ventricular dilatation to increase the stroke volume due to bradyarrhythmia or it can also be due to the ventricular asynchrony due to right ventricular pacing alone. It is seen in 10% of cases and the mortality is higher in the neonates presented early with CHB than presenting after birth. CHF is rarely seen in CHB presenting after birth.

Structural heart disease has been reported occasionally in association with NLE. However, caution is needed in interpreting such reports because the inflammatory fibrosis of conduction system occurs usually after the organogenesis is complete (after first trimester) and some structural abnormalities may cause heart block per se (e.g., L-transposition of the great vessels with a single ventricle, ostium primum type atrial septal defect, and rarely ventricular septal defects). Out of all these anomalies, only VSD has been reported in association with NLE. The commonest among these are ASD, PDA and VSD [Buyon, 1998; Falcini, 1998; Houssiau, 1986].

Other congenital structural cardiac anomalies have also been observed in association with NLE (persistent patent ductus arteriosus, patent foramen ovale, pulmonary stenosis, pulmonary regurgitation, coarctation of aorta, tetrology of Fallot, hypoplastic right ventricle, anomalous pulmonary venous drainage, pulmonary valvular dysplasia, fusion of chordae tendinae of the tricuspid valve, TR, MR, and ostium secundum type atrial septal defects [Table 1].

NLE with CHB has been associated with endocardial fibroelastosis (EFE). In a report of 13 affected children, seven had EFE at presentation (four fetal and three postnatal), and six developed EFE weeks to as long as five years after the diagnosis of complete heart block. Eleven either died or underwent cardiac transplantation because of the EFE. EFE has also been reported in the absence of a conduction defect in infants with maternal anti-Ro and anti-La antibodies [Nield, 2002].

6.3 Hematological manifestations

They are commonly asymptomatic in the form of thrombocytopenia (frequently associated with splenomegaly), anemia (Coombs-positive hemolytic anemia or microangiopathic hemolytic anemia), leucopenia, neutropenia (in up to 25% of NLE) and rarely aplastic anemia. The thrombocytopenia and anemia very rarely can be so severe requiring blood transfusions and sterioid therapy. Lymphopenia, which is commonly seen in adult lupus, is not usually seen in neonatal lupus [Wolach, 1993].

6.4 Hepatic and gastrointestinal manifestations

They are seen in 10-25%. Three types of liver manifestations were observed. Liver failure, with histological features of neonatal iron storage disease, occurring in utero or shortly after birth and resulting in fatality; cholestasis with conjugated hyperbilirubinemia and minimal transaminase elevations occurring a few weeks after birth and eventually resolving; and mild or moderate transaminase elevations occurring a few weeks or months after birth and resolving. Rarely patients can have cirrhosis and gastrointestinal hemorrhage. The pathology resembles idiopathic neonatal giant cell hepatitis [Silverman, 2010; Izmirly, 2010].

6.5 Neurological manifestations

They are seen in less than 1% of patients in the form of myelopathy, aseptic meningitis, seizures with or without hypocalcaemia, myasthenia gravis (transient) [Kaye, 1987], hydrocephalus, microcephaly, macrocephaly, non- specific white matter changes, calcification of basal ganglia, vasculopathy and neuropsychiatric dysfunction/attention deficient disorders [Boros, 2007].

6.6 Other rare manifestations

They can be in the form of pulmonary (Pneumonia), renal (nephritis or nephritic syndrome), bony (chondrodysplasia punctata) [Silverman, 2010] or multiple thrombosis due to maternal cardiolipin antibodies [Tabbut, 1994].

The NLE occurring in the subsequent pregnancies after a lupus child is up to 36%, out of which 12.8% were complicated by cardiac NL and 23.1% by cutaneous NLE. There were no significant differences in the following maternal risk factors for having a subsequent child with cardiac or cutaneous NLE: age, race, ethnicity, anti-SSB/La status, diagnosis, use of non-fluorinated steroids, or breastfeeding. The sex of the subsequent fetus did not influence the development of cardiac or cutaneous NL [Izmirly, 2010].

The manifestation of anti-RNP positive is a rare occurrence. It was noted that infants affected with NLE from anti-RNP antibodies developed only cutaneous lesions and were all male [Boh, 2004].

The transient hematologic abnormalities and skin disease of the neonate reflect the effect of passively acquired auto- antibodies on those organ systems that have the capacity of continual regeneration, in contrast to the heart, which apparently lacks this capability, because, to date, third-degree heart block is irreversible [Buyon, 2007].

7. Diagnosis

The diagnosis of NLE is made when a fetus or newborn of a mother with anti-SSA/Ro and/or anti-SSB/La, or anti-RNP, antibodies develops heart block and/or the typical rash, hepatic or hematologic manifestations, in the absence of other causes. The following recommendations for prenatal screening and postnatal diagnosis are based upon the potential cardiac manifestations of neonatal lupus (NLE) and their associated morbidity and mortality.

7.1 Prenatal screening (antibodies)

Prenatal screening for anti-SSA/Ro and anti-SSB/La antibodies is warranted for women who are known to be at risk of having a pregnancy complicated by NLE. Women who are more likely to have anti-SSA/Ro and anti-SSB/La antibodies include those with lupus, Sjogren's syndrome, an undifferentiated autoimmune disease, or NLE in a previous pregnancy. Women with these identifiable risk factors should be tested before conception or early pregnancy as soon as possible.

7.2 Intra-natal diagnosis

CHB in an offspring can be the first sign in the mother that has anti-SSA/Ro and anti-SSB/La antibodies. These antibodies are not part of routine prenatal testing in asymptomatic women.

7.2.1 Fetal echocardiography

Women who test positive for SSA/Ro and SSB/La auto antibodies may benefit from more intense assessment for fetal heart block with frequent fetal echocardiographic testing during pregnancy. There are no formal guidelines for the type or the frequency of testing to detect fetal heart block, but performing weekly pulsed Doppler fetal echocardiography from the 16th through the 26th week of pregnancy and then every other week until 32 weeks should be strongly considered. The most vulnerable period for the fetus is during the period from 18 to 24 weeks gestation. Normal sinus rhythm can progress to complete block in seven days during this high-risk period. New onset of heart block is less likely from 26 to 30 weeks, and it rarely develops after 30 weeks of pregnancy.

7.2.2 Pulsed Doppler echocardiography

Less-advanced degrees of heart block can be detected in utero by this technique [Glickstein, 2000]. And it depends upon measurement of the mechanical PR interval as determined from the onset of atrial contraction (initiation of mitral valve movement) to ventricular contraction (aortic pulsation). It is generally accepted that women with low titer antibodies are less likely to have offspring with cardiac NLE than women with high titers. The problem is that laboratories have different cutoff values and most women with these antibodies have high titers.

7.2.3 Fetal auscultation (fetoscope) / fetal ultrasound

Complete heart block (and usually second-degree block) results in fetal bradycardia that can be detected by even routine fetal auscultation or ultrasonography (sonogram). The use of echocardiographic monitoring may present a way to more selective use interventions to prevent or reverse the development of more advanced heart block. Fetal monitoring may include a biophysical profile and non-stress test [Vesel, 2004; Sonesson, 2004].

7.2.4 Biophysical profile

A biophysical profile (BPP) score is calculated to assess the fetus' health. It consists of five components which include non-stress testing and ultrasound measurement of four fetal parameters: fetal body movements, breathing movements, fetal tone (flexion and extension of an arm, leg, or the spine) and measurement of the amniotic fluid levels. Each component is scored individually, with two points given for a normal result and zero points given for an abnormal result. The maximum possible score is 10. The amniotic fluid level is an important variable in the BPP because a low volume (called oligohydramnios) may increase the risk of umbilical cord compression and may be a sign of changes in the blood flow between the baby and mother. Amniotic fluid levels can become reduced within a short time period, even a few days.

7.2.5 Non-stress testing

Non-stress testing is done by monitoring the baby's heart rate with a small device that is placed on the mother's abdomen. The device uses sound waves (ultrasound) to measure the baby's heart rate over time, usually for 20 to 30 minutes. Normally, the baby's baseline heart rate should be between 110 and 160 beats per minute and should increase above its baseline by at least 15 beats per minute for 15 seconds when the baby moves. The test is considered reassuring (called "reactive") if two or more fetal heart rate increases are seen within a 20 minute period. Further testing may be needed if these increases are not observed after monitoring for 40 minutes.

7.3 Postnatal diagnosis

Testing for maternal anti-SSA/Ro antibodies should be performed in any neonate with heart block, because these antibodies account for 80 to 95 percent of reported cases of CHB in the

fetus and neonate. Infants up to eight months of age with an annular or polycyclic rash and/or any degree of heart block should be tested for anti-SSA/Ro and anti-SSB/La antibodies. A positive test in the child or mother fulfills the diagnostic criteria for NLE [Buyon, 2001, Jaeggi, 2002, Johansen, 1998].
An infant diagnosed with NLE who has compatible clinical manifestations and detectable auto antibodies (i.e., anti-SSA/Ro and/or anti-SSB/La in the mother or infant), but no electrocardiographic evidence of heart block of any degree at birth, is at very low risk of subsequently developing conducting system disease. However, there have been rare cases of isolated cardiomyopathy reported.

8. Differential diagnosis

8.1 Differential diagnosis of cutaneous neonatal lupus

Polycyclic Skin Lesions	Isolated Annular Erythematosus
Urticaria Erythema marginatum Tinea Seborrheic dermatitis Ichthyosiform genodermatosis	Erythema annulare centrifugum Familial annular erythema Erythema multiforme Infantile epidermodysplastic erythema Pityrosporum (Malassezia species) dermal infection Annular erythema of infancy Erythema gyratum atrophicans

Table 2. Differential diagnosis of cutaneous neonatal lupus
(Data adopted from Lee LA, 1997)

The differential diagnosis includes various rashes seen in the newborn period. These other rashes are not associated with maternal anti-SSA/Ro, anti-SSB/La, or anti-RNP antibodies or with congenital heart block [Table 2].

8.2 Differential diagnosis of cardiac neonatal lupus

Differential diagnosis of congenital CHB [Jaeggi et al, 2002]
Although neonatal lupus is responsible for 95% of congenital CHB in neonate but it is a cause for CHB after birth in only 5% of the children. The other causes of CHB are:

- Myocarditis
- Various structural cardiac defects
- Congenitally corrected transposition of the great arteries,
- Atrioventricular discordance,
- Polysplenia with atrioventricular canal defect.
- Several hereditary disorders

In complicated congenital lesions such as transposition of great vessels it is difficult to say whether it is due to NLE or due to the cardiac defect itself.
The patients who present with congenital CHB can be differentiated from other causes of CHB by early presentation (20-24wks of gestation) as fetal bradycardia and/or fetal PR interval and may have additional structural cardiac abnormalities commonest being VSD & endocardial fibroelastosis along with presence of antibodies to SSA/SSB. They may also

have complications due to CHB like hydrops fetalis, endocardial fibroelastosis, pericardial effusion, and spontaneous intrauterine fetal death.

9. Treatment

9.1 Treatment of congenital heart block

Prenatal testing for anti-SSA/Ro and anti-SSB/La antibodies is being done only in high risk women, like women with SLE, Sjogren's syndrome, or other systemic rheumatic diseases (UCTD or UAS) and previous child with NLE where the risk is up to 25%. Careful monitoring during gestation with fetal ultrasound and echocardiography from 16th week of pregnancy is to be done. The best treatment for CHB is prevention as once CHB is diagnosed medical treatment seems to be unsuccessful. Testing for candidate antibodies is important prior to initiating therapy for a presumed case of neonatal cardiac lupus, because there are cases of heart block not associated with anti-SSA/Ro and SSB/La antibodies.

9.1.1 Preventive therapy

As the incidence of congenital heart block is only 2% in the offspring of unselected anti-Ro antibody positive mothers the preventative therapy cannot be advocated for this group.

However, in women with a previous child with congenital heart block the risk is greater, in the region of 17-19%. Graham Hughes has proposed that in this group of patients, maternal administration of intravenous immunoglobulins (IVIG) may reduce the risk of recurrences.

A multinational open label study is currently underway based at The Lupus Unit, St. Thomas' Hospital, London, UK [Gordon, 2007] to confirm or refute the efficacy of IVIG in preventing congenital heart block.

Another potential strategy to prevent recurrence in subsequent pregnancies was immune-suppression with fluorinated steroids, which cross the placenta. However, the toxicity of these agents precludes their use as a preventative therapy. Serious effects on the fetus such as spontaneous abortions, stillbirth, IUGR, low birth weight, mild adrenal insufficiency, left ventricular myocardial hypertrophy and delayed psychomotor development were noticed with these drugs apart from the adverse effects on the mother [Gordon, 2007]. A case control study suggests that hydroxychloroquine, a Toll-like receptor (TLR) inhibitor the usage of which carries minimal risk to the mother and fetus, may decrease the risk of neonatal cardiac lupus related to anti-SSA/SSB antibodies. But prospective studies are needed for its confirmation [Izmirly, 2010].

9.1.2 Care of neonates at risk for complete heart block

Careful observation of infants whose second-degree atrioventricular block has been reversed in utero is necessary in the postnatal period, as there is still a risk of progression to a higher degree heart block, even with clearance of maternal auto antibodies. If prenatal screening or fetal monitoring has detected any degree of heart block in utero, consultation with a pediatric cardiologist should be obtained. Some infants with complete heart block will require insertion of a cardiac pacemaker, especially if the heart rate at delivery is less than 55 beats per minute [Izmirly, 2010].

An electrocardiogram (ECG) should be performed in all neonates born to mothers with anti-SSA/Ro and/or anti-SSB/La antibodies to detect first-degree heart block; infants with first-degree heart block are at risk of postnatal progression to higher degree block [Lawrence,

2000]. A normal ECG is reassuring. However, even a normal EKG at birth cannot exclude the subsequent development of second degree heart block. There are reports of anti-Ro antibody associated cardiomyopathy also, in the absence of heart block [Gordon, 2007].

9.1.3 Treating of fetal heart block

Complete heart block is irreversible even with glucocorticoid therapy [Saleeb, 1999]. Second-degree heart block may be reversible, but it also may progress to complete heart block despite therapy [Yamada, 1999]. The clinical relevance of first-degree heart block is unclear, since progression from first-degree block to more advanced heart block in untreated fetuses has not been reported.

Fluorinated glucocorticoids such as dexamethasone and betamethasone, which are not inactivated by placental 11-beta hydroxysteroid dehydrogenase, may suppress the associated pleuro-pericardial effusion or hydrops and may improve outcomes. Fluorinated glucocorticoids are also considered for signs of a more global cardiomyopathy. However, the effectiveness of these agents in the treatment of endocardial fibroelastosis is unknown. Maternal dexamethasone in conjunction with transplacental β-adrenergic stimulation for bradycardia in fetus with HR of <55 beats/mt was reported to be effective in CHB [Jaeggi et al, 2010).

Many children with congenital heart block (33–53%) require pacing as newborns. Due to the long-term risk of sudden death the vast majority of patients are paced by the time they reach adult life. Data from several studies suggest that right ventricular apex pacing may cause left ventricular dysfunction secondary to asynchronous right and left ventricular contraction and relaxation. Thus, late onset cardiomyopathy, in at least some congenital heart block patients, may be due to right ventricular apex pacing rather than the underlying disease process. Pacing at earlier age and higher rate of pacing may accentuate this problem [Lawrence, 2000].

A prolonged QTc is a recognized feature of congenital heart block and occurs in 15–22% of patients. Due to the risk of torsades de pointes these patients should be paced and treated with a beta-blocker. A prolonged QTc has been reported to occur in isolation in children born to anti-Ro positive mothers, although prospective studies do not suggest this as a common occurrence [Gordon, 2007].

Prolonged in-utero exposure to fluorinated glucocorticoids (e.g., betamethasone or dexamethasone) can lead to adrenal hypoplasia and result in neonatal adrenal insufficiency [Costedoat-Chalumeau, 2003]. This is a rare complication that can be anticipated and tested for. Neonatal hypotension that potentially results from adrenal insufficiency should be treated empirically with hydrocortisone in addition to standard supportive care.

9.1.4 Laboratory evaluation and management (Buyon, 2001)

1. ELISA- If this initial screening test is negative for anti-SSA/Ro and anti-SSB/La antibodies the pregnancy has no known risk for CHB. If positive,
2. Immunoblot testing to be done to stratify the risk into low, moderate and high.
   a. Negative immunoblot defines low risk pregnancy (<2% probability of CHB)
   b. Positive 52kD and 60kD Ro and La antibodies is moderate risk (2-5% probability of CHB)
   c. Positive 52kD and 60kD Ro and La antibodies with previous NLE child is high risk pregnancy (15-20% probability of CHB)

Monitoring

Low risk- Fetal echo alternate weeks from 16-36wks & continuous auscultation
Moderate risk- Fetal echo every week from 16-26 wks and then alternate weeks from 26-36 Wks & Continued auscultation
High risk- Fetal echo weekly from 16-36 wks & continued auscultation

If echo shows prolonged mechanical PR interval or advanced degree block then follow the therapeutic approach which depends on degree of block and fetal morbidity at presentation [Jaeggi et al, 2004].

1a. III° AVB >2wks from detection=serial echo, fetal US, no therapy initiated
1b. III° AVB <2wks from detection=start oral dexamethasone-4mg/day for 6wks
If no change taper the dose
If reversed to II° AVB or less continue till delivery, and then taper
1c. Alternating III° AVB with II° AVB = start oral dexamethasone-4mg/day for 6wks
If it progress to III° AVB taper the dose
If reversed to II° AVB or less continue till delivery, and then taper
1d. II° or I° AVB =start oral dexamethasone-4mg/day till delivery, and then taper
If it progress to III° AVB give for 6 wks, and then taper
2. Heart block with signs of myocarditis, CHF, and/of hydropic changes
Start oral Dexamethasone until improvement, and then taper
3. Severe hydrops fetalis= start oral dexamethasone-4mg/day +
+Plasmapheresis (to remove the antibodies rapidly)
+Deliver if the lungs are mature

Fluorinated steroids cross the placental barrier, therefore dexamethasone or betamethasone is chosen for treatment. However, data during the same period at Guy's Hospital, London, has not supported the hypothesis that the improved survival can be attributed to dexamethasone therapy. As such a prospective study is needed to establish the role of routine dexamethasone therapy in congenital heart block.

At present, given the potential toxicity of dexamethasone to the fetus it is perhaps advisable to take a conservative approach and reserve the use of fluorinated steroids for cases where there is evidence of hydrops, poor ventricular function, or both. In compromised fetuses with a heart rate below 55 bpm maternal administration of β-sympathomimetic agents may be considered. New ultrasound methods allow measurement of the fetal atrioventricular time interval which provides a 'mechanical' PR interval and therefore it is now possible to detect first-degree heart block *in utero.*

If the natural history of congenital heart block involves the development of lesser degrees of heart block progressing to complete congenital heart block, detection of first-degree congenital heart block could theoretically provide a window of opportunity where therapeutic intervention is beneficial, either reversing the heart block or preventing progression to complete congenital heart block. The PRIDE (PR interval and dexamethasone evaluation) study is assessing this possibility by frequent measurement of the mechanical PR interval, weekly from 16 to 26 weeks gestation and then biweekly until 34 weeks, in pregnancies where the mother is anti-Ro antibody positive [Gordon,2007].

Thus even with intense monitoring lesser degrees of heart block are frequently not detected prior to the development of complete congenital heart block, providing little opportunity for

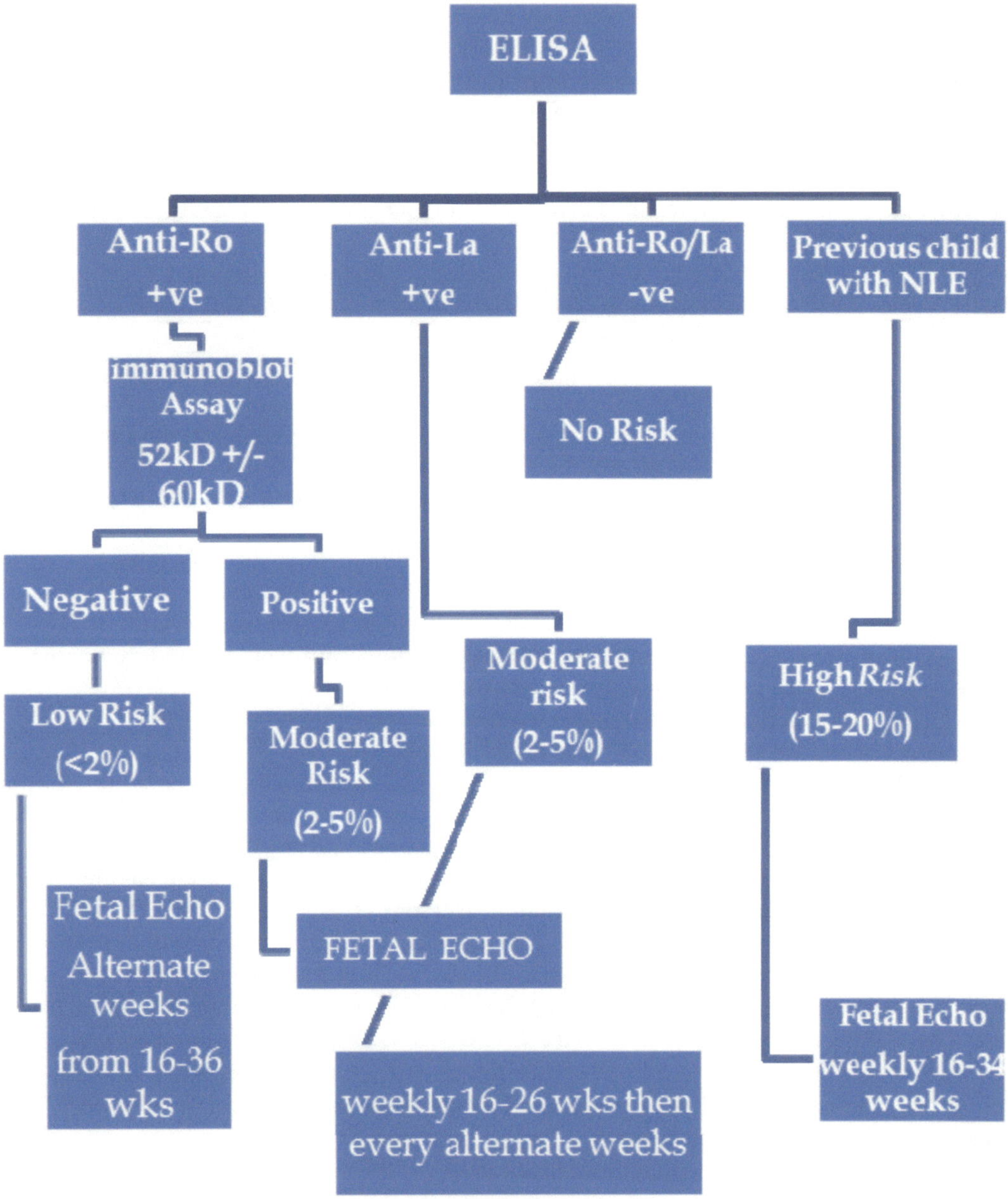

Fig. 3. Decision tree for diagnosis & management of CHB [Buyon, 2000]

intervention. Second-degree heart block detected *in utero* responds to treatment with fluorinated steroids. Whilst first-degree heart block detected *in utero* resolves following fluorinated steroid therapy, however its natural history is unclear with many cases resolving spontaneously.

Management of congenital heart block in utero and in the perinatal period can include

- steroid therapy if associated with anti-Ro/SSA and anti-La/SSB antibodies, and
- isoproterenol (β- sympathomimetic stimulation)

- And/or pacemaker insertion immediately postpartum.

The principal therapeutic decision after the immediate perinatal period involves the need for pacemaker placement. Most patients ultimately have a pacemaker inserted, regardless of the time of onset of the syndrome. Even patients who are free of symptoms at age 15 remain at risk for syncope or sudden cardiac death. And pacemaker is usually inserted in at least 90 percent by age 60 [Michaëlsson M, 1995].

Pacemaker: The type of pacemaker implanted is often based upon physician preference; either a ventricular (with rate responsiveness) or dual chamber pacemaker can be used. However, most physicians prefer physiologic dual chamber pacing in young patients as right ventricular pacing alone can cause ventricular asynchrony, which over long period of time can itself lead to cardiomyopathy. In addition if patient is not paced the bradyarrhytmia itself try to compensate with ventricular dilatation to increase the stroke volume which also can lead to heart failure.

In general implantation of permanent pacemaker in advanced second or third degree heart block which is either intermittent or permanent is in one of any of the following:

- Symptomatic bradycardia (syncope or presyncope)
- Ventricular dysfunction or low cardiac output
- A wide QRS escape rhythm
- Complex ventricular ectopy
- In an infant, ventricular rates <55 beats per minute or <70 beats per minute when associated with congenital heart disease

However any patient with CHB is at the risk of syncope or presyncope with stokes- Adam attacks and sudden death, therefore they need a pacemaker.

9.2 Treatment of neonatal cutaneous lupus

It does not require much therapy beyond avoidance of sun exposure and use of sun block and hydrocortisone cream. Systemic steroids are usually not required and systemic antimalarials are not advised due to slow onset of action in a transient illness and because of its potential toxicity in infants [Lee La, 1997].

10. Course

10.1 Early outcome

The rash of neonatal lupus (NLE) generally does not cause scarring or atrophy and disappears within six to eight months. Appearance of NLE skin lesions postnatally is independent of breastfeeding [Klauninger, 2009]. Thus, breastfeeding is not contraindicated in mothers with anti-SSA/Ro and/or anti-SSB/La antibodies.

There is little risk of later cardiac involvement in patients who had no evidence of heart block of any degree at birth or who had non-cardiac manifestations of NLE (rash or hematologic/liver abnormalities) at the time of diagnosis. However, infants with non-cardiac manifestations of NLE should at least have an ECG, and possibly an echocardiogram, since first-degree block is clinically silent and can progress postnatally. There have been no reported cases, nor has the Research Registry for Neonatal Lupus recorded the occurrence, of subsequent development of heart block following a normal electrocardiogram. As noted previously, second-degree block detected in utero and first or second degree heart block found at birth, can progress to complete heart block [Askanase, 2010].

10.2 Childhood mortality

The early outcome in infants with congenital complete heart block had a mortality of 43% if diagnosed in utero but only 6% for cases diagnosed at birth and among survivors 89% were paced [Jaeggi, 2010]. Therefore the mortality is higher for CHB diagnosed in utero than at birth. Late mortality may occur from arrhythmias, pacemaker failure or CHF. Mortality due to refractory heart failure is about 10% while the average mortality due to CHB is up to 20%.

The majority of the deaths occur in utero and first three months of life. And one year mortality is up to 41% (12%-41%) out of which 27% die within the first week of birth and 9% in the first three month but the mortality is only 3% for cases diagnosed after birth. Predictors of early mortality include a fetal heart rate<55 beats/min, delivery prior to 34 weeks and hydrops. The mortality is 3% in the 2nd year and another 3% in the 3rd year and no deaths related to cardiac lupus after three years in a study by Buyon and his colleagues. The main cause of early death is cardiac failure secondary to cardiomyopathy particularly in children between 2 and 4 years.

These children developed late onset cardiomyopathy despite early pacing. Survival also depends on the gestational age of birth. The earlier they are born the more the mortality is. The children born before 34 weeks the mortality is 52% than children born later in whom the mortality is only 9% [Buyon, 1998].

10.3 Long-term prognosis of the child

Infants and young children with complete heart block who are asymptomatic usually remain well until later childhood, adolescence, or adulthood. However, exercise limitation and even death are possible in the absence of pacing. The prognosis following pacemaker implantation is excellent for most children, although development of heart failure may occur.

Children who have had NLE may be at increased risk of developing an autoimmune and/or rheumatic disease, although it is rare. They are usually SLE, Juvenile RA, Sjogren's syndrome, undifferentiated connective tissue disease (UCTD), Hashimoto thyroiditis, Psoriasis, Iritis, type 1 DM, Raynaud's phenomenon or nephritic syndrome. Probably the longer the follow up period the higher the incidence of autoimmune disease in the child with NLE but, it is usually around 10% [Martin, 2007].

10.4 Maternal health & long-term outcome of mothers

At least 50% of the mothers with NLE had rheumatologic disease at presentation. Out of which 10% have SLE, 20% Sjogren's syndrome and 20% undifferentiated (UCTD). And 50% of the remaining asymptomatic patients developed disease in 20 year follow-up period mainly Sjogren's syndrome, SLE, UCTD, and others. Greater proportion of mothers has rheumatologic disease whose children have cutaneous NLE than CHB.

The development of lupus nephritis in mothers of children with NLE is relatively uncommon. In a review of the database of the Research Registry for Neonatal Lupus, 50 percent of mothers had some progression of their health status toward development of autoimmune (rheumatologic) symptoms. These asymptomatic mothers had a 19 percent risk of developing SLE and a 28 percent chance of developing probable or definite Sjogren's syndrome within 10 years. The NLE manifestations were not predictive of maternal disease progression.

The incidence of hypothyroidism is increased in women with anti-SSA/Ro antibodies, which is about 10% and the incidence of CHB in these mothers with hypothyroidism is higher than those without (56% Vs 13%). Therefore evaluation of thyroid disorders is warranted in any mother of an infant with neonatal lupus who complains of hair loss or fatigue [Askanase et al, 2006).

11. Conclusion

Neonatal lupus is due to passive transplacental transfer of maternal IgG auto-antibodies to SSA/Ro, SSB/La or U1RNP. It is seen in 1-2% of these neonates. The incidence is higher if the mother also has autoimmune disease. The incidence increases 5-10 folds in mothers who already have a child with neonatal lupus. The pathogenesis is mainly due to fibrosis of the atrioventricular node with or without cardiomyopathy caused by auto antibodies.

It can cause cutaneous lupus which is transient and self-limiting which usually do not require treatment. It can also present with complete heart block which is usually permanent requiring permanent pacemaker in most of the patients. They are prone for cardiomyopathy either as a result of the disease or due to right ventricular pacing which also contributes to mortality at least by 10%. The diagnosis is made by detecting auto-antibodies to SSA or SSB or U1 RNP and the CHB is made mainly in utero by periodic fetal echocardiography from 16 weeks onwards.

Fluorinated glucocorticoids (oral dexamethasone 4 mg per day or betamethasone 3 mg per day) are given for mothers of fetuses with second-degree heart block, cardiomyopathy or hydrops. It is not effective in CHB and not recommended in first degree heart block as they do not progress to advanced heart block and the adverse side effects of the drugs also limit its use.

The mortality is high in children who were detected of having CHB in utero than that detected after birth and it is mainly high in the first year and more so in the first three months of life. Many aspects of its pathogenic mechanisms are revealed but still research is needed as many questions are unanswered which could help in the preventive and therapeutic aspects of these patients.

12. Acknowledgment

The work to produce this chapter was supported by Alzaidi's Chair of research in rheumatic diseases- Umm Alqura University.

13. References

Agarwala B, Sheikh Z, Cibils LA. (1996). Congenital complete heart block. *J Natl Med Asso,* 88:725-729.

Askanase AD et al. (2006). Hypothyroidism and antithyroglobulin and antithyroperoxidase antibodies in the pathogenesis of autoimmune associated congenital heart block. J Rheumatol, 33:2099.

(2010). Frequency of neuro-psychiatric dysfunction in anti-SSA/SSB exposed children with and without neonatal lupus. *Lupus,* 19:300.

Bennion SD, Ferris et al. (1990). IgG subclasses in the serum and skin in sub acute cutaneous lupus erythematosus and neonatal lupus erythematosus. *J Invest Dermatol,* 95: 643–646.

Boh, E. (2004). Neonatal lupus erythematosus due to anti-RNP. *Clin Dermatol,* 22: 125–128.

Borda E, Sterin-Borda L. (2001). Auto-antibodies against neonatal heart M1 muscarinic acetylcholine receptor in children with congenital heart block. *J Autoimmun,* 16: 143–150.

Boros, Christina et al. (2007). Hydrocephalus and macrocephaly: New manifestations of neonatal lupus erythematosus. *Arthritis & Rheumatism,* 57(2) *Arthritis Care & Research,* 261-266.

Botard N, Sainte-Marie D et al. (2000). Cutaneous neonatal lupus erythematosus: discordant expression in identical twins. *Ann Dermatol venereal,* 127(10):814-817.

Brucato A et al. (1995) Isolated congenital complete heart block: long-term outcome of children and immonogenetic study. *J Rheumatol,* 5;22:541-543.

(2010). Ghidoni S. Arrhythmias presenting in neonatal Lupud. [Review] *Scandinavian Journal of Immunology,* 72(3):198-204.

Buyon JP et al. (1998). Autoimmune-associated congenital heart block: demographics, mortality, morbidity and recurrence rates obtained from a national neonatal lupus registry. *J Am Coll Cardiol,* 31:1658.

(2001). Anti-Ro/SSA antibodies and congenital heart block: necessary but not sufficient. *Arthritis Rheum,* 44:1723.

(2005). Neonatal Lupus: Basic research and Clinical perspectives *Rheum Dis Clin N Am,* 31:299–313

(2007). Neonatal Lupus, In: *Dubois' Lupus Erythematosus* (7th Edition).

Wallace, Daniel J Hahn et al. Lippincott Williams & Wilkins Clancy RM et al. (2005). Maternal antibody responses to the 52-kd SSA/RO p200 peptide and the development of fetal conduction defects. *Arthritis Rheum,* 52:3079.

(2006). Impaired clearance of apoptotic cardiocytes is linked to anti-SSA/Ro and -SSB/La antibodies in the pathogenesis of congenital heart block. *J Clin Invest,* 116: 2413.

Costedoat-Chalumeau N, Amoura et al. (2003). Questions about dexamethasone use for the prevention of anti-SSA related congenital heart block. *Ann Rheum Dis,* 62: 1010.

Eftekhari P, Roegel JC, et al. (2001). Induction of neonatal lupus in pups of Mice immunized with synthetic peptides derived from amino acid sequences of the serotoninergic 5-HT4 receptor. *Eur J Immunol,* 31:573–579.

Eronen M, Siren et al. (2000). Short and long- term outcome of children with congenital completer heart block diagnosed in utero or as a newborn. *Pediatrics,* 106:86-91.

Falcini F, De Simone et al. (1998). Congenital conduction defects in children born to asymptomatic mothers with anti-SSA/SSB antibodies: report of two cases. *Ann Ital Med Int,* 13:169.

Friedman DM, Llanos, et al. (2010) Evaluation of fetuses in a study of Intravenous immunoglobulin as preventive therapy for congenital heart block: Results of a multicenter, prospective, open-label clinical trial. *Arthritis Rheum*, 62:1138.

Garcia S, Nascimento et al. (1994). Cellular mechanism of the conduction Abnormalities induced by serum from anti-Ro/SSA-positive patients in rabbit hearts.*J Clin Invest*, 93:718.

Glickstein JS, Buyon et al. (2000). Pulsed Doppler echocardiographic assessment of the fetal PR interval. *Am J Cardiol*, 86:236.

Goldsmith DP. (1989) Neonatal rheumatic disorders. View of the pediatricians. *Rheum Dis Clin North Am,* 15:287-305.

Gordon PA. (2007). Congenital heart block: Clinical features and therapeutic approaches. Lupus, 16:642-646.

Hornberger LK. Al Rajaa . (2010). Spectrum of cardiac involvement in neonatal lupus. [Review] *Scandinavian Journal of Immunology*, 72(3):189-97.

Houssiau FA, Lebacq. (1986). Neonatal lupus erythematosus with congenital heart block associated with maternal systemic lupus erythematosus. *Clin Rheumatol,* 5:505.

Izmirly PM et al. (2002). Outcome of children with fetal, neonatal or childhood diagnosis of isolated congenital atrioventricular block. A single institution's experience of 30 years. *J Am Coll Cardiol*, 39:130.

(2007). Neonatal Lupus Syndromes. *Rheum Dis Clin N Am*, 33:267–285

Jaeggi E et al. (2010). Evaluation of the risk of anti-SSA/Ro-SSB/La antibody-associated cardiac manifestations of neonatal lupus in fetuses of mothers exposed to hydroxychloroquine. *Ann Rheum Dis*, 69:1827.

(2010). Cutaneous manifestations of neonatal lupus and risk of subsequent congenital heart block. *Arthritis & Rheumatism*, 62(4):1153-1157

(2010). The importance of the level of maternal anti-Ro/SSA antibodies as a prognostic marker of the development of cardiac neonatal lupus erythematosus. *J Am Coll Cardiol*, 55:2778

Johansen AS, Herlin T. (1998). Neonatal lupus syndrome. Association with Complete congenital atrioventricular block. *Ugeskr Laeger*, 160:2521.

Kaye EM, Butler IJ, Conley S. (1987). Myelopathy in neonatal and infantile lupus erythematosus. *J Neurol Nourosurg Psychiatry*, 50:923.

Klauninger R, Skog A, Horvath et al. (2009). Serologic follow-up of children born to mothers with Ro/SSA autoantibodies. *Lupus*, 18:792

Lee LA et al. (1993). Neonatal lupus liver disease. *Lupus*, 2:333-338.

(1994). The autoantibodies of neonatal lupus erythematosus. *J Invest Dermatol*, 102:963–966.

(1996). The recognition of human 60-kDa Ro ribonucleoprotein particles by antibodies associated with cutaneous lupus and neonatal lupus. *J Invest Dermatol*, 107:225–228.

(1996). Special considerations concerning the cutaneous manifestations of rheumatic diseases in children. In: Sontheimer, RD,Provost, TT, (eds), *Cutaneous manifestations of rheumatic diseases*, 2nd ed. P. 323-344. Baltimore, Maryland: Williams & Wilkins;

(1997). Cutaneous Lupus erythematosus during the neonatal and childhood periods. *Lupus,* 6:132-138.

(2009). The clinical spectrum of neonatal lupus. Archives of Dermatological Research. 301(1):107-110.

(2010). Cutaneous lupus in infancy.*Lupus,* 19, 1112–1117.

Lawrence S, Luy et al. (2000). The health of mothers of children with cutaneous neonatal lupus erythematosus differs from that of mothers of children with congenital heart block. *Am J Med,* 108:705.9.

Maddison PJ, Lee L, Reichlin M, et al. (1995). Anti-p57: a novel association with neonatal lupus. *Clin Exp Immunol,* 99: 42–48.

Martin V, Lee LA, Askanase AD, et al. (2002). Long-term followup of children with neonatal Lupus and their unaffected siblings. *Arthritis Rheum,* 46:2377.

McCuiston, C, Schoch, E Jr. (1954). Possible discoid lupus erythematosus in newborn infant; report of a case with subsequent development of acte systemic lupus erythematosus in mother. *AMA Arch Derm Syphilol,* 70: 782–785.

Miranda-Carús ME, Askanase AD, et al. (2000). Anti-SSA/Ro and anti-SSB/La Autoantibodies bind the surface of apoptotic fetal cardiocytes and promote secretion of TNF-alpha by macrophages. *J Immunol,* 165:5345.

Michaëlsson M, Engle MA. (1972). Congenital complete heart block: an international study of the natural history.Cardiovasc Clin,1972;4:85

Michaëlsson M, Jonzon A, Riesenfeld T. (1995). Isolated congenital complete atrioventricular block in adult life. A prospective study. Circulation 1995; 92:442.

Miyagawa S, Yanagi K, et al. (1998). Neonatal lupus erythematosus: maternal IgG antibodies bind to a recombinant NH2-terminal fusion protein encoded by human alpha-fodrin cDNA. *J Invest Dermatol,* 111:1189–1192.

Neiman, A, Lee, L, Weston, W, Buyon, J. (2000). Cutaneous manifestations of neonatal lupus without heart block: characteristics of mothers and children enrolled in a national registry. *J Pediatr,* 137: 674–680.

Nield LE, Silverman ED, Taylor GP, et al. (2002). Maternal anti-Ro and anti-La antibody-associated endocardial fibroelastosis. *Circulation,* 105:843.

Niewold, Timothy B, Rivera et al. (2002). Interferon in neonatal lupus. *Arthritis & Rheumatism,* 58(2):541-546.

Niewold, Timothy B ; Rivera, et al. (2008). Serum type I interferon activity is dependent on maternal diagnosis in anti-SSA/Ro-positive mothers of children with neonatal lupus. *Arthritis & Rheumatism,* 58(2):541-546.

Peñate Y, Guillermo et al. (2009). Histopathologic characteristics of neonatal cutaneous lupus erythematosus: description of five cases and literature review. *J Cutan Pathol,* 36:660.

Pisoni CN, Brucato A, Ruffatti A, et al. (2010). Failure of intravenous immunoglobulin to prevent congenital heart block: Findings of a multicenter, prospective, observational study. *Arthritis Rheum,* 62:1147.

Plant RK Steven RA. (1945). Complete AV block in fetus. Case report. *Am Heart J,* 30:615-618.

Saleeb S, Copel J, Friedman D et al. (1999). Comparison of treatment with fluorinated glucocorticoids to the natural history of autoantibody-associated congenital heart block: *Arthritis Rheum,* 42:2335.

Salomonsson S, Dörner T, *Theander* E, et al. (2002). A serologic marker for fetal risk of congenital heart block. *Arthritis Rheum*, 46:1233.

Shimosegawa M, Alaska T, Matsuta M. (1997). Neonatal lupus erythematosus occurring in identical twins. *J Dernatol*, 24: 578-582.

Silverman ED et al. (1995). Autoantibody response to the Ro/La particle may predict outcome in neonatal lupus erythematosus. *Clin Exp Immunol,* 100:499.

(2010). Non-cardiac manifestations of Neonatal Lupus Erythematosus. *Scandinavian Journal of Immunology*, 72(3):223-225.

Singsen BH, Nevon P, Wang G, et al. (1986). Anti-SSAand other anti-nuclear antibodies (ANA) in healthy pregnant women and in newborn cord blood (Abstract) *J Rheumatol,* 13:984

Spalding, T Hennon, J Dohar and T Arkachaisri. (2007). A case report-Neonatal lupus erythematosus complicated by mucocutaneous and visceral hemangiomas. *Lupus,* 16, 904-907

Sonesson SE, Salomonsson et al. (2004). Signs of first-degree heart block occur in one-third of fetuses of pregnant women with anti-SSA/Ro 52-kd antibodies. *Arthritis Rheu,* 50:1253.

Sontheimer RD, Nguyen TQ, Buyon JP, et al. (1996). Clinical correlations of autoantibodies to a recombinant, hYRNA-binding form of human calreticulin. *J Invest Dermatol,* 106: 938

Spence D, Hornberger et al. (2006). Increased risk of complete congenital heart block in infants born to women with hypothyroidism and anti-Ro and/or anti-La antibodies. *J Rheumatol,* 33:167.

Tabbut S, Griswold WR, Ogino MT, et al. (1994). Multiple thromboses in a premature infant associated with maternal antiphospolipid syndrome. *J perinatol,* 14:66-70.

Vesel S, Mazić U, Blejec T, Podnar T. (2004). First-degree heart block in the fetus of an anti-SSA/Ro-positive mother: reversal after a short course of dexamethasone treatment. *Arthritis Rheum,* 50:2223.

Waltuck J, Buyon JP. (1994). Autoantibody-associated congenital heart block: outcome in mothers and children. *Ann Internal Med,* 120:544.

Wang D, Buyon JP, Zhu W, Chan EK. (1999) Defining a novel 75-kD a Phosphoprotein associated with SS-A/Ro and identification of distinct human autoantibodies. *J Clin Invest,* 104: 1265–1275.

Watson RM, Braunstein BL, Watson AJ, et al. (1986). Fetal wastage in women with anti-Ro/SSA antibody. *J Rheumatol,* 13:90-94.

White, P, Eustis, R. (1921). Congenital heart block. Am J Dis Child, 22:299.

Wisuthsarewong, Wanee M.D. et al. (2011). Neonatal Lupus Erythematosus: Clinical character, investigation, and Outcome. *Pediatric Dermatology,* 28(2):115-121

Wolach B, Choc L, Pomeranz A, et al. (1993). Aplastic anemia in neonatal lupus erythematosus. *Am J Dis Child,* 147:941.

Xiao GQ, Hu K, Boutjdir M. (2001). Direct inhibition of expressed cardiac l-and t-type calcium channels by igg from mothers whose children have congenital heart block. *Circulation,* 103:159

Yamada H, Kato EH, Ebina Y, et al. (1999). Fetal treatment of congenital heart block ascribed to anti-SSA antibody: case reports with observation of cardiohemodynamics and review of the literature. *Am J Reprod Immunol,* 42:226.

Yazici Y, Onel K, Sammaritano L. (2000). Neonatal lupus erythematosus in triplets. *J Rheumatol,* 27(3):807-809.

24

Maternal SLE Influence in Fetal Development: Immune and Endocrine Systems

Emma Rodriguez[1], Juan Gabriel Juarez-Rojas[1] and Luis Felipe Montaño[2]
[1]*Instituto Nacional de Cardiologia*
[2]*Universidad Nacional Autonoma de Mexico*
Mexico

1. Introduction

Pregnancy markedly alters the normal physiology of the women and immune response mechanisms. During normal pregnancy the immune system is reinforced to maintain the well-being of the mother and fetus by modifying the manner that a mother responds to the environment, in such a way that recognition, communication, trafficking and repair mechanisms are all uniformly regulated. In spite of the fact that the fetus could be considered a stranger to the mother´s immune system, maternal tolerance develops; the latter could be the result of the integration of numerous mechanisms promoted by different cells present in the decidua.

Autoimmunity even in the absence of clinically manifest autoimmune disease can affect each event of pregnancy and can induce fetal and maternal complications as well as adverse outcomes. The effect pregnancy has on the course of systemic lupus erythematosus (SLE) remains speculative. Elevated levels of auto-antibodies are frequently are associated with lost pregnancy, as they can cross placental barrier and make contact with blood vessels. Fetal endothelial cells make the first encounter with maternal cells or molecules that cross the placental barrier and this initial contact induces some primary regulation on endothelial cell activity thereby modifying inflammatory response or vascular tone, amongst others. If maternal antibodies cross the placental barrier, this could induce the expression of proinflammatory molecules, such as TNF-alpha, IL-6 or IL-8 (Yazici et al., 2001), by endothelial cells or could induce the formation of immune complexes that can cause fetal damage. Pregnant lupus patients are susceptible to preeclampsia, especially if they suffer lupus nephritis, and also to steroid-induced hypertension and hyperglycemia. At the same time fetuses are susceptible to placental insufficiency if antiphospholipid antibodies or other procoagulant states are present, and to neonatal lupus in the presence of anti-Ro/La antibodies (Lockshin & Sammaritano, 2003). The study of the physiology and immunology of pregnancy in SLE mothers may enhance our understanding of SLE and the possible consequences on the child development and quality of life.

2. Objective

To describe the effects of maternal SLE on the development of the immune and endocrine systems of the fetus during pregnancy and their postnatal consequences.

3. Immune system deregulation in SLE pregnant women

Systemic lupus erythematosus may remain silent, even undiagnosed, during many years in some women, but in others it may become more aggressive during pregnancy, placing both the mother and the fetus at risk. In general, active inflammation from rheumatic or autoimmune diseases poses a stronger threat to the well-being of both the mother and fetus than many immunosuppressant medications. Therefore, continued immune-suppression could be useful to allow for the most optimal pregnancy outcomes. Autoantibodies are a hallmark in autoimmune diseases but the real problem is the diminishing of their clearance and the subsequent immune complex formation that alters immune responses. Furthermore, the altered production of sexual hormones has an influence on immunity, since sexual dimorphism related to SLE development exists.

3.1 Pro-inflammatory molecules

The placenta serves as an immunologic barrier between the maternal and fetal circulations in normal situations. This barrier prevents the potential damage of maternal immune responses, since the fetus is considered a semiallogeneic graft. The trophoblast is the fetal tissue in most intimate contact with the maternal deciduas and it is crucial to the development of the normal placenta; it participates in the regulation of maternal immune responses but the mechanisms involved are still not clear. The placental barrier is continuously changing during pregnancy but the first hurdle between the invasive trophoblast and the circulating cells of the maternal immune system is the maternal endothelium of local vessels. Therefore, specialized mechanisms may exist regulating leukocyte extravasation into the deciduas, implicating an interaction between trophoblast antigens and maternal leukocytes.

Leukocyte recruitment is mediated by specialized cell adhesion molecules on the surface of circulating cells and their counterreceptors or ligands on the endothelium, especially integrins. The a4b7 integrin, for example, is a lymphocyte homing receptor for the mucosal vascular addressin MAdCAM-1 (mucosal addressin cell adhesion molecule 1), which is expressed by high endothelial venules (HEV) in mucosal lymphoid tissues. Another integrin, a4b1, binds to the vascular cell adhesion molecule 1 (VCAM-1), which can be induced in diverse sites of inflammation (Butcher et al., 1999). The major change in the end-term pregnant uterus is that the decidua basalis contains remarkably few maternal leukocytes in the lumina of the maternal vessels and in the tissue, suggesting decreased recruitment at this stage and it is associated with a loss of selectivity from trophoblast and maternal endothelial cells (Kruse et al., 2002).

Inflammatory cytokines and cell adhesion molecules (CAM) appear to be centrally involved in the pathogenesis of autoimmune diseases. During pregnancy it is possible that placental dysfunction may account for some complications. Hopefully in SLE pregnancy an inflammatory state where TNF-alpha, IL-1 or IL-6 could be elevated, is present. These cytokines can stimulate endothelial cells to express cell adhesion molecules like E-Selectin or P-Selectin, VCAM-1 and/or ICAM-1 to promote leukocyte migration. It has been observed that TNF-alpha may increase the level of IL-6 in human vein endothelial cells (HUVEC) both in SLE and normal mothers, without difference, but E-Selectin, VCAM-1 and ICAM-1 are reduced (Rodriguez et al., 2008). Therefore it is possible that the immune response in the offspring of SLE mothers could be diminished because endothelial cells of corial *villi* might not be activated or be noncompliant to stimulus, or in the SLE mother it could be diminished because there are increased levels of VCAM-1 and ICAM-1 in maternal serum related with a endothelial cells activation and those may contribute to an increased migration of leukocytes into placenta. Although circulating maternal concentration of soluble cell adhesion molecules showed differences between SLE patients and controls, no differences were observed when placental tissues were immunostained with the same cell adhesion molecule antibodies (Lakasing et al., 2000).

Antiphospholipid antibodies have been associated with thrombosis and endothelial cell activation, so they can enable the increased expression of CAMs and other cytokines by the endothelium, thus enhancing a proinflammatory state. TNF-alpha levels are increased in some diseases related to miscarriage. It is known that TNF-alpha modulates endothelial cells through the activation of NF-kappaB, a transcription factor which activates genes of proinflammatory molecules such as CAMs, but also prothrombotic factors such as tissue factor (TF), thrombomodulin and plasminogen activator inhibitor (PAI-1) (Scarpati & Sadler, 1989). This proinflammatory state would contribute to the malformation of the placenta, miscarriage and fetal circulating system alterations. TF expression on endothelial cells, monocytes and neutrophils is a hallmark of inflammatory conditions, such as sepsis, atherosclerosis, inflammatory bowel disease and systemic lupus erythematosus (Girardi et al., 2008).

3.2 The complement system

This system has a crucial role as an effector mechanism in placental and fetal damage that conduce to ill-fated pregnancy outcomes. In normal pregnancies there are many potential sites where the complement system could be activated as the intervillous space or deciduas, by interaction with the trophoblast. It has been suggested that complement activation during placentation should be highly regulated by locally expressed membrane-bound complement regulators, such as DAF, MCP and CD59, providing protection to the fetus (Girardi et al., 2011).

The complement is part of the innate immune system and can be activated through one of three pathways: the classical, the alternative, or the mannose-binding lectin. Central to each of these pathways is the cleavage of C3, resulting in the production of C3a and C3b. Upon its generation, C3b attaches covalently to cells and has binding affinity for a variety of circulating and cell-bound proteins, meanwhile C3a contributes to inflammatory responses such as leukocyte accumulation and enhancement of vascular permeability occurring in various infectious and noninfectious states. The final stage of complement activation by any pathway, is the formation of C5b by C5-convertase, where C3b is an important component. C5b, together with other complement molecules, form an attack complex bound to the membrane that destroys cells.

Girardi, et al. (2011) have proposed that the activation of complement system during placental and fetal injury is produced by antiphospholipid-autoantibodies, lack of regulatory proteins or activated T-cells. In patients with SLE, recurrent miscarriage, fetal growth restriction and intrauterine fetal death are frequently occurring complications of pregnancy, and it is highly possible that the auto-antibodies produced in SLE form an immune complex recognized by C1, which is the triggering of the complement system classical pathway. C1q, a component of C1, deserves special consideration for its role promoting trophoblast invasion of deciduas, a crucial step in normal placental development (Bulla, 2008). But, in human placenta of women with SLE, immunohistochemically stained for C4d and C1q, the presence of both molecules was observed and the presence of C4d was strongly related to adverse fetal outcome in the setting of SLE. The excessive deposition of C4d supports the concept of severe autoantibody-mediated injury at the fetal-maternal interface (Cohen et al., 2011).

The role of C3a in the pathogenesis of SLE has not been defined, but it has been found that the inhibition of complement activation at the level of C3-convertases significantly reduced renal disease in MRL/*lpr* mice (Bao et al., 2003). Given that inhibition of C3-convertases prevents generation of C3a (as well as C3b, C5a, and C5b-9), it is conceivable that the use of C3-convertase inhibitors, which limit C3a generation, might be of invaluable therapeutic benefit (Bao et al., 2005). One of the possible mechanisms that damage the developing placenta is through the action of anaphylotoxin C5a, which promotes neutrophil infiltration into the deciduas, leading to fetal death (Girardi et al., 2003). In some, but not in all, mice models of antiphospholipid syndrome (APS), complement activation plays a major role in pregnancy loss, with a massive accumulation of C3 in the placenta. Interestingly, C3 deficient mice do not show fetal reabsorption. Based upon these findings, anti-phospholipid antibodies and complement activation (via C3a, C5a, and MAC) may cooperate in the triggering a local inflammatory process, eventually leading to placental thrombosis, hypoxia, and neutrophil infiltration (Tincani et al., 2010).

3.3 Th1 and Th2 responses

Cytokines secreted by the embryos and cells within the uterus are important for the implantation process, but they can also be responsible for causing miscarriages. The activity of cytokines has been characterized as proinflammatory and anti-inflammatory depending on whether they are secreted by Th1 or Th2 T cells. Prolonged exposure to Th1 cytokines is detrimental to pregnancy, while Th2 cytokines are necessary to stimulate the invasion of the blastocyst and the formation of blood vessels during the implantation period. Trophoblastic cells, as well as uterine epithelium and maternal immune cells, secrete cytokines, which promote immunotolerance. Some of these cytokines are transforming growth factor beta, progesterone-induced blocking factor, and regeneration and tolerance factor. The sources of proinflamatory cytokines, such as interleukins, chemokines and TNF-alpha, are macrophages and NK cells, which infiltrate the implantation sites thus favoring pregnancy loss (Cerkiene et al., 2010).

The immune response is regulated by components of the innate immunity, including antigen-presenting cells (APCs) such as monocyte/macrophage and other phagocytic cells, as well as by components of the acquired immunity such as T helper (Th) cells, subdivided into subclasses Th1 and Th2. Th1 cells produce the cytokines interleukin IL-2, IL-12, interferon (IFN)-γ and tumor necrosis factor-alpha (TNF-alpha) and TNF-beta, whereas Th2 cells produce the cytokines IL-4, IL-6, IL-10 and IL-13. These Th1- and Th2-mediated immune responses are mutually inhibitory, and to some extent opposing (Elenkov & Chouosos, 1999). A strong, maybe deregulated Th1 response is often found in autoimmunity and there is compelling evidence for a third effector Th pathway, so-called Th17 T cells that secrete IL-17A and IL-17F, two cytokines not synthesized by either Th1 or Th2 CD4+ T cells (Saito 2010). Healthy pregnant women have a predominant TH1 response (Lit, 2007; Muñoz-Valle et al., 2003), whereas SLE pregnancy is accompanied by a TH2 response, especially through IL-10, that promote antibody production by B cells. (Viallard et al., 1999). This change could explain protection to the fetus from maternal Th1-cell attack, but a predominant Th2 type immunity in recurrent abortion cases has been observed. So it is not sufficient to know the Th1/Th2 relationship in order to explain the pathogenesis mechanisms in autoimmune diseases. Treg cells play a central role for induction of tolerance because they inhibit proliferation and cytokine production in both CD4+ and CD8+ T cells. An overstimulation of Th1 or Th2 immunity might be harmful for successful pregnancy. IL-17, a proinflammatory cytokine, has been observed in peripheral blood and deciduas in spontaneous abortion patients; moreover, Treg and Th17 cells can be inversely regulated by IL-6, which blocks the development of Treg cells and induces differentiation of Th17 cells (Saito et al., 2010). Auto-antibodies may induce secretion of IL-6 in mesangial cells (Bobst et al., 2005) and enhance IL-6 concentration in serum (Arslan et al., 2004), therefore they could be related to pregnancy loss.

If auto-antibodies cross the placenta, they would stimulate fetal endothelial cells to produce proinflammatory molecules like IL-6, so the Th1/Th2 immune balance could be modified in the offspring. Indeed, two transcription factors, T-bet (for Th1) and GATA-3 (for Th2), have been found to play an important role in the organogenesis of the immune system of the mice offspring during the perinatal period (Yamamoto et al., 2009). It is possible that autoantibodies of SLE mothers exert some modulation on the above mentioned transcription factors and they may induce some immune suppression on the new born child.

4. Hormonal levels in SLE+ pregnant women

Endocrine and immune systems work very closely to allow and maintain the development of gestation by means of hormones, cytokines and its receptors. These molecules can stimulate or suppress the activity both of them. Therefore, the regulation of autoimmnity by hormones or the alteration of hormone levels by immune responses happen during the reproductive age. The increase of progesterone and estrogens during normal pregnancy allow the regulation of implantation and placentation in order to avoid the rejection of the embryo and fetus.

Serum levels of steroid hormones vary during pregnancy in SLE patients, depending upon disease activity being increased in the second trimester and decreased in the third. However, estradiol and progesterone serum concentrations were found significantly reduced in SLE patients compared with controls (Doria, et al., 2002, 2004). The increase in sexual hormones during normal pregnancy boosts the humoral response and leads to a more efficient clearance of auto-antibodies. But in SLE women there is an increment of circulating auto-antibodies which is associated with a decrease of serum estrogen in the third trimester of pregnancy. Sex hormones are considered as major regulators of the immune response in SLE patients (Doria et al., 2006).

4.1 Estrogens

Estrogens are able to modulate immune response exerting specific effects on T and B cells, dendritic cells (DC) and peripheral blood mononuclear cells (PBMC), enhancing IL-10, IL-2, and IFN-gamma production, inhibiting TNF-alpha secretion by PBMC, stimulating antibody production by B cells, and decreasing apoptosis of DC and macrophages (Zen et al., 2010).

17-beta estradiol induces anti-apoptotic effects in monocyte and macrophage cell lines by interfering with NF-kB activities (Catelo et al., 2005). In consequence, if estrogens are reduced, the activity of NF-kB is augmented; therefore there will be a larger expression of cell adhesion molecules favoring a proinflammatory condition. Estrogen treatment induces an increase in the production of IL-10 and a decrease in that of TNF-alpha by PBMCs of patients with SLE, but not in healthy subjects (Evans et al., 1997). Because of the TNF-alpha regulatory function on apoptosis, the failure to maintain the production of this cytokine might alter the apoptosis of activated immune cells in SLE patients exposed to high estrogen concentrations, as it occurs in pregnancy.

The serum concentration of soluble adhesion molecules is higher in women with SLE than in normal women, but the placental values are identical (Abd-Elkareem et al., 2010, Lakasing et al., 2000). However, endothelial cells of umbilical cordons of SLE mothers express several times less CAMs (E-Selectin, VCAM-1, ICAM-1) compared with healthy mothers (Rodriguez, 2008). Even if a relationship between diminished serum estrogen and augmented serum CAMs levels exists in SLE patients, maternal estrogen does not exert any deleterious effect on the fetus endothelial cells (FEC). That may be possible if FEC could exhibit immunotolerance or lack estrogen receptors. It is assumed that estrogen regulation upon the immune system uses different pathway in the fetus compared with the SLE mother.

4.2 Androgens

Sexual dimorphism has been shown in SLE diseases since women are more affected than men. In fact, androgens seem to act in counter part to estrogens modulating the immune response; because of that, they have been used as therapy on SLE patients (Gordon et al., 2008). However, it has been shown that androgens can favor adverse effects on circulating lipids increasing the risk of atherosclerosis (Nutall et al., 2003).

Some favorable effects of androgens on immunity are to inhibit Il-1b and IL-6 secretion by PBMC, enhance IL-2 secretion by T cells and inhibit antibody secretion by B cells. Testosterone also exerts pro-apoptotic effects and reduces macrophage proliferation, and inhibits IL-1b and IL-6 secretion by PBMC (Zen et al., 2010).

Testosterone and related steroid hormones have a variety of effects on the immune system. Dehydroepiandrosterone (DHEA), the major product of the adrenal glands in both men and women, whose sulphated (DHEA-S) molecule is its inactivated form, stimulates IL-2 production (Dillon, 2005) and reduces IL-10 (Chang et al., 2004) in normal T cells, therefore favoring the Th1 pathway. But in SLE patients a significant finding is that serum levels of DHEA-S and other adrenal androgens and cortisol are decreased (Zen et al., 2010). Decreased adrenal production, increased conversion or conjugation to downstream hormones are the most likely causes of inadequately low serum levels of adrenal hormones in SLE (Straub 2004). It is believed that lower levels of androgen is a cause of proinflammatory events. In SLE pregnant women, differences in androgen levels compared with normal pregnant women have not been found (Doria, et al., 2002).

4.3 Progesterone

Progesterone is the most important hormone during pregnancy reaching its higher levels at the third trimester of pregnancy. All throughout the sexual cycle, progesterone modulates immune responses generating protection to the female tract against microorganisms. Progesterone can act enhancing IL-4, IL-5, IL-6, and IL-10 production, and inhibiting IFN-gamma secretion by PBMC, stimulating antibody generation by B cells, and decreasing T cell proliferation. Also, it induces the secrection of a 34-kD protein, named "Progesterone-induced blocking factor" (PIBF), which is known to regulate humoral and cell-immune responses in several ways (Beagley & Gockel, 2003), including the induction of a Th2-dominant cytokine profile (Lashley et al., 2011). During pregnancy Th2 polarization occurs both in the systemic circulation and at the feto-maternal interface, enhancing IL-3, IL-4, IL-5 and IL-10 production. Thus, high progesterone levels might contribute to successful pregnancy, favoring feto-allograft tolerance (Zen et al., 2010).

Disproportional changes of progesterone levels in pregnant women are associated with different manifestations of autoimmune pathologies since Th1-related diseases such as rheumatoid arthritis tend to improve, whereas Th2-related diseases may get worse (Tait 2008). Lower production of progesterone is seen during SLE pregnancy, especially in the third trimester compared with normal pregnancies (Doria eta al., 2004).

Progesterone plays a key important role at many levels including control of neuroendocrine responses to stress, procuring required immune balance and controlling placental and decidual function. A lack of progesterone can explain many unwanted consequences (Douglas 2010). It is possible to speculate that lack of progesterone in SLE mothers could cause damaging effects in the offspring's future development.

4.4 Prolactin

Different to steroids hormones, prolactin is a peptide produced by the adenohypophysis but also by neurons, endothelium, mammary epithelium, leukocytes and thymocytes. Prolactin has pleiotropic effects on the immune system and it appears to stimulate both humoral and cell-mediated immune responses, through enhanced IL-1, IL-2, IL-12, and IFN-gamma secretion by PBMC. It also stimulate antibody secretion, decreases B cell apoptosis, and T cell proliferation (Vera-Lastra et al, 2002), but it specifically promotes the survival of the T-cell-dependent autoreactive follicular B-cell subset, and enhances the development of antigen presenting cells expressing MHC class II and costimulatory molecules CD40, CD80, and CD86 (Matera et al., 2001). The effect of prolactin on antigen presentation and on B-T cells interaction results in increased response to MHC presented auto-antigens, leading to the loss of self tolerance. The interaction between CD40 on B cells and CD40L on T cells up-regulates the expression of the antiapoptotic molecule Bcl-2 leading to autoreactive B cell rescue from negative selection which reduces tolerance to self (Peeva et al., 2003). Thus, hyperprolactinaemia has been found to be a risk factor for the development of autoimmunity by favoring Th1 immunity.

High levels of serum prolactin have been found in a subset of SLE patients associated with active disease, promoting deficiency of dendritic cell functions, suggesting a lack of induction of T and B cell activity (Jara et al., 2008). Hyperprolactinaemia is associated with several autoantibodies involved in SLE such as antinuclear antibodies (ANA), anti-double stranded DNA (anti-dsDNA), anticardiolipin, and hypocomplementaemia (Zen et al, 2010).

4.5 Hormone receptors

The effects of sexual hormones are mediated through membrane receptors independent of their isoform or the tissue and physiological condition of the host. The relationship between estrogens and its receptor (ER) may play an important role in the pathogenesis of SLE. Results obtained from a mouse model of lupus (NZB/NZW) suggest that ER-alpha activation exerts a stimulatory effect on the endocrine response whereas ER-beta activation appears to induce a slightly immunosuppressive effect on the disease (Li & McMurray, 2007). It has also been reported that ER-alpha mRNA expression is increased and ER-beta mRNA expression decreased in PBMC (Inui et al., 2007) as well as CD4+ T cells (Phiel et al., 2005) of SLE patients.

The presence of estrogen receptors on the cells involved in the immune response, namely thymocytes, macrophages and endothelial cells is well recognized. Estrogens modulate cytokine production by target cells, through interference with their transcriptional activity. The effect of estrogens on the expression of protooncogenes and oncosuppressor genes involved in apoptosis might also be relevant to human autoimmunity (Cutolo et al.,, 1995). It is possible that different polymorphisms of the ER-alpha gene, are involved in SLE development and apparently they are related to sex, age at the onset of the disease, and the appearance of some clinically relevant symptoms, suggesting that these polymorphisms might contribute to SLE susceptibility (Johansson et al., 2005).

Gonadotropin releasing hormone (GnRH) is a hypothalamic and pituitary hormone known to exert immune actions. GnRH administration has been associated with gender-specific alterations in mRNA expression of the GnRH and IL-2 receptors, after 2 weeks of treatment. These differences might be attributable to gender differences in response to gonadectomy. GnRH and GnRH receptor mRNA levels vary dynamically with the estrous cycle in lymphoid organs in the intact female mouse thus contributing to gender differences in the development and activity SLE patients (Jacobson et al., 1999). Interestingly, it has been recently shown that prolactin exerts a regulatory influence on GnRH through dopamine and LH (Hodson et al., 2010).

5. Auto-bodies in SLE pregnant women

Autoimmunity originates after breaking self-tolerance of the immune system, a process that involves many different molecules and yet poorly understood processes. It remains an open question whether bacterial or viral pathogens contribute to the initiation of these diseases as major causative agents (Borchers et al., 2010). The presence of autoantibodies has been mainly associated with pathologic states, probably because they were first described as a hallmark of autoimmune diseases. Indeed, endothelial cell autoantibodies (AECA) are often reported in conditions where pathologic autoantibodies bind to activated or damaged endothelial cells.

5.1 Non active SLE

Although it is increasingly recognized that autoimmunity, even in the absence of clinically manifest autoimmune disease, can affect every aspect of pregnancy (starting with fertilization) and can contribute to maternal complications and adverse fetal outcomes, (Cervera & Balasch, 2008) the risk of lupus flare is not as great as many people used to think and flares, when they do occur, are not necessarily severe. The best prevention of SLE flares during pregnancy is the delay of conception until a woman has had quiescent SLE for at least 6 months. In many situations, however, this is not possible and the continuation of medications for SLE helps to prevent flares.

In the past, patients stopped all their therapy when they discovered that they were pregnant. This may very well have contributed to the increased risk of disease flare during pregnancy, especially in patients with a history of renal involvement and other forms of serious lupus disease. Patients should now be counseled before becoming pregnant, and in early pregnancy, about the use of appropriate drugs. (Gordon, 2004)

Many women with SLE take hydroxychloroquine (HCQ) (Plaquenil) prior to pregnancy. This medication decreases the risk of SLE flare, improves the prognosis of SLE nephritis, and prevents death. (Kasitanon et al., 2006) It is also very well tolerated with arguably the best side-effect profile of any medication available to treat SLE. An expert panel, comprised of 29 international leaders in research and care of women with SLE, recently recommended the continuation of HCQ during pregnancy. (Ostensen et al., 2006) Among over 300 pregnancies described in the literature that were exposed to HCQ for the treatment of autoimmune disease, no elevation of fetal anomalies was identified. When chloroquine is taken at supratherapeutic doses, there may be ocular or auditory damage. However, no such changes were seen among 133 babies exposed to HCQ *in utero*. (Costedoat-Chalumeau, 2003).

In non-pregnant SLE patients, the cessation of HCQ is associated with a 2-fold risk of SLE flare within the following 6 months. Among pregnant SLE patients, the risk for flare also increases when HCQ is discontinued. In the Hopkins Lupus Pregnancy Cohort, 38 women discontinued HCQ just prior to or early in pregnancy due to concerns about fetal exposure whereas 56 women continued HCQ throughout pregnancy (Clowse et al., 2006) Among those who discontinued the medication, the risk for increased lupus activity, whether measured by the absolute physician's estimate of activity or the SLEDAI scale was significantly increased. More of these women required corticosteroid therapy at higher doses than those who continued HCQ treatment. Within this cohort, as in other reports, there was no increase in fetal abnormalities after HCQ exposure. The pregnancy outcomes among women who continued and discontinued HCQ were similar. This likely reflects the type of SLE activity that women who discontinued HCQ suffered: they did not have increased rates of lupus nephritis, anemia, or thrombocytopenia. Instead, women who discontinued HCQ had increased incidence of fatigue and joint symptoms. Though these symptoms are uncomfortable, they are generally not life-threatening nor require cytotoxic therapy. They may, however, prompt the initiation or the increase of corticosteroid therapy in mid-pregnancy. Again, little data is available about the use of azathioprine in inactive SLE pregnancy. In the Hopkins Lupus Pregnancy Cohort, 31 pregnancies were exposed to azathioprine. (Ostensen et al., 2006) Among the women who conceived while taking azathioprine and continued it through pregnancy, 2 out of 13 ended in pregnancy loss, both women had developed active SLE in pregnancy. Among the 10 women who maintained low lupus activity and azathioprine throughout pregnancy, all gave birth to live newborns at 34 weeks or greater gestations. Based on these data, azathioprine treatment should be continued throughout pregnancy, especially if the woman required it prior to pregnancy to treat her lupus (Clowse, 2007). It is also recommended to switch women from mycophenolate mofetil (MMF) to azathioprine prior to conception to avoid the teratogenic effects of the MMF.

5.2 Active SLE

Mild activity SLE can be treated with low dose prednisone (under 20mg per day) as required. The side effects include increased risk for hypertension and diabetes, just as in a non-pregnant woman. There may be a 2-fold increased risk for cleft lip or palate with systemic corticosteroid use, though the absolute risk for this remains low (about 20 per 10,000 babies with corticosteroid exposure) (Pradat et al. 2003).

Nonsteroidal anti-inflammatory drugs (NSAIDs) can be used during the late part of the first trimester and during the second trimester. There is evidence, in a murine model, that COX enzymes are important for embryo implantation, which may explain the increased risk for early miscarriage in women taking NSAIDs around the time of conception. (Clowse, 2007). NSAIDs are considered fairly safe in the second trimester, though they may decrease fetal

renal excretion and therefore promote oligohydramnios. (Holmes and Stone, 2000). NSAIDs should be stopped in the third trimester for 2 reasons: they can prolong labor and may promote premature closure of the ductus arteriosis. (Ostensen et al., 2006).
Moderate lupus activity can also be treated with higher doses of corticosteroids, including pulse-dose steroids. Only a small percentage of each dose of prednisone and prednisolone crosses the materno-fetal barrier. However, fluorinated glucocorticoids, such as dexamethasone and betamethasone, easily transfer to the fetus. These steroids can be helpful in treating the fetus, in particular in promoting fetal lung maturity prior to a preterm delivery. However, they have also been associated with lasting adverse effects on the offspring. Children exposed to these corticosteroids may have increased blood pressure and cognitive deficits. (Velíšek, 2011, Rothenberger et al., 2011) Therefore, dexamethasone and betamethasone should not be used to treat lupus activity during pregnancy.
The commencement of azathioprine in mid-pregnancy for a lupus flare may be risky. There is little data published on the use of azathioprine in lupus pregnancy. However, in the Hopkins Lupus Pregnancy Cohort there was an increase in pregnancy loss among woman who used azathioprine to treat a moderate to severe flare. Of the 8 pregnancies treated with azathioprine, 5 (63%) resulted in pregnancy loss, whereas only 1 out of 9 (11%) without azathioprine had a misscarriage (p=0.02). (Clowse, 2007)
Another option for the treatment of lupus in mid-pregnancy is intravenous immunoglobin (IVIg). IVIg can be particularly helpful in controlling hematologic and renal disease (Friedman et al., 2010). There are no published series of IVIg use in pregnancy for lupus patients, however there are multiple reports of IVIg use to prevent recurrent miscarriage. In these cases, the primary outcome is live birth, and there is no change in this rate with the use of IVIg. Little has been published on the effects of IVIg on the offspring, but cell count levels seem to be stable and no congenital anomalies have been reported. IVIg´s that contain sucrose can prompt renal insufficiency, but this has not held back the treatment of non-pregnant women with lupus nephritis (Micheloud, 2006). Some women will develop headaches, rigors, or fevers with IVIg therapy, but more severe side effects are rare.
Cyclophosphamide (Cytoxan) and mycophenolate mofetil (Cellcept) should be avoided during pregnancy. First trimester exposure to cyclophosphamide causes fetal abnormalities in a significant minority of patients. Exposure in the second and third trimesters does not increase the risk for fetal anomalies among women treated for breast cancer during pregnancy. Of the 3 SLE pregnancies with cyclophosphamide treatment during mid-pregnancy reported in the literature, only one resulted in a live birth. (Clowse et al, 2005b). Cyclophosphamide should only be used when all other options are exhausted and a forthright discussion about the risk for pregnancy loss has been discussed with the mother. The data on the use of mycophenolate mofetil in pregnancy are scarce but worrisome. There appears to be an elevated risk for both fetal anomalies and pregnancy losses especially in SLE mothers.

6. Placental barrier and auto-antibody transfer

During pregnancy the placenta plays a very important role in the mechanism that regulates and maintains a suitable communication between the mother (matro-environment) and the fetus (micro-environment). The placental barrier, mainly constituted by syncytiotrophoblast, cytotrophoblast, mesenchyma and endothelium, is continuously changing while the gestation progresses, in such a way that the placental barrier becomes, at the third trimester, a thin layer constituted by syncytiotrophoblast and chorionic-vessels endothelium. These morphological changes affect the traffic of cells and molecules through the placenta that could affect fetal development. Endothelial cells control the traffic of molecules and cells across the vessel wall and play an active role in hemostasis, inflammatory reactions, and immunity. The vascular cells dynamically respond to molecular signals, actively regulating many aspects of vascular homeostasis, including metabolic and cellular events, and executing a major role in the modulation of immune–inflammatory responses.

6.1 Maternal auto-antibodies and its effect on the developing fetal immune system

Immunoglobulins with the ability to bind to endothelial cell surface antigens are commonly known as AECA, and are often reported in conditions where potentially pathologic autoantibodies bind to activated or damaged endothelial cells (Salomonsson, 2010). However, natural AECA of both the IgG and IgM classes have been described. These antibodies, present in the serum of healthy individuals, are strictly controlled in terms of antigen specificity, and their expression may be regulated by the idiotypic network (Vazquez-del Mercado, 2006). This control is lost in SLE (Dhar & Sokl, 2006) in which IgG-AECA display quantitative and qualitative modifications and exert proinflammatory effects on cultured endothelial cells (Munther, 2006). So far, little work has been done on AECA expression in pregnant healthy subjects and in pregnant SLE patients.

6.2 Maternal auto-antibodies and its effect on the development of the embryonic and fetal heart

Complete atrioventricular block (AVB), in 91% of affected neonates, results from neonatal lupus erythematosus, a disease associated with transplacental passage of maternal anti-Ro/SSA and/or anti-La/SSB antibodies (Salomonsson, 2010). The mothers of these neonates are commonly diagnosed with SLE, Sjögren syndrome (SS), or other rheumatic diseases, although many are asymptomatic. Complete fetal AVB, which usually develops during gestational weeks 16 to 24, conveys a significant fetal mortality (15% to 30%) and morbidity rate, where two thirds on the affected offspring will require permanent pacing (Dhar & Sokol, 2006). It has been suggested that complete AVB may result from unresolved wound healing and scarring subsequent to transdifferentiation of cardiac fibroblasts into proliferating myofibroblasts, initiated by the specific maternal antibodies (Buyon et al., 1996). The process that leads to AVB may rarely progress postnatally. Given the high recurrence in neonates of SLE mothers (18% to 25%), complete AVB could be expected to occur in approximately 1-3 of the every 70 newborns whose mothers have anti-SSA/Ro or anti-SSB/Lb antibodies (Rein AJJT, 2009).

Membrane-associated LA protein is required for the in vivo normal maintenance of the inner cell mass (ICM) of the blastocyst, thus demonstrating that nullizygous disruption of the LA gene leads to early embryonic lethality, consistent with the observed critical defect in the ICM of the blastocyst observed during blastocyst outgrowth. (Park JM, 2006). One difficulty in identifying a pathogenic effect of an autoantibody is accounting for the heterogeneity of that effect. Congenital heart block (CHB) is a paradigmatic example in that not only is the injury seemingly rare, but the degree of injury varies along a spectrum from clinically inconsequential first-degree block through third-degree (complete) block and even, in some cases, an associated cardiomyopathy that is often fatal. Identification of a necessary or essential factor is only part of the challenge in defining the pathology of CHB, since recurrence rates from one pregnancy to the next are 18%, not 100%, and identical twins are, with rare exception, discordant for the disease. Antibodies to the 52-kd SSA/Ro protein (Ro 52) are found in 80% of mothers whose children have CHB (Clansy RM, 2005) and it has been suggested that the core of the problem is that SSA/Ro or SSB/LA antigens translocate and then there is surface binding by maternal autoantibodies, and then through a TGF-beta mediated mechanism, scaring and blockade is initiated.

7. Anomalies in newborns from SLE positive mothers

In addition to causing pregnancy complications and adverse pregnancy outcomes, transplacental passage of maternal autoantibodies of the IgG isotype can result in a variety of neonatal diseases. Among the best known of these is the neonatal lupus syndrome (NLS), which can appear as cutaneous lesions resembling those of SLE (16–50%), life-threatening congenital complete heart blockade (CCHB, 1–2%), and hematological (~26%) and hepatobiliary manifestations (9–24%) (Hoftman et al. 2008). The prevalence of anti-SSA/SSB antibodies varies considerably in different ethnic groups. Overall, ~1–2% of women are thought to have anti-SSA/SSB antibodies, and estimates of the risk of them having a child affected by NLS range between 2% and 52% in prospective studies (Brucato, 2001). Only 1–2% of anti-SSA/SSB antibody positive mothers will give birth to a child with CCHB. The large variation stems from differences in the thoroughness with which the various (and frequently asymptomatic) manifestations of NLS are determined and the length of follow-up since some of the NLS symptoms, including the cutaneous lesions, are not always obvious at birth. The risk that a second child is affected ranges between 15% and 20%. The fact that not all children of women with anti-SSA/SSB antibodies develop NSL indicates that other factors, probably including fetal ones, play a role. NLS is almost invariably associated (in 95% of cases) with maternal antibodies against Ro/SSA alone or in conjunction with anti-La/SSB. Anti-U1-RNP (ribonucleoprotein) antibodies are associated exclusively with the cutaneous manifestations of NLS. All of these antibodies are found primarily in women with SLE. Interestingly, there are some suggestions that infants of mothers with SLE are more rarely affected by CCHB than those of mothers with Sjögren's syndrome or with undifferentiated connective tissue disease (Borchers, 2010). In contrast, there are indications that the presence of hypothyroidism increases the risk of CCHB, but not NLS overall, in infants of anti-SSA-positive mothers regardless of whether they have an underlying autoimmune disease or are asymptomatic. Of particular note, a recent report on the long-term follow-up of 49 children with NSL indicated that definitive autoimmune diseases were already present in 6 of 49 affected children (5 of them female) at a mean age of 14.8 years, but in none of the 45 unaffected siblings or the 53 unrelated controls (Martin et at., 2002) . Similarly, it has been reported that children and adolescents diagnosed with autoimmune thyroid disease had been exposed to maternal thyroid peroxidase antibodies in utero more frequently than randomly selected control children (Svensson, et al 2006). This strongly suggests that, in addition to inheritance of susceptibility genes from an affected mother, transplacental exposure to maternal autoantibodies predisposes one to the development of autoimmune diseases.

7.1 Cardiovascular

A frequent outcome in newborns of SLE mothers is fetal intrauterine growth retardation, which is associated with long-term medical complications such as adult-onset hypertension.

Maternal immune deregulation may play a role in the appearance of diseases such as myocarditis, autoimmnunity and probably atherosclerosis. Cardiac injury is presumed to be dependent on the transplacental passage of maternal IgG autoantibodies via Fc receptor-bearing trophoblasts and the target antigens of the antibodies have been molecularly cloned and identified as three separate proteins: 52 kDa SSA=Ro and 60 kDa SSA=Ro, which share no sequence homology, and 48 kDa SSB=La (Tincani et al, 2010). Sera containing anti-Ro and anti-La antibodies can induce atrioventricular block and inhibit L-type calcium currents in ventricular myocytes in vitro. The developing myocardium appears to be particularly sensitive to the effects of these antibodies because Ro and La are localized in the surface blebs of apoptosing myocytes. (Tseng et al., 1999)

The more severe condition of congenital heart blockade was bradycardia which was observed in 53% of the pregnancies between weeks 16 and 24, in 24% of pregnancies between weeks 25 and 30 weeks and in 23% of pregnancies after week 30. Congenital heart block may be associated with myocarditis, but clinical heart failure is fortunately uncommon. Lesser degrees of heart blockade are sometimes detected prior to the development of congenital third-degree heart blockade and may reverse with fluorinated steroids such as dexamethasone. Heart failure associated with myocarditis and first- and second-degree block may be reversible with steroids. As prednisolone does not cross the placenta, dexamethasone should be used. (Gordon, 2004) There is no evidence to date that established third-degree heart blockade can be reversed with dexamethasone, but in cases where there is strong suspicion that the blockade has developed within the past few days, it may be worth a therapeutic trial. Over half of the children with congenital heart blockade will require a pacemaker by the age of 1 year-old, sadly about one-third will need it within the first month of life. Some of the remaining children will require pacemakers by the age of 12. Up to 20% of children with congenital heart block die in infancy (Gordon, 2004).

In order to identify heart blockade as early as possible, when treatment may be beneficial, mothers with anti-Ro antibodies should have the fetal heart rate assessed weekly from the week 16 onwards by auscultation, and by ultrasound scans monthly, including a detailed scan looking for cardiac abnormalities at 20 weeks of pregnancy. An ECG should be performed after delivery as some neonates develop more severe degrees of blockade after birth. (Askanase et al., 2002). About half the cases of neonatal lupus syndrome will occur in children whose mothers do not have confirmed systemic connective tissue diseases; at least half of these children will develop Sjogren's syndrome or mild lupus over the following 10 years. If a mother has delivered a child with congenital heart blockade, the risk of this recurring in subsequent pregnancies is about one in five (Tseng & Buyon, 1997).

7.2 Immune response

Maternal tolerance of the fetal allograft could be the result of the integration of numerous mechanisms promoted by different cells present in the decidua. Decidual macrophages and dendritic cells, which are found in close association with T lymphocytes are the most potent activators of T lymphocyte responses and could play a sentinel function for the immune system, initiating antigen-specific T cell responses to fetal antigens. T cell cytokines produced in response to fetal molecules could have a role in the maintenance or in the failure of pregnancy. The levels of LIF, IL-4, IL-10 and macrophage colony stimulating factor produced by decidual T cells of women suffering from unexplained spontaneous abortion are lower than those of normal pregnant women indicating that these cytokines may contribute to the maintenance of pregnancy. T cells from the cumulus oophorus surrounding the blastocyst produce LIF and IL-4. These findings suggest that cytokines produced by maternal T cells create a suitable microenvironment for the proper implantation process and further development of the placenta (Piccinni MP, 2005).

From the early developmental stages onward, the secretory activity of placenta cells clearly contributes to increased local, as well as systemic levels, of cytokines and inflammatory molecules. Two aspects of the progression of the immune response have been thoroughly investigated: the highly regulated process of throphoblast invasion and blastocyst implantation, and the induction of preterm labor associated with infections. With the progression of pregnancy, the physiological role of most placental cytokines is uncertain, since many of them are similar to adipose tissue derived cytokines. It is possible that they contribute to the low grade systemic inflammation that develops during the third trimester of pregnancy.

Maternal transmission of IgG antibodies to the fetus usually occurs between weeks 16 and 32 (Tseng & Buyon 1997), but an autoimmune condition in the neonate may not be diagnosed until after delivery. The best-recognized condition is neonatal lupus syndrome due to the transmission of anti-Ro and/or anti-La antibodies to the fetus from a mother with lupus, primary Sjogren's syndrome or an undifferentiated connective tissue disease. There are three reports of neonatal cutaneous vasculitis in infants born to mothers with cutaneous polyarteritis nodosa (PAN) that appeared early after delivery and resolved with treatment soon after birth, with no neonatal deaths. (Borrego et al., 1997). A case of hypersensitivity vasculitis that deteriorated in pregnancy and postpartum, and that was associated with an identical vasculitis rash in the newborn, has been reported, it was almost certainly associated with the transmission of a maternal autoantibody, although none was identified (Morton, 1998). Neonatal thrombocytopenia is a well recognized consequence of the transmission of anti-platelet antibodies from the mother to the fetus and the transmission of anti-phospholipid antibodies has also been reported. However, most infants born of thrombocytopenic mothers with SLE have normal platelet counts. IgG Coombs' hemolytic antibody may also be transmitted to the fetus and can cause hemolysis in the fetus and newborn. Antiphospholipid antibody causes placental insufficiency, intrauterine growth restriction and fetal death but does not usually cause abnormalities in the infant, although fetal thrombosis has been detected (Tincani et al., 2003). IgG1 and IgG3 antiphospholipid antibodies not only affect the placental barrier but reach the fetus (Sammaritano et al., 1997) and induce the secretion of TF and other inflammatory cytokines by FEC thus favouring a prothrombotic state. Infants do not usually develop APS from maternal antibodies, but exceptions do occur in women with anti-SSA/Ro or anti-SSB/La antibodies, where neonatal lupus development is a risk (Buyon & Clancy, 2003). In all cases of neonatal transmission of autoantibodies, the disease in the neonate usually resolves over 3–6 months as maternal antibodies are gradually destroyed in the infant. But there are many questions to be solved still, such as: What do these maternal antibodies do to the newborn? Do they initiate an early proinflammatory signaling pathway? Do they induce immune complex formations that eventually lead to tissue damage? Do they induce immune tolerance?

The two main determinants of fetal outcome in patients with autoimmune diseases are the degree of active disease at conception and the presence of anti-phospholipid antibodies. The two main outcomes are fetal loss and premature delivery. The term 'fetal loss' includes spontaneous abortions under 10 weeks, miscarriages between 10 and 24 weeks, and stillbirths from 24 weeks onwards. Fetal loss occurs in about 20% of pregnancies in women with lupus (Petri, 2004). Retrospective studies have shown that active disease at conception and a history of renal disease are associated with a higher risk of fetal loss, but more recent prospective studies do not support this conclusion and show that the main predictor of fetal loss is the presence of high concentrations of anti-phospholipid antibodies. (Meroni et al., 2010). Anti-phospholipid antibodies are also associated with intrauterine growth retardation and pre-eclampsia that may result in premature delivery. These complications are the result of uteroplacental dysfunction, but the mechanisms involved are poorly understood. Early pregnancy loss may result from a failure of placentation owing to the effects of anti-phospholipid antibodies on anionic phospholipids and the co-factor B2-glycoprotein 1 on trophoblasts (Serdiuk, 2008). Second- and third-trimester losses are more likely to result from the damage to the uteroplacental vasculature since histological data reveals massive infarction of the decidual and placental vessels in human and experimental APS. Platelet deposition, prostanoids imbalance and spiral artery vasculopathy may contribute to fetal hypoxia which would lead to fetal death. In stillbirth, the most common predisposing factor to prematurity in SLE mothers, are IgG isotype antibodies (Motta et al. 2009). There is evidence that active SLE at conception, a history of renal disease and maternal high blood pressure increase the risk of a prematurity (Shah et al., 2001). Premature babies, irrespective of the underlying cause, may suffer from complications such as pulmonary immaturity, infection and feeding problems and developmental abnormalities all of which may cause neonatal death. To induce the rapid maturation of the lungs whose hallmark is a shortage of surfactant, a short course of dexamethasone is usually given over 48 hours to the mother if a premature delivery is considered likely because of maternal disease, poor fetal growth or signs of pulmonary distress. Use of antenatal dexamethasone in premature babies to promote lung maturity may significantly diminish the incidence of respiratory distress syndrome and additionally, mortality (5.7% versus 14.8%) and use of the neonatal intensive care unit (12.9% versus 21.1%) were reduced (Nayeri et al., 2005). Therefore, use of corticosteroids during gestation or perinatally could be beneficial to the fetus and SLE mother outcomes.

The most typical feature of neonatal lupus syndrome is a photosensitive rash on the face and scalp, usually erythematous, annular or elliptical (Tseng & Buyon, 1997), that is often precipitated by exposure to sunlight in the first couple of months after delivery or following ultraviolet light exposure if the newborn developed neonatal jaundice. This rash may be accompanied by purpura caused by thrombocytopenia or by haemolytic anaemia. These haematological manifestations may result from the transmission of anti-platelet or anti-erythrocyte antibodies. Other possible manifestations of neonatal lupus include hepatosplenomegaly and abnormal liver function tests without evidence of biliary tract obstruction. Neurological manifestations such as aseptic meningitis and myelopathy are very rare.

7.3 Central nervous system

The central nervous system (CNS) is susceptible to suffer damage during embryo and fetal development. Although in autoimmune diseases, such as SLE, antibodies react with double-stranded DNA forming immune complex that affect several organs including the brain, spinal cord and nerves, the mechanisms involved are not fully understood.

Antibodies and maternal autoantibodies that cross the placental barrier are believed to be responsible of almost all the fetal alterations in NLE, specially the autoantibodies against ribonucleoproteins SSB/La, SSA/Ro and SSA/Ro. Although the most severe and frequent manifestation of neonatal lupus is third-degree heart blockade, which usually begins during the second trimester of gestation, there are other manifestations such as rash, present in 15-

25% of children with NLE, asymptomatic elevation of liver function tests seen in 10-25% of cases, or some neurological manifestations like hydrocephalus, non-specific white matter changes and alterations of brain vessels (Silverman, 2010).

Less evident alterations during development of CNS could be associated to behavior and movement. There are reports that mothers of individuals with autism have antibodies that react with brain proteins and when these antibodies are passively transferred to pregnant non-human primates or rodents the offspring has behavioral and nervous system changes. It is still not clear whether the antibodies found in mothers of individuals with autism actually play a role in the disease. More studies need to be performed to identify the proteins recognized by the antibodies and to determine how these could affect development, behavior and changes within the CNS (Libbey, 2010). Besides, the high incidence of learning disorders in children born to mothers with SLE may be due to the passage of antibodies, mainly IgGs, through the brain barrier. Given that the blood brain barrier is not fully formed in utero, the pathogenic antibodies in maternal circulation represent a risk factor for fetal brain development (Lee, 2009).

Maternal antibodies that pass from the mother to the fetal circulation could interact with proteins or cell receptors to produce organ and tissue damage during gestation. In a murine model of lupus, NP-SLE, it has been shown that nervous system involvement can include seizures, stroke and other cerebrovascular events, psychosis, cognitive dysfunction, and notably a very high incidence of mood disorders, particularly anxiety and depression (Gulinello, 2011). Actually, it has been reported that the involvement of 5-HT4 receptors in congenital heart blockade associated to a systemic autoimmune response in the mother. 5-HT4 receptor isoforms can be expressed in both central and peripheral organs and it is possible that they are important in order to maintain the normal cellular activity (Eftekhari, 2000). Also 5-HT4 receptors have been reported to be involved in memory and learning as well as in gastrointestinal function, although almost nothing is known about its role in embryogenesis. The importance of the embryonic serotoninergic system in central nervous and cardiovascular functions has been largely described [Lambert, 2001; 15-20]. In early mouse embryogenesis, maternal serotonin (5-HT) activates different 5-HT receptors to control gene expression, migration and proliferation of neuronal crest and neuronal-crest derived cells (Kamel, 2007).

When disease manifestations are not so apparent it is too hard to make a diagnostic or an association with a specific pathology, which is the case for SLE. The main alterations could be related with CNS. However, it is not possible to discard environmental factors modulating the interactions of maternal antibodies and autoantibodies with the treatment used. According to Tincani, et. al. (2006), children with complete CHB need permanent pacing, but apparently do not have neuropsychological problems. Nevertheless, their neuropsychological development shows an increased number of learning disabilities, even in children with normal intelligence. The need to consider fetal consequences when the SLE mother is being treated should always be considered thus preferentially choosing non teratogenic drugs, but the withdrawal of medications just because the patient is pregnant should be avoided to protect of SLE flares.

8. Conclusion

Newborns from SLE mothers can have a myriad of silent or openly clear manifestations in several organs, tissues and systems of the newborn, some of which are secondary to the transfer of maternal autoantibodies through the placenta as well as the brain barrier, that

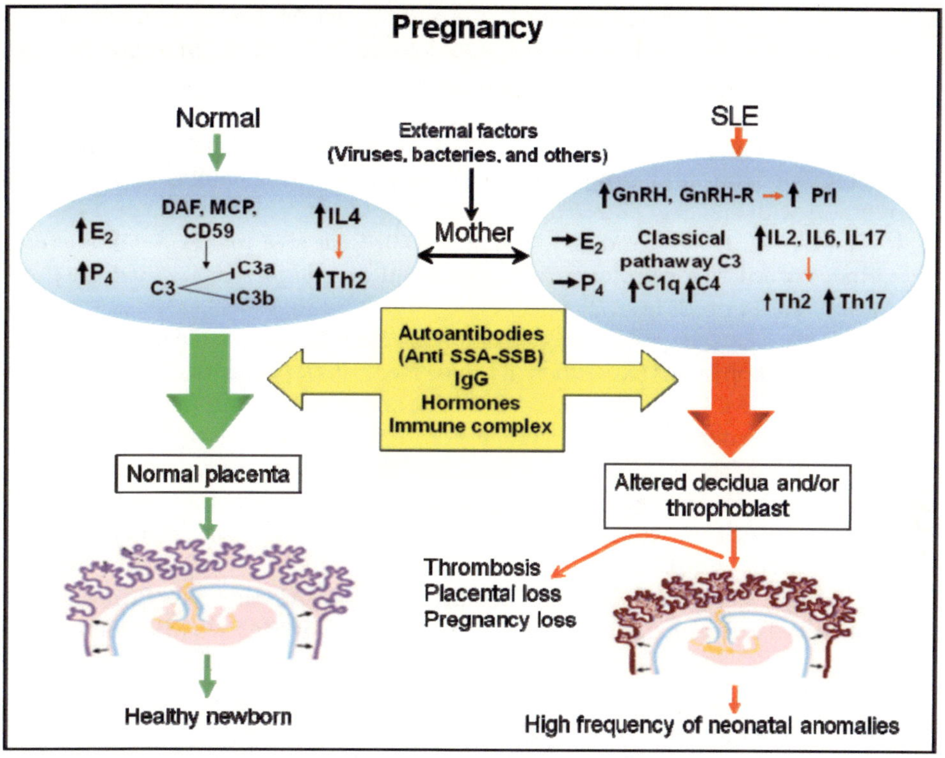

Fig. 1. Represent the two main outcomes of a pregnancy. A normal outcome, shown in the left of the figure, can results even in the presence of maternal autoantibodies the condition being that the quantity and isotype is below a threshold yet to be defined, when there is an excess and the mother has a clear SLE condition, the outcome is shown in the right side of the figure.

react with several fetal proteins (glycoproteins, lipoproteins, or lipids), but there is also the possibility that some of the alterations might be the consequence of drugs used to treat the mother in order to avoid SLE flares. All these should be clearly present within the medical community related to the diagnosis, treatment and follow up of offsprings from SLE mothers, since it is highly possible that these children will manifest some of the pathologies associated with maternal SLE, mainly those of the immune system.

9. Acknowledgment

This work was partially supported by CONACyT grant ID 00000008965 and a special grant from the Instituto Nacional de Cardiologia "Ignacio Chávez", SS, México. Special thanks to Ian David Daugs from Banner Sun Health Research Institute, Sun City, AZ for language review.

10. References

Abd-Elkareem MI, Al Tamimy HM, Khamis OA, Abdellatif SS, Hussein MR. (2010). Increased urinary levels of the leukocyte adhesion molecules ICAM-1 and VCAM-1 in human lupus nephritis with advanced renal histological changes: preliminary findings. *Clinical and Experimental Nephrology*, Vol. 14, No. 6 pp. 548-57.

Arslan E, Colakoglu M, Celik C Gezqinc K, Acar A, Capar M Aköz M, Akyürek C. (2004) Serum TNF-alpha, IL-6, lupus anticogulant and anticardiolipin antibody in women with and without a past history of recurrent miscarriage. *Archives of Gynecology and Obstetric,*Vol. 260 pp. 227-9.

Askanase AD, Friedman DM, Copel J, Dische MR, Dubin A, Starc TJ, Katholi MC, Buyon JP. (2002). Spectrum and progression of conduction abnormalities in infants born to mothers with anti-SSA/Ro-SSB/La antibodies. *Lupus,* Vol. 11, No. 3 pp.145-51.

Bao, L., J. Zhou, V. M. Holers, and R. J. Quigg. (2003). Excessive matrix accumulation in the kidneys of MRL/lpr lupus mice is dependent on complement activation. *J. Am. Soc. Nephro,* Vol.14 pp. 2516–2525.

Bao L, Osawe I, Haas M, Quigg RJ.(2005). Signaling through Up-Regulated C3a Receptor Is Key to the Development of Experimental Lupus Nephritis1. *J Immunol,* Vol. 175 pp. 1947-55.

Beagley KW, Gockel CM. (2003). Regulation of innate and adaptive immunity by the female sex hormones oestradiol and progesterone. *FEMS Immunol Med Microbiol,* Vol, 38 pp. 13-22.

Bobst SM, Day MC, Gilstrap LC 3rd, Xia Y Kellems RE. (2005). Maternal autoantibodies from preeclamptic Patients activates angiotensin receptors on human mesangial cells and induce inteleukin-6 and plasminogen activator inhibitor-1 secretion. *Am J Hypertens,* Vol. 18, No. 3 pp. 330-6.

Borchers AT, Naguwa SM, Keen CL and Park JM, Kohn MJ, Monique W. Bruinsma, Vech C, Intine RV, Fuhrmann S, Grinberg A, Mukherjee I, Love PE, Ko MS, DePamphilis ML, Maraia RJ. (2006) The Multifunctional RNA-Binding Protein La Is Required for Mouse Development and for the Establishment of Embryonic Stem Cells. *Molec Cell Biol.,* Vol. 46 pp. 1445–1451.

Borrego L, Rodríguez J, Soler E, Jiménez A, Hernández B. (1997) Neonatal lupus erythematosus related to maternal leukocytoclastic vasculitis. *Pediatr Dermatol,* Vol. 14, No. 3 pp. 221-5.

Branch DW. (2004) Pregnancy in patients with rheumatic diseases: obstetric management and monitoring. *Lupus.* Vol. 13, pp. 696-98.

Brucato A, Frassi M, Franceschini F, Cimaz R, Faden D, Pisoni MP, et al. (2001). Risk of congenital complete Herat block in newborns of mathers with anti. Ro/SSA antibodies deteted by counterimmunoelectrophoresis - a prospective study of 100 women. *Arthritis Rheum,* Vol. 44, pp. 1832-5.

Butcher EC, Williams M, Youngman K, Rott L, Briskin M. (1999). Lymphocyte trafficking and regional immunity. *Adv Immunol,* Vol. 72, pp.209–253.

Buyon JP. (1996). Neonatal lupus: Bedside to bench and back. *Scand J Rheumatol,* Vol. 25, pp. 271-6.

Buyon JP, Clancy RM. (2003). Neonatal lupus: review of proposed pathogenesis and clinical data from the US-based Research Registry for Neonatal Lupus. *Autoimmunity,*Vol. 36, pp.41-50.

Catelo M, Capellino M, Motagna, P Ghiiorzo P, Sulli A, Villagio B. (2005). Sex hormones modulation of cells growth and apoptosis of the human monocyte/macrophage cell line. *Arthritis Res Ther,* Vol. 7, pp. R1124-R-1132.

Cerkiene Z, Eidukaite A, Usoniene A. (2010). Immune factors in human embryo culture and their significance. *Medicina (Kaunas),* Vol. 46, No. 4, pp. 233-9.

Cervera R, Font J. Carmona F, Balasch J. (2002). Pregnancy outcome in systemic lupus erythematosus: good news for the new millennium. *Autoimmune Reviews*, Vol. 1, No. 6, pp. 354-9.

Cervera R, Balasch J. (2008). Biderectional effects on autoimmunity and reproductions. *Human of Reproduction Update*, Vol. 14, pp. 359-66.

Chandran V, Aggarwal A, Misra R. (2005). Active disease during pregnancy is associated with poor foetal outcome in Indian patients with systemic lupus erythematosus. *Rheumatol Int*, Vol. 27 pp.152-6.

Chang DM, Chu SJ, Chen HC, Kuo SY, Lai JH. (2004). Dehydroepiandrosterone suppresses interleukin 10 synthesis in women with systemic lupus erythematosus. *Ann Rheum Dis*, Vol. 63, pp.1623–1626.

Clancy RM, Buyon JP, Ikeda K, Nozawa K, Argyle DA, Deborah M. Friedman DM, Chan EKL. (2005). Maternal Antibody Responses to the 52-kd SSA/Ro p200 Peptide and the Development of Fetal Conduction Defects. *Arthritis Rheumatism*, Vol. 52, No.10, pp. 3079–3086.

Clowse ME, Magder LS, Petri M. (2005). The impact of increased Lupus activity on obstetric outcomes. *Arthritis Rheumatism*, Vol. 52, No. 2, pp. 514-21.

Clowse ME, Magder LS, Petri M. (2005). Cyclophosphomide for lupus during pregnancy. *Lupus*, Vol. 14, No. 8, pp. 593-97.

Clowse ME, Magder L. Witter M. (2006). Hydroxychloroquine in lupus pregnancy. *Arthritis Rheum*, Vol. 54, No. 11, pp. 5640-47.

Clowse, ME. (2007). Lupus activity in pregnancy. *Rheum Dis Clin North Am*, Vol. 33, No. 2, pp.237-v. doi 10.1016/j.rde.2007.01.002.

Cohen D, Buurma A, Goemaere NN, Girardi G, le Cessie S, Scherjon S, Bloemenkamp KW, de Heer E, Bruijn JA, Bajema IM. (2011). Classical complement activation as a footprint for murine and human antiphospholipid antibody-induced fetal loss. *J Pathol.* Mar 10. doi: 10.1002/path.2893. [Epub ahead of print] Abstract

Costedoat-Chalumeau N, Amoura Z, Duhaut P, Huong DL, Sebbough D, Wechsler B, Vauthier D, Denjoy I, Lupoglazoff JM, Piette JC. (2003). Safety of hydroxychloroquine in pregnant patients with connective tissue diseases: a study of one hundred thirty-three cases compared with a control group. *Arthritis Rheum*, Vol. 48, No. 11, pp. 3207-11.

Cutolo M, Sulli A, Seriolo B, Accardo S, Masi AT. (1995). Estrogens, the immune response and autoimmunity. *Clin Exp Rheumatol*, Vol. 13, No. 2, pp. 217-26.

Dhar JP, Sokol RJ. (2006). Lupus and Preganancy: Complex Yet Manageable. *Clin Med Res*, Vol. 4, No. 4, pp. 310-21.

Dillon JS. (2005). Dehydroepiandrosterone, dehydroepiandrosterone sulfate and related steroids: Their role in inflammatory, allergic and immunological disorders. *Curr Drug Targets Inflamm Allergy*, Vol. 4, pp. 377–85

Doria A, Cutolo M, Ghirardello A, Zampieri S, Vescovi F, Sulli A, Giusti M, Piccoli A, Grella P Gambari PF. (2002). Steroids hormones and disease activity during pregnancy in systemic lupus erythematosus. *Arthritis Rheuma*, Vol. 47, pp. 202-9.

Doria A, Iaccarino L, Sarzi-Puttini P, Ghirardello A, Zampieri S, Arienti S, Cutolo M, Todesco S. (2006). Estrogen in pregnancy and systemic lupus erythematosus. *Am N Y Acad Sci*, Vol. 1069, pp. 247-57.

Douglas AJ. (2010). Baby on board: do responses to stress in the maternal brain mediate adverse pregnancy outcome? *Front Neuroendocrinol*, Vol. 31, pp. 359-76.

Draca S. (2002). Is pregnancy a model how we should control some autoimmune deseases? *Autoimmunity*, Vol. 35, pp. 307-12.

Eftekhari P, Salle L, Lezoualc'h F, Mialet J, Gastineau M, Briand JP, Isenberg DA, Fournie GJ, Argibay J, Fischmeister R, Muller S, Hoebeke J. (2000). Anti-SSA/Ro52 autoantibodies blocking the cardiac 5-HT4 serotoninergic receptor could explain neonatal lupus congenital heart block. *Eur J Immunol*, Vol. 30, pp. 2782-90.

Elenkov IJ, Chouosos GP. (1999). Stress, cytokine patterns and susceptibility to diseases. Bailliere´s Best Pract *Res Clin Endocrinol*, Vol. 13, pp. 583-95.

Evans MJ, MacLaughlin S, Marvin RD, Abdon NI. (1997). Estrogen decreases in vitro apoptosis of peripheral blood mononuclear cells from women with normal mestrual cycles and decreases TNF alpha production in SLE, but not in normal cultures. *Clin Immunophatol*, Vol. 82, pp.258-62.

Friedman DM, Llanos C, Izmirly PM, Brock B, Byron J, Copel J, Cummiskey K, Dooley MA, Foley J, Graves C, Hendershott C, Kates R, Komissarova EV, Miller M, Paré E, Phoon CK, Prosen T, Reisner D, Ruderman E, Samuels P, Yu JK, Kim MY, Buyon JP. (2010). Evaluation of fetuses in a study of intravenous immunoglobulin as preventive therapy for congenital heart block: Results of a multicenter, prospective, open-label clinical trial. *Arthritis Rheum*,Vol. 62, No. 4, pp. 1138-46 PubMed PMID: 20391423.

Girardi G, Berman J, Redecha P, Spruce L, Thurman JM, Kraus D, Hollmann TJ, Casali P, Caroll MC, Wetsel RA, Lambris JD, Holers VM, Salmon JE. (2004) (2003). Complement C5a receptors and neutrophils mediate fetal injury in the antiphospholipid syndrome. *J Clin Invest*, Vol. 112, No. 11, pp. 1644–54.

Girardi G. Mackman N. (2008). Tissue factor in antiphospholipid antibody-induced pregnancy loss: a pro-inflammatory molecule *Lupus*, Vol. 17, NO. 10, pp. 931–36.

Girardi F, Prohászka Z, Bulla R, Tedesco T, Scherjon S. (2011). Complement activation in animal and human pregnancies as a model for immunological recognition. *Mol. Immunol*. doi:10.1016/j.molimm.2011.04.011 (in press)

Gordon, C. (2004). Pregnancy and autoimmune diseases. *Best Practice Research clinical Rheumatology*, Vol. 18, pp. 359-79.

Gordon C, Wallace DJ,Shinada S, Kalunian KC, Forbess L , Braunstein GD, WeismanMH. Testosterone patches in the management of patients with mild/moderate systemic lupus erythematosus. Rheumatology 2008; 47: 334–338.

Gulinello M, Putterman C. (2011). TheMRL/lpr Mouse Strain as a model for neuropsychiatric systemic lupus erythematosus. *J Biomed Biotechol*, 2011; Vol., Article ID 207504, 15 pages, pubmed

Hodson DJ, Townsend J, Gregory SJ, Walters C, Tortonese DJ. (2010). Role of prolactin in the gonadotroph responsiveness to gonadotrophin-releasing hormone during the equine annual reproductive cycle. *J Neuroendocrinol*, Vol. 22, No. 6, pp. 509-17.

Hoftman AC, Reañades MI, Lee KW, Stiehm ER. (2008). Newborn illnesses caused by tranplacental antibodies. *Advances in Pediatric*, Vol. 55, pp. 271-302.

Holmes RP, Stone PR. (2000). Severe olygohydramnios induced by cyclooxygenase-2 inhibitor nimesulide. *Obstet Gynecol*, Vol. 96, pp. 810-811.

Inui A, Ogasawara H, Naito T, Sekigawa I, Takasaki Y, Hayashida Y, et al. (2007). Estrogen receptor expression by peripheral blood mononuclear cells of patients with systemic lupus erythematosus. *Clin Rheumatol*, Vol. 26, pp. 1675–8.

Jacobson JD, Ansari MA, Kinealy M, Muthukrishnan V. (1999). Specific Exacerbation of Murine Lupus by Gonadotropin-Releasing Hormone: Potential Role of Gaq/11. *Endocrinology*, Vol. 140. No. 8, pp. 3429-37.

Jara LJ, Benitez G, Medina G. (2008). Prolactin, dendritic cells, and systemic lupus erythematosus. *Autoimmun Rev*, Vol. 7, pp. 251–5.

Johansson M, Arlestig L, Moller B, Smedby T, Rantapaa-Dahlqvist S. (2005). Oestrogen receptor alpha gene polymorphisms in systemic lupus erythematosus. *Ann Rheum Dis*, Vol. 64 pp. 1611–7.

Kamel R, Garcia S, Lezoualc'h F, Fischmeister R, Sylviane Muller S, Hoebee J, Eftekhari P. (2007). Immunomodulation by maternal autoantibodies of the fetal serotoninergic 5-HT4 receptor and its consequences in early BALB/c mouse embryonic development. *BMC Developmental Biology*, Vol 7, pp. 34.

Kassi EN, Vlachoyiannopoulos PG, Moutsopoulos HM, Sekeris CE, Moutsatsou P. (2001). Molecular analysis of estrogen receptor alpha and beta in lupus patients. *Eur J Clin Invest*, Vol. 31, pp. 86–93.

Khamashta MA. (2006). Systemic lupus erythematosus and pregnancy. *Best Practice ans research clinical rheumatology*, Vol. 20, No. 4, pp. 685-94.

Kruse A, Martens N, Fernekorn U, Hallmann R, Butcher EC. (2002). Alterations in the Expression of Homing-Associated Molecules at the Maternal/Fetal Interface During the Course of Pregnancy. *Biol Reprod*, Vol. 66, pp. 333–345.

Lakasing L, Campa JS, Parmar K, Poston R, Hunt BJ, Poston L. (2000). Normal expression of cell adhesion molecules in placentae from women with systemic lupus erythematosus and the antiphospholipid symdrome. *Placenta*, Vol. 21, No. 2-3, pp. 142-9.

Lambert HW, Weiss ER, Lauder JM. (2001). Activation of 5-HT receptors that stimulate the adenylyl cyclase pathway positively regulates IGF-I in cultured craniofacial mesenchymal cells. *Dev Neurosci*, Vol. 23, pp. 70-7.

Lashley LE, van der Hoorn ML, van der Mast BJ, Tilburgs T, van der Lee N, van der Keur C, van Beelen E, Roelen DL, Claas FH, Scherjon SA. (2011). Changes in cytokine production and composition of peripheral blood leukocytes during pregnancy are not associated with a difference in the proliferative immune response to the fetus. *Hum Immuno*, Jun 12. [Epub ahead of print] Abstrat

Lee JY, Huerta PT, Zhang J, Kowal C, Bertini E, Volpe BT, Diamond B. (2009). Maternal lupus and congenital cortical impairment. *Nat Med*, Vol. 15, pp. 91-96.

Li J, McMurray RW. (2007) Effects of estrogen receptor subtype-selective agonists on autoimmune disease in lupus-prone NZB/NZW F1 mouse model. *Clin Immunol*, Vol. 123, No. 2, pp. 219–26.

Libbey JE, Fujinami RS. (2010). Role for antibodies in altering behavior and movement. *Autism Res*, Vol. 3, No. 4, pp. 147-52.

Lit LC, Wong CK, like, Tam LS, Lam CW, Lo YM. (2007). Elevated gene expression of Th1/Th2 associated transcription factors is correlated with disease activity in patients with systemic lupus erithematosus. *J Rheumatol*, Vol. 34, pp. 89-96.

Lockshin MD, (2003). Sammaritano LR. Lupus pregnancy. *Autoimmunity*, Vol. 36, pp. 33-40.

Marshall D, Dangerfield JP, Bhatia VK, Larbi KY, Nourshargh S, Haskard DO. (2003). MRLulpr lupus-prone mice show exaggerated ICAM-1-dependent leucocyte adhesion and transendothelial migration in response to TNF-alpha. *Rheumatology*, Vol. 42, pp. 929–934.

Martin V, Lee LA, Askanase AD, Katholi M, Buyon JP. (2002). Long-term followup of children with neonatal lupus and their unaffected siblings. *Arthitis Rheum*, Vol. 46, pp. 2377-83.

Matera L, Mori M, Galetto A. (2001). Effect of prolactin on antigen presenting function of mononocyte derived dendritic cells. *Lupus*, Vol. 10, pp. 728–34.

Meroni PL, Tedesco F, Locati M, Vecchi A, Di Simone N, Acaia B, Pierangeli SS, Borghi MO. (2010). Anti-phospholipid antibody mediated fetal loss: still an open question from a pathogenic point of view. *Lupus*, Vol. 19, No. 4, pp. 453-6.

Micheloud D, Nuño L, Rodríguez-Mahou M, Sánchez-Ramón S, Ortega MC, Aguarón A, Junco E, Carbone J, Fernández-Cruz E, Carreño L, López-Longo FJ. (2006). Efficacy and safety of Etanercept, high-dose intravenous gammaglobulin and plasmapheresis combined therapy for lupus diffuse proliferative nephritis complicating pregnancy. *Lupus*, Vol. 15, No. 12, pp. 881-5. PubMed PMID: 17211995.

Molad Y, Borkowski T, Ben-Haroush A, Sulkes J, Hod M, Feldberg D, Bar J. (2005). Maternal and fetal outcome of lupus pregnancy: a prospective study of pregnancies. *Lupus*, Vol. 14, pp. 145-51.

Motta M, Rodriguez-Perez C, Tincani A, Lojacono A, Nacinovich R, Chirico G. (2009). Neonates born from mothers with autoimmune disorders. *Early Hum Dev*, Vol 85, No. 10 Suppl, pp. S67-70.

Mork CC, Wong RW. (2001). Pregnancy in systemic lupus erythematosus. *Postgrad Med J*, Vol. 77, pp. 157-65.

Morton MR. (1998) Hypersensitivity vasculitis (microscopio polyangiitis) in pregnancy with transmisión to the neonato. *British Journal of Obstetrics and Gynaecology*, Vol. 105, pp. 928-930.

Munther AK. (2006). Systemic lupus erythematosus and preganacy. *Best Practice and Research Rheumatology*, Vol. 20, No. 4, pp. 685-94

Muñoz-Valle JF, Vazquez-del Mercado M, Garcia-Iglesias T, et al. (2003). T(H)1/T(H)2 cytikine profile, metalloprotease-9 activity and hormonal status in pregnant artritis and systemic erytemathosus patients. *Clin Exp Immunol*, Vol. 131, pp. 377-84.

Nayeri F, Movaghar-Nezhad K, Assar-Zadegan F. (2005). Effects of antenatal steroids on the incidence and severity of respiratory distress syndrome in an Iranian hospital. *East Mediterr Health J*, Vol. 11, No. 4, pp. 716-22.

Nuttall SL, Heaton S, Piper MK, Martin U, Gordon C. (2003). Cardiovascular risk in systemic lupus erythematosus–evidence of increased oxidative stress and dyslipidaemia. *Rheumatology*, Vol. 42, pp. 758–62

Ostensen M, Khamashta M, Lockshin M, Parke A, Brucato A, Carp H, Doria A, Rai R, Meroni P, Cetin I, Derksen R, Branch W, Motta M, Gordon C, et al. (2006). Anti-inflammatory and immunosuppressive drugs and reproduction. *Arthritis Res Ther*, Vol. 8, No. 3, pp. 209.

Peeva E, Michael D, Cleary J, Rice J, Chen X, Diamond B. Prolactin modulates the naive B cell repertoire. J Clin Invest. 2003; 111:275–83.

Petri M. (2004). Prospective study of systemic lupus erythematosus pregnancies. *Lupus*. Vol. 13, pp. 688-9.

Phiel KL, Henderson RA, Adelman SJ, Elloso MM. (2005). Differential estrogen receptor gene expression in human peripheral blood mononuclear cell populations. *Immunol Lett*, Vol 97, pp. 107–13.

Piccinni MP. (2005). T cells in pregnancy. *Chem Immunol Allergy*, Vol. 89, pp. :3-9.

Pradat P, Robert-Gnasia E, Di Tanna GL, Rosano A, Lisi A, Mastroiacovo P. (2003). First trimester exposure to costiscosteroids and oral clefs. Birth Defects Res A *Clin Mol Teratol*, Vol. 67, No. 12, pp. 968-70. Abstract

Rein AJJT, Mevorach D, Perles Z, Gavri S, Nadjari M, Nir A, Elchalal U. (2009). Early Diagnosis and Treatment of Atrioventricular Block in the Fetus Exposed to Maternal Anti-

SSA/Ro-SSB/La Antibodies: A Prospective, Observational, Fetal Kinetocardiogram-Based Study. *Circulation*, Vol. 119, pp. 1867-72.

Rider V, Li X, Peterson G, Dawson J, Kimler BF, Abdou NI. (2006). Differential expression of estrogen receptors in women withsystemic lupus erythematosus. *J Rheumatol*, Vol. 33, No. 6, pp. 1093–101.

Rodriguez E, Guevara L, Paez A, Zapata E, Collados MT, Fortoul TI, Lopez-Marure R, Masso F, Montaño LF. (2008). The altered expresión of inflammatory-related molecules and secretion of IL-6 and IL-8 by HUVEC from newborns with maternal inactive systemic lupus erythematosus is modified by estrogens. *Lupus*, Vol. 17, pp. 1086-95.

Rothenberger SE, Resch F, Doszpod N, Moehler E. (2011). Prenatal stress and infant affective reactivity at five months of age. *Early Hum Dev*, Vol. 87, No. 2, pp. 129-36.Epub 2010 Dec 30. PubMed PMID: 21194854. Abstract

Ruiz-Irastorza G, Khamashta MA. (2004). Evaluation of lupus erythematosus activity during pregnancy. *Lupus*, Vol. 13, pp. 679-82.

Saito S, Nakashima A, Shima T, Ito M. (2010). Th1/Th2/Th17 and regulatory T-cells paradigm in pregnancy. *Am J Reprod Immunol*, Vol. 63, No. 6, pp. 601-10.

Salomonsson S, Strandberg L. (2010). Autoantibodies associated with congenital heart block. Scand *J Immunol*, Vol. 72, No. 3, pp. 185-8.

Sammaritano LR, Ng S, Sobel R, Lo SK, Simantov R, Furie R, Kaell A, Silverstein R, Salmon JE. (1997). Anticardiolipin IgG subclasses: association of IgG2 with arterial and/or venous thrombosis. *Arthritis Rheum*, Vol. 40 No. 11, pp. 1998-2006.

Scarpati EM, Sadler JE. (1989). Regulation of endothelial cell coagulant properties. Modulation of tissue factor, plasminogen activator inhibitors and, thrombomoduline by phorbol 12.myristate 13-acetate and tunor necrosis factor. *J Biol Chem*, Vol. 264, No. 34, pp. 20705-13.

Serdiuk GV, Selivanov EV, Barkagan ZS. (2008). [Significance of the determination of B2-glycoprotein-1 antibodies in recognizing the thrombogenicity in antiphospholipid syndrome]. *Klin Lab Diagn*. Vol. Mar, No. 3, pp. 38-9. Russian. PubMed PMID: 18453060. Abstrat

Silverman E, Jaeqqi. (2010). Non-cardiac manifestation of neonatal lupus erythematosus. *Scand J Immnunol*, Vol. 72, No. 3, pp. 223-5.

Shah V, Alwassia H, Shah K, Yoon W, Shah P. (2011). Neonatal outcomes among multiplebirths ≤ 32 weeks gestational age: Does mode of conception have an impact? A Cohort Study. *BMC Pediatrics*, Vol. 11, pp. 54. In process.

Straub RH, Weidler C, Demmel B, Herrmann M, Kees F, Schmidt M, Scho¨lmerich J, Schede J. (2004). Renal clearance and daily excretion of cortisol and adrenal androgens in patients with rheumatoid arthritis and systemic lupus erythematosus. *Ann Rheum Dis*, Vol. 63, pp. 961–968.

Shuey DL, Sadler TW, Lauder JM. (1992). Serotonin as a regulator of craniofacial morphogenesis: site specific malformations following exposure to serotonin uptake inhibitors. *Teratology*, Vol. 46, pp. 367-78.

Svensson J, Lindberg B, Ericsson Ub, Olofsson P, Ivarsson SA. (2006). Thyroid antibodies in cord blood sera from children and adolescens with autoimmune thyroiditis. *Thyroid*, Vol. 16, pp. 79-86.

Tait AS, Butts CL, Sternberg EM. (2008). The role of glicocorticoids and progestins in inflammatory, autoimmune and infectious diseades. *J Leukoc Biol*, Vol. 84, pp. 924-931.

Tasitanon N, Fine DN, Haas M, Magder IS, Petri M. (2006). Hydroxichloroquine use predicts complete renal remission with i2 months among patients treated with mycophenolate mofetil therapy for membraneous lupus nefritis . *Lupus*, Vol. 15, No. 6, pp. 366-70.

Tincani A, Balestrieri G, Danieli E, Faden D, Lojacono A, Acaia B, Trespidi L, Ventura D, Meroni PL. (2003). Pregnancy complications of the antiphospholipid syndrome. *Autoimmunity*, Vol. 36, pp. 27-32.

Tincani A, Cavazzana I, Ziglioli T, Lojacono A, De Angelis V, Meroni P. (2010). Complement activation and pregnancy failure. *Clin Rev Allergy Immunol*, 39, No. 3, pp. 153-9).

Tseng CE, Buyon JP. (1997). Neonatal lupus Syndromes. *Rheumatic Disease Clinics of North America*, Vol. 23, pp. 31-54

Tseng CE, Miranda E, Di Donato F, Boutjdir M, Rashbaum W, Chan EK, Buyon JP. (1999). mRNA and protein expression of SSA/Ro and SSB/La in human fetal cardiac myocytes cultured using a novel application of the Langendorff procedure. *Pediatr Res*, Vol. 45, No. 2, pp. 260-9.

Vazquez-del Mercado M, Martin-Marquez BT, Petri-Marcelo H, Martinez-Garcia EA, Muñoz-Valle JF. (2006). Molecular mechanisms in normal pregnancy and rheumatic diseases. *Clin Exp Rheumatol*, Vol. 24, pp. 707-12.

Velíšek L. (2011). Prenatal corticosteroid exposure alters early developmental seizures and behavior. *Epilepsy Res*, Vol. 95, No. 1-2, pp. 9-19. Epub 2011 Mar 22.PubMed PMID: 21429712. Abstrat

Vera-Lastra O, Jara LJ, Espinoza LR. (2002). Prolactin and autoimmunity. *Autoimmun Rev*, Vol. 1, pp. 360–4.

Viallard JF, Pellegrin JL, Ranchin V, Schaeverbeke T, Dehais J, Longy-Boursier M, Ragnaud JM, Leng B, Moreau JF. (1999). Th1 (IL-2, interferon gamma (INF-gamm) and Th2 (IL-10, IL-4) cytokine production by peripheral blood mononuclear cells (PBMC) from patients with systemic lupus erithematosus (SLE). *Clin Exp Immunol*, Vol. 115, No. 1, pp. 189-95.

Yamamoto S, Tin-Tin-Win-Shwe, Yoshida Y, Kunugita N, Arashidani K, Fujimaki H. (2009). Children´s immunology, what can we learn from animal studies (2): Modulation of systemic TH1/TH2 immune response in infant mice after prenatal exposure to low-level toluene and toll like receptor (TLR) 2 ligand. *J Toxicol Sci*, Vol 34, pp. SP341-SP348.

Yazici ZA, Rashi E, Patel A, et.al. (2001). Human monoclonal anti-endothelial cell IgG-derivated from systemic lupus erythematosus patient binds and activated human endothelium in vitro. *Int immunol*, Vol. 13, pp. 349-57.

Zen M, Ghirardello A, Iaccarino L, Tonon M, Campana C, Arienti S, Rampudda M, Canova M, Doria A. (2010). Hormones, immune response, and pregnancy in healthy women and SLE patients. *Swiss Med Wkly Review*, Vol. 140, pp. 187-201.

Živilė Čerkienė, Audronė Eidukaitė, Audronė Usonienė. (2010). Immune factors in human embryo culture and their significance. *Medicina (Kaunas)*, Vol. 46, No. 4, pp. 233-9